THE ENCYCLOPEDIA OF

THE MUSCLE AND SKELETAL SYSTEMS AND DISORDERS

THE ENCYCLOPEDIA OF

THE MUSCLE AND SKELETAL SYSTEMS AND DISORDERS

Mary Harwell Sayler

Foreword by
Lori Siegel, M.D.
Associate Professor and Medical Education Director
The Finch University of Health Science/
The Chicago Medical School

Facts On File, Inc.

The Encyclopedia of the Muscle and Skeletal Systems and Disorders

Facts On File, Inc.
132 West 31st Street
New York NY 10001

Library of Congress Cataloging-in-Publication Data
Sayler, Mary Harwell.
The encyclopedia of the muscle and skeletal systems and disorders / Mary Harwell Sayler ; foreword by Lori Siegel.
p. ; cm.
Includes bibliographical references and index.
ISBN 0-8160-5447-9 (hard cover : alk. paper)
1. Musculoskeletal system—Diseases—Encyclopedias. 2. Musculoskeletal system—Encyclopedias. [DNLM: 1. Musculoskeletal System—Encyclopedias—English. 2. Musculoskeletal Diseases—Encyclopedias—English. WE 13 S275e 2005] I. Title.
RC925.5.S29 2005
616.7'003—dc22
2003026606

Facts On File books are available at special discounts when purchased in bulk quantities for businesses, associations, institutions, or sales promotions. Please call our Special Sales Department in New York at (212) 967-8800 or (800) 322-8755.

You can find Facts On File on the World Wide Web at http://www.factsonfile.com

Text and cover design by Cathy Rincon

Printed in the United States of America

VB FOF 10 9 8 7 6 5 4 3 2 1

This book is printed on acid-free paper.

To my husband, Bob, who gives a great massage
and to my chiropractor, Dr. David Nelson,
who literally saved my neck

CONTENTS

FOREWORD

Stand Up for What You Believe in . . . or *Can* You?

There is always an argument about which organ system is most important. Some say it is the heart. Without the heart, the brain would not get nourishment and survive. Some say it is the brain. Although the heart can beat without a brain, to do more than merely exist an organism needs to have some degree of consciousness and purpose. I would argue that both the heart and the brain are important. However, the musculoskeletal system is the most important because it allows us to act, react, and be human! That is not to diminish the importance of the heart and brain. As is very clear, the former provides nourishment for the musculoskeletal structures while the latter controls the complex movements of which the structures are capable. If not for our musculoskeletal system, we would be amorphous blob creatures unable to do the exquisite activities that we do like dance, run, show expression, and communicate. The brain allows thought, and the musculoskeletal system allows follow-through and expression of the thought.

The musculoskeletal system is complex and composed of many different types of tissues and cells. A malfunction of any part of these components can ultimately affect the structures around it and cause pain, deformity, and progressive physical impairment. When assessing a patient with a potential problem in the musculoskeletal system, the health care professional must be cognizant of all the structures and their intimate relationships. Although it may appear overwhelming, a logical and organized approach is essential. A strong background in the normal is imperative before diagnosing and managing a variation from that apparent normalcy.

With all the basics of the anatomy of the musculoskeletal system and its structures in check, diagnosing and treating patients with musculoskeletal problems is not an easy task. However, it can be organized into a logical and sequential approach. The health care provider must view each individual as a unique person whose concerns may not be organized in the manner in which the health care provider was trained. The patients do not "read the book" or truly understand what is happening where and for what reason, although they are often able to explain their symptoms and come up with their own diagnosis, which can be quite creative. It is incumbent on the health care provider to put the pieces of the puzzle together.

In order to solve the puzzle appropriately, one must have decision trees that guide the diagnosis and then ultimately the treatment. When someone begins to describe a musculoskeletal symptom, the first decision is whether the symptom is truly a joint process or an area around the joint or soft tissue. If there is a true joint problem, the patient is likely to experience a diffuse achiness and not be able to pinpoint an exact location of the pain. Also even though the pain may seem to be coming from a specific area, more often than not the offending joint is proximal to where the pain is felt. Also with true joint problems, the patient will experience a decreased passive range of motion as he or she is examined.

The pain and discomfort of a soft tissue process comes from inflammation or irritation of a bursa, tendon, muscle, or nerve entrapment. In these conditions, the pain is more localized to the irritated area and the passive range of motion is not impaired although it may be painful. When a local condition such as these is identified, it is important to figure out what repetitive movements may be causing this or what is off balance in the body that is straining these supportive structures. The primary treatment is correcting the imbalance and stopping the offending movement. When this is not possible due to vocational aspects, heat and ice may help along with a carefully outlined plan of muscle strengthening and stretching. Consultation with a physical therapist or exercise specialist is important so that other parts of the body do not become stressed while repairing the initial pain. Along with the above treatments, consideration may be given to anti-inflammatory medications as well. Although these may be found over the counter, side effects are common and may involve the stomach, kidneys, and blood. It is important the patient ask his or her primary care practitioner about their safety especially if on other medications. Sometimes these soft tissue conditions may respond to a local injection of a corticosteroid and/or local analgesic. This would also require a consultation with the appropriate specialist. Nontraditional remedies are also helpful in combination with traditional therapies, and therefore acupuncture or massage would be of little harm and may help.

Other conditions that may cause pain but are not truly articular are fibromyalgia, myofascial pain syndromes, hypermobility syndromes, and nerve entrapments. The patient with fibromyalgia hurts all over, and regular physical examination and laboratory testing are within the normal range. There is usually a history of trauma and lack of sleep, and the patient develops tender points that are often diagnostic. The treatment for this condition is difficult because of a common psychiatric overlay, but this is not always the case. Moderate exercise, sleep-restoring medication, and reassurance is most helpful. The road to recovery may be long. However, if a patient keeps a journal, it will reveal progress otherwise overlooked.

Myofacial pain is similar to fibromyalgia in that all the tests are normal. In contrast, the pain is confined to a specific reason and is usually a result of overuse of that area or poor posture when lifting or during prolonged immobility. Treatment is attention to proper muscle alignment and stretching with either heat or cold application.

Hypermobility syndromes are a unique group of diseases that involve the musculoskeletal tissues at many levels. However, the benign hypermobility syndrome (BHMS) causes the most musculoskeletal complaints. People with BHMS often have strained ligaments and tendons and also traumatic lesions. Their laboratory evaluation is usually unrevealing. Patients may have associated clinical manifestations such as hyperextensible skin, striae, mitral valve prolapse, and stress fractures because of increased bone fragility. Keys to this condition are hyperextension of the elbows or knees, apposition of the thumb to flexor aspect of the forearm and passive dorsiflexion of the fifth metacarpal phalangeal joints (knuckles of the fist) to 90 degrees, and forward flexion of the trunk placing the hands flat on the floor with knees extended. The treatment focuses on education and reassurance that the patient does not have a deforming or crippling disease. Stretching and muscle strengthening will help stability.

Nerve entrapments also present as musculoskeletal problems and may be clouded by the sensation of joint swelling and stiffness. The classic syndrome is carpal tunnel syndrome, which is impingement of the median nerve. This is a condition in which the patient's hands actually sleep better than they do. There may be numbness and tingling of the fingers with eventual weakness. Upon hearing these complaints, the health care professional should look for the cause of the condition. The most commonly associated problem is that of overuse. However, anyone with carpal tunnel syndrome, especially those with bilateral conditions, should be evaluated for underlying diabetes, thyroid disorders, and autoimmune disorders and also be up-to-date on their routine health screens for malignancy. The underlying problem is dealt with either by treatment of the disease or by ergonomic alteration of the environment. Splints are useful, but only if they are actually worn. Local injections may also help and, depending on any evidence of weakness or atrophy, surgical intervention may be indicated.

If, however, there is concern that the pain is indeed initiated by an articular process, then other thoughts and decisions must be made. First the health care professional must determine if there is any degree of inflammation. Inflammatory conditions of the joints usually have some degree of morning joint stiffness lasting longer than 30 minutes. The joints feel better with movement but tend to relapse after periods of inactivity. The joints may also have signs of inflammation such as redness, heat, swelling, and tenderness. When an inflammatory process is likely, consideration must be given as to how many joints are involved and what is the pattern of involvement. If less than three joints are involved, the diagnostic possibilities are most commonly infectious arthritis, crystal-induced arthritis (gout or pseudogout), or traumatic arthritis. If four or more joints are involved and they are symmetrically distributed, then rheumatoid arthritis, viral arthritis, or systemic lupus erythematosus need to be considered. If the distribution of joint involvement is asymmetrical or involves the knuckles at the end of the fingers, the diagnostic possibilities are ankylosing spondylitis, reactive arthritis, psoriatic arthritis, or inflammatory bowel associated arthritis. In peri- or post-menopausal women, erosive osteoarthritis is a concern.

These conditions do require consultation with a specialist or someone who is well educated on these topics. The treatment basics include appropriate education about the condition, physical therapy for muscle strengthening and joint movement, occupational therapy for home and social adjustment, heat and/or ice, and finally medications. The medications used are often quite strong. They suppress the immune system so it no longer fights against itself. Many of these agents have potentially strong side effects, so they must be taken with close follow-up by an experienced practitioner.

If the joints involved do not demonstrate much inflammation, aside from a little "water on the joint" and the stiffness of the joints in the morning lasts less than 30 minutes, then the most likely underlying condition is osteoarthritis (OA). This type of arthritis gets worse with activity or exercise and may fall on top of a joint already vulnerable from other types of trauma or arthritis. Other terms for this arthritis are "old age arthritis," "rheumatism," or "degenerative joint disease." Generalized OA primarily involves the spine and weight bearing joints. Crepitation, joint instability, and deformity may be noted. Laboratory evaluations are not usually helpful, and any finding may reflect another concomitant disease. Radiographs may show asymmetrical joint space narrowing and bone spurs or osteophytes. The degree of radiographic involvement may not correlate well with the clinical symptoms. The patient's symptoms are treated, not the X-ray!

Treatment of OA is to make certain that there is no underlying disease predisposing the patient to more aggressive or early OA. Then exercise and range of motion are important. Muscle strengthening helps pain, joint stability, and alignment. Anti-inflammatory medications started at an analgesic dose are often helpful and may need to be titrated upward. Analgesics such as acetaminophen or tramadol are also useful. Viscosupplementation is helpful in OA of the knee. This is a series of joint lubricant injections into the knee that will help calm down the condition. Some evidence suggests this aids in cartilage repair. Ultimately, if the joint pain is too high and conservative measures are unsuccessful, surgery may be indicated. Arthroscopic procedures may repair underlying abnormalities, and joint replacements are often successful.

Another group of diseases that affect the musculoskeletal system are a group of autoimmune diseases called connective tissue diseases. These are groupings of symptoms and signs along with laboratory tests that signal a hyperactive immune system targeted at an individual's own proteins. Detailed discussion of these is beyond the scope of this book. However, people need to be aware that these conditions exist and, if experienced, they should be referred to a specialist. The various diagnoses are made primarily via a thorough history and physical with laboratory data supporting the diagnosis. A fishing expedition into these laboratory tests to "look" for possible disease will only stir the water and create confusion and distress since the tests would be most likely false positive. Unless one has a high suspicion of any connective tissue disease, the laboratory tests are better not ordered! Some of the diseases in this category include Raynaud's phenomenon, systemic lupus erythematosus, systemic sclerosis, inflammatory myopathies, and vasculitis. Most of these involve many organs all at once, and the need to solve the big puzzle is the medical challenge.

The musculoskeletal system not only provides diagnostic and treatment challenges but also challenges for the future of treating these conditions even more successfully. Much of the management involves controlling the symptoms but not reversing the disease process itself. Over the past decade, a wealth of information about the molecular biology and biochemistry of these diseases has been revealed. New treatments targeting the specific components of the inflammatory process and the use of biologically active medications have been revolutionary in rheumatoid arthritis, psoriatic arthritis, and Crohn's disease. As more molecules are understood and the vast cascade of chemical signals are identified and labeled, they can be targets for pharmacological alteration. Genetic coding of disease predisposition and identifying areas of modification make the field of proteomics hopeful for those who suffer from complications of an altered musculoskeletal system. We have a long way to go, both figuratively and literally. However, our musculoskeletal system will help us get there—with the help of our heart and our brain.

—Lori B. Siegel, M.D.
Associate Professor and Director,
Undergraduate Medical Education,
The Finch University of Health Science/
The Chicago Medical School

PREFACE

These bones are mine.
I cling to them.

In the heart of bone,
   the marrow
deepens.
Humors flow,
and blood cells
breed.

But how
will I circumvent
those times the joints
   articulate
no movement?

Who best can
   answer
the spine's
   ongoing question
as an aching back
finally finds
its rest?

ACKNOWLEDGING YOU, THE READER—AND OTHER THANKS

Muscles and bones shape major regions of the human body and major fields of health, both of which encompass numerous categories and specialties of medicine—not to mention hundreds and hundreds of body parts! Nevertheless, I wanted to include as many aspects and approaches as possible with longer discussions reserved for areas that more greatly interest the reader. I cannot speak for everyone, of course. However, the topics and issues consistently addressed in the media revealed most people's primary concerns to be the same as mine—concerns about understanding the bodies we have been given, building our muscles, protecting our bones, managing pain, finding the most effective treatments, and, yes, aging with energy, mobility, ingenuity, and strength.

As you can imagine, the potential sources for this in-depth muscle research became bone-boggling with expert perspectives in such diverse disciplines as rheumatology, orthopedics, osteopathy, podiatry, chiropractics, nutritional therapy, physical therapy, occupational therapy, sports medicine, nursing, physical training, and various types of surgical specialties. I could merely glean from and report on these fields in the attempt to make this work as accurate and well-rounded as an overwhelming amount of information allowed. To keep an equitable balance also meant weighing and sorting the voluminous data from specialists or practitioners trained in the use of herbs, massage, acupressure, acupuncture, and other ancient arts. Since this is the 21st century, however, I am particularly indebted to technology and the Internet for making readily available so many outstanding libraries and archives of medical colleges, government sites, and foundations devoted to ongoing research and informational assistance.

Most of those sites proved so helpful that I have included a list at the end of this book with gratitude for each organization in providing us with places to find more information and answers about specific conditions or disorders. Before you search elsewhere though, I hope you will start here, perhaps leafing through this book to get an idea of the wonderfully intricate workings of muscles and bones as the body aims for balance—that healthy state of homeostasis for which we can all be thankful whenever it arrives.

On a more personal note, I want to thank Dr. Lori B. Siegel for reviewing this manuscript, writing the foreword, and offering her excellent expertise. Special thanks also go to my writer-friend Dana Cassell, a veteran author for Facts On File and founder of Cassell Network/FL Freelance Writers Association, who encouraged this work. I am grateful, too, to my responsive editor at Facts On File, James Chambers, and my supportive husband, Bob, for being open to the unique connections between poetry writing and encyclopedia writing—the muscles and bones of my work.

—Mary Harwell Sayler, Lake Como, Florida

INTRODUCTION

Form, Structure, and Hope

In the absence of bone, we would look like jellyfish. Without muscle, we would be like stick figures, rising from a preschooler's drawing pad. Yet neither of these systems has to do with appearances only for there is more to everybody's body than meets the eye.

Beneath the smooth surfaces and contours of our skin lie bones—not as dead matter to be disposed of in a sarcophagus but as living organs in a constant state of remodeling themselves. With nutrients and fluids supplied by food, water, and sunshine, our cells and blood actively participate in building bone, though not necessarily as we might choose. Factors such as health and heredity come into play as newborn cartilage ossifies, gradually hardening into the size and shape of bone that is needed to perform a particular task. For instance, the springiness and arched vault of the rib cage is exactly what is required to protect the vital organs of our heart and lungs. In contrast, this would not be a workable form for, say, sitting in a chair or writing with a pen.

For the latter, the bones in our hands, wrists, and arms need to articulate—a word with connotations similar to the typical definition of communicating with other people. In this case, *articulating* refers to the cooperation between the bones that comprise our joints. Why is such a joint effort needed? Because every bone in the body connects with another one, except for the hyoid bone, which, amusingly, anchors the tongue but has no articulation with any other part of the human skeleton.

Excluding this notoriously "loose tongue," our bones join at the joints where protective fluids, connective tissue, and collagen-empowered cartilage offer us ease of movement. There, shiny bands of whitish fibrous tissue known as ligaments hold our bones and cartilage in place, not too snugly but with enough strength and flexibility to give each joint full range of motion. Without our muscles, however, our bones would stand woodenly still. Therefore, to get us up and moving, our bones need corresponding muscles attached by strong fibrous tendons that come in a variety of lengths and widths, depending on their locations or the specific jobs they have been given to do.

Our muscles also have unique tasks and compositions with diverse shapes and types relating to their placement and function. In our skeletal muscles, for example, fine thin threads or myofilaments comprise the long striated fibers that house our capillaries. These capillaries then supply oxygen and nutrients via our blood, thus providing our muscles with energy for action. We need, however, a different type of muscle for our body organs to function involuntarily. Therefore, our highly specialized cardiac muscle fibers pump our hearts while our smooth muscles aid our internal organs. Fortunately, those functions take place without our ever having to recall or reschedule such vital matters. For each task involving our musculoskeletal systems, though, we think about our actions before they can occur. Even if the ensuing movement becomes commonplace enough to seem automatic, it really is not. We still alert our brains to drive the car, write a note, or walk across a room without bumping into the furniture. Then, when our brains have even vaguely decided what to do, our senses heighten, and our bodies prepare to move.

To make this coordinated effort possible, our skeletal muscles come in pairs, with opposites causing almost every action. As a result, one muscle (the agonist) relaxes as its antagonist contracts, and in less than a microsecond, that action reverses as our muscles switch jobs—back and forth, back and forth—relaxing and contracting. With our bones acting as levers and our joints allowing movement, our counterbalanced sets of muscles apply alternating forces to get us moving or to hold us upright, opposing gravity.

Going against the Earth's gravitational pull takes strength and balance. It also takes good timing and high levels of organization for us to have such flexible, mobile bodies. No matter how small or insignificant a cell or fiber seems to be, each part plays a part in bringing our muscles and bones closer to homeostasis—that state of equilibrium we find in optimal health. Therefore, our bodies work best when our cartilage, tendons, ligaments, and joints stay in comfortably close alliance and alignment, enabling every one of our 206 bones (give or take those three tiny ossicles in each ear) to cooperate well with our 600-plus muscles. Then, our innumerable muscle cells and fibers will relax and contract according to what is needed at that immeasurable moment. If we want speed or power, our muscles prepare for action. If we seek flexibility and grace or endurance and strength, our muscles comply, assuming, of course, they can.

What Goes Wrong and Why?

Unfortunately, accidents happen. Stress fractures and strokes occur. Bacterial and viral impostors invade the body disguised as normal cells. Genetic codes secretly pass from one generation to another, allowing abnormalities to begin before birth. Also passed on to us are environmental factors and cultural or personal ways of doing things—subtle influences that, nevertheless, sway our opinions and affect our muscles, bones, and the least-considered cellular parts of our bodies. We may not like to think so. We may try to argue or defend the familiar ways we have known as being harmless enough to once keep our ancestors going. Nevertheless, our musculoskeletal conditions reportedly impair one of us in every seven—with an estimated cost to our society of $254 billion each year.

For those of us who have now passed age 50, half of the women and one in eight of the men will have an osteoporosis fracture before this lifetime ends. Yet young people experience impairments too. Of those 18 and older, 18.4 million will incur some type of problem with the back or spine. Every year, 28.6 million Americans of all ages will acquire some sort of musculoskeletal injury. With so many problems involving the muscles and bones of so many people, all 50 states and some 60 health care organizations have joined forces and resources in proclaiming the National Bone and Joint Decade from 2002–11. In March 2002, President Bush officially added the U.S. government's support of this organized effort that goes forth in hopes of developing unbiased research, performing clinical trials, raising public awareness, and allowing each of us to decide for ourselves about the medical care and type of treatments we most want or need.

These choices are ours, yet they begin long before anything goes wrong. They do not start with a national number but with each person's everyday decisions about simple matters relating to what we will do or will not do in the course of a day or evening. We choose for ourselves what we eat, drink, or wear. Sometimes, though, we do so automatically with little deliberation and, perhaps, with little recollection of how our bodies work. For example, we might prefer to choose high-heeled pumps or cowboy boots because they make our legs look great or make us taller or make us feel cool and then later wonder why we have bunions or our backs ache or our vertebral disks show signs of disintegration. We get a sweet tooth, and instead of choosing energizing fruit, we buy candy. If we do not feel too well, we select over-the-counter medicines and synthetic vitamins to get healthy, even though unneeded additives, such as food coloring, make them more enticing. Seldom do we know those appealing colors have been shown by some to ooze into the no-zone areas, breeching the blood-brain barrier or crossing into a placenta's normally protected environment.

We are not what we eat and drink, but those choices certainly shape our bodies. We are much more than our food preferences or selections. However, many of us may be a whole lot more with added pounds compressing our hips, legs, ankles, and other weight-bearing bones. That is not true for everyone, of course. Sadly, some of us may feel so fed up with life, we eat almost nothing, not knowing our muscles and bones will maintain us if given no choice about the nutrients supplied by feeding off their own tissue. Most of us, however, are hungry for something, so we grill choice cuts of beef. We fry delicious chicken with the crispy skin intact, scoop up big bowls of ice cream, and overcook our too-few vegetables with bacon grease, globs of butter, or too much of the normally healthful choice of olive oil. For many of us, we do not decide what nutrients we need so much as what our palates have been culturally trained to appreciate and accept. Yet our inconspicuous arteries clog for lack of fiber—both the soluble and insoluble kinds needed to mop up glops of cholesterol and sponge the excess fats far from our systems. We bake or buy cakes, glazed doughnuts, and breads made of heavily processed white sugar and white flour with many of the natural nutrients in cane and whole grain stripped away, convincing ourselves it is probably OK since artificial vitamins and minerals have been added back into the batter. Yet no one really knows for sure what imbalances have occurred in the food processing or what micronutrients may be as yet unidentified and missing like a Jane or a John Doe. To make up for the added calories, however, we drink diet sodas. With artificial sweeteners defying what the body knows of nature, we consume large quantities of carbonated soft drinks, pouring excess phosphorus into our systems then often dispense too much salt to get a heightened taste. Ultimately, these choices become habits that imbalance the calcium in our bodies, and, with too few signs telling, we may wonder where our bones have gone.

We thirst for something. Yet we drink too little water to keep the natural wastes and artificial additives successfully washed away, or we drink unfiltered water and add other unknowns to our previously unbalanced systems. We hear that one glass of red wine for women and one and a half for men have been shown to reduce our cholesterol and our stress, so we drink three or four, thinking more is best. We smoke, so our children smoke and dry more bones and tissue. We spray our lawns with pesticides because our neighbors do. With assurances of these neighboring numbers, all seems well, and euphoria says, "We are invincible. We do not need to wear the seat belts in our cars or those extrasturdy helmets on our two-wheelers to protect our bones from breaking," but still they break and buckle.

Such choices bring no lecture, for surely I am "we" too, with my 30 percent clogged arteries, extra 10 pounds, and bones slimming as we speak. Yet my task at hand is to assess what can go askew without our even noticing that the spine has shifted, the feet have gone flat, the muscles are tense, or the arteries are too congested. For each of us, the specific causatives and solutions will most likely differ. For each, though, our questions remain the same. What gets us out of balance? More importantly, what can we do to gain not just good-looking or well-sculpted bodies but measurably healthier muscles and bones? Since I am neither a physician nor desirous of replacing yours, I cannot answer for you. However, I can and have compiled a larger perspective that encompasses what medical experts, equitable studies, and continuous research on muscles and bones have consistently suggested: with the aid of the following pages and any other information required to clarify, our bodies can and will inform us.

Ultimately, the signs and symptoms we notice are meant to serve a useful purpose in helping us to identify with greater precision what needs to be corrected—preferably, before our bones dissolve and our muscles waste. Some of the symptoms that signal an imbalance or a disorder of our musculoskeletal systems include these common signs:

- pain, tenderness, or stiffness
- inflammation, heat, or swelling
- muscle weakness, tingling, or numbness
- limited range of motion

What causes our bodies to protest? Why do our muscles and bones present such a strong case for gaining our attention? Frankly, many of us work too long and too hard or we get too tense. We forget to rest and move around or jump playfully onto that empty swing in the nearby park. If economic considerations offer us few constraints, it is often easier to hire someone to do the yard work or the housecleaning and then go to a nearby gym to pump iron, with no thought of the irony building. Yet stretching a bit to reach the top of the venetian blinds with a duster or squatting to weed a garden or pushing a lawn mower until our freshly opened pores spill forth sweat and release unwanted toxins may be just what we need to circulate our body fluids, pump our muscles, and build our bones.

Unfortunately, some of the factors that contribute to our slow and inconspicuous acquisition of musculoskeletal problems cannot be prevented or avoided. Yet, some can. Shall we find out which is which? In fair warning, this resolve may require audacity! Being honest with ourselves or mustering the courage needed to listen to our bodies as they speak is tough, especially when we do not like what they have to say about the way we have been treating them. Nevertheless, this can change. Like young children, our wonderfully human bodies show characteristic signs of adapting and forgiving. Even if genetic factors prove to be irreversible or damages remain beyond our quick undoing, our bodies have mysterious mechanisms set to rebalance themselves. Additionally, we have a tremendous selection of up-to-the-minute technology, new pharmaceuticals, innovative treatments, and medical expertise available to assist. With our muscles and bones—and undoubtedly, our minds—set on healing, we may find more medical alternatives and traditional options for our health care than we deemed possible. We may even get to know ourselves and the remarkably adjusted bodies we carry with us through every choice we make.

ENTRIES A–Z

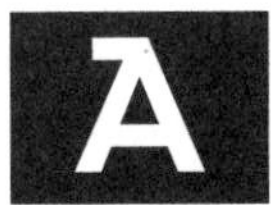

abasia The Greek roots that form this word also define the abasic or abatic condition as *not step.* Muscles and bones do not pull their weight together, so mobility suffers and balance becomes impossible or impaired. Abasia may involve trembling or may stiffen the legs and lock the joints in a type of paralysis that is psychologically induced, for instance, if one becomes "frozen with fear." As a chronic condition, however, abasia may present itself as extreme awkwardness, acute lack of coordination, or an inability to walk.

abdominal muscles These amazing groups of muscles come from various directions in sets and layers intent on holding internal organs in place and enabling the torso to bend, twist, turn, or stretch. Straplike pairs of rectus abdominus muscles straddle either side of an imaginary line drawn down the front of the body, from the upturned V of the ribs through the navel and above the pubic bone. On either side of that midline, the internal oblique muscles stretch diagonally, pointing downward toward the outer edges of the hips as external oblique muscles extend diagonally in the opposite direction, completing the top layer of an X. Across the midriff and lower abdomen, horizontal transversus abdominis muscles create a girdle effect meant to control protrusion or sagginess. When that is not done to a person's satisfaction, though, attention often focuses on the abs rather than on the weight loss that is typically needed.

In evaluating the effectiveness of exercise on abdominal muscles, a 2001 study completed by Dr. Peter Francis of the Biomechanics Lab at San Diego State University and sponsored by the American Council on Exercise indicated that all ab exercises do not necessarily offer uniform results. Traditional, reverse, and vertical leg crunches work well as do crunches on an exercise ball. However, a favored exercise for strengthening abs is the bicycle maneuver done while lying on the back with hands at the head and knees at a 45-degree angle. As the legs rotate in a slow cycling motion, the left elbow aims for the right knee then the right elbow for the left knee while breathing remains natural and relaxed.

Selecting a variety of ab exercises helps a person to maintain posture, lessen back pain, and improve athletic performance. Since the same workout will often become counterproductive after two or three months, one exercise can be replaced with another of similar purpose or increased intensity. In general, an effective ab exercise will move the breastbone toward the frontal pelvic area while keeping the lower back naturally arched to avoid undue strain. For example, sit-ups done on a regular basis will give the large rectus abdominis muscles a workout that strengthens the abdominal region, which, in turn, aids normal breathing movements, enhances muscular support of the spine, and tucks the abdominal organs nicely into place.

In the presence of vertebral problems, however, sit-ups can be a pain in the neck! To avoid strain, the neck needs to stay relaxed and supported in its natural curve by both of the hands or by a small, rolled hand towel. A doctor's advice is the first exercise to undertake in any program, though, and pregnant women especially will want to ask about their optimal levels for strengthening abdominal muscles. Too much ab exercising, for instance, can inhibit the natural expansion required to accommodate the last weeks of pregnancy. However, too little can result in back pain or other problems associated with weak abdominal muscles that have become burdened by additional weight.

See also EXERCISE; NUTRITION.

Murphy, Myatt. "Get Abs Fast." *Men's Fitness* (March 2002): 23a.

Wilkins, Rob. "Phenomenal Abdominals in 8 Weeks or Less!" *Natural Muscle* (September 2002): 22–23.

abducens muscle Like all other parts of the body, eyes have muscles too. Of the four short muscles accompanying each eyeball, the abducens muscles enable a person's sight to turn outward, away from visual contact with the nose.

abductor muscles These muscles move part of the body from center to side as in raising an arm, spreading the toes, or shifting the eyes from a midpoint of reference. In the exercise jumping jacks, for example, limbs go out during abduction. During adduction, they return.

See also RANGE OF MOTION.

abnormality In musculoskeletal systems, an abnormality includes malformations or malfunctions caused by an accident, injury, disease, or birth defect. The word denotes something other than average or normally expected, thus flawlessly sculpted or artificially enhanced muscles offer examples of abnormality at the opposite extreme.

abrachia With this congenital condition, a baby is born without arms. Although causatives may remain unclear, some type of disruption most likely occurred during the developmental stage when embryonic arms would normally appear.

See also BIRTH DEFECTS.

absorptiometry Used to measure bone mineral density, the particular choice of instruments in this type of test will depend on what is to be examined. Single-energy X-ray absorptiometry (SXA), for instance, measures the density of small areas of bone, such as those found in the wrist, whereas dual-energy X-ray absorptiometry (DXA or DEXA) may be used to test larger areas of the body or the whole skeleton.

absorption Although this term frequently refers to the movement of nutrients through the digestive tract, absorption also includes the passage or incorporation of a substance into the body through the membranes, mouth, nose, or skin. As it relates to bone, the absorption and dispersal of waves during an ultrasound test reveal bone mass. Additionally, absorption refers to the loss of minerals as happens in osteoporosis or in joint damage where bone rubs against bone, wearing the bones away and transporting minute particles into the bloodstream.

accessory muscles Every good plan has a backup system, including muscular systems. In normal breathing, for instance, the muscles of the diaphragm and abdomen expand on inhalation and contract on expiration. If anything disturbs that flow, accessory muscles along the back, the neck, and the shoulders assist the person in getting enough air to breathe. Some factors causing respiratory muscles to work harder than usual may include a supine sleeping position, aerobic exercise, or a sudden change of elevation from sea level to a high altitude. Neuromuscular diseases involving some type of abnormality in ventilatory control can impede normal breathing patterns, as can the use of alcohol or drugs that suppress the action of respiratory muscles. In addition, fractured ribs, surgery in the chest area, and muscle damage in the diaphragm or abdomen may stress respiratory muscles to their maximum, thus requiring the use of accessory muscles to ease a person's breathing. A significant factor will then be if previous conditioning around the neck and shoulders or the person's overall health allows the functional ability needed to enable the accessory muscles to perform. Nevertheless, when an obstacle of any kind hinders one's breathing ability even for a moment, most people become frightened or panicked, thereby constricting the air passage even more. The treatment depends, of course, on the cause of respiratory distress, but a low voice and a soothing approach usually provide a calming effect. Repositioning the body may also help. For instance, standing up, placing both hands flat on a table or countertop, and leaning forward may make breathing easier. After some types of surgery, such as a heart bypass that opens the chest and rib cage, patients can be encouraged to lean forward and cradle a pillow to lessen pain while performing the deep-breathing and coughing exercises needed to hasten recovery.

See also RESPIRATORY MUSCLES.

accidents In a 2002 press release by the American Medical Association, Dr. Donald J. Palmisano said, "Patients with severe trauma injury have one 'golden hour' to get care," with the odds of a full recovery diminishing as time lapses. This causes particular concern if a trauma center has a poor doctor-to-patient ratio or is located outside an optimal driving area. Although swift transportation helps accident victims improve the likelihood of healing, vehicles also initiate the top cause of accidental deaths among children, while unintentional injuries of all kinds rank fifth as the cause of death for adults.

See also SAFETY.

CDC National Center for Health Statistics. "Deaths: Leading Causes for 2000." *National Vital Statistic Reports*. Available online. URL: http://www.cdc.gov/nchs/releases/02Facts/Final2000.htm Updated on January 3, 2004.

acetabulum This saucer-shaped hollow of the hip bone articulates with the femur (thighbone). Its ball-and-socket rotation is second only to the shoulder joint in the potential range of motion. Because of its mobility and its ability to bear body weight, the acetabulum experiences wear and tear and can provide an easy access for damage to occur.

See also HIP; INJURY.

achalasia For unknown reasons, this condition occurs when a muscle valve or ring of muscle, such as the stomach sphincter, fails to loosen or relax. As a disease of the esophagus, achalasia affects one child in 10,000 before age 15 according to statistics from the Vanderbilt Medical Center in Nashville, Tennessee. At the University of Miami School of Medicine, suggested treatments for achalasia include injections of a muscle relaxant at the site, stretching the muscular canal of the esophagus, or surgery. To avoid the latter, however, some medical centers now use botulinum toxin type A—better known as Botox—injected into the area when relaxation of the involved nerves is warranted. This does not offer a permanent solution nor has there been adequate research to ascertain the long-term effects. Nevertheless, the majority of patients find the treatment effective enough to return when help may be needed once again.

ache If asked to define an ache, most people think of a headache—probably because 45 million Americans will be pained by recurring ones in the course of a year, according to The National Headache Foundation. Regardless of the location, an ache differs from a pain both in its persistence and intensity. Generally dull and unremitting, aches range from mild muscular discomfort to a slight throb with the treatment depending on the cause. An allover body ache, for instance, may indicate a fever, while a headache can result from sinus pressure or tension, and an aching back can be from stress or strain. "Most simple aches and pains are the result of overexertion," says Dr. Randy Braith of the University of Florida. "Achiness in medical terms is known as 'delayed onset of muscle soreness,' and that passes quickly." If not, a doctor's diagnosis should be sought.

See also ACUTE PAIN; CHRONIC PAIN; DELAYED ONSET MUSCLE SORENESS; HEADACHE; PAIN MANAGEMENT.

Cassey, John. "Oh, My Aching Body." Available online. URL: http://content.health.msn.com/content/article/61/67337.htm?printing=true Downloaded on April 2, 2003.

Achilles tendon The largest tendon in the body, the Achilles attaches the calf muscle to the vulnerable heel where ill-fitting shoes or strenuous running can readily cause swelling or discomfort. The Achilles tendon is particularly vulnerable to tendinitis, an inflammation or soreness of the tendon. As a July 2002 press release from the American College of Foot and Ankle Surgeons (ACFAS) reports, "Heel pain among weekend sports participants, runners, and those beginning exercise programs is reaching epidemic proportion." Eventually, tendinitis hinders range of motion, and, with additional stress, the tendon itself may rupture, as is often discerned by a popping sound.

For most people, problems can usually be prevented with warm-ups that gently stretch the Achilles tendon and calf muscles before rigorous activity begins. Proper footwear guards against injury too. Aside from those injuries produced by a direct blow or a hard misstep, Achilles tendinitis can come about from paralytic conditions, congenital problems concerning the structure of the foot, poor posture, or stresses that come from wearing high-heeled boots or shoes. Suddenly lowering the heel by walking barefoot or wearing flat shoes, however, can exacerbate contractures of the Achilles tendon. However, stretching exercises and a gradual change in choice of footwear can often help.

Even with a good walking or running shoe, though, problems can occur. In another 2002 press release by ACFAS entitled, "The Right Shoe Can Prevent Achilles Tendon Injuries," Dr. Michael K. Lowe, a foot and ankle surgeon in Utah, says, "Athletic shoes that bend in the midfoot area lack proper support and put more pressure on the heel and Achilles tendon." He goes on to explain, "When the middle of the sole in an athletic shoe collapses, pressure is transferred from the midfoot area to the heel, which can stretch the Achilles tendon too much." Replacing worn shoes avoids this. For runners, Dr. Lowe suggests replacements every 350–400 miles.

If tendinitis does occur, home treatment typically begins with an ice pack on the area for up to a half hour several times a day. Shoes, such as an open-back sandal, should be chosen even more carefully to relieve direct pressure and stress on the heel. If the Achilles tendon has ruptured, however, immediate medical attention will be needed. Usually, the patient can tell the difference between tendinitis and a rupture by assessing the level of pain. Tendinitis causes swelling and discomfort, but a rupture of the Achilles tendon will often be indicated by the sudden onset of very sharp pain immediately followed by difficulty in walking or even standing. That is an appropriate response by the body, too, since the person should not put weight on an injured foot anyway. In such cases, surgery may be needed to repair the tendon. Regardless, a cast or splint on the foot will most likely be needed for about six weeks with a little weight bearing sometimes possible after a couple of weeks.

See also FOOTWEAR; TENDINITIS OR TENDONITIS.

achondroplasia This inherited disorder impedes development of cartilage and bone. It results in the most common type of dwarfism characterized by shortened limbs and a disproportionately large head as compared with adults without dwarfism. Adults with achondroplasia reach an average height of four feet unless spinal stenosis and vertebral compressions produce health problems as the person ages. Torso size, intelligence, and life expectancy, however, remain within the ranges generally tabulated as normal for all people.

See also DWARFISM.

acro- When combined with varying suffixes, this prefix indicates either an extreme condition or a body extremity, such as a toe. Acroagnosis, for example, means no awareness of one's limbs. Acrodolichomelia refers to unusually long hands and feet. Acrokinesia denotes severe movement of the extremities.

acromegaly In this chronic disease, growth hormones begin to overproduce during middle age, causing muscular pain and headaches as facial features gradually coarsen and enlarge. The jaw expands. Teeth begin to have gaps between them, and the hands and feet get noticeably bigger.

Muscular weakness also occurs and, occasionally, diabetes. More commonly, joint pain results—sometimes with degenerative arthritis that may become crippling. In children, a similar set of circumstances would produce gigantism, but in an adult 30–50 years old, the growth plates have closed, thus resulting in malformations of the bones. In either case, treatment may include radiation therapy and medications in an attempt to lower overproduction of growth hormones.

See also GROWTH HORMONES.

acromioclavicular joint Stabilized by two sets of ligaments, the acromioclavicular (AC) joint occurs where the acromion part of the shoulder blade (scapula) meets the collarbone (clavicle) with cartilage between for ease of movement. If that cartilage disappears, as happens with arthritis, or if the ligaments stretch or snap, as can occur in a collision sport, treatment hinges on the severity of the trauma. In its patient guide, John Hopkins University suggests, "The more the joint hurts the more ice be used," with surgery preferably reserved for "high caliber athletes." Indeed, the statistics in "What Affects AC Joint Stability?" in the November 2001 *Sports Medicine Reports* say that approximately 45 percent of all shoulder injuries suffered by athletes involve the AC joint. How those injuries affect the potential of individual ligaments to resume normal movement after surgery remains less clear. When a surgical procedure is warranted, careful preservation and repair of the AC joint capsule may significantly help to avoid long-term pain and limited movement.

Sports Medicine Reports. "What Affects AC Joint Stability?" Available online. URL: http://www.findarticles.com/cF_0/mOKHT/11_3/80305481/print.jhtml Downloaded on May 11, 2003.

action potential This is not an assessment of one's ability to move but, instead the movement of electrical charges or nerve impulses within a muscle leading to its contraction. In the heart muscle, for example, action potential can last 10–30 times longer than in skeletal muscle.

activator In the body, an activator is one substance that stimulates the action of another. In the mouth, it is an orthodontic device that passively transmits force from oral muscles to teeth. In a chiropractor's office, an Activator is an instrument used to initiate a light, controlled thrust with such rapidity that the muscles have little time to tense up and resist, thereby receiving an adjustment with reportedly more precision and a minimum of strain.

activity An ability to move about and perform the functions that meet daily needs can be the deciding factor between good health and diminished capacity, yet people may not accurately assess how sedentary they have become. To see if discrepancies existed between estimated and actual movements, researchers furnished pedometers to a group of healthy adults of various ages to count the steps each typically took throughout the day. Results showed that the expectations and less-taken realities of activities had little in common.

Besides causing a person to move around, exercise and physical activity may also have little in common. Exercising usually involves a specific goal, such as engaging in a sport or strengthening a particular part of the body, whereas activity means a movement of any kind. This can be carrying groceries (an activity that increases strength), dancing around while dusting (aids flexibility), or taking the stairs (endurance) instead of passively riding an elevator. Although moderate activity may be described as an ability to walk two miles in a half hour, 30 minutes a day of any activity lessens the risk of heart disease.

A report by the surgeon general entitled "The Link Between Physical Activity and Morbidity and Mortality" indicates that regular activity throughout the week reduces the risk of premature death; controls body weight; maintains the strength of bones, muscles, and joints; and enhances a person's outlook in general. That optimal view, in itself, can strengthen. Not only does activity lessen fatigue, it boosts the immune system and, as indicated in studies of cancer patients, increases the rate of survival. In addition, physical activity affects overall body functions, such as the production of hormones and the normalization of body composition and metabolism, thereby reducing cancer risks.

A November 29, 2001 report by the American Accreditation HealthCare Commission states, "Physical activity can increase the basal metabolic rate by approximately 10%" for up to 48 hours after the activity ceases. To take advantage of this in a weight loss program, the commission recommends considering variables, such as the time spent on an activity, the weight of the person involved, and the pace of performance. A 45-minute walk, for example, burns more calories than 20 minutes of walking unless the pace picks up during the shorter time. Also, a heavier person uses more energy than a lighter-weight person walking the same amount of time at the same pace.

Because a sedentary life increases morbidity and loss of functional capacity, the Centers for Disease Control and Prevention encourage childrens' guardians to establish good patterns that children can readily carry into adulthood. Safe play areas, flexible curricula, and extracurricular activities help children of all types to develop the motor skills and the social patterns needed to maintain active lives at any age. Unfortunately, children who are nearing or entering their teen years may spend only eight to 10 minutes a day in heightened activity. A study of children, age 10–16, showed that their belief in the benefits of physical activity did not help to increase their actual movements. However, when the children engaged in high-level physical movements, their confidence levels increased, thus activating further interest in pursuing additional activities.

Batty, David. "Does Physical Activity Prevent Cancer?" Available online. URL: http://findarticles.com.cf_0m0999/7274_321/68863611/print.jhtml Downloaded on April 4, 2003.

Centers for Disease Control and Prevention. "Physical Fitness and Activity in Schools." Available online. URL: http://findarticles.com/cf_0/m0950/5_105/62193569/ print.jhtml Downloaded on April 4, 2003.

Jet. "Daily Physical Activity is Key to Good Health." Available online. URL: http://findarticles.com/cf_0/m1355/23_100/80309329/print.jhtml Downloaded on April 4, 2003.

Reiff, Michael. "Psychosocial Correlates of Physical Activity in Healthy Children." Available online. URL: http://findarticles.com/cf_0/mOHVD/6_22/81596908/print.jhtml Downloaded on April 4, 2003.

Squires, Sally. "The Lean Plate Club: Taking Steps to Move More." *The Washington Post.* Available online. URL: http://www.washingtonpost.com/ac2/wp-dyn/A22313-2003feb17?Language-printer.htm Downloaded on February 18, 2003.

activity, limitations of With the potential sources of activity limitation too numerous to list, medical evaluations generally focus on a particular condition. For example, to determine the motor and sensory involvement following an injury to the spine, the American Spinal Injury Association (ASIA) developed the ASIA Impairment Scale, which gauges results from complete impairment to normal function. The gradual limitations due to normal aging may be more difficult to access. However, therapists in care facilities for the elderly typically work to improve mobility, balance, and the practical activities of daily life.

A 2002 National Center for Health Statistics report, *Chartbook on Trends in the Health of America,* acknowledges a discrepancy in health surveys. Despite the variances, though, chronic musculoskeletal conditions, such as arthritis, limit activity consistently with almost one-fifth of adults 75 and older requiring assistance for everyday routines. In children, the numbers fluctuate because of a wide range of developmental differences, but chronic conditions that limit activities are twice as likely among boys.

In very young children, delayed development further limits activity as babies and preschoolers who have been previously hindered from self-initiating movement begin to restrict themselves through lack of interest. Caretakers can help children increase activity, however, by providing the opportunities and equipment that encourage more mobility in crawling, walking, and exploring a safe environment.

Wright-Ott, Christine A., et al. "Encouraging Exploration." Available online. URL: http://www.rehabpub.com/Features/672002/3.asp Downloaded on April 16, 2003.

acupressure Also known as contact healing, acupressure applies pressure at potent points throughout the body to release muscular tension, alleviate pain, and stimulate the body's curative devices. In the absence of bruising or broken bones, acupressure can be applied by pressing directly into an ache with a thumb or knuckle or, for hard-to-reach knots, the padded tip of a cane. In his book *Acupressure's Potent Points,* Michael Gach, founder of the Acupressure Institute in Berkeley, California, explains, "Tension tends to concentrate around acupressure points. When a muscle is chronically tense or in spasm, the muscle fibers contract due to the secretion of lactic acid. . . ." Dr. Gach goes on to say, "As a point is pressed, the muscle tension yields to the finger pressure, enabling the fibers to elongate and relax, blood to flow freely, and toxins to be released and eliminated."

Kallen, Ben. "Acupressure for the Active Guy." Available online. URL: http://www.findarticles.com/cF_0/m1608/9_17/80309807/print.jhtml Downloaded on April 7, 2003.

acupuncture Based on the theory of energy flowing through the body, this ancient form of treatment addresses imbalances or blockage as the primary source of disease in the body. A very thin needle inserted at specific points along an energy pathway or meridian can be used to anesthetize an area prior to surgery or to alleviate pain, nonsurgically, in musculoskeletal conditions, such as tendinitis, osteoarthritis, or carpal tunnel syndrome.

Since about 300 B.C.E., classical Chinese practices generally accepted acupuncture charts as pointing to specific areas of the skin surfaces that were thought to connect to corresponding organs, but later charts became guides to principal meridians of the body. In this country though, researchers have often puzzled over explanations that might fit the Western mind. Recently, such studies proposed a correlation between the acupuncture meridians and the technologically explicable planes of connective tissue indicated by ultrasound or other means. The resulting tests on a cadaver's arm, for instance, found that the majority of acupuncture points and meridian intersections coincided with identifiable intermuscular or intramuscular planes of the body.

To apply traditional treatment, a trained acupuncturist inserts and then rotates a thin needle of gold or stainless steel until a "needle grasp," similar to the tug of a fish on a line, signals that a connection has been made with an optimal acupuncture point. As the acupuncturist twirls or lightly pulls and pushes the inserted needle, the adjacent tissue adheres slightly and then winds around the needle, altering the tissue's pattern of response. As an important aspect of this procedure, stainless steel needles have been a frequent choice because of the safety factors in disposability. However, recent study indicate that a sterilized gold needle encourages the winding process, potentially bringing about a continuum of more effective cellular responses along the connective tissue plane.

See also MEDICAL ALTERNATIVES.

Langevin, Helene M. and Jason A. Yandow. "Relationship of Acupuncture Points and Meridians to Connective Tissue Planes." Available online. URL: http://www.Interscience.wiley.com Downloaded May 12, 2003.

acute pain Intense but of relatively short duration, "Acute pain is often associated with an identifiable injury or trauma as a known antecedent, responds to therapeutic options, and resolves in less than 1 to 3 months."

See also CHRONIC PAIN; PAIN MANAGEMENT.

Barkin, Robert L. and Diana Barkin. "Pharmacologic Management of Acute and Chronic Pain." *Southern Medical Journal* 94, no. 8, (August 2001): 756–763.

ad- or -ad Whether adhering as a prefix or a suffix, ad- means *toward.*

adductor muscles Having the opposite task of abductors, these muscles bring an arm, leg, finger, toe, or eye toward its common center, such as when dropping one's arms to the sides.

See also RANGE OF MOTION.

adhesive capsulitis Also known as frozen shoulder, adhesive capsulitis severely limits a person's range of motion—a condition that medical author Dr. William C. Shiel Jr., speaking for the University of Miami School of Medicine, warns can become permanent unless treated with anti-inflammatory medication, cortisone injections, or therapy. Any related injury can lead to frozen shoulder, but the syndrome often occurs through scarring or other source of thickening around a joint. Sedentary patients with arthritic, diabetic, or cardiac conditions may be especially prone to developing secondary adhesive capsulitis.

Although primary adhesive capsulitis usually affects people over age 40, the two to three percent of the population who experience frozen shoulder can also include children. Regardless of age, the syndrome progresses in three stages. The first stage, the painful onset, lasts three to eight months and includes stiffness and muscle spasms. The second or adhesive stage lasts four to six months with pain diminishing but stiffness increasing. In the final or recovery stage, minimal pain occurs, but limited movement may continue for another one to three months.

Siegel, Lori B. "Adhesive Capulitis: A Sticky Issue." Available online. URL: http://www.findarticles.com/cF_O/m322517_59/54591719/print.jhtml Downloaded on March 7, 2003.

adult Still's disease As occurs in juvenile rheumatoid arthritis, symptoms of this systemic form of chronic arthritis include fever, rash, and joint pain. X-rays and blood tests provide a diagnosis with the treatment generally similar to that for other arthritic conditions.

See also ARTHRITIS.

adynamic bone disease Recognized in the 1980s, this disorder shows a reduction of bone turnover typical of aluminum intoxication and dialysis. As reported in "Types of Bone Disease that Can Occur in People with Kidney Diseases" by the U.K.'s National Kidney Foundation, "Normally bone is quite active with constant reabsorption of bone and laying down of bone," but adynamic bone disease slows this healthy process.

U.K. National Kidney Foundation. "Types of Bone Disease that Can Occur in People with Kidney Disease." Available online. URL: http://www.kidney.org.co.uk/Medical-Info/Calcium-Phosphate/bone-disease.html Downloaded on April 8, 2003.

aging, effects of As a person ages, physiological changes decrease the body's circulation, thereby lessening the distribution of hormones, blood, oxygen, liquids, lipids, and other nutrients needed for maximal function. Muscles and tendons gradually lose their elasticity and strength, creating conditions for strains or injuries to occur more easily, particularly in the absence of regular exercise or warm-up times. During the two decades between a person's midforties and sixties, muscle mass may diminish by 30 percent.

Aging bones also encounter problems. Statistics vary, but according to data from the U.S. Administration on Aging, 49 percent of the elderly cope with arthritis while various orthopedic impairments affect another 18 percent. Bone losses occur, too, in both men and women as hormonal fluxes increase bone resorption without a corresponding increase in the formation of bone. While attempting to understand this common occurrence, one study shows that aging reduces plate density rather than bone thickness, with structural changes beginning long before any symptoms have manifested themselves.

As bones wear, so does the shock-absorbing tissue between them. "More precisely, the spaces between the thirty-three vertebrae that constitute the spine compress," states Curtis Pesman. This translates into loss of height. As a result, without regular exercise, such as stretching and abdominal crunches, a six-foot-tall 30-year-old man may be a quarter-inch shorter by age 40. He will not, however, be alone. In the U.S. in 2000, the 60-year-old and over population stood at 16 percent with expectations of 28 percent by 2050. By that same year, the United Nations projects that the fastest-growing 80 and older age group will comprise one-fifth of the world's population.

Administration on Aging. "A Profile of Older Americans: 2001." Available online. URL: http://www.usdhhs.gov Downloaded on April 8, 2003.

American Academy of Orthopaedic Surgeons. "The Effects of Aging on Your Body." Available online. URL: http://orthoinfo.aaos.org/fact/thr_report.cfm?Thread_ID=224+topcategory=wellness Downloaded on April 14, 2003.

Kanapaux, William. "Healthy Aging: Confront a Worldwide Challenge." Available online. URL. http://www.geriatrictimes.com Downloaded on May 2002.

Parfitt, A. M., C. H. Mathews, A. R. Villanueva, M. Kleerekoper, B. Frmae, and D. S. Rao. "Relationship Between Surface, Volume, and Thickness of Iliac Trabecular Bone in Aging and in Osteoporosis. Implications for the Microanatomic and Cellular Mechanisms of Bone Loss." *The Journal of Clinical Investigation* 72, no. 4 (October 1983): 1,396–1,409.

Pesmen, Curtis. "How a Man Ages." *Esquire* (May 2002): 77–88.

Albright's disease Medically referred to as polyostotic fibrous dysplasia, this genetic disorder of bone and cartilage may be discernible in young infants or may show little signs in older children who, otherwise, seem to be in good health. Depending on the severity and progression of the disease, the person may become fracture prone, thus contributing further to potential deformities often involving the legs, arms, and skull. In addition, endocrine abnormalities, such as early puberty, may occur as well as thyroid dysfunctions that cause goiters, nodules, and cysts to form. Irregular pigmentation of the skin and an overproduction of growth hormones can generate other concerns. With no known treatment to control the progression of this disorder, supplements of calcium and vitamin D may prove beneficial. Also, surgery can correct fractures with pinning or grafting and offer reconstruction of bones to improve the person's appearance.

-algia With an identifying prefix, this suffix points to pain.

allograft This transplanted tissue from human beings may not be as safe as an AUTOGRAFT from one's own body. However, a February 2003 report by the American Academy of Orthopaedic Surgeons says the benefits of musculoskeletal allografts outweigh risks in receiving human tissue from donors. Processed for transplant within 24 hours, allografts stabilize joints, restore bone, and assist spinal fusions with only one in 1.6 million affected by viral contamination.

American Academy of Orthopaedic Surgeons. "Benefits of Musculoskeletal Allograft Tissue Outweigh Risks." Available online. URL: http://www.newswise.com/articles/2003/2/TISSUE.OSR.html Downloaded on February 14, 2003.

alternative medicine See MEDICAL ALTERNATIVES.

amputation The accidental loss of a limb or other part of the body can be caused by diverse equipment or activities that are often work related or associated with mechanical devices left in unguarded areas. Hazards generally decrease with adequate training in the safe use of equipment or tools. However, if no measures are taken to protect employees, complaints can be made by calling OSHA's toll-free number, (800) 321-OSHA (6742).

For conditions such as diabetes, medical amputation can often be prevented with therapeutic footwear and prompt treatment of ulcerations or other circulatory concerns. As the American Podiatric Medical Association reports, 60–70 percent of diabetics have varying degrees of nerve damage that impairs hands and feet, necessitating more than 86,000 amputations each year and making diabetes the leading cause of lower extremity amputations in the U.S.

See also PROSTHESIS; SAFETY.

American Podiatric Medical Association. "Facts on Diabetes and the Foot." Available online. URL: http://www.apma.org/dm_faqs_printable.html Downloaded on February 15, 2003.

amyoplasia In this rare congenital disorder, muscle fails to develop due to thickening of the joint tissues, which results in contractures. In the May 2002 issue of the *Journal of the Indian Medical Association,* Dr. Nilesh Banker of Karasad, India, presented case notes which said, in part, "Here, amyoplasia was marked by multiple flexion and extension contractures of all extremities notably at the hips, knees, elbows, and spine. In advanced cases, muscle fibres are lacking and replaced by collagenous scar tissue." Although this particular case presented severe symptoms at the child's birth, signs of the disorder may not be apparent until a few months later. The disease's etiology remains unknown. However, Dr. Banker classifies occurrences of amyoplasia as either a neuropathic form involving nerve damage or myopathic in which joint deformities result from womb crowding and the fetus's subsequent lack of movement.

See also ARTHROGRYPOSIS; BIRTH DEFECTS.

Journal of the Indian Medical Association. "Case Note: Amyoplasia Congenita Nilesh Banker." Available online. URL: http://www.jimaonline.org/May2002/print_casenote2.htm Downloaded on June 24, 2003.

amyotonia Weak muscles or lack of tone demonstrate this condition, sometimes called floppy infant. When originally recognized, amyotonia may have encompassed a number of disorders that manifest similar symptoms that have since been identified and classified with greater precision, thus leaving this term somewhat obsolete. If, for example, a primary defect presents itself in the newborn's spinal cord, the resulting weak muscle condition may be known as infantile spinal amyotrophy. With numerous origins to consider, health information from Johns Hopkins University suggests that amyotonia congenita might best identify the occurrence of a nonprogressive condition in which the primary abnormality resides in the muscles. Although therapeutic treatment would, most likely, involve physical therapy, specific procedures would depend on a thorough physical examination and medical tests intent on locating the source, which then can be addressed.

OMIM-Online Mendeliau Inheritance in Mau, Johns Hopkins University. "#205000 Amyotonia Congenita." Available online. URL: http://www.ncbi. nlm.nih.gov/entre3/query.Fcgi?cmd=Retrieve+db=omim+dopt=Detailed Downloaded on June 24, 2003.

amyotrophic lateral sclerosis Also named Lou Gehrig's disease for the 20th-century baseball star who died of amyotrophic lateral sclerosis (ALS), this degenerative disease of the nervous system hinders the adult's neurological impulses until stiffness of limbs, spasticity, and minor muscular weakness become full abasia. Initially, symptoms affect only one side of the body as the fatigued patient becomes increasingly unsteady. As ALS progresses, difficulties in speaking and swallowing also occur and, within three to five years, death.

Although causes remain unclear, more than 5,000 people in the U.S. annually contract ALS, the majority of whom are men in their mid-40s to mid-60s. At Johns Hopkins, where the first known center for ALS research began, investigations include such issues as stem cell regeneration, the involvement of specific types of protein, and factors responsible for the death of motor neurons. At present, various forms of therapy increase an ALS patient's quality and duration of life. As researchers learn more about the mechanisms of this disease, new therapies should be forthcoming.

See also ABASIA.

Shurkin, Joel. "In the Name of Lou Gehrig." Available online. URL: http://www.hopkinsmedicine.org/hmn/sp00/Feature 1.html Downloaded on February 4, 2004.

angular As one of the four possible movements of the joints, angular action occurs between long bones, such as those in the leg or arm, as the angle increases or decreases.

ankle Located between the foot and leg, the ankle bone (talus) articulates with the fibula (calf bone) and the second longest bone in the body, the tibia. With its hinged joint held in place by rubber band–like ligaments, the healthy ankle moves the foot up or down in a motion just right for walking and running. Below that hinged joint, a ball-and-socket joint allows the foot to wiggle back and forth unless a sprain or torn ligament skews that plan.

With ankle sprains the most common athletic injury in the U.S. each year, about one-half of those four million or so sprains are fracture free but involve a significantly higher number of women than men. Regardless of gender, statistics from the American College of Foot and Ankle Surgeons say that 85 percent of ankle sprains, from mild to severe, situate on the outside of the ankle joints and heal within three to eight weeks. X-rays may be needed to identify dislocations or fractures and an MRI to show details of soft tissue and bone. Recommended treatment usually begins with the RICE method of rest, ice, compression, and elevation. If left untreated, however, a sprain can weaken an ankle indefinitely.

In high school and college sports, a recent trend has been to tape ankles prior to an event in hopes of eliminating sprains, strains, and other injuries. After 10 minutes of activity, athletic tape loses 40 percent of its support with a corresponding loss of consistency in strength. Factors such as perspiration or the expertise of the person applying the tape also contribute to variations. Adjustable ankle braces have an advantage in that they can be adapted throughout a game and, if used regularly during sports events, can be less expensive than forever buying multiple rolls of tape. As a long-term practice, however, bracing or taping can prevent muscles from strengthening naturally, thus weakening the ankle overall.

In addition to sprains, bangs, and other injuries, ankles can be fractured. Since osteoporosis has frequently been cited as a cause of bone breaks, assumptions may have been made about the ability of thinning bones to contribute to spontaneous fractures found in the lower extremities. Although research does reveal that low bone density and physical inactivity create a climate for quickly fracturing one's foot, the recent findings on ankles do not fall into the same category. According to a report in the May 2003 *Journal of Bone and Joint Surgery,* a 10-year study monitored a group of 9,700 or more women age 65 and older. Those who experienced a fractured foot during that time proved to be the older and less active participants of the group who, indeed, had lower bone density as expected. On the other hand (or, perhaps, foot), the younger, more physically active, and overweight participants were shown to be the group most likely to succeed in fracturing an ankle.

American College of Foot and Ankle Surgeons. "Ankle Sprains and Treatments." Available online. URL: http//www.acfas.org/brank/tr.html Downloaded on February 15, 2003.

Comeau, Matthew J. "Bracing vs. Tape." Available online. URL: http://www.rehabpub.com/features/220002/8.asp Downloaded on April 16, 2003.

Journal of Bone and Joint Surgery. *Focus on Healthy Aging* newsletter. Pg. 2.

Ottaviani, Robert A., James A. Ashton-Miller, and Edward M. Wojtys. "Inversion and Eversion Strengths in the Weight Bearing Ankle of Young Women." Available online. URL: http://www.findarticles.com/cf_0/m0918/2_29/74482806/p1/article.jhtml Downloaded on April 16, 2004.

ankylosing spondylitis Like other rheumatic diseases in the spondylarthropathies group, ankylosing spondylitis (AS) attacks the spine, sometimes hindering a diagnosis since the symptoms often mimic common back problems. For women, a diagnosis may be further delayed since three times more men suffer from AS, making the disease less suspect in women. Regardless of gender, over 90 percent of the patients exhibit antigens in their bodies, indicating an underlying problem with their immune systems. Studies also show a tendency among family members to acquire the disease even though the specific causes remain unknown.

According to a fact sheet from the American College of Rheumatology, AS most often strikes adolescent or young adult males with 129 persons in 100,000 affected in the U.S. Initially, the patient may periodically complain of low backaches on waking or after prolonged inactivity with the pain sometimes accompanied by signs of fever, fatigue, decreased appetite, or reddened eyes. As the disease progresses, joint movement and range of motion become of greater concern than the pain. Treatment often focuses on retaining posture and hip movement. Otherwise, chronic inflammation of the spine eventually leads to inactivity and vertebral fusion until spinal mobility is lost. However, anti-inflammatory medication, hydrotherapy, and muscle-strengthening exercises that aid flexibility and deep breathing can slow debilitation and provide a more functional outcome. The support of a firm mattress and good nutrition offer additional help.

American College of Rheumatology. "Ankylosing Spondylitis." Available online. URL: http://www.rheumatology.org/patients/factsheet/as.html Downloaded on February 17, 2003.

anorexia and bone loss A fact sheet, "Skeletal Effects of Anorexia," from the National Institutes of Health Osteoporosis and Related Bone Diseases National Resource Center states, "Bone loss is a well-established consequence of anorexia," with spinal density well below healthy range and recovery of bone mass unlikely if the disorder goes unchecked. Very low weight causes the body to cease producing hormones needed for healthy growth, making male and female adolescents especially vulnerable to nutritional deficiencies and bone loss.

Osteoporosis and Related Bone Diseases National Resource Center. "Skeletal Effects of Anorexia." Available online. URL: http://www.osteo.org/newfile.asp?doc=r709I+doctitle=Skeletal+Effects+of+anorexia Downloaded on February 19, 2003.

anterior cruciate ligament injury Of the seven ligaments connecting the bones at the knee, the anterior cruciate ligament (ACL) has the primary role of stabilization and so will usually be most adversely affected by sports involving a speedy change of direction. If ACL tearing occurs, the knee may give out with a pop, causing many people to opt for surgery. From the U.K., however, Dr. Nicola Maffulli prefers to reserve surgery for "skeletally mature patients" with functional instability caused by a torn ACL but, even then, only if six to 12 weeks of intensive rehabilitation have failed.

A sports tip sheet, "The Injured ACL," provided by the American Orthopaedic Society for Sports Medicine and the National Athletic Trainers Association, says the question of surgery varies from one person to the next with many factors to be considered by the patient and physician. "These factors include the activity level and expectations of the patient, whether there are associated injuries, and the amount of abnormal knee laxity, or looseness." A leisurely walker, for example, may do better by elevating the leg, icing, and then bracing the knee until swelling has subsided and stability increased. Then, a professionally designed course of therapeutic exercises can strengthen the supportive muscles around the knee until normal range of motion and balance have returned. To return to professional play, however, an athlete may require arthroscopic or another type of surgery.

The results of an X-ray or MRI (magnetic resonance imaging) may be the deciding factor by clarifying the extent of an injury and showing, for example, whether the ACL has unraveled like a rope. If so, the damaged ligament may be replaced with tissue taken from a nearby tendon, such as a strip of hamstring. The surgeon then threads the fibers together and, in the process, repairs whatever else may need to be secured. In discussing such procedures in the October 2000 fact sheet "ACL Reconstruction," the American Academy of Orthopaedic Surgeons (AAOS) says the physicians in this country see more than 95,000 ACL tears per year with about 50,000 receiving various types of ligament reconstruction. Of these surgeries, AAOS reports a success rate of 85–92 percent but, to increase the likelihood of those good odds, a patient may want to look for a surgeon who has successfully performed dozens of similar procedures every year.

See also JOINT REPLACEMENT; KNEE; KNEE SURGERY.

American Academy of Orthopaedic Surgeons. "ACL Reconstruction." Available online. URL: http://orthoinfo.aaoss.org/fact/thr_report.cfm?Thread_ID=216+topcategory=knee Downloaded on July 15, 2003.

American Orthopaedic Society for Sports Medicine and the National Trainers Association. "The Injured ACL." Available online. URL: http://www.sportsmed.org/Publications/Stips/ACL.htm Downloaded on July 5, 2003.

Maffulli, Nicola, M.D., "Anterior Cruciate Ligament Tears: Not All Patients Need Reconstruction." *Isakos Newsletter* 4, no. 2 (Winter 2001): 11.

appendicular skeleton To provide balance and assist movements of the axial skeleton, the appendicular consists of arms, legs, and other bony structures of the shoulders and pelvic regions with 64 bones included in the upper extremities and 62 in the lower. For discussion of these well-coordinated parts, see the individual entries, such as FINGER OR FINGERS, FEET OR FOOT, and HAND.

See also Appendix I.

apraxia Indicative of a neurological disorder, apraxia is the inability to initiate or direct movement even though the corresponding muscles show no impairment. With ocular motor apraxia, for example, the person has trouble controlling eye movements on a horizontal plane. With oral apraxia, the muscles of the mouth fail to coordinate, making coughing, swallowing, or pursing the lips difficult. With verbal apraxia or apraxia of speech, unpredictable muscle control makes speaking an effort with several attempts sometimes needed to pronounce a word in the correct sequence of sounds or syllables. Apraxia can also involve the fine muscle coordination required to hold a fork or to write. Although developmental apraxia may be present from the start of life, acquired apraxia often results from an injury, stroke, brain tumor, or infection. For either type of the disorder, however, the treatment depends on the specifics and severity of the impairment. Generally speaking, rhythmic activities, such as hand clapping, may be beneficial as will allowing the person plenty of time to get out the words or to concentrate on the task at hand.

arch This bidirectional curve in the underside of the foot cushions an active body from jolts, but that unique shape makes the arch sometimes need cushioning itself. Shoes with unyielding sides and custom molding at the instep help to support the arch and sidestep backaches.

See also FLATFOOT OR FLATFEET.

arm or arms Most people think of arms as the limbs extending from the shoulders to the hands. However, the anatomical classification goes from the shoulder to the elbow in a single bone—the humerus. For medical distinction, the forearm has two bones—the radius and ulna—both of which extend from the elbow to the wrist. Since females come equipped with an increased carrying angle over their straighter-armed male counterparts, arms bear secondary sex characteristics that can be used to determine gender—a factor that undoubtedly helps law enforcement teams and forensic investigators identify skeletal remains.

At birth, an arm can be missing due to the presence of a genetic defect, a chronosomal abnormality, or the use of certain drugs, such as thalidomide, which was sometimes taken by women in the mid-20th century to combat morning sickness during the first trimester of pregnancy. Other malformations can occur because of constriction in the womb, which may cause a misshapen limb to form. Although some children can become quite adept at using a smaller or shrunken arm, others may require an artificial limb for ease of use.

Weakness or potential paralysis can also occur to one or both of a baby's arms if the nerves sustain damage during an unusually difficult birth. Special care must then be taken in lifting or moving the infant to avoid further injury during the weeks of healing. Rarely will an arm be broken in the delivery room, but this can certainly happen as a child becomes actively mobile or if an injury occurs at any age.

When weakness or debilitation occurs in an elderly patient's arms after surgery or a stroke, recovery of function can be the deciding factor between independent living and assisted care. In either case, an occupational therapist can work with the patient in developing exercises intended to restore mobility, improve overall coordination of the arm and hand, and increase the strength needed to perform one's daily activities.

See also FRACTURES; PROSTHESIS.

arth- or arthro- When combined with a clarifying suffix, this prefix has some connection to the joints of the body. For example, arthrography brings an X-ray to a joint, whereas arthrocentesis refers to the procedure known as JOINT ASPIRATION, and ARTHRALGIA has to do with joint pain.

arthralgia A pain in one or more joints, arthralgia occurs for many reasons, including fever, arthritic conditions, injury, or lead poisoning. Therefore, locating the specific cause of the problem will offer the most relevant treatment options. For example, compression arthralgia (called *compression pains* by the "U.S. Navy Diving Manual") occurs when external oceanic pressures surround a diver, causing deep aching pains usually improved by reversal of the dive or by decompression or recompression. If caused by toxins, detoxing the system with an herbal cleansing or prescribed medication can be beneficial. If arthralgia results from pain or fever, anti-inflammatory medication may relieve the discomfort. The addition of cold therapy and an elastic or compression-type bandage may further reduce the stress on a joint after an injury.

See also ASCORBIC ACID; INJURY.

Campbell, Ernest, M.D. "Compression Arthralgia." Available online. URL: http://www.scuba-doc.com/cmprarth.html Downloaded on June 14, 2003.

arthritis According to October 2002 statistics from the Centers for Disease Control and Prevention, nearly 70 million adults in the U.S. (one in three) have arthritis or chronic joint symptoms as compared with the one in seven previously estimated. These statistics show arthritis to be the leading cause of work-related disabilities, with nearly two times more women affected than men. Children suffer from arthritis, too, with juvenile arthritis one of approximately 100 types of arthritic conditions, each of which relate to inflammation of the joints. Because the prognosis and treatments vary for each type, early evaluation by a rheumatologist or an arthritis specialist should offer the most accurate diagnosis and workable treatment plan.

Initially, arthritis exhibits pain and swelling, with most types accompanied by increased stiffness and decreased range of motion. In general, recommended treatments combine rest, anti-inflammatory medication, personalized programs of exercise, physical therapy, and application of heat or cold. As a further preventative, maintaining a low-to-normal body weight will relieve undue stress on achy joints. Early medical assessment, such as a blood test for the rheumatoid factor, can help to clarify the specific type of arthritis and, therefore, the specific treatment. For example, the fact sheet "Arthritic Disorders and Treatments," published by the American College of Foot and Ankle Surgeons, defines osteoarthritis as a degenerative disease with "pain and stiffness caused by cartilage destruction," whereas rheumatoid arthritis is "a 'systemic' disease that can affect the entire body."

A 2003 study by the Arthritis Foundation shows that the body is not all that arthritis affects. In this country alone, the economic impact on society tallies $124.8 billion a year. Dr. Dorothy D. Dunlop of Northwestern University's Feinburg School of Medicine says, "Vigorous physical activity could reduce disability among older adults with arthritis by 5–10 percent." In its 2000 fact sheet "Exercise and Arthritis," the American College of Rheumatology recommends three types of exercise with low-impact movements for flexibility, muscle conditioning for strength and endurance, and aerobic conditioning for duration and intensity. The best choices or combinations depend on a doctor's assessment of an individual's needs, while the best time of day to exercise will depend on the person's daily cycle. For 75 percent of arthritis patients, however, midafternoon works well for exercise since pain and stiffness often reach maximum intensity prior to rising or just before going to bed.

Besides exercising during the times of the day when symptoms typically reduce, other suggestions appear in the article "Exercising for Arthritis," published by the Mount Sinai School of Medicine's July 2003 issue of *Focus on Healthy Aging*. For instance, moist heat or a very warm shower can help to minimize pain prior to beginning the day's exercise with a stretching exercise. With specific recommendations by a physician or a physical therapist, exercises can be developed in consideration of the degree of joint pain or inflammation. If discomfort increases for more than an hour after a workout, the exercises may be too strenuous. If, however, the pain would have likely persisted anyway, continuing with an appropriately designed exercise program offers other benefits, such as increased energy and endurance, improved quality of sleep, and better-maintained bones and cartilage. If aerobics can be safely added, this can offer additional paybacks in improving circulation and respiration. Should stress on the weight-bearing joints prove too uncomfortable, an aquatic exercise program may offer a workable solution. Not only does walking in water alleviate strain on achy ankles and knees, it also provides resistance and typically a water temperature that helps to soothe arthritic joints.

In addition to exercise programs and standard allopathic treatment, nutritional support can bring a flavorful taste of relief. For instance, turmeric rubbed into fish or other foods before cooking purportedly eases the symptoms of arthritis. A dash of celery seeds to season couscous or vegetables, such as carrots and peas, has been lauded as helpful too. Hot or cold beverages containing a spoon each of apple cider vinegar and honey can lessen arthritic deposits in the joints, whereas capsules of devil's claw and echinacea may bring anti-inflammatory assistance.

Care must be taken, though, to avoid combining an herb with a medication used for the same or similar purpose. Also keep in mind that these remedies are based on the general consensus among herbalists and have not been subjected to scientific studies. Prescription drugs can be inhibited or overly enhanced by some herbs too. So any contraindications mentioned on the medicine's informational sheet become even more important and must be double-checked before using a particular herb. Also, herbs have the ability to trigger an allergic response, as can occur with many foods. For example, the black walnut recommended by many herbalists as an effective way to detox an arthritic system would itself be a poison to those allergic to nuts.

See also HERBS FOR MUSCLES AND BONES; NUTRITION.

American College of Foot and Ankle Surgeons. "Arthritis Disorders and Treatment." Available online. URL: http://www.acfas.org Downloaded on February 17, 2003.

American College of Rheumatology. "Arthritis More Widespread than Previously Reported." Available online. URL: http://www.rheumatology.org/press/am2002/pr10.asp Downloaded on February 25, 2003.

American College of Rheumatology. "Exercise and Arthritis." Available online. URL: http://www.rheumatology.org/patients/factsheet/exercise.html Downloaded on February 17, 2003.

Dunlop, Dorothy. "The High Cost of Pain." Available online. URL: http://www.arthritis.org/Resources/DisplayScreamingNews.asp?id=293 Downloaded on February 26, 2003.

Mount Sinai School of Medicine. "Exercising for Arthritis." *Focus on Healthy Aging* (July 2003): 3–4.

arthrodesis Arthrodesis surgically fuses and stabilizes a joint to decrease pain and repair damage. A number of possible techniques are available.

See also SURGERY.

arthrogryposis A muscle disorder apparent in one of 3,000 births, arthrogryposis is often attributed to anything that prevents an unborn baby from moving in the womb. Although causatives are not entirely clear and opinions vary, some factors may include genetics, abnormal nerve or muscle development, and possibly prenatal environmental conditions, including the presence of drugs in the unborn infant's system. Regardless of the causes, joint contractures usually occur at birth. If no other medical condition exists, however, range of motion can improve with physical therapy and other types of interventions intent on improving function and mobility, rather than appearances. Because of the complexity of the musculoskeletal issues and concerns, a multidisciplinary team can be most effective as the pediatrician, neurologist, orthopedic surgeon, physical therapist, and occupational therapist work together in assisting the child toward ambulation and increased autonomy.

arthroplasty Also known as joint replacement surgery, arthroplasty can be used for any joint, with the most common occurrences in weight-bearing locations receiving high stress, such as the hip or knee.

See also JOINT REPLACEMENT; KNEE SURGERY.

arthroscopy To scope out a joint, arthroscopy inserts needlelike probes with tiny optical fibers to get a picture that helps determine whether surgery is needed. It reveals tiny bone fragments or other particles that can then be removed during an arthroscopic procedure. A well-lit tube about the width of a pencil assists the surgeon in viewing the interior of a joint and assessing the damage before proceeding with arthroscopic repair of the cartilage or a reconstruction of the torn ligaments. Arthroscopic surgery on the knee, for instance, inserts a camera with a diameter of less than one-quarter inch through an incision in the knee joint, allowing the surgeon to see inside. With saline pumped into the area to expand the joint and control the bleeding, a surgeon may then make one to four other tiny incisions to allow other surgical instruments to gain entry. According to the National Institutes of Health (NIH) July 11, 2002 fact sheet on knee arthroscopy, "Commonly used instruments include a blunt hook to pull on various tissues, a shaver to remove damaged or unwanted soft tissues, and a burr to remove bone." When surgery has been completed, the saline solution is then drained from the knee, the incisions are closed, and a dressing is applied. If the surgery involves repairing a meniscal tear in the crescent-shaped cartilage of the knee, the NIH reports that full recovery can be expected. Indeed, for most patients, arthroscopic surgery requires less time with less complications but with a faster recovery rate than other procedures. However, the presence of arthritis changes the effectiveness of arthroscopy so that "up to 50 percent of patients may not improve post-operatively." For patients with rheumatoid arthritis though, "Arthroscopic removal of the synovium (arthroscopic synovectomy) can be of great benefit."

See also KNEE SURGERY.

National Library of Medicine. "Knee Arthroscopy." Available online. URL: http://www.nlm.nih.gov/medlineplus/print/ency/article/002972.htm Downloaded on July 5, 2003.

arthrosis Sometimes called osteoarthritis, arthrosis can refer to any abnormal or degenerative condition of a joint but also to the joint itself. As a synonym for the healthy joint, an arthrosis consists of articulating bones held in place by cartilage and fibrous connective tissue that permit flexibility and ease of movement.

See also JOINT.

articular cartilage injury Also known as the surface of a joint, articular cartilage protects the end of bones with resilient tissue that, nevertheless, wears out with disease, injury, or time. Unfortunately, the damage does not stop there since pain radiates as bone chafes bone. The American Academy of Orthopaedic Surgeons expresses hope in the ability of new techniques to ease thousands of annual sufferers of articular cartilage injury. For example, autografts of a patient's own cells and tissue can repair cartilage, while research suggests that stem cells harvested from the individual's bone marrow can develop additional cartilage to be used to restore a site.

articulation Where two or more bones come together, their articulation creates a joint. Suture joints, for example, occur where the fixed bones of the skull articulate.

See also JOINT.

artificial disk A January 2003 press release from the internationally known Cedars-Sinai Medical Center in California announced an increased availability of artificial replacements for damaged disks in the spine. Compared with previous methods of disk removal or fusion, the newer procedure requires less time and avoids disrupting large muscles of the back since the artificial disk enters below the navel to take the place of the damaged bone.

See also DISK OR DISC; SURGERY.

artificial limb See PROSTHESIS.

ascorbic acid Also known as vitamin C, bones and connective tissue use this essential nutrient in fighting infection, shielding cells and tissue from oxidation, protecting arteries from the formation of plaque, and developing bones, blood vessels, and skin. Because it is water soluble, vitamin C washes out of the body each day. However, fresh fruits and vegetables make it easy enough to replenish—unless one happens to be awash at sea without citrus or some other vitamin C–rich food to prevent scurvy. Of more concern today, ascorbic acid helps to heal cuts and bruises, lower the risk of eye problems, and rid the body of toxins, such as lead and the histamines produced by allergens. Vitamin C also assists the body in activating folic acid, increasing absorption of iron and calcium, and producing collagen, a protein vital to the health of bones, cartilage, and joints.

Besides citrus fruits like oranges, vitamin C comes in all colors of berries, rose hips, melons, and vegetables, such as red peppers, yellow peppers, carrots, and greens. Copper pots and heat—especially boiling water—destroy vitamin C's nutritional value, but canning usually does not. If fresh produce is not available, vitamin C supplements can be taken according to the recommended dose on a product label unless contraindicated as shown on the information given with prescription drugs. An individual's sensitivity must also be considered since large amounts of ascorbic acid can irritate the stomach and skin. To cleanse the body intentionally, however, a vitamin C flush can be undertaken. It concludes with diarrhea as the person ingests a supplement and lots of water every hour to rebalance an out-of-sorts system—an old herbal remedy that is finding current use in drug and alcohol rehabilitation centers. For regular use though, the body can only take so much vitamin C at a time. To maintain a constant supply, particularly in the presence of a fever, smoke, stress, baking soda, sulfa drugs, allergies, and estrogen therapy, a minimal dosage every four hours can help. However, fresh produce and other natural sources, such as wheat germ, come more highly recommended.

See also COLLAGEN; NUTRITION.

athletes, considerations for A July 10, 2002 press release from the American College of Sports Medicine warns athletes about stiffness and destabilization of the spine when benched on backless seats after warm-ups or during game play. For athletes off the bench and on to the Swifter, Higher, Stronger creed of the Olympics, sports psychologists recommend enhancing physical regimens with mind-toughening techniques of goal setting, relaxation training, positive self-talk, and visualization of reaching for the gold.

See also EXERCISE; INJURY.

American College of Sports Medicine. "Fact Sheet." Available online. URL: http://www.acsm.org/publications/newsreleases2002/BenchRestLumbar.html Downloaded on April 14, 2003.

Ward, Scott. "Swifter, Higher, Stronger, More Mentally Touch?" Available online. URL: http://www.acsm.org Downloaded on July 20, 2004.

atlas The first vertebra in the neck, the open ring-shaped atlas supports the skull.

See also SKULL; VERTEBRA.

atrophy The opposite of hypertrophy, disuse atrophy occurs in muscles due to lack of exercise. In temporary conditions, such as fractures or sprains requiring immobilization, muscle strength usually resumes with activity. However, muscular atrophy can result if disuse atrophy goes on too long or if nerves have suffered damage, whereas physiological atrophy may result from natural aging processes that weaken muscle tissue. In spinal muscular atrophy, physical therapists use mechanical means of exercise, massage, heat, light, and electrical impulses to stimulate movement but warn against overfatigue. If needed, a brace or walker may be recommended to assist movement.

Robison, Jenny. "Physical Therapy for Spinal Muscular Atrophy," (Fall/Winter 1998): Available online. URL: http://www.fsma.org/physio_02.shtml. Downloaded on April 14, 2003.

autograft Unlike an ALLOGRAFT, which is also transplanted tissue used to stabilize or repair a joint, an autograft makes use of tissue harvested from the person's own body.

automated twitch-obtaining intramuscular stimulation ATOIMS mechanically stimulates muscles to alleviate pain or spasm. For only two seconds or less, according to information from the University of Pennsylvania Health System, a tiny, sterilized pin oscillates in the muscle, causing mere pinprick pain to lessen excruciating conditions.

UPHS Health Care. "Fact Sheet." Available online. URL: http://pennhealth.com/health/hi_Files/rehab_med/atoims_etoims/how_work.html Downloaded on April 12, 2003.

axial skeleton A combination of 80 bones centrally located in the cranium (skull), sternum (breastbone), vertebral column (spine), and rib cage, the axial skeleton forms the center axis of the body, shielding vital organs and lending structure to the skeletal frame. Classified separately from the protective axial skeletal, the appendicular skeleton assists the body in gaining support, balance, and mobility.

See also Appendix I; CRANIUM; VERTEBRA.

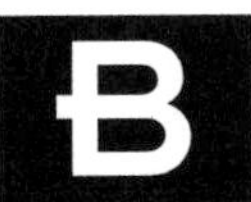

back The posterior region from the neck to the pelvis consists of the spinal vertebrae including the sacrum and coccyx (tailbone) plus the many pairs of nerves, muscles, ligaments, and tendons needed to hold all of the above together. Between each vertebrae, resilient disks cushion the backbone and keep it flexible, enabling the torso to bend, stretch, twist, turn, or remain upright and ready to carry a reasonable load. To assist weight bearing and balance further, a series of natural curves in the neck and back absorb the pressures and impacts of a typically mobile life.

See also SPINE; VERTEBRA.

backache With its complex network of muscles, bones, nerves, and connective devices, the back has a lot of strength and flexibility—and a lot that can go wrong. Therefore, the best remedy for a backache is to avoid one. To strengthen the torso, the American Academy of Orthopaedic Surgeons suggests leg raises, leg swings, partial sit-ups, and wall slides. For the latter, the back stays against a wall as the person slides from standing to crouching with knees bent at a 90-degree angle for a count of five with five repetitions recommended.

Stretching, walking, and weight lifting offer good options for exercise too, but other important preventatives include moving correctly and using brains over brawn to lift. For instance, as a person squats beside an object and draws it near the body, the legs should do most of the work in lifting. Wearing low-heel, ergonomically balanced shoes also helps to curtail backaches as does sitting on an upright chair, frequently shifting positions, keeping joints neutral, or sleeping on a firmly supportive mattress.

Despite the preventatives, backaches rank second only to headaches in being a recurrent pain. According to the American Academy of Physical Medicine and Rehabilitation, back discomforts trouble 80 percent of the people in this country. They are the second most likely reason (next to the common cold) for missing work. Statistics from the American College of Rheumatology (ACR) say that about half of those employees return to their jobs with 70 percent recovering within a month. For about 4 percent, backaches continue beyond six months.

The ACR also reports that approximately 10 percent of the cases involving back pain can be attributed to systemic illness. Because so many possibilities exist, a physician or specialist, such as a rheumatologist, will need to discover if the pain emanates from muscle and bone or from another system of the body, perhaps signaling a serious medical condition. When considering the latter, the Mayo Clinic advises immediate medical attention if back pain occurs in conjunction with fever, numbness, tingling, abdominal pain, or injury.

Most often, low back pain results from musculoligamentous strain. Acute pain in the lumbosacral region lasts up to a month, subacute pain lasts up to 12 weeks, and chronic low back pain lasts more than three months. When predicting an individual's recovery time, a good estimate includes psychological factors, such as depression or anxiety; psychosocial factors, such as job satisfaction; physical demands of the work; and personal factors, such as age, income, or general health habits. Conversely, little or no expectation of recovery can cause patients to lose patience with pain that could conceivably go on forever, thus making surgical options more appealing.

According to the American Academy of Orthopaedic Surgeons, a slipped disk creates occasion for the most common surgery on the lower back. Likewise, the Mayo Clinic reports that one of the most often performed surgeries in the U.S. involves removal of a herniated disk with little risk but beneficial results similar to less invasive treatments. For most backaches, physicians suggest over-the-counter pain relievers, massage, and alternating applications of cold or heat, usually for 15–20 minutes every two hours or so. A good, old-fashioned bath with Epsom salts may also help. If there is no reason to suspect a bone fracture, chiropractic maneuvers or spinal manipulations by an osteopath may bring relief as can the limited use of a back brace or corset. However, extended use of those supportive devices can have a counterproductive effect by further weakening the back muscles.

American Academy of Orthopaedic Surgeons. "Back Pain Exercises." Available online. URL: http://orthoinfo.aaos.org/Fact/thr_report.cfm?Thread_ID=17+topcategory=spine Downloaded on February 17, 2003.

American Academy of Orthopaedic Surgeons. "Low Back Pain." Available online. URL: http://orthoinfo.aaos.org/brochure/thr_report.cfm?Thread_ID=10+topcategory=spine Downloaded on March 6, 2003.

American Academy of Physical Medicine and Rehabilitation. "Hot Story Topics." Available online. URL: http://www.aapmr.org/media/htstory.htm Downloaded on February 25, 2003.

American College of Rheumatology. "Back Pain." Available online. URL: http://www.rheumatology.org/patients/factsheet/backpain.html Downloaded on March 6, 2003.

Ferguson, Sue A., Purmendu Gupta, M.D., William S. Marras, and Catherine Heaney. "Predicting Recovery Using Continuous Low Back Pain Outcome Measures." *Spine Journal* 1, no. 1 (2001): 57–65.

Huffman, Grace Brooke. "Acute Low Back Pain Is Rarely Due to a Serious Problem." Available online. URL: http://www.findarticles.com/cf_0/m3225/6_64/78437343/print.jhtml Downloaded on April 8, 2003.

backbone See VERTEBRA.

backpack safety A flyer, "Pack It Light, Wear It Right," published in 2002 by the American Occupational Therapy Association addresses proper ways to load and wear a backpack, beginning with decisions about whether an item is even necessary. With the total load no more than 15 percent of the person's body weight, the heaviest objects need to be located closest to the wearer's back with other items snuggly in place to avoid shifting and sliding. Besides keeping the backpack's contents in balance, wearers can also keep themselves balanced with both of the padded shoulder straps on and adjusted so the pack hangs loosely with the belt lightly around the lower back curve.

American Occupational Therapy Association. "Pack It Light, Wear It Right," Available online. URL: http://www.aota.org/general/sitesearch.asp?qu=Backpack+Strategies Downloaded on July 23, 2003.

balance Fear of falling probably exceeds fear of flying and rightly so as sports injuries compromise stability, arthritis lessens mobility, and muscle and bone grow less flexible with age. In the January 2003 article "Falls in the Elderly," Dr. Ian Maclean Smith, emeritus professor at the University of Iowa Hospital and Clinics says, "Sway decreases from age 6–9, remains stable till 50 then increases thereafter until sway in an 80-year-old equals that in a 6-year-old." Since too much sway results in loss of balance and potential falls, certain types of exercise help to increase stability—especially exercises in which a person slowly extends performance time in standing on one foot and then on the other.

Exercises themselves can cause a fall if done too quickly or too soon, but exercising in an area with nothing around except a padded floor and a sturdy grab bar provides one option. Another is exercising in water. Aquatic surroundings lessen the fear of falling on a hard surface, thus encouraging a person's confidence in increasing movements that ultimately strengthen limbs and improve overall balance.

Salzman, Andrea. "Nowhere to Fall." Available online. URL: http://www.rehabpub.com/Features/122002/2.asp Downloaded on April 16, 2003.

Virtual Hospital. "Aging Begins at 30; Falls in the Elderly." Available online. URL: http://www.vh.

org/adult/patient/internalmedicine/aba30/2003/Falls.html Downloaded on March 6, 2003.

ball-and-socket joint In this type of synovial joint, one bone cradles the round end of another, allowing the widest range of motion, as in a shoulder or hip joint.

See also JOINT.

bent finger See FLEXION CONTRACTURE.

biceps A quick reference to *biceps* usually means the biceps brachii or flexor muscles that bend and flex the arm in a show of strength. The biceps femoris, however, falls into the hamstring group, flexing the portion of the leg equipped with the hamstring nerve and allowing the knee to bend. Regardless of location, *biceps* refers to a muscle with two heads, which is better than one in lifting, dancing, hugging, or delivering a powerful punch. For many men, but for more and more women, building biceps builds confidence and positive attitudes. According to Caroline Knapp, "With arms, we get the pairing of sexuality with strength instead of frailty, with power instead of passivity."

Knapp, Caroline. "The Right to Bare Arms." *Savonhealth* (Spring 2003): 36–40.

biofeedback In conjunction with traditional medical treatment, this noninvasive method offers complementary forms of therapy approved by the National Institutes of Health. A trained professional interprets and relays information from various monitoring devices, thus enabling patients to be aware of their own bodily responses to pain, which they can then alter through conscious effort. For example, an electromyogram (EMG) set to monitor muscular tension allows the patient to notice the point at which muscles begin to tighten. With a flashing light or beep to indicate increasing tautness, patients work to slow those reactions, thereby breaking cycles that perpetuate pain or injury. Conversely, a biofeedback machine can also assist those suffering from paralysis by signaling even the smallest activity within an affected limb, subsequently encouraging patients to repeat and increase strengthening movements instead of believing that none are possible.

biomechanics This study of human movement provides useful information to improve efficiency and performance or to correct faults, such as postural imbalances or awkward positions that cause injuries. In an office, biomechanical faults can arise in poor working conditions for repetitive tasks or improper seating, both of which are usually correctable with ergonomics. Pelvic tilt or legs of unequal length may show abnormal biomechanics by uneven wear on the heel of a shoe. Adjustments may include orthotics, chiropractic manipulation, osteopathic maneuvers, or surgery. If left unchecked, though, an out-of-balance body will find ways to compensate. According to Chris McGibbon, Ph.D., "Although the impairment may directly affect only a single joint, the loss of function may involve the whole body's response to the impairment. As a result, to better understand loss of function, we need to focus on biomechanical measurements that can link multi-segment movements to one another."

McGibbon, Chris A. "Biomechanics in Disability Research." Available online. URL: http://www.geriatrictimes.com/go20823.html Downloaded on February 4, 2003.

biopsy In this type of test, a sample is taken from the area being evaluated to determine the presence of malignant cells, bacteria, fungi, deposits, or other abnormalities. Usually, the procedure requires a local anesthetic before removal of a tiny piece of muscle or other tissue through a hollow needle. If cells are not accessible by aspiration, an endoscope or tube with forceps on the end may be inserted into the body to obtain the sample.

birth defects In 2002, the March of Dimes Perinatal Data Center reported that every three-and-a-half minutes in this country alone, a baby is born with a birth defect. Generally, these physical abnormalities fall into three categories: structural/metabolic, congenital infections, and other conditions. The first group categorized as other conditions includes muscular or skeletal concerns in one of every 130 births. In the United States, congenital malformations, deformations, and chromosomal abnormalities accounted for 20.5 percent of total infant deaths, making this the number one cause of infant mortality.

Two common birth defects often occurring together are cleft lip and cleft palate, present in one of 930 births and frequently caused by lack of folic acid. Spina bifida has also been attributed to folic acid deficiency. A sore, red tongue indicates that a woman of childbearing years needs foods such as beef, barley, brewer's yeast, or brown rice before pregnancy commences. Because of folic acid's crucial role in regulating normal embryonic formation and development, the U.S. has—since the late 1990s—required packagers of bread, cereal, pasta, and other grain foods to fortify those products.

Although nutritional deficiencies cause some birth defects, other contributing factors include genetic disposition, chemical exposure, prenatal injury, adverse response to medication, or crowding in the uterus, with the latter particularly significant in conditions affecting muscle and bone. For example, pigeon toes and other hip-related problems can occur if an unborn child has no turning room in the womb. Most children outgrow minor bone displacements without corrective devices. However, the American Academy of Family Physicians says, if needed, a soft Pavlik harness can brace a baby's knees in a corrective position and alleviate many hip problems in three to six months.

American Academy of Family Physicians Information from Your Family Doctor. "Hip Problems in Infants." Available online. URL: http://www.familydoctor.org/handouts/444.html Downloaded on April 22, 2003.

Anderson, Robert N. "Deaths: Leading Causes for 2000." *National Vital Statistics Reports* 50, no. 16 (September 2002): 1–11.

March of Dimes. "Quick Stats for the U.S." Available online. URL: http://www.marchofdimes.com Downloaded on April 22, 2003.

birth injury From minor bruises to broken bones, traumas may occur in a labor room or neonatal unit. Although malpractice can certainly be a cause of birth injuries, the use of forceps or the need for a cesarean section comes with risks that may have to be taken to ease a dangerous delivery. Additionally, the moment in which a birth injury occurs may be impossible to isolate. For example, cerebral palsy results from loss of oxygen, but this can come about because of neglectful treatment after a baby arrives or because of unavoidable difficulties experienced in the birth canal.

During normal delivery, a newborn's head receives 40–70 pounds of pressure. Yet, according to Dr. Adam Kerzner, the mere weight of a dime can "significantly change the functioning of a nerve and, therefore, the functioning of whatever that nerve controls, whether a muscle, an organ, or an immune system." To alleviate a potential source of dysfunction between the spine and nervous system, a gentle chiropractic maneuver of a newborn reportedly uses only a few ounces of pressure to help the tiny body adjust to new surroundings.

Kerzner, Adam. "Educating Parents." Available online. URL: http://www.worldchiropracticalliance.org/tcj/2002/jau/jau2002icpa.htm Downloaded on February 13, 2003.

Warner, Stuart. "Adjusting Newborns." Available online. URL: http://www.worldchiropracticalliance.org/tcj/2002/jau/jau2002icpa.htm Downloaded on February 13, 2003.

bleph- When combined with other words, this has to do with conditions of the eyelid. For instance, blepharospasm, usually caused by eye pain, results in spasms of the eyelid, while blepharism results in continual blinking.

bone A bone is a living thing—half water, half solid matter, porous, and light. Although each bone is a separate organ, each has a distinctive place in the musculoskeletal system. The different sizes (long or short) and diverse shapes (flat or irregular) make each bone well suited for its specific task. With the help of tendons, muscles, arteries, and nerves, the bones work together in protecting vital organs or in giving a person his or her individual form. For example, both the flat and the irregular bones of the skull protectively cradle the brain, but they also shape the face and create the locations for the eyes, ears, nose, and mouth. As they connect the skull to the body, irregular bones of the vertebrae enable movement and protect the spinal cord through which neural messages can be rapidly transmitted, back and forth, from brain to body. To shield the heart, lungs, liver, and spleen, the flat but bowed bones of the ribs provide a protective cage, while pelvic bones cradle organs crucial to the digestion and utilization of nutrients or to the reproduction of human life.

In addition to protecting, supporting, and moving the body, living bones store minerals, such as calcium and phosphorus, for use as needed. If an excess exists, minerals might leave unwanted deposits on bones or joints. However, if supplies dip too low, the body takes what it needs from the bones. If kept in beneficial measure, however, bones store around 97 percent of the body's calcium—a mineral needed to harden compact bone and make its exterior as beautiful as ivory yet stronger than steel of equal weight.

Inside the dense form of compact bone, hollow channels hold blood vessels, nerves, and cancellous or spongy bone. The spaces inside spongy bone fill with hivelike trabecular bone and marrow—the fat of yellow marrow and the blood cell–breeding ground of red marrow. In the red marrow, 2.6 million red blood cells come to life every second, totaling around 200 million red blood cells each day. To fight infection and assist with clotting, white blood cells also form within the marrow of the spongy, cancellous bone.

In all parts of the body, similar cells come together to form tissues, and the tissues combine to form organs. The same occurs with bones. Yet each tiny cellular unit has purpose and distinction. Bone cells, for example, come in three types. Osteoclasts clear away old cells in the remodeling process. Osteoblasts make repairs, create new tissue, and line a bone's interior with collagen to provide flexibility. Osteocytes transport nutrients and wastes. Together these ongoing actions keep healthy bone alive and actively participating in the well-being of the living body.

bone break See FRACTURES.

bone bruise Like other types of bruising, a bone bruise reveals discoloration but no break in the skin. This suggests the area received enough pressure to cause some type of damage, perhaps indicating additional injury, such as a stress facture of trabecular bone.

bone cancer During a state of metastasis, cancer can spread to bone through lymphatic channels or the bloodstream. The resulting secondary bone cancer can be more dangerous than primary tumors as metastatic cancer cells overrun normal cells and tissue throughout the body. Cancer in central positions of the body, such as the breast, prostate, kidneys, and thyroid, frequently metastasize in bone as the cancerous cells facilitate bone resorption, creating a place that tumor cells then fill. Understanding this series of events, however, presents one therapeutic aim of inhibiting bone resorption by finding ways to restrain the osteoclast cells that normally break down bone cells prior to remodeling.

Unlike secondary bone cancer, primary bone cancer originates at a bone site where it can be detected by X-ray, CAT scan, MRI, or bone scan. A biopsy must then be taken to confirm the presence of malignancy rather than another bone disease. In 2003, the American Cancer Society (ACS) expected about 2,400 di[illegible]es of cancer in the bones or joints with half or more resulting in death. Of the existing cases, osteosarcoma accounts for about 35 percent of the recorded bone cancers, with chondrosarcoma at 26 percent and Ewing's Sarcoma at 16 percent.

Internal factors, such as genetics, can initiate the uncontrolled spread of abnormal cells typical of all types of cancer. However, external factors, such as exposure to infectious organisms, chemicals, or radiation, can also be responsible. Sometimes more than one causal factor exists. Again, according to the ACS, about one-third of the deaths due to cancer relate to obesity, inactivity, or nutrition as a body loses its healthy balance between cellular production and cellular loss.

Regardless of the cause, treatment generally consists of radiation, chemotherapy, and/or surgery. To determine the prognosis and course of action, the most commonly used system—developed by the American Joint Committee on Cancer—classifies cancer according to stages. In stage I and II bone cancers, for example, most patients have bone tumors surgically removed with approximately an inch of normal tissue included to assure elimination. When that is not possible, radiation therapy and/or chemotherapy begin after surgery, although some surgeons prefer this to be done before surgery to shrink a tumor and to increase the likelihood of its complete eradication.

In addition to regular medical treatment, the ongoing support of exercise and nutrition programs carefully designed for the individual can boost the patient's outlook and quality of life. Generally speaking, fresh food sources of vitamins A, C, E help to prevent cancer cells by protecting normal cellular activity. Also, the body often continues to assimilate active enzyme foods, such as pineapple, papaya, alfalfa, or bean sprouts. During a convalescent period after surgery, however, a broth made of excess water skimmed from cooked barley has restorative value in helping a patient regain strength.

Cancer Care agrees that a healthy diet can be particularly crucial to overall health when combating bone metastases. Information provided by their Web site further suggests limiting salt, increasing calcium to 1,000–1,500 mg a day for women and 1,000 for men under age 50 or 1,200 mg thereafter with 400–800 IU each day of vitamin D and moderate amounts of protein—44 g per day for women and 56 g per day for men. To disrupt the acceleration of bone breakdown, intravenous bisphosphonates therapy can also work with other cancer treatments in addressing problems associated with bone loss. These problems include spontaneous fractures and what can be excruciating pain, especial during the middle of the night when sleep will not come with the discomforts. Once again, however, Cancer Care takes an assertive approach by exhorting patients to "know your body, and listen to it." Besides taking control of one's own health while cooperatively working with a physician or cancer specialist in developing an individualized exercise program, Cancer Care offers this advice, "Don't let symptoms scare you. See them as a signal to get more information and take action." Undoubtedly, that is an excellent attitude to maintain when combating any disease.

Cornelius, J. F., Van Noorden, et al. "Metastasis." Available online. URL: http://www.americanscientist.org/articles/98articles/vintro.html Downloaded on February 13, 2003.

Martin, T. John. "Manipulating the Environment of Cancer Cells in Bone: a Novel Therapeutic Approach." *The Journal of Clinical Investigation* 110, no. 10 (November 2002): 1,399–1,401.

bone development With girls reaching 90 percent of their peak bone mass by age 18 and boys by age 20, the strength of a child's bones can determine skeletal quality for life. Therefore, development of healthy bone affects not only the child's present strength but lessens the likelihood of future concerns, such as osteoporosis.

From the beginning, bone growth carries significance as a distinguishing factor in the womb. In the first few weeks following conception, embryonic limbs bud forth like a flower, then toes and fingers form. When bone cells appear around the eighth week, the embryo leaps into the category of fetus at which time all 206 bones of the body have arrived in their initial stages. Ossification or the hardening process occurs in most bones after the infant has been born.

Although flat and round bones have the capacity for development throughout a person's life, long bones lengthen only until the child reaches maximum height. How tall a child becomes, of course, depends on numerous factors, such as genetic disposition and race. Not surprisingly, underdeveloped countries produce underdeveloped children whose bone length and width may be greatly diminished by nutritional loss. Additionally, the development of strong bones depends on their continual employment and exercise.

Studies consistently show that healthy bones accommodate the increasing loads placed on them, making weight-bearing exercise more developmentally constructive than other activities. Walking, running, jumping rope, and climbing stairs fall into the weight-bearing category as do impact sports, such as volleyball, thus encouraging most research to focus on young athletes. To assess the effects of daily activities on bone accretion in younger children, however, the Iowa Study found, "The implication is that more active children will have greater bone mass even before adolescence and early adulthood when physical activity is assumed to be most influential on bone development."

At any age, bones need nutrients to aid their development in the remodeling process. For women, 1,200–1,500 mg of calcium come especially recommended, but for men, about half that amount may be preferable. Although products from cereal to orange juice have been supplemented with calcium, nonfat dairy still provides the best source since the body absorbs it well and, most of the time, the vitamin D that aids calcium absorption has been added. If calcium comes from other sources, vitamin D supplements may be needed for those who do not see light of day—or who use enough sunscreen to block the skin's natural ability to produce vitamin D from the sun's rays.

See also GROWTH AND DEVELOPMENT IN CHILDREN; NUTRITION.

Janz, Kathleen F. "Physical Activity and Bone Measures in Young Children: The Iowa Bone Development Study." Available online. URL: http://www.findarticles.com/cf_0/m0950/6_107/7556/210/print.jhtml Downloaded on April 28, 2003.

National Institutes of Health. Publication 02-5186, *Kids and Their Bones: A Guide for Parents.* Bethesda, Md.: National Institute of Arthritis and Musculoskeletal and Skin Diseases. August 2002.

Staff. "What You Need to Know About Calcium." *Harvard Health Letter* 28, no. 6 (April 2003): 1–2.

bone graft See GRAFT OR GRAFTING.

bone health With the National Bone and Joint Decade (2002–11) well underway, the surgeon general convened a national meeting to compile data on bone health from a broad range of perspectives. These included scientific research, health care, public health, and foundations and also individuals experiencing bone disease. Discussions included diagnosing and treating osteoporosis and other bone disorders, collecting data on minorities, considering prevention strategies, promoting public awareness, and improving availability of health services with participants asked to identify the issues they deem most important for bone health.

bone infection A generic term for bone infection, *osteomyelitis* appears as a separate entry to discuss specific types. In most cases, though, it comes from microorganisms, such as bacteria or fungi, introduced into a bone. How this happens often depends on the infection site. For instance, the spread of a middle ear infection, usually caused by streptococcus or staphylococcus bacteria, can affect the mastoid bone. Prompt treatment with an antibiotic can avoid serious complications, such as mastoiditis, loss of bone, or meningitis. Mastoid infections generally present early evidence, however, as swelling pushes the ear forward with pain, redness, fever, and sometimes drainage.

Sinusitis or sinus infections can also inflame cavities in the skull or facial bones, filling them with mucus, producing pressure, and creating an ideal environment for fungi and bacteria to flourish. Upper respiratory infections and allergies—initially mistaken for colds but lasting beyond a week—can lead to fever with yellowish or green discharge, signaling infection. Merely touching facial bones can be uncomfortable as sinuses fill. To assess the pressure visually, a flashlight inside the mouth lights up normal, airy cavities but not mucus. For acute and chronic sinus infections, an X-ray or scan can show what treatment may be needed beyond antibiotics, saltwater washes, or herbs like eyebright and goldenseal. Gargling with the face aimed at the ceiling thrusts a weak saline solution into the facial cavities and out the nose to alleviate phlegm. Alternating gargles of warm water and a pinch of echinacea with cold, watery pineapple juice every few hours quickly rids sinuses of excessive phlegm too, which makes this not recommended for dry sinuses or a dry cough when a cup of hot tea with honey would be more effective. To open clogged sinus passages, inhaling steam with rosemary, thyme, or camphor can also help. If a fungal infection or an anatomical reason for the sinus condition worsens, corrective surgery may be needed. However, in the presence of allergies, less radical measures consist of identifying and eliminating irritants, such as dust, dander, pollen, or food. For the latter, the most likely allergens include wheat and dairy products.

bone loss Banking bone—developing as much bone mass as possible—in youth can help to prevent osteoporosis and carry adults through normal bone losses as people age. However, a fact sheet from the National Institutes of Health (NIH) reports bone losses due to prolonged bed rest, immobilization, and weightlessness even when nutritional support, such as calcium, has been added. Although the long-term effects of space travel on bones have yet to be proven, related studies go back to 1892 when Wolff established his theory concerning the negative impact on bones receiving less and less gravitational pull or mechanical loading. To correct this imbalance, mechanical stress must surpass whatever level the bone has adjusted to or previously endured. Then, in an otherwise healthy individual, bone mass generally improves once the person steadily increases weight-bearing loads.

Although little research has focused on dental risks, another NIH fact sheet, "Oral Manifestations of Bone Loss," expresses concern over the relationship between bone loss, periodontitis, and ultimate loss of teeth. Hormonal and chemical factors also affect losses and gains. For example, the decline of estrogen in postmenopausal years weakens bones, making them more prone to injury. This occurs because hormonal losses affect the health of the osteoblast cells needed to build new bone. Although some researchers found that the statins used to lower cholesterol proved effective in gaining bone strength or reducing fractures, others believe they do not show the potential of anabolic alternatives in rousing the osteoblast cells. Indeed, statins aim to assist the liver, not bone. However, the bisphosphonates typically used to treat osteoporosis give the strongest indication of binding to bone surfaces, thereby lessening the risk of fracture.

See also BONE DEVELOPMENT.

National Institutes of Health. "Oral Manifestations of Bone Loss." Available online. URL: http://www.osteo.org/newfile.asp?doc=r704;+doctitle=Oral+Manifestations+of+Bone+Loss Downloaded July 1999.

National Institutes of Health. "Weightlessness, Bed Rest and Immobilization: Factors Contributing to Bone Loss." Available online. URL: http://www.osteo.org/newfile.asp?doc=r999+doctitle=Weightlessness%2C+Bed+Rest Downloaded on February 19, 2003.

Watts, Nelson, M.D. "Bisphosphonates, Statins, Osteoporosis, and Atherosclerosis." *Southern Medical Journal* 95, no. 6 (June 2002): 578–582.

Whitfield, James F. "Statins and the Stimulation of Bone Growth—Do They or Don't They?" Available online. URL: http://www.geriatrictimes.com/go20423.htm Downloaded on February 4, 2004.

bone marrow Hidden in the heart of bone, this soft, organic tissue comes in red and yellow marrow, with the latter consisting primarily of fat. Inside the long bones of the body, spongy red marrow forms more widely in children than in adults but, in either case, produces various cells that bring forth red blood cells, white blood cells, and platelets.

Unfortunately, bone marrow may also produce abnormalities that give rise to cancer cells or leukemia. To test for these or other conditions, the pelvis provides ready access to marrow. The hip bone also offers a common site for bone marrow donors to give tissue in hopes of boosting someone's immune system, replacing diseased bone marrow, or restoring healthy cellular activity, such as the white blood cells' fight against infection, the red blood cells' transportation of oxygen, or the platelets' task of allowing blood to clot after a cut or injury. However, a technique known as peripheral blood stem cell transplantation allows stem cells to be processed and skimmed from the patient's own blood for bone marrow transplant.

In bone marrow research, other promising events have occurred. A 2003 report published by the National Institute of Neurological Disorders and Stroke states, "This study shows that some kind of cell in bone marrow, most likely a stem cell, has the capacity to enter the brain and form neurons." While cautioning against premature expectations regarding application in treatment, hope remains that bone marrow–derived stem cells may travel, as Dr. Mezey reportedly said, into an "area of need."

National Institutes of Health. "Bone Marrow Generates New Marrow in Human Brains." Available online. URL: http://www.nind.nih.gov/news_and_events/pressrelease_bone_marrow_neurons.htm? Downloaded March 2003.

bone mass During adolescence, most people reach 60 percent of the total bone mass acquired in their first two decades of life, with peak bone mass achieved when an individual arrives at his or her own maximum. A report, "Peak Bone Mass in Women," from the National Institutes of Health, Osteoporosis and Related Bone Diseases, says genetics may account for 60–80 percent of bone mass with environmental factors accountable for the rest. Males, for instance, usually achieve greater bone mass than females, while Caucasian women in this country often have less bone mass than African-American women. Despite these factors of inheritance, most people can increase bone mass through nutrition, physical activity, and mechanical loading of bone.

Somewhere between genetics and those environmental factors that one can control, hormonal influences continue to affect bone throughout life. Much has been reported on the role estrogen plays in regulating bone resorption, thus slowing bone loss in women, but less research has focused on hormonal factors in men. In cooperation with the U.K.'s Northern General Hospital, researchers from the Mayo Clinic and Mayo Foundation studied the effects of declining levels of testosterone and estrogen in aging men. They concluded that both hormones contribute to bone formation, but, as occurs in women, adequate estrogen levels in men hold bone resorption in check and bone mass within normal bounds.

See also BONE DEVELOPMENT; EXERCISE; NUTRITION.

Falahiti-Nine, Alireza, et al. "Relative Contributions of Testosterone and Estrogen in Regulating Bone Resorption and Formation in Normal Elderly Men." *The Journal of Clinical Investigation* 106, no. 12 (December 2000): 1,553–1,560.

National Institutes of Health. "Peak Bone Mass in Women." Available online. URL: http://www.osteo.org/newfile.asp?doc=r70li+doctitle=Peak+Bone+Mass+In+Women Downloaded on July 1999.

bone mineral density (BMD) Bone mass measurement assesses bone density with painless, noninvasive tests using either ultrasound or absorptiometry techniques. With several machines available for BMD tests, the choice often relates to the part of the body examined. For example, dual-energy X-ray absorptiometry (DXA) scans bone mass in the full body or weight-bearing areas, such as the hip or spine, while peripheral dual-energy X-ray absorptiometry (pDXA) assesses the finger, wrist, or heel. For the shinbone and kneecap, quantitative ultrasound uses sound waves to measure bone mass, and quantitative computed tomography (QCT) commonly assesses the spine.

Once a test has been completed, the t-score shows the results as compared with a standard of young, healthy individuals. The normal range established by the World Health Organization remains above -1.0 with below -2.0 signaling a need for regular monitoring, but some doctors prefer monitoring under 1.5 to develop a long-range plan for preventing bone loss or to begin early treatment. According to a *Southern Medical Journal* report of highlights of the 2001 conference on osteoporosis, general treatments include medication and adequate vitamin D intake, with 400–600 IU recommended daily. The need for calcium fluctuates from person to person, and several factors must be considered. However, for postmenopausal women not on hormonal replacement therapy, 1,500 mg is often the recommended daily amount.

Besides nutritional support and weight-bearing exercise, therapeutic efforts to conserve or increase bone mass usually include the bisphosphonates prescribed by physicians. Since its discovery in the 1960s, the 32-amino acid peptide calcitonin has also been shown to aid conservation of bone mass by its physiological function of controlling bone resorption. As an added plus, calcitonin has an analgesic component of reducing pain.

Staff. "Highlights of the Fourth Annual Conference on Osteoporosis, Amelia Island, Florida, February 22–24, 2001." *Southern Medical Journal* 94, no. 6 (2001): 561–568.

Zaidi, Mone, et al. "Calcitonin and Bone Formation: A Knockout Full of Surprises." *The Journal of Clinical Investigation* 110, no. 12 (December 2002): 1,769–1,771.

bone paste Unlike the bone wax used in surgery to control bleeding in cranial or other types of bone, bone paste hardens in minutes and sets as hard as bone within hours. A mixture comprised of substances natural to the body, such as bone matrix, bone chips, or combinations of calcium, carbon, phosphorous, and hydrogen, create the bone paste used to fill fissures or restore injured bone with minimal risk of rejection. Biodegradable bone cement injected into bone sites has also been developed with a year-long study showing good results in controlling degradation by cross-linking matter and lowering pH.

Staff. "Degradation of Network Can Be Controlled By Crosslinking Density." Available online. URL: http://www.mindbranch.com/reports/pdfs/N244_032 Downloaded on April 29, 2003.

bone scan To get a clear picture of what is happening in the skeleton, a bone scan finds problem areas long before an X-ray would, revealing sources of pain and making possible prompt treatment of infections, injuries, or tumors. Although the test itself takes only about an hour, the procedure begins three hours prior as the patient receives an injection of a radioactive substance that collects in active bone sites. The person then lies very still as the scanner moves across the body, reproducing images of hot spots onto a paper chart or film. About 90 percent of the time, the bone scan will detect malignant tumors and inflammatory changes in bones caused by conditions such as arthritis.

Because the radioactive material of a bone scan adversely affects a fetus or breast-fed baby, even potentially pregnant and lactating women must delay this procedure. For others, additional scans are considered safe after two or three days since the body eliminates the radioactive material within 36 hours. To assist this purging, the apple pectin found in juice, jelly, or fresh apples helps to rid the body of radioactive material as does a soothing warm bath with salt and baking soda.

Lipari, Audrey. "Bone Scan Safety." Available online. URL: http://www.findarticles.com/cf_0/m1189/4_274/87706211/print.jhtml Downloaded on April 30, 2003.

bone spur These bony overgrowths just do not belong between bones or on the ends of bones where, nevertheless, they collect and cause discomfort or hard pain. If left untreated, a bone spur may ulcerate skin or push the affected part out of alignment to the point of deformity, at which time surgery may be needed to remove the spur. Unfortunately, surgery cannot remove the cause for its existence. To address the source of the problem directly means looking at whatever causes one bone to rub against another bone or something equally hard. For instance, loss of cartilage in osteoarthritis eliminates the protective cushion between bones. However, excessive stress—as in high-activity sports or high-energy dancing—can also produce spurs, particularly in weight-bearing bones or joints. Ill-fitting shoes cause bone spurs to form, too, especially on the heel.

Regardless of their location, most bone spurs are a pain. Chiropractic maneuvers, physical therapy, and anti-inflammatory medication may alleviate discomfort as do properly fitted shoes and lessened stress on the affected area. In cases involving vertebrae, an X-ray or computer-assisted tomography (CAT) scan of the spine may be needed. To check for abnormalities around disks, a physician may order a magnetic resonance imaging (MRI) or electromyography (EMG) to pinpoint painful involvement of the nerves.

bone syphilis When acquired in the womb or at birth, this congenital infection reaches the fetus through the placenta. Lesions occur in long bones, such as the tibia, and show almost total lack of osteoblasts needed for bone formation. When acquired later in life, bone syphilis can also affect long tubular bones in addition to the skull and vertebrae.

brachi- or bracho- When combined with either a prefix or a suffix, *brachi-* or *bracho-* pertains to the arm.

breastbone See STERNUM.

brittle bone disease See OSTEOGENESIS IMPERFECTA.

Brodie's abscess An accumulation of pus located at the head of a bone characterizes this type of infection or osteomyelitis. The typical treatment requires an antibiotic and surgical drainage.

bunion A painful condition of the foot, bunions come about because of heredity, a degenerative bone or joint disease, or a biomechanical alteration. For example, ill-fitting shoes that unevenly distribute body weight will stress the large toe joint, causing a bunion to form. This bony enlargement at the base of the joint then pushes the large toe toward the smaller ones instead of straight forward, eventually deforming the foot in an unnaturally pointed position. According to the fact sheet "Bunion Deformities and Treatment," published by the American College of Foot and Ankle Surgeons, correction depends on the severity of the condition, but an untreated bunion will continue to worsen. Shoes with ample toe room come highly recommended, with padding or shoe inserts as needed. Ultrasound treatments and whirlpool baths can also provide temporary relief. However, if moderate measures fail, surgery may be needed to remove the bunion and reposition the toe joint.

American College of Foot and Ankle Surgeons. "Bunion Deformities and Treatment." Available online. URL: http://www.acfas.org/brbundef.html Downloaded on February 15, 2003.

bursitis Between bones, muscles, and tendons, saclike bursas assure smooth gliding of the joints. When one or more of these bursas becomes irritated by injury or inflamed with infection, bursitis results in a painful condition that may be erroneously assumed to be arthritis. Although X-rays do not show dryness or other disruptions of bursas, they can rule out arthritic involvement or abnormality of bone. If bursas remain chronically inflamed, however, calcium deposits can build up, resulting in calcific bursitis that can then be viewed with an X-ray or magnetic resonance imaging (MRI).

According to the National Institute of Arthritis and Musculoskeletal and Skin Diseases, bursitis, tendinitis, and shoulder impingement syndrome can occur alone or can accompany one another with pain slowly rising in the upper arm or shoulder. Overuse, injury, or the poor biomechanics that typically cause bursitis can be assessed with a physical examination and medical history. However, the doctor or rheumatologist may also look for underlying causes, such as rheumatoid arthritis or diabetes.

In the absence of disease, treatments usually consist of applying ice compresses, taking anti-inflammatory medication, and resting the injured area. For persistent problems, a physician may recommend physical therapy, drainage, cortisone injections, or surgery to get the involved joint moving again.

For minor concerns, home remedies for bursitis usually include a compress or poultice of some kind. For instance, apple cider vinegar boiled with cayenne pepper can be applied as a compress, although the pepper may irritate sensitive skin. A poultice of cabbage leaves—cooked, mashed, and spooned between layers of cheesecloth—can bring warm relief too, assuming the odor does not annoy the nose.

National Institute of Arthritis and Musculoskeletal and Skin Diseases. "Health Topics." Available online. URL: http://www.niams.nih.gov/hi/topics/shoulderqa.htm Downloaded on February 5, 2004.

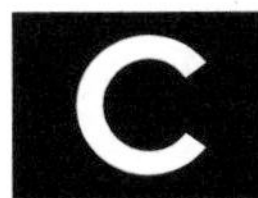

calcaneovalgus This most common type of foot deformity points the foot up and outward at such a sharp angle that the top of the foot may brush the shin. Despite this extremity, a fact sheet by the March of Dimes classifies this birth defect as mild and often self-resolving with treatment seldom required.

March of Dimes. "Clubfoot and Other Foot Deformities." URL: http://www.marchofdimes.com/printableArticles/681_1211.asp?printable=true Downloaded on April 22, 2003.

calcaneus bone The largest tarsal bone, the calcaneus or heel bone articulates with the ankle talus and cuboids of the foot.

See also HEEL.

calcitonin Secreted by the thyroid, this hormone regulates calcium in the blood. It aids bone strength by inhibiting osteoclast cells from breaking down tissue while promoting osteoblast cells in building new bone. Patients with osteoporosis or with Paget's disease—a dysfunction of the bone-remodeling process—may benefit from calcitonin injections under the skin or into a muscle. Uncommon side effects, such as nausea, usually subside as the body adapts to treatment.

See also BONE MINERAL DENSITY.

calcium As a primary structural element of bones and teeth and a regulator of normal muscle function, inadequate supplies of calcium (hypocalcemia) can weaken bones, trigger muscle cramps, cause tingling or numbness, and make a person cranky. Too much calcium (hypercalcemia) can adversely affect the body, too, causing bone pain, flaccid muscles, drowsiness, headaches, depression, or confusion. Hypercalcemia can also elevate blood levels to a potential danger point and interfere with the absorption of medications. Usually, the latter can be prevented by delaying a calcium supplement for three to four hours—something seldom done when taking products containing calcium carbonate to control stomach acidity. Ironically, regular use of those initially helpful products has been known to increase stomach acid production over time, rather than relieve it.

Safe levels of calcium vary according to a person's age and physical needs. The National Institutes of Health (NIH) suggests 1,000–1,500 mg per day to lessen the bone loss that normally occurs in aging. Because supplements can easily produce a buildup, the safest sources of calcium come from dietary items such as yogurt, milk, mozzarella, Swiss cheese, dried figs, fortified orange juice, canned sardines or salmon with the soft bones left in, ricotta, cheddar cheese, and broccoli—in that sequence—with far less calcium than one might expect in sour cream, cream cheese, or butter.

The intake of calcium alone, however, does not address other crucial factors, such as calcium balance. For example, vitamin D—found in fatty fish, eggs, fortified foods, and direct sunlight—increases calcium absorption whereas caffeine slows it down. A fact sheet, "Nutrition and the Skeleton," from the NIH says a couple of tablespoons of milk in coffee will remedy the calcium-caffeine imbalance but warns that typical salt intakes in the United States distort the calcium-sodium balance. For those on low-salt diets, though, calcium needs should proportionately diminish.

Oxalates also interfere with calcium absorption. However, this does not occur when eating different foods as much as when eating a single food containing both, such as spinach. Phosphorous, including the phosphoric acid found in cola, also inhibits calcium absorption, while the protein needed to build and repair muscles and bones increases the body's elimination of calcium. Another NIH fact sheet on the calcium crisis places children in their growth years at risk for various imbalances affecting bone, primarily because of a tendency to replace milk products or whole-fruit beverages with nutritionally impoverished soft drinks.

See also NUTRITION.

Harmon, Kimberly G. "Banking on Strong Bones for Life," Available online. URL: http://www.physportsmed.com/issues/2002/03_02/harmon_pa.htm Downloaded on February 14, 2003.

National Institutes of Health. "'Calcium Crisis' Affects American Youth." Available online. URL:http://www. nichd.nih.gov/new/releases/calcium_crisis.cfm Downloaded on April 22, 2003.

National Institutes of Health. "Nutrition and the Skeleton: The Role of Calcium and Other Nutrients." Available online. URL: http://www.osteo.org/newfile.asp?doc=r708I&doctitle=Nutrition+and+the+skeleton+doct. Downloaded on February 19, 2003.

cancellous bone Lacy, spongy, and latticelike tissue describe healthy cancellous bone. In contrast, broad mosaic-type patterns in cancellous bone often indicate disease. In a paper presented at the 2001 annual meeting of the Orthopaedic Research Society, doctors from Aarhus University Hospital in Denmark suggested that investigations of mid to late stages of osteoarthrosis provide little information about the deterioration of cancellous bone in early stages of the disease when changes in structural patterns may be better indicators of bone loss than measurements of bone density. With the bone pattern being key, the normal structure of needlelike spicules assists new cells in forming after a bone graft of porous cancellous bone, while grafts of densely packed compact bone may develop less rapidly.

Ding, M., et al. "Deterioration in the Quality of Tibial Cancellous Bone in Early Stage Human Osteoarthritis." *47th Annual Meeting, Orthopaedic Research Society,* February 25–28, 2001, San Francisco, Calif.

capsaicin This powerful compound kindles the fire in chili peppers, including capsicum or cayenne, with 80 percent of the potency found in the membranes and seeds. Just touching those peppery parts produces a burning sensation on the skin that is not only painful but dangerous if in contact with eyes, nasal membranes, or other body part linings. A good pair of gloves, good hand washing, and good sense, however, prevent the occurrence of such problems. Since they are a source of vitamins A, C, and E—a combination able to combat free radicals and prevent cellular damage—hot peppers can fight fire with fire. Once the initial burning subsides, topical capsaicin ointment or cream can temporarily numb the pain in joints and muscles nearest to skin surfaces. To keep these medicinal creams from creaming other areas though, a cotton covering can help to hold the fieriness in check.

cardiac muscle In the heart, muscle fibers branch and curve around nuclei with a design similar to knotty pine but rhythmically alive and unique. Like skeletal muscle, some heart muscle forms a striated pattern. Like smooth muscle, it is involuntarily controlled with special intercalated disks allowing free passage of ions from cell to cell. If one cardiac muscle cell reacts, so do all—with the action potential lasting up to 30 times longer than in skeletal muscle. Indeed, the heart contains the most durable muscle fibers in the body.

As cardiac fibers contract (systole), chambers of the heart get smaller, expelling blood into the pulmonary artery or the aorta. As the fibers relax (diastole), blood from the atria again fill the heart chambers. This occurs somewhere around 100,000 times each day as about 1,000 gallons of blood course through a 60,000-mile network of blood vessels. For this pumping action to continue smoothly, though, the heart must release calcium as the cardiac muscles contract so that, with each beat, the calcium levels rise to approximately 10 times the concentration found when the heart is at rest.

If anything impairs the calcium release, the heart's muscular contractions subsequently decrease. Likewise, hindering calcium removal thwarts the heart's ability to relax. In his discussion of this process in "Calcium and the Heart: A Question of Life and Death" in the March 2003 issue of *The Journal of Clinical Investigation,* Dr. Andrew R. Marks of the Center for Molecular Cardiology at Columbia University suggested that "the obvious experiment required to address this important issue is to measure calcium in heart muscle cells from failing hearts." Since heart failure remains the number one cause of death in industrialized nations, further study of calcium's role in pathological heart conditions will hopefully be forthcoming.

cardi-, cardia-, or cardio- Regardless which of those prefixes begins a word, the suffix pins down its specific reference to the heart. For example, a cardiogram refers to the electrical activities of the heart muscle as charted on an electrocardiograph machine, also known as an ECG or EKG (German version). Cardiomalacia indicates softened heart muscle, while cardiomyoplasty surgically repairs the heart with skeletal muscle implants.

cardiomyopathy This chronic disease of the heart muscle affects children as well as adults. Symptoms appear as centralized chest pain, breathlessness, dizziness, sudden loss of consciousness, or, most seriously, cardiac arrest. Causes can be due to inheritance, a virus, alcoholism, or unknown factors. Since the type of cardiomyopathy and the personal limitations encountered vary for each person, a cardiologist should be consulted prior to beginning any physical activity. Some patients require complete bed rest with passive, range-of-motion exercises administered to maintain joint mobility and avoid atrophy of skeletal muscles. For almost all cardiomyopathy patients, however, competitive sports, aerobics, or other strenuous activities must cease. General treatments include medication, weight control, and a nutritious diet devised for the individual's unique needs.

carpal bones Classified as part of the appendicular skeleton, two rows of wrist bones comprise the carpus or carpal bones with the metacarpals consisting of the long bones that fan out and frame the palm of the hand.

carpal tunnel syndrome Beneath the elastic ligament that binds the hand to wrist, the carpal tunnel protectively houses the median nerve controlling the thumb, index finger, and parts of the adjacent fingers. If excessive vibrations, cumulative trauma, injury, or repetitive movements cause lesions or inflammation, the median nerve can become compressed or entrapped. Resultant pain, weakness, tingling, or numbness often extend from the fingertips, up the arm, and into the neck or spine. Shaking the affected limb may bring temporary relief. However, if repetitive motion has caused the problem, the person will need to reassess the use of equipment or consider ways to keep the wrist joints in neutral positions. For instance, awkward hand posturing while driving, typing, sewing, or performing other tasks—from woodworking to holding a cigarette with the hand cocked to one side—can usually be corrected, avoiding a loss of dexterity and preventing the muscles around the thumb from wasting away.

In some instances, carpal tunnel syndrome (CTS) may be caused by an endocrine disorder, such as a thyroid condition, diabetes, malignancy, or a disease of the connective tissue. Women may be particularly at risk for CTS during the last trimester of pregnancy or in the weeks following childbirth. Treatments vary according to the cause and the severity of the problem, but a conservative allopathic approach will consider ergonomic changes, carpal tunnel splints, and corticosteroid injections into the carpal tunnel. If needed, an occupational therapist can demonstrate proper body mechanics and suggest exercises to increase the patient's dexterity and reduce the overall symptoms. Alternative treatments include chiropractic adjustments to normalize bone placement and to alleviate pressure on the median nerve. Acupressure and acupuncture treatments can also help alleviate pressure and pain as can nutritional support, such as vitamin B_6.

Older studies indicated a lack of vitamin B_6 in CTS patients, but recent investigations cast doubt on this belief. Either way, B vitamins—known for strengthening the nerves of the body—seem to be the most effective when taken as a B complex group rather than as individual nutrients since the body apparently robs its own stores when B vitamins get out of balance. A safer and more wholesome choice would be to consume foods, such as bananas, carrots, brown rice, lentils, wheat germ, whole wheat, salmon, and tuna, that come naturally packed with B_6.

When other possibilities have been exhausted, a physician may suggest carpal tunnel release surgery performed by endoscopy or incision. A study done in May 2001 and reported in *Arthritis and Rheumatism* found that two-thirds of patients having carpal tunnel release surgery remained satisfied with the results almost three years later. Doctors Robert A. Weber and Malcolm J. Rude of Temple, Texas, reported similar findings in the November/December 2002 issue of *The Journal of Hand Surgery* on the effectiveness of carpal tunnel release surgery in patients age 65 and older. Although controversies abound on the recovery of older patients, 80 percent of the test group expressed satisfaction with results.

Staff. "Focus." Available online. URL: http://www.acatoday.com/publications/jaca/back-issues.shtml Downloaded on February 20, 2003.

Weber, Robert A. and Malcolm J. Rude. "Abstract." *The Journal of Hand Surgery* 27, no. 6 (November/December 2002): 43–44.

cartilage The tip of the nose gives a feel of the cartilage found throughout the body as either a fibrous or elastic but tough type of tissue capable of protecting and cushioning the joints. Fibrous cartilage, for instance, forms the disks between spinal vertebrae, while elastic cartilage shapes the outstanding back part of the external ear. Since cartilage contains no nerves or blood flow, exercise and collagen keep the gel-like, gristly, and/or rubbery substance in repair, especially with the help of foods naturally containing zinc and vitamins A, C, and E. Other compounds, such as the flavonoid molecules that bring red-black or blue-black color to cherries and berries, also support collagen in shielding osteoarthritic or aging joints.

In younger patients suffering knee injuries, cartilage transplantation uses cells cloned from the person's own knee with cultured cartilage cells injected into the site. Significant data have not yet been collected. However, the success rate of such surgeries appears to be promising. In older adults, surgical procedures like allograft, arthroscopy, or knee replacement can presently be considered with future treatments likely to involve gene therapy or genetic engineering. Until then, surgery can sometimes be postponed with the injection of synthetic hyaluronic acid into the knee. For most people and most types of cartilage, however, preventative measures often work well. By including fresh fruit and berries in a well-balanced diet and warming up with gentle stretching exercises before engaging in sports or physical activities, one's cartilage should keep bouncing back.

CAT scan or CT scan See COMPUTED TOMOGRAPHY OR COMPUTERIZED AXIAL TOMOGRAPHY SCAN.

cervical disk herniation Because of their cushy location between the first seven vertebrae of the spinal column, these flat, round disks of the neck usually receive far less force than disks in the lower back or lumbar region. When herniation does occur, treatment often begins with anti-inflammatory medication and bed rest for a day or two. Conservative treatment may also include an osteopathic adjustment, chiropractic manipulation of the neck, physical therapy, or manual traction to reduce any pressure on painfully affected nerves. Additionally, severe pain lasting beyond a couple of weeks may require oral steroids to lessen the inflammation. If relief does not arrive within six to 12 weeks, the herniated disk may require surgical removal followed by insertion of a bone graft or an artificial replacement disk.

cervical spine injury Usually caused by blunt trauma, a suspected cervical spine injury (CSI) will first be accessed by X-ray even though the Agency for Healthcare Research and Quality says those images may miss up to 40 percent of cervical spine fractures. A computed tomography (CT or CAT) scan may then be required to identify or further clarify bone injury, whereas magnetic resonance imaging (MRI) more accurately distinguishes injury to soft tissue or the spinal cord.

Agency of Healthcare Research and Quality. "Researchers Assess the Performance of Radiographic Imaging of Spinal Injuries." Available online. URL: http://www.ahrq.gov/research/dec02 Downloaded on February 5, 2004.

cervical spondylosis An old neck injury increases the likelihood of this degenerative disorder of cervical vertebrae that, otherwise, has to do with aging. As a fact sheet from the University of Maryland Medicine reported, 70 percent of the women and 85 percent of men x-rayed by age 60 showed at least some evidence of cervical spondylosis, also referred to as cervical osteoarthritis. During this disorder's typically slow progress, cervical disks wear down, and spinal bones acquire overgrowths or spurs that stiffen the neck or compress the nerves in the cervical vertebrae, causing pain, tingling, or numbness of limbs. Muscle relaxants, moist heat, and anti-inflammatory medication may relieve the symptoms. To address the disorder directly, cervical manipulation by a chiropractor or osteopath, therapeutic exercise, traction, and other preventative measures can help to avoid additional compression or vertebral collapse. Most physicians will want magnetic resonance imaging (MRI) or a myelogram to establish the severity of the condition and to determine whether hospitalization or surgery is warranted.

See also OSTEOARTHRITIS.

Charcot-Marie-Tooth disease (CMT) With the name derived from the three doctors who discovered it, CMT begins as a neurological disorder with extremities weakened by the affected nerves so that high arching of the foot typically presents as the first sign. According to information provided by the Charcot-Marie-Tooth Association, foot deformities occur as the disease progresses and, eventually, result in an unusually high gait or other problems of mobility and balance. Symptoms widely vary, but fine hand movements, such as buttoning clothes or writing, become difficult as muscles continue to atrophy. The unaccommodating shape of shoes also adversely affects feet with blistering or chafing. In time, feet and hands of CMT patients lose the sense of touch and the ability to distinguish hot from cold. Because inherited factors may be associated with this disease, primary physicians need to know of the possibility to avoid misdiagnosis. No cure presently exists, but symptoms experienced by the 150,000 or so Americans with CMT can be reduced with individually determined combinations of physical therapy, moderate exercise, and orthotics or other devices. In some cases, corrective surgery may help a patient maintain mobility.

See also GENETIC FACTORS.

Staff. "What is CMT?" Available online. URL: http://www.charcpt-marie-tooth.org/site/content/ what_is_it_cmt.asp Downloaded on February 28, 2003.

charley horse See CRAMP.

child development See GROWTH AND DEVELOPMENT IN CHILDREN.

children See BONE DEVELOPMENT; GROWING PAINS; PEDIATRIC STUDIES; SAFETY.

chiropractics After a decade of joint lobbying, the American Chiropractic Association and the Association of Chiropractic Colleges announced in

October 2000 that legislation now mandates the availability of chiropractics for active military personnel. This landmark—and the increasing inclusion of chiropractic care in insurance and health coverage—may help to legitimize the importance of this medical discipline by promoting research and detailed documentation of individual studies and patient response times. "We have a lot of theories," says Dr. Joel Pickar of the Palmer Center for Chiropractic Research, quoted in a December 2002 "Focus" article in the *Journal of the American Chiropractic Association.* To give an example, Dr. Pickar continued, "There are theories of altered sensory discharge affecting central facilitation, or what's called segmental dysfunction." One area of Dr. Pickar's research investigates the corrective responses of muscle spindles to therapeutic manipulation. Elsewhere, clinical studies concern aspects as diverse as physiological motions, neuron encoding, and practical matters. These include how many chiropractic adjustments are needed to realign a spine and effectively hold bones in a corrected position.

Sometimes referred to as a philosophy, a science, and an art, chiropractic care has been shown to help those with musculoskeletal problems encompassing everything from bad backs and tendinitis to temperomandibular joint (TMJ) problems. Consistently, help comes through spinal manipulation to bring the body into proper alignment. Now, the interest of government and insurance agencies may help to bring chiropractics itself into alignment with ensuing interests in clinical studies, private research, and statistical data regarding nonsurgical relief for pinched nerves, sore muscles, and achy bones.

See also MEDICAL ALTERNATIVES.

Staff. "Focus." Available online. URL: http://www.acatoday.jaca/backissues.shtml Downloaded on February 24, 2003.

chocolate Why would a book about muscles and bones list an entry for chocolate? As cocoa lovers probably know, pure chocolate (natural, not artificial) comes packed with flavonoids—a plant substance with antioxidant and platelet reduction properties *plus* anti-inflammatory effects similar to those found in aspirin. This means chocolate can provide pain relief. According to "The Chocolate Paradox," released June 2000 by the Public Information Committee for The American Society for Nutritional Sciences *and* The American Society for Clinical Nutrition, the bitter substance can lower risks of blood clots too. Although exceptions must be made for those allergic to chocolate—and everyone else just has to keep in mind that large, medicinal doses of chocolate are *not* recommended—consuming amounts somewhat bigger than a baby aspirin would surely do each day.

Public Information Committee for the American Society for Nutritional Sciences and the American Society for Clinical Nutrition. "The Chocolate Paradox." Available online. URL: http://www.faseb.org/ascn/july00pr.htm Downloaded on May 5, 2003.

chondral, chondric, or chondro- These terms and suffix—and longer words including them—refer to cartilage. For example, chondrodysplasia refers to the abnormal development of cartilage in various types of dwarfing, such as the achondroplasia previously discussed. Originally, the primary definition of hypochondriac referred to the specific region beneath cartilages of false ribs—a central location in the body with connections capable of radiating pain most likely felt by those who fret about their health.

chondrosarcoma The second most common form of primary bone cancer, this affects cartilage cells, usually in the pelvis and bones of the arms or legs. It occurs uncommonly in young adults and children with greater cartilage strength. Chondrosarcoma has more prevalence among men and women past their growth years but less than 75 years old. Initial symptoms appear as a mass in the pelvic region. Treatments may involve anticancer drugs, chemotherapy, surgery, or amputation, depending on the rapidity of progress. To slow the growth of cancer cells, antioxidants, such as vitamin C, may be beneficial.

chordoma This rare type of primary bone cancer usually presents as a tumor at the base of the skull or bones of the spine. Unfortunately, surgery and therapy encounter difficulties because of the close proximity of the spinal cord and nerves.

See also BONE CANCER.

chorea Although a number of variations exist in this nervous condition, most involve involuntary twitches of muscles in the face or limbs. Medications may calm the irregular or writhing movements, but nutritional support, such as B complex vitamins, may also bring some benefit.

chronic pain Unlike the acute pain usually associated with injury, chronic pain just does not go away. According to Mary Lou Fairchild of the Department of Physical Therapy at the University of Iowa Hospitals and Clinics, chronic pain continues for one of two reasons. Either the problem cannot be alleviated with treatment, or—as often happens—the nerves continue to send pain messages even though adverse stimulation has ceased. In the latter case, exercise and physical therapy can reeducate the body, perhaps in a manner similar to the kinetic memory that assists a person in touch dialing a familiar phone number without having to think about it. Still another factor takes into account the logical and medically sound inclination after injury to back off from activities involving that portion of the body so it can rest and heal. Once this has been accomplished and the acute pain has diminished, however, many patients continue to favor the area, avoiding movements that could ultimately prove strengthening.

Besides pain medication and exercise, other treatments include chiropractic or osteopathic adjustments, massage therapy, hydrotherapy, acupressure, and acupuncture. Soothing baths and ointments, such as capsaicin cream, rubbed into an area may lessen surface pain long enough to encourage additional movements that, subsequently, help to break the pain cycle.

Apparently this cycle is not uncommon. In autumn 2000, Congress passed a law declaring the Decade of Pain Control and Research. In January 2001, the Joint Commission on Accreditation of Healthcare Organizations issued mandates requiring health care professionals to inquire about or measure pain as routinely done for pulse, blood pressure, or body temperature. As a result, some medical colleges soon added pain management courses to their curriculum with most states now enacting legislation and guidelines on the subject. Reporting on this in an editorial for the August 2001 issue of *Southern Medical Journal,* Dr. Ronald C. Hamdy referred to surveys showing that 37 percent of men and 46 percent of women with arthritis endure chronic pain with about 50 percent of cancer patients acknowledging inadequate relief. The unfortunate use of painkillers for nonmedical purposes has made physicians wary of prescribing pain medication, yet today's choices of analgesics lessen pain more effectively for longer periods of time with fewer side effects than in years past.

See also PAIN MANAGEMENT.

Hamdy, Ronald C. "The Decade of Pain Control and Research." *Southern Medical Journal* 94, no. 8 (August 2001): 753–754.

circumduction One of the four ways in which some joints can move, circumduction encompasses actions such as rolling the eyes or swinging an arm in a circular motion. For this to work, the head of a bone fits into an articular cavity with the end or distal part free to encircle the joint in a movement resembling the shape of a cone.

clavicle Commonly known as the collarbone, the clavicle lies horizontally above the first rib where it connects the sternum (breastbone) with the scapula—the triangle-shaped bone of the shoulder blade. Where the clavicle joins the sternum, the sternoclavicular joint occurs while articulation with the acromion of the shoulder creates the acromioclavicular joint—famous for its high incidence of sports injuries.

Because of its position with the shoulder, the collarbone often takes the impact of a blow or fall, making it one of the most commonly broken bones in the body. As author Amy E. Abbot says in her May 2001 article "Stress Fracture of the Clavicle in a Female Lightweight Rower," in the *American Journal of Sports Medicine,* "Clavicular fractures typically result from a traumatic event in which the force of a blow to the shoulder exceeds the critical buckling force of the bone." Comparatively, stress fractures of the clavicle rarely arise with the first case reported in a rower caught in the current during intensive training. In that particular instance, the athlete circumnavigated surgery by ceasing the activity and engaging in physical therapy to improve shoulder stability and strength.

For collarbones injured in more common ways, hard pain and swelling usually accompany the incident. Holding the arm close to the body or in a sling is recommended to immobilize the arm and shoulder with ice applied for 15–20 minutes every two hours to reduce swelling until medical treatment can be obtained. Then, X-rays can pinpoint the severity and location of the break. Unfortunately, a very severe break may be obvious to the eye in the form of a newly created angle of bone not present before the fall or injury. Multiple fractures of the clavicle may take longer to heal than those with fewer fragments. According to patient guide information from staff at Johns Hopkins Orthopaedic Surgery, broken collarbones in adults usually mend within four months whereas children under eight years of age may only take four to five weeks to heal.

When considering the clavicle, its historical use in diagnosing medical problems is interesting to note. As reported in the July 2001 issue of *Chest,* Dr. Robert S. Crausman, director of the Memorial Hospital Internal Medicine Residency Program in Rhode Island, laments "the lost art" of chest percussion, which relies, in part, on sounds emanating from the collarbone. Without this once-common bedside skill, doctors must now depend on ultrasonography and the hands of a radiologist in locating and then removing superfluous chest fluids through an extraction procedure known as thoracocentesis. However, a physician's well-trained ear can locate troublesome lung-filling fluids before beginning an extraction at the patient's bedside. Unless bleeding or another hindrance exists, the doctor initiates chest percussion by tapping the clavicle and then using a stethoscope to listen. In a state of health, sounds resonate through air-filled lungs to the posterior chest wall. If fluid has replaced air though, a corresponding loss of sound characteristically follows.

Abbot, Amy E. "Stress Fracture of the Clavicle in a Female Lightweight Rower." Available online. URL: http://www.findarticles.com/cf_0/m0918/3_29/75561138/print.jhtml Downloaded on May 12, 2003.

Crausman, Robert S. and Amanda Crausman. "Clavicle Tapping and Auscultation as an Alternative to Chest Percussion When Performing Thoracocentesis." Available online. URL: http://www.findarticles.com/cf_0/m0984/1_120/76994093/pl/article.jhtml Downloaded on February 5, 2004.

McFarland, Edward G., et al. "Patient Guide to Clavicle (Collarbone) Fractures." Available online. URL: http://www.hopkinsmedicine.org/orthopedicsurgery/sports/clavicle.html Downloaded on May 12, 2003.

cleft lip and palate When clefts occur in the oral-facial region, the hard palate (bony roof of the mouth), soft palate (back of the mouth), and/or lip reveal a separation or fissure in the structural pattern. Of 400 or so types, cleft lip and/or cleft palate are most common, either together or separately, but sometimes with additional defects apparent on physical examination at birth. Other problems arise if a baby experiences difficulty in swallowing or sucking with adequate force. Although the infant's health and severity of cleft must be considered, many surgeons prefer to repair a cleft lip within three months and cleft palate in nine to 18 months with additional surgery sometimes required as the child continues to grow.

In studying prenatal influences, recipients of grants from the March of Dimes identified a gene causing a rare cleft lip/palate syndrome that possibly contributes to more common types. Additional research focuses on identifying what effects inheritance, maternal illnesses, and the use of drugs, alcohol, cigarettes, and nutrients have on fetal development. Although each factor has an influence, studies indicate that consuming foods or multivitamins with folic acid prior to conception and throughout the first trimester of pregnancy may keep clefts from forming since a fetus's lip closes five to six weeks after conception and the palate by 10 weeks. Care should be taken, though, to avoid a surfeit of oil-based vitamins stored by the body. For instance, excess retinoids derived from vitamin A may be associated with the formation of oral-facial clefts.

See also BIRTH DEFECTS.

clubfoot Apparent at birth, this common congenital disorder affects around one in 750 babies with one in three having both feet clubbed. Depending on the location of shortened ligaments or tendons, the foot usually turns down or inward but signifies neither pain nor likelihood of other defects. If left uncorrected, however, all sorts of bone problems would arise if the growing child had to learn to walk atop the feet. Therefore, treatment begins early with gentle stretches of the foot toward a corrected position that a cast then holds in place. Usually, the first cast comes off within a week, and the foot is again stretched and worked toward proper positioning before another cast is applied. X-rays document this progress. During the casting period, a primary concern would be awareness of a change in skin coloration or temperature that might indicate any kind of circulatory impediment. Otherwise, the process of serial casting gradually eases foot bones into alignment within four months, at which time braces or special shoes may be needed until the child can walk unhindered. According to a press release, "Infant Clubfoot Can Be Corrected Without Surgery" from the American College of Foot and Ankle Surgeons, nine in 10 infants respond well enough to avoid surgery. With or without surgery, though, the foot often remains a size or so smaller than one in no need of correction.

American College of Foot and Ankle Surgeons. "Infant Clubfoot Can Be Corrected Without Surgery." Available online. URL: http://www.acfas.org/prinfant clubfoot.html Downloaded on February 25, 2003.

coccydynia This painful condition of the coccyx or tailbone occurs through a congenital defect or, more commonly, a trauma sustained during a blow or fall. Unless pain in this bony prominence fails to resolve without surgery, treatment usually consists of avoiding tailbone sitting, padding a seat, and relieving inflammation with medication. Spontaneous eruptions of pain in the coccygeal region may indicate an infection, cyst, or sciatica with appropriate tests required to identify the cause. However, medical treatment itself may be the culprit. A review of pressure ulcers in the May 2001 issue of *RN* states that up to 45 percent of surgical patients develop pressure ulcers —sometimes in as little as two-and-a-half hours—with the coccyx involved for reasons as varied as the quality of the mattress, unnatural positioning during prolonged tests, or devices used to keep the patient from moving during surgery.

Staff. "Pressure Ulcers Can Develop Despite Your Best Efforts." Available online. URL: http://www.find articles.com/cf_0/m3235/5_64/74829210/print.jhtml Downloaded on May 13, 2003.

coccyx or coccygeal The coccygeal or coccyx bone ends the lowest part of the spine in small, taillike vertebrae varying in numbers from three to five.

cold therapy With most types of minor injuries, a bag of frozen corn or peas grabbed from the freezer can bring speedy relief and keep swelling, bleeding, and bruising to a manageable minimum. For more clinically correct occasions, cold therapy consists of applying cold compresses, ice water, cooling fluids, or bags of crushed ice to relieve the pain caused by injury, inflammation, bruising, or swelling in the muscles or joints. Since care must be taken to avoid a state akin to frostbite on already damaged tissue, treatments usually last 15–20 minutes at about two-hour intervals. As a precaution against dangerously dropping the patient's body temperature to a point of hypothermia, cold therapy rarely addresses large areas of the chest or stomach. With sudden back pain, however, cold can often be applied with positive results. Exceptions to this general rule include those who show sensitivity to cold or who have circulatory problems as occurs in diabetes. In such instances, the person will probably not respond well to any form of cold therapy.

Although some controversy exists on the effectiveness of cold versus heat, the latter should seldom be used for therapy until 24–48 hours after an injury or when the bleeding and swelling have ceased. Not only does ice slow blood flow, but, as reported in the October 2001 issue of *The Back Letter,* ice "reduces the metabolic rate in injured muscles." This reduction could be bad or good, depending on varying factors, at which time varying opinions also arrive. For instance, the same report in *The Back Letter,* "Scientific Evidence on Icing Simply Chilling," notes that, in consulting 28 textbooks, all gave advice about ice but with no consensus on its therapeutic aspects. Still other concerns deal with the long-term effects of icy liquids and compresses on soft tissue, particularly if cold has been copiously used after a sport injury. Inadequate time given to assess the water content of body tissue or the thickness of fat and muscle in the areas adjacent to an injury can also be sources of caution before applying cold therapy.

An innovative study conducted at Vanderbilt University Medical Center focused on ice water cryotherapy applied continuously for two hours in an effort to drop, not the surface, but the intra-articular temperature in patients with various conditions leading to knee surgery. After 120 minutes, the average temperature dropped three degrees. In contrast, the test group who did not have cryotherapy experienced a rise of five degrees in the first hour, creating a discrepancy of seven plus degrees between the groups.

As the report maintains, other studies need to test other regions before broadly applying these findings. Some questions also remain as to whether ice suppresses a body's natural inflammatory responses to pain and injury at a time when warmth and rising temperatures could be needed to mend. In managing the pain and swelling that follows most injuries, muscular strains, sprains, and overuse, however, most medical professionals and therapists agree that cold therapy will provide immediate relief.

See also HEAT THERAPY.

Martin, Stephanie S. "Cryotherapy: An Effective Modality for Decreasing Intraarticular Temperature after Knee Arthroscopy." Available online. URL: http://www.findarticles.com/cf_0/m0918/3_29/7556/123/print.jhtml Downloaded on May 14, 2003.

Staff. "Scientific Evidence on Icing Simply Chilling." Available online. URL: http://www.findarticles.com/cf_0/m0670/10_16/80299506/print.jhtml Downloaded on May 14, 2003.

collagen As the main protein found in cartilage, connective tissue, tendons, bones, muscle, and skin, collagen provides protective strength and elasticity as far-reaching as the cornea of the eye. Collagen's other duties include creating scar tissue to cover wounds, strengthening the walls of arteries, and laying a protein base for healthy teeth.

Although collagen forms tissue throughout the body, it needs vitamin C to assist the essential amino acid lysine in its own formation. Therefore, one does not ingest collagen but precursors to collagen development, such as lysine-rich foods like meat, eggs, or dairy products plus fruits and vegetables high in ascorbic acid. Additionally, the flavonoids found in blue-black and red-black berries and the amino acids in wheat germ, gelatin, and other high-fiber foods assist in collagen production. Conversely, alkaloids found in nightshades, such as tomato, potato, peppers, or eggplant, restrain collagen from repairing joints, so those foods may advisedly be excluded from the diets of people suffering from arthritis and other inflammatory joint or cartilage conditions.

Although meant to be the most abundant protein in the body, dire lack of collagen has unfortunate results as seen in osteogenesis imperfecta (brittle bone disease) caused by an error in the body's ability to metabolize collagen. Similarly, impaired metabolism can be seen in the eyes in such complications as glaucoma and retinal detachment. Indeed, collagen's effect on connective tissue can be felt throughout the body.

Besides natural benefits, collagen has been used to plump lips in cosmetic surgery and to speed healing with patches applied at an implant or bone graft site. In a December 15, 2001 report for *Science News,* J. Gorman discussed experiments at the University of California focusing on bone resilience resulting from the strength of bonds of collagen fibers. By better understanding the potential of this natural polymer, researchers and scientists may soon be able to improve synthetic polymers for tooth and bone repair.

See also NUTRITION.

Gorman, J. "Bonds Make a Sacrifice for Tough Bones." Available online. URL: http://www.findarticles.com/cf_0/m1200/24_160/81827788/print.jhtml Downloaded on May 14, 2003.

collarbone See CLAVICLE.

combat stress A lengthy report, *Combat Stress,* published by the U.S. Marine Corps on July 20, 2000, discusses the tactics and techniques needed to identify, prevent, and manage combat stress, which may be encountered during military operations other than war. Combat stress includes mental and emotional tension as well as physical concerns. For the latter, combat stress generally reveals itself through fatigue, tremors, or muscular tension of the head or spine. The continuation of tension leads to exhaustion since muscles must relax to maintain a natural flow of blood, nutrients, and body wastes. Sleep, rest, and realistic goals help to manage this syndrome as do recognizing and admitting one's fears and concerns rather than practicing denial. In the absence of immediate physical danger, muscle relaxation, deep breathing, and other exercises may help the person regain equilibrium.

Rhodes, J. E. and B. J. Smith. *Combat Stress. PCN 143 000083 00* Washington, D.C.: Department of the Navy, July 20, 2000.

compact bone Not unlike a crosscut tree showing its inner core, compact bone looks alive because of its pattern. Elongated cylinders known as osteons unite in structural formations that can withstand the weight and mechanical stresses placed on the body's limbs, yet this is no solid mass. Through the center of each osteon runs a canal with its blood vessel and nerve comprising just one of the haversian systems that make up bone matrix. Nutrients also pass through the haversian canal to osteocytes—the mature cells whose metabolic activities help to keep bone alive. To assure health and strength further, a thin membrane (periosteum) encompasses compact bone with additional supplies of nerves and blood to nourish and innervate all but the softer ends that articulate as joints with other bones.

compartment syndrome A broad range of categories covers this condition in which swelling and increased pressure hinder nerves, vessels, and tendons running through that particular compartment or body space. This can mean anything from compression of the median nerve in carpal tunnel syndrome to the pressure of a too-tight wound dressing or cast. After an accident or injury, acute compartment syndrome presents a medical emergency since excessive pressure can result in loss of life or limb. In such cases, surgical decompression may be needed to repair nerves or tissue and correct blood flow before an affected bone or muscle has time to wither or die.

In chronic compartment syndrome, no emergency exists since the condition is ongoing—usually due to overuse or overexertion. Therapy may consist of correcting abnormal biomechanics or applying therapy to the involved muscles or soft tissue, but more severe cases could require surgical intervention.

complementary medicine See MEDICAL ALTERNATIVES.

computed tomography or computerized axial tomography scan More commonly known as a CT or CAT scan, this procedure enables multiple X-rays to become a three-dimensional image that shows a cross section of tissue. Since different body tissues have varying densities, a CT can help a physician gather diagnostic information about a patient's bones, organs, and blood. The level of radiation stays within the range of an X-ray too, but a CT scan offers far greater resolution, thus enabling a trained technologist to detect even tiny lesions in need of treatment or repair. According to 2003 information from the Radiological Society of North America, however, a CT does not show the very fine details of soft tissue in the knee or shoulder since nearby bones may obscure the view, thereby making the technology of magnetic resonance imaging (MRI) preferable in such situations. Also, pregnant women and nursing mothers should delay having a CT. For most people though, this painless, noninvasive, and fairly fast procedure can identify normal and abnormal structures, clearly showing even very small bones and surrounding muscles. This makes a CT particularly valuable in assessing spinal problems, injuries to the hands or feet, and the overall health of the musculoskeletal structures throughout the body. Additionally, a CT can be used to measure bone density, making it a helpful tool in the early detection of osteoporosis.

Staff. "Computed Tomography (CT)—Body." Available online. URL: http://www.radiologyinfo.org Downloaded May 2003.

connective tissue As the name implies, connective tissue links parts of different sizes to one another, creating an amazing maze of interconnections throughout the body and then covering them with skin. More abundant than other types of tissue, connective tissue comes in various forms, including liquid, webs, and honeycombs. As blood, connective tissue transports nutrients where needed. As a series of delicate webs, it provides flexible structure for internal organs. When rubbery, it comes together as cartilage or, if tough and hard, as bone. Whatever lolls between its cells comprises matrix—whether the fluid matrix of blood or the rigid matrix of compact bone. When it is between nonconnective tissues or organs, connective tissue may be fibrous and loose or, if beneath the skin, show itself as honeycombs of adipose tissue capable of storing fat and adding padding to that part of the body. Because connective tissue has so many connections, diseases involving it, such as rheumatoid arthritis, may be especially difficult to cure. However, scientific research, innovative technology, and nutritional support continuously conceive of possibilities.

contraction When a muscle tightens or shortens in moments of tension or movement, it draws up or contracts. If a muscle contracts too much too soon, a cramp may follow, especially if calcium or another key nutrient is out of balance.

Normally, muscular contraction begins when the brain sends electrical impulses through the spinal cord by way of motor neurons heading for voluntary muscles. The motor neurons or nerve cells then release chemicals that, in turn, stimulate muscle cells to release calcium ions. The calcium activates proteins (actin and myosin) in movements that shorten muscle cells until the whole muscle contracts. Individual muscle fibers then reinstate the calcium and let loose the proteins as the muscle again relaxes.

Because so many elements come together to produce this natural but complex series of movement, any disruption can hasten or lessen the muscular response. When occurring normally, however, isometric contractions allow tension to increase without altering muscle length, while isotonic contractions maintain a steady tension with muscle length changing during motion. Therefore, isotonic and isometric contractions can provide productive forms of exercise, depending on the results desired.

contracture A contracture differs from a contraction in that a contracture remains. Whether by scarring, injury, illness, or chronic lack of exercise, something causes a tendon or muscle to shorten or permanently contract until the contracture results in deformity. For instance, joint contractures of weight-bearing hips and knees often affect inactive persons as they age, whereas fibrotic contractures arise when fibrous tissue replaces more flexible muscle tissue, perhaps after an injury. Consequently, treatment depends on the type and cause.

coxa See HIP.

cramp Riding a charley horse may cramp leg calves, but other contractures can appear as suddenly, bolting by in the form of a muscle spasm that jolts the whole body. Although some types can signify muscular disease, most cramps come unarmed by any underlying disorder. Broadly ranging from a light flutter to a hard contraction, cramping can be instigated by unaccustomed activity, prolonged exercise, dehydration, anemia, metabolic disorders, imbalances of nutrients (specifically calcium, potassium, sodium, and magnesium), or exposure to cold. Depending on the cause, a muscle cramp can be sudden and excruciatingly intense, yet go away in minutes. If this happens too often without addressing the source of the problem, permanent contracture can occur. In most cases though, gently massaging then lightly stretching the muscle will restore it to normalcy. Also helpful are filtered water, fresh fruit, nonfat dairy products, and, if needed, natural multivitamin supplements. When muscle cramping begins after heavy activity or profuse perspiration, rehydration may alleviate the problem. For example, a reliable home remedy suggests melting a tablespoon of honey in a little warm water, adding a tablespoon of natural apple cider vinegar, then filling the glass with ice water for a restorative drink.

crani- or cranio- Words including these forms refer to some aspect of the cranium or skull. For example, the thickening of skull bones in the rare disorder craniodiaphysial dysplasia results in deformities as portrayed in the movie *Mask.* In craniosynostosis, cranial sutures close too soon, impeding normal expansion of a baby's developing brain.

cranium The part of the skull that protects the brain, the cranium consists of 28 bones, which do not include the face but add to the axial skeleton. The platelike bones of the cranium consist of the frontal (forehead), parietal (top with bulging sides), temporal (lower sides behind ears), occipital (back of head), plus the sphenoid and the ethmoid bones located in or around the eyes, ears, and nose or sinus cavities. The outer edges of these predominately flat bones articulate as sutures rather than movable joints. In a newborn, what will eventually be suture joints initially appear as six fontanels or soft spots that take 18–24 months to fuse. This happens so the bony plates of the cranium can accommodate the rapid growth of the brain during the first year or so.

To allow easier passage through the birth canal, many bones—particularly in the head and shoulders—do not ossify or harden until a baby nears the second birthday. The most obvious instances occur in the cranium as the infant arrives with what appears to be an elongated or flattened head but that usually rounds itself within a day or two. Any misshapenness coming later often indicates positional molding—correctable by changing the child's position while lying down. For newborns and smaller or weaker infants unable to lift the head, however, stomach positioning has been associated with sudden infant death syndrome. Caretakers with any concerns at all about such matters should remain beside the crib when placing an infant on the stomach in an effort to avoid further flattening the back of the head. A towel rolled lengthwise can also prop an infant in a safer side position. However, if these changes do not correct the baby's head shape, a pediatrician may suggest using a helmet or other head device—sometimes for a year but frequently for only a few days.

See also FACE; HEAD; SKULL.

creatine supplements See ERGOGENICS.

crossover toe In a February 21, 2003 press release, "Seniors: Repair Crossover Toe to Stay Active," the American College of Foot and Ankle Surgeons advocated outpatient surgery for this common problem as well as its underlying cause. For instance, bunions or hammertoes make the second toe more apt to cross over by slowly extending, particularly as a person ages. Generally, symptoms first present as pain in the ball of the foot as the joint capsule wears and ultimately tears, allowing the toe to slide. Since the resultant pain and misalignment hinder the patient's ability to walk, mobility quickly lessens, increasing the likelihood of serious health risks linked to inactivity. With successful surgery, however, patients can often be comfortably on their feet within a few weeks.

Staff. "Seniors: Repair Crossover Toe to Stay Active." Available online. URL: http://www.acfas.org/prcrossovertoe.html Downloaded on February 25, 2003.

cumulative trauma disorder See REPETITIVE MOTION DISORDERS.

curvature of spine See SCOLIOSIS.

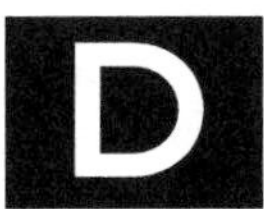

degenerative disk disease (DDD) Usually associated with aging, degenerative conditions may not be noticed until middle age or beyond, but events leading to DDD often begin in the teen years. As reported in the September 2002 issue of *The Back Letter,* Dr. Norbert Boos of Switzerland found in his Volvo–award-winning study, a reduced blood supply to spinal disks during adolescence "appears to initiate tissue breakdown." In considering over 20,000 variables involving lumbar disks, Dr. Boos and his colleagues classified the tiny microscopic changes that indicated early evidence of structural problems. This does not mean that teens will need surgical repairs sometimes required by older adults with DDD. However, further studies will likely focus on relevant causal factors, such as the postural or sedentary conditions that can encumber blood flow to the spine, particularly during the formative growth years.

At any age, injury or obesity can bring genetically disposed DDD to light as disks receive stronger forces than they can handle. A characteristic lack of cushioning in DDD also impacts the ligaments that hold the vertebrae in place and attach spinal bones to corresponding muscles, so the entire region reacts with numbing shock or pain. If in the neck, the condition may be referred to as cervical disk disease or spondylosis. In the midback, it is thoracic disk disease. In the lumbar spine, it might be called lumbago or, in the joints, degenerative arthritis or osteoarthritis.

By any name, a conservative course of treatment includes rest, anti-inflammatory medication, heat therapy (unless an injury causes bleeding or swelling in the adjacent tissue), rehabilitative exercise, and nutritional programs intent on maintaining cartilage and keeping a person's weight within optimal range. X-rays may be also needed, but findings do not always correspond with a patient's symptoms. For instance, some pain may not be identifiable by one radiograph while another may show a problem when no pain exists. However, if a physician suspects a compression of the spinal cord or the involvement of some type of nerve damage, a computed tomography (CT) scan or magnetic resonance imaging (MRI) can determine if surgery is needed. More importantly, such tests can help to locate the precise disks in question.

In the February 17, 2001 *British Medical Journal,* P. I. Bentley authored the report "Degenerative Cervical Disc Disease Causing Cord Compression in Adults Under 50"—highlighting a condition doctors may not initially consider since problems with mobility seldom bring the neck to mind. Yet all three of the cases cited in the article corresponded with this author's experience of back pain and weakness of limbs misdiagnosed and incorrectly treated until MRI assessment of the spine revealed cord compression originating in the cervical disks. In each instance, though, the neck pain typically symptomatic of cervical disk prolapse or cervical disk degeneration did not present itself.

Such exceptions aside, DDD presented as lower back pain usually does involve the lower back or lumbar region. In July 2, 2002, the U.S. Food and Drug Administration announced in *FDA Talk Paper* their approval of the first lumbar fusion device using a genetically engineered protein to treat DDD. The manufacturer—Medtronic Sofamor Danek of Memphis, Tennessee—will continue to observe long-term effects. However, as the present FDA report warns, "The InFUSE Bone Graft/LT-CAGE lumbar tapered fusion device should not be used if patients are pregnant or suspected to be pregnant since potential adverse effects of the genetically engineered human protein (rhBMP-2) on a developing fetus are currently not well understood." Other risks relate to the common concerns of spinal surgery—a topic that hospitals and research centers persistently address.

An April 29, 2003 medical update from Johns Hopkins University and Health System in Baltimore, Maryland, discusses disk options available at their hospital and outpatient clinic. For many years there and elsewhere, the solution to lower back pain in DDD patients has been surgical fusion with bone grafts. This brought pain relief about 90 percent of the time but generated other problems, such as tissue damage and weakened muscles, because of the large incision and rib removal required to get to the damaged disk. As a less-invasive outpatient alternative, intradiscal electrothermal annuloplasty (IDET) allows the surgeon to insert a wire through a catheter into the disk space where the coiled wire can then be heated long enough to cauterize the tiny nerves that kindle pain. Although IDET can presently be used for only one to two disks showing no evidence of herniation or fusion, 80 percent of the DDD patients experience instant relief. As orthopedic surgeon Dr. Khaled Kebaish, who performs the outpatient procedure at Johns Hopkins, said, "This gives you more room to do something that is not irreversible. You don't sacrifice the disc."

The Chicago Institute of Neurosurgery and Neuroresearch lauds yet another possibility. A press release from NewsRx.com appearing in the February 10, 2003 issue of *Clinical Trials Week* reported on the ongoing assessment of new artificial lumbar disk replacement surgery. While speaking for the institute, neurosurgeon Dr. Fred H. Geisler said, "The artificial disk is really the next generation of treatment and appears to be an excellent alternative to fusion." As he explained, the artificial disk does not immobilize the joint, as occurs with fusion, but restores "normal height, motion, and angulation." After a hospital stay of one to three days, patients immediately begin rehabilitation and regular activity. To qualify for the procedure at present, however, patients must be between 18 and 60 years old with a single degenerative disk producing lower back pain for a minimum of six months. Despite those limiting factors, an estimated 400,000 or more DDD patients in the U.S. could be helped when conditions for FDA approval have been met, hopefully by 2006.

Bentley, P. I. "Degenerative Cervical Disc Disease Causing Cord Compression in Adults Under 50." Available online. URL: http://www.findarticles.com/cf_0/m0999/7283_322/71350557/print.jhtml Downloaded on May 19, 2003.

Boos, Norbert. "Volvo." Available online. URL: http://www.findarticles.com/cf_0/m0670/9_17/92588485/print.jhtml Downloaded on May 17, 2003.

Clinical Trials Week. "First Came the Artificial Hip, Then the Artificial Knee, Now the Artificial Disk." Available online. URL: http://www.NewsRx.com Downloaded February 10, 2003.

Johns Hopkins University and Health System. "An Alternative to Spinal Fusion." Available online. URL: http://www.jhintl.net/English/Patients/An%20Alternative%20%20Spinal%20Fusion.asp Downloaded on April 29, 2003.

Logan, Gary. "For Some Disc Problems, An Alternative to Spinal Surgery." Available online. URL: http://www.hopkinsmedicine.org/hmn/W02/medupdates.html#alternative Downloaded on April 29, 2003.

U.S. Food and Drug Administration (FDA). "FDA Approves First Device to Utilize Genetically Engineered Protein to Treat Degenerative Disc Disease." Available online. URL: http://www.fda.gov/bbs/topics/ANSWERS/2002/ANSO1155.html Down-loaded on May 17, 2003.

degenerative joint disease See OSTEOARTHRITIS.

dehydration See HYDRATION.

delayed onset muscle soreness That old adage, "No pain, no gain," needs revising to something sensible like, "No workout spurt, no hurt," or maybe, "Refrain from pain; don't strain." Physical fitness and sports enthusiasts are not the main ones with muscle soreness, though. It happens to almost everyone. The garage or attic cleaning turns into an all-day project of moving boxes and stretching for new storage space. A neighborhood Frisbee game goes on too long, or an hour of lawn mowing turns into an afternoon of manicuring the yard. What is a body to do but hurt?

As Amanda E. Vogel said in her July 2002 article in *Muscle & Fitness/Hers,* "Exercise physiologists identify two kinds of acceptable discomfort from intense exercise: 1) lactic acid buildup, which occurs during a workout, and 2) a post-exercise sensation called delayed-onset muscle soreness." The former generates a natural but uncomfortable burning in the muscles that lasts a few hours until lactic acid clears. However, with delayed onset muscle soreness (DOMS), symptoms may not even begin until a day or two later when a temporary loss of muscle strength occurs due to the previous microscopic tearing of muscle fibers.

Although DOMS usually resolves itself within a week, continuing to strain the muscle before healing transpires may gain only pain with a potential loss of long-term muscle function. Even though rest and ice alleviate present symptoms, future ones can be avoided by adequately warming up, regularly exercising with a wide range of motion involving each joint, and slowly building those very muscles most people forget they have.

Vogel, Amanda E. "Hurts So Good: For Effective Workouts, Learn to Distinguish Between Productive Discomfort and the Pain of Injury." Available online. URL: http://www.findarticles.com/cf_0/m0KGB/ 4_3/ 98641147/print.htm Downloaded on February 5, 2004.

depression Regarding bone, this movement of a joint lowers an associated part of the body, as when opening the mouth drops the jaw. Regarding the emotions, depression can affect every part of everybody. In the article "The Melancholy Body" in the December 16, 2002 issue of *U.S. News & World Report,* Marianne Szegedy-Maszak discussed depression as a serious risk factor for osteoporosis. The National Institute of Mental Health (NIMH) concurs, saying that "abnormally elevated stress hormone levels may contribute to bone loss." With results still forthcoming, NIMH instituted a one-year study comparing the bone loss of women diagnosed with depression with that of their nondepressed counterparts.

Szegedy-Maszak, Marianne. "The Melancholy Body." *U.S. News and World Report* (December 16, 2002): 48–49.

diabetes, effects on hands and feet With a 33 percent increase of diabetes in the United States in the 1990s, foot problems have also been on the rise. Because of circulatory risks associated with this disease, preventative measures center on selecting shoes that avoid frictional stress and orthotics that support normal foot biomechanics. A fact sheet from the American Orthopaedic Foot and Ankle Society (AOFAS) further suggests buying shoes later in the day when feet are apt to swell and then keeping them on at all times—indoors or outside. The AOFAS also cautions against open-toe footwear, such as slippers or sandals, that allow potential irritants to chafe the skin. White socks come especially recommended as do professional pedicures with no accompanying foot soak.

Because abnormalities of glucose metabolism affect peripheral neuropathy, diabetic patients may also suffer from increasing difficulties with mobility and balance. As the disease progresses, small-fiber dysfunctions reduce the patient's sensitivity to touch or temperature, while large-fiber neuropathies diminish reflexes, sensitivity to vibration, foot placement, and/or muscle strength. Nerve entrapment commonly involves the hands or feet with about 30 percent of diabetic patients experiencing carpal tunnel syndrome. When nerve entrapment occurs as tarsal tunnel syndrome, the patient may experience lessened gait speed, which is especially hazardous when crossing a street or responding to physical danger. Since diabetic patients encounter so many variables, treatments must be carefully adapted to each individual's needs.

Another musculoskeletal condition solely confined to diabetic patients can occur in diabetic cheiroarthropathy, symptoms including a general stiffening of the joints. As scar tissue rapidly forms, the regions of the hands, hips, and shoulders may be most noticeably affected. Treatments typically include therapeutic exercises that help to increase the patient's range of motion. Also, the use of gentle analgesics or other anti-inflammatory medications approved by the primary physician can assist in relieving pain and getting the joints working again.

See also AMPUTATION.

Charrette, Mark N. "Diabetes and Orthotic Therapy." Available online. URL: http://www.worldchiropracticalliance.org/tcj/2002/jun/jun2002charrette.htm Downloaded on February 13, 2003.

Vinik, Aaron. "Diabetic Neuropathy, Mobility and Balance." Available online. URL: http://www.geriatrictimes.com/go30213.html Downloaded on April 1, 2003.

diskitis or discitis Unlike a bone infection, diskitis occurs between, rather than in, the spinal vertebrae. About half of the cases result as bacteria invades a disk, often from an infection elsewhere, such as in the pelvic region. Unsanitary needles in drug use can also put a person at risk for diskitis and other possible complications, such as endocarditis (an inflammation of the lining of the heart), which can be particularly life threatening if not promptly treated with a full course of antibiotics. Viral, fungal, or postoperative infections can produce diskitis, too. Regardless of the causes, most cases affect children of all ages. Because diskitis can eventually cause the spinal vertebrae to fuse, early diagnosis can help to prevent abnormal growth patterns, such as the tilting or curvature of the spine that characteristically occurs with kyphosis—commonly known as a humpback.

Most of the time, preventative measures work best with active treatment of any conditions that could conceivably compromise the disks. Also, a diagnosis of diskitis may be delayed until distinguishing characteristics become apparent—especially since initial symptoms apply to other conditions, such as vertebral osteomyelitis. However, a study from Baylor College of Medicine in Houston, Texas, indicates that radiographs of the spine usually verify diskitis while magnetic resonance imaging (MRI) reveals vertebral osteomyelitis. Additionally, this comparative study suggests consideration of the patient's age as a determining factor.

Once a diagnosis of diskitis has been confirmed, antibiotic treatments may last four to six weeks with the specific choice of medications depending on what caused the disks to become infected. Since staphylococcus is a frequent culprit, that is the usual assumption. However, other possibilities, such as anaerobic bacteria, can be identified only by properly collecting, transporting, and cultivating causative organisms. With the disease, its cause, and the extent of the damage made known, therapy consists of "eradicating the infection, relieving pain, preserving or restoring neurological function, improving nutrition, and maintaining spinal stability," according to the research by Dr. Bobby Tay and his associates.

Brook, Itzhak. "Two Cases of Diskitis Attributable to Anaerobic Bacteria in Children." Available online. URL: http://www.pediatrics.org/cgi/content/Full/107/2/e26 Downloaded on May 21, 2003.

Fernandez, M., et al. "Discitis and Vertebral Osteomyelitis in Children: An 18-Year Review." *Pediatrics* 105, no. 6 (June 2000): 1,299–1,304.

Tay, Bobby K-B, et al. "Spinal Infections." Available online. URL: http://www3.aaos.org/jaaos/abstr/v10n3a5.cfm?articles=N Downloaded on May 21, 2003.

disk or disc Regardless of the spelling, these small pads of cartilage come as relatively flat, round fibrous tissue covering a gelatinous center. Specific types of disks refer to locations in the body. For instance, the articular disks occur in the temporomandibular joint (TMJ) renowned for aggravations of TMJ dysfunction. With the exception of the first two vertebrae of the spine (the atlas and the axis, respectively), intervertebral disks rest between each vertebral bone like little shock absorbers or gel-stuffed cushions. Since each disk attaches to the individual vertebrae above and below, it does not slip as once supposed but can tear, bulge, herniate, rupture, disintegrate, or just wear out. Should any of those possibilities happen, treatment depends on the type of damage and the surrounding conditions. A bulging disk, for example, will remain intact but misshapen enough to press nerves and bone, causing pain and swelling. Disk tearing allows the inner jellylike fluid to leak until the fibrous cover flattens, losing its cushiony effect. A herniated disk both bulges and ruptures, while a dried-out, desiccated disk wears away until bone touches bone, ultimately fusing. With a prolapsed disk, part of the actual disk matter can dislodge as a free-floating fragment.

See also DEGENERATIVE DISK DISEASE; EXERCISE; HERNIATED DISK; NUTRITION; OSTEOARTHRITIS.

dislocated joint Unlike subluxation or partial shifting of the bone, a dislocated joint fully dislodges one bone from another at the point of articulation, including the jaw. In older children and adults, weak tendons or a sudden jolt can cause a joint to bolt or slip out of place. Restoration by a doctor or professional attendant prevents further damage to surrounding the nerves and tendons. If medical attention is obtained within a half hour, the anesthesia usually needed after an area has had time to swell is avoided.

Often, a dislocated joint takes on a misshapen look, but with infants, a tendency toward dysplasia may not be obvious. According to guidelines from the American Academy of Pediatrics (AAP), one to one-and-a-half of 1,000 newborns suffer from joint instability with special concern noted for babies born breech. Since dislocation will not always be apparent in new infants, the AAP refers to the condition as developmental dysplasia rather than congenital dysplasia and suggests screening by physical examination at birth followed by careful monitoring over the next few weeks. Cautions also come regarding use of triple diapers, which can exacerbate weakened areas of a baby's hips.

Regarding children and adolescents, a fact sheet from the American Academy of Orthopaedic Surgeons (AAOS) identifies the elbow as the most common site of dislocation with indicative signs of pain and swelling. As with other dislocated joints, immobilization remains the first course of treatment with a trip to the doctor's office or emergency room. X-rays may also be needed to ascertain nerve damage or fracture. If the joint requires stabilization, splinting may last a few weeks with anti-inflammatory medication for pain.

If dislocation occurs too easily or a joint receives recurring injury, the growth plates of children can be impacted even more than the obviously involved tendons and ligaments. In a February 13, 2002 press release from the AAOS entitled "High School Athletic Injuries Merit More Attention," spokesperson Dr. Joseph A. Bosco III expressed concerns about growing tissue, especially since 1 million children annually participate in high school sports. The common practices in orthopedics, however, have primarily been developed as aggressive treatment for professional adult athletes.

For all ages, any injury involving the head, neck, back, or spine must be treated with high caution, keeping the person still and unmoved until professional medical help arrives. If this simply is not possible because of some greater danger, immense care must be taken to immobilize the neck to avoid disrupting partially dislocated vertebrae, potentially injuring the spinal cord, or inadvertently causing disability or paralysis.

Once a joint has been properly restored to its correct position, rehabilitation can often begin right away. Therapeutic movements encourage healing and strengthen the involved muscles, bones, and tendons. Stressful motions or sports activities, however, must be limited until the area completely heals to avoid reinjuring the joint. For those chronically weak joints or ones that spontaneously dislocate, surgery may be needed to tighten surrounding ligaments in hopes of preventing recurrence.

American Academy of Orthopaedic Surgeons. "Dislocated Elbow." Available online. URL: http://www.orthoinfo.org/fact/thr_report.cfm?Thread_ID=174&topcategory=Arm Downloaded on May 21, 2003.

American Academy of Orthopaedic Surgeons. "High School Athletic Injuries Merit More Attention." Available online. URL: http://www.newswise.com/articles/2002/2/SCHLATHL.OSR.html Downloaded on May 21, 2003.

dorsiflexion In this joint movement, toes point upward toward the front of the leg. If the Achilles tendon has been injured, dorsiflexion of the ankle joint will increase the pain.

dowager's hump A type of kyphosis commonly known as a humpback affecting the neck vertebrae, dowager's hump curves the upper spine and creates a bulge that people once considered the exclusive property of dowagers—i.e., elderly widows with monetary means and social esteem. Today, the opposite might be true since the hump results from untreated conditions marked by bone loss and spinal fractures to the point of disfigurement.

See also BONE LOSS; OSTEOPOROSIS.

dual X-ray absorptiometry (DEXA or DXA) Of the various methods and types of equipment used to measure bone mineral density, the dual X-ray absorptiometry (DEXA or DXA) test offers the highest level of precision with a 1 percent error rate. Comparatively speaking, the amount of radiation and time required to take the test (about 20 minutes) remains minimal too. The high-resolution of DEXA detects early signs of stress fracture, bone resorption, and even collagen strength. In an effort to identify those at greatest risk for bone loss, the U.S. Preventative Services Task Force released a September 16, 2002 bulletin recommending routine screening of osteoporosis for women age 65 and older.

U.S. Preventative Services Task Force. "Osteoporosis Screening." Available online. URL: http://www.ahcpr.gov/clinic/uspstf/uspsoste.htm Downloaded on September 16, 2002.

Dupuytren's contracture Named for the 19th-century surgeon who first documented this disease, Dupuytren's contracture begins beneath the skin of the palm with scarring that progressively worsens. The cause remains undetermined. However, genetics seem most likely with a less severe type linked to diabetes.

Initially, a minor lump appears at the base of the ring finger but could arise below other fingers in either or both hands. As scar tissue continues to form, the finger pulls or flexes downward until impossible to straighten by placing on a rigid surface or flattening with the opposite hand. Information from Johns Hopkins recommends warming before self-massaging the palm and fingers to increase flexibility. If surgery cannot be postponed, the thick band of scarring will be removed, the finger(s) extended into a normal position, and the hand splinted. About three days later, range-of-motion exercises usually begin—an important factor in avoiding surgical repetition in five to 10 years. As a fact sheet from the American Association for Hand Surgery reports, up to 50 percent of the patients require the same surgery again, often because of a lack of rehabilitative effort. Less commonly, a skin graft may be needed if insufficient skin remains at the site. Even more uncommon, however, is any association of this disease with pain.

American Association for Hand Surgery. "Dupuytren's Contracture FAQ." Available online. URL: http://www.handsurgery.org/dupuytrencont.pdf Downloaded on February 6, 2003.

dwarfism The Little People of America (LPA) defines dwarfism "as a medical or genetic condition that usually results in an adult height of 4'10" or shorter, among both men and women, although in some cases a person with a dwarfing condition may be slightly taller." Of an estimated 200 types, achondroplasia represents about 70 percent of all cases of dwarfism and, like other common types, remains untreatable. Proportionate dwarfism, however, results from a hormonal deficiency that can be medically addressed. If an adult develops the common problem of spinal stenosis, surgery may be needed to alleviate the pain or numbness. For healthy persons with dwarfism, though, elective surgery to length bones involves great controversy and much pain with no real guarantee of results. As LPA advises, it can be "far more useful to build a dwarf child's self-esteem."

With derogatory terms, such as midget, arising from the unfortunate freak show era of the 1860s, children with dwarfism may encounter inappropriate responses from an uninformed public. Being compared with other individuals also generates problems, particularly if a couple with dwarfism produces a child who does not have this condition or vice versa. For the latter, LPA expresses concern for prospective parents, stating, "Genetic testing carries with it frightening implications for a whole range of issues, including a person's right to obtain medical and other forms of insurance." In an effort to inform the public and the medical community of the "truths of life with short stature," LPA identifies the main challenges as the same environmental concerns experienced with other disabilities. Yet, apart from secondary conditions, people with dwarfism live ordinary lives as teachers, physicians, artists, lawyers, engineers, and other typically productive members of society.

See also ACHONDROPLASIA.

The Little People of America, Inc. "FAQ." Available online. URL: http://www.lpaonline.org/resources_faq.html Downloaded on March 15, 2003.

dys- Words in combinations with this prefix usually have connotations of some type of pain, adversity, or abnormality as perceived by a general public. For example, dysphagia indicates difficulty in swallowing, often due to constrictions of bones or muscles around the esophagus. Dysplasia involves abnormal development of tissue, whereas dysstasia refers to difficulties in standing.

dystonia The National Institute of Neurological Disorders and Stroke (NINDS) describes the various types of dystonia as "movement disorders in which sustained muscle contractions cause twisting and repetitive movements of abnormal postures." These involuntary and sometimes painful actions can affect a single muscle, a muscle group, or the whole body. Early detection can be noted in tremors or difficulty in carrying out ordinary tasks, such as writing or walking. Causes include birth injury, infections, reactions to drugs, stroke, or other types of trauma. In about half the cases, primary or idiopathic dystonia results from hereditary factors. Genetic research continues. At NINDS laboratories, scientists have also been studying muscle patterns and neurotransmitters in the brain to assess how cells communicate in producing movement.

Since no cure has been discovered, the Dystonia Medical Research Foundation says that treatment typically attempts to lessen the symptoms of spasm, pain, and postural disturbances or muscular dysfunction. Several types of medication and complementary therapies can often reduce symptoms, according to the individual's needs. For many dystonia patients, one promising treatment injects just enough botulinum toxin into the muscles to weaken the actions producing spasm yet not enough to produce paralysis. When conservative treatments show little or no improvement, however, surgery may be considered, usually in an attempt to interrupt involuntary movements and contractions.

National Institute of Neurological Disorders and Stroke (NINDS). "NINDS Dystonias Information Page." Available online. URL: http://www.ninds.nih.gov/health_and_medical/disorders/the_dystonias.htm?format Reviewed July 1, 2001.

Staff. "Dystonia Defined." Available online. URL: http://www.dystonia-foundation.org/defined Downloaded on March 17, 2003.

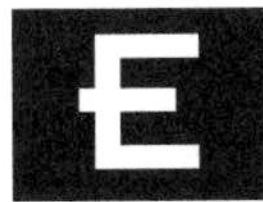

ear Between the outer ear and middle ear, the tympanic membrane stretches like a thin drumhead, creating an instrument appropriately referred to as the eardrum. Sound waves brush against the surface, vibrating the tympanic membrane with sensations received by three tiny bones or ossicles of the middle ear. Most commonly called the hammer, anvil, and stirrup respectively, the malleus, incus, and stapes carry externally produced sounds deeper into the inner ear's key organ—the sensory organ of Corti. There, inside the snail-shaped cochlea, hairlike cells respond to varying frequencies of sound, converting the vibrations into impulses that the cochlear nerve fibers then transmit to the brain. If too much noise bombards the ear for too long a time, however, the hairlike cells die, causing the type of hearing loss that often comes as people age.

Such a complex sound system conducted by so many minuscule muscles and bones allows other breakdowns in orchestration too. According to a fact sheet from the National Association of the Deaf, hearing loss typically results from illness in childhood or pregnancy, injury, extended exposure to noise, heredity, or aging. Regarding the latter, presbyacusis comes on gradually with high-pitched sounds, such as a ringing telephone, that are especially difficult to hear. In their health information page "Hearing and Older People," the National Institute on Aging says one-third of Americans age 65–74 and one-half of those 85 and older have hearing problems. Most likely, the hearing losses of middle age begin unnoticed in earlier years of listening to blaringly loud music or being around intense or prolonged noise without adequate ear protection. To get a baseline for future reference of a person's hearing ability, an audiologist can perform a variety of diagnostic tests while an otolaryngologist will look for progression of underlying medical factors.

Since 1995 researchers have identified over a dozen genes as the basis of isolated deafness, yet about 90 percent of the children with genetically determined conditions have no family history of hearing impairment. About one in 1,000 children under three have hearing difficulties prior to developing language skills with about 30 percent of the cases of prelingual deafness related to genetic factors. Recurrent inflammations and infections of the middle ear in young children can also cause hearing loss. However, a May 12, 2003 news release confirmed the findings of a study funded by the National Institute of Child Health and Human Development and the National Institute on Deafness, saying that infants who sleep on their backs have fewer ear infections than those placed onto their stomachs.

Although frequent infections of the middle ear can be a primary source of hearing loss in very young children, the common cause for older adolescents or young adults is otosclerosis—a hereditary condition where bone overgrowth stops the stirrup (stapes) from transmitting sound. Surgery can sometimes reactivate the stapes, but often, this tiny bone will be removed and a prosthesis inserted to restore full or partial hearing.

Andrews, Linda Wasmer. "Hear Today, Gone Tomorrow." *Mature Outlook* (April 2001): 42–46.

Jeng, Linda Bone. "Progress in Understanding the Genetics of Impaired Hearing." *Contemporary Pediatrics* (June 2002): 44–48.

National Association of the Deaf. "What is the Difference Between a Deaf and a Hard of Hearing Person?" Available online. URL: http://www.nad.org/infocenter/infotogo/dcc/difference.html Downloaded on May 24, 2003.

National Institute on Deafness. "Study Confirms Safety of Placing Infants to Sleep on Their Back. Infants Who Sleep on Back Have Fewer Fevers and Ear Infections." Available online. URL: http://www.nidcd. nih.gocv/news/releases/03/05_12_03.asp Downloaded on May 12, 2003.

National Institutes of Health Age Page. "Hearing and Older People." Available online. URL: http://www.aoa.dhhs.gov/aoa/pages/agepages/hearing.html Downloaded on May 26, 2003.

ectro- In combination with other word forms, *ectro-* usually denotes congenital absence, such as the absence of all or part of a finger in ectrodactylism. With ectrosyndactyly, however, one or more fingers may be missing at birth while others remain fused together.

elbow As the long humerus bone of the upper arm articulates with the radius and ulna bones of the forearm, the elbow comes together as a hinge joint. More like a hinged drop lid than a door, the elbow allows the forearm to open and close against the upper arm with normal range of motion confined to flexion and extension with no shifting side to side. Along the back of the arm, the ulnar nerve sits close to the skin surface, producing an unamusing tingle if something should happen to tap this "funny bone." The location also allows entrapment of the vulnerable ulnar nerve due to causes similar to carpal tunnel syndrome when chronic inflammation follows injury or repetitive use. Repetitive but inept use of drug needles will eventually damage areas around the elbow, too, as scar tissue replaces muscle fiber.

Among children under five, injuries of the elbow range from bruises to fractures with nursemaid's elbow, a common occurrence in the past when an uninformed attendant might snatch a child by the arm. Today, such incidents probably occur when playtime gets too rowdy or when someone automatically grabs a child's arm to avoid an accident or fall. Then, a slight pop and the child's immediate reaction of pain indicates a need for medical treatment before swelling hinders the joint from being returned to its correct position. If, though, a child has fallen and landed on an elbow, a fracture may be likely. Therefore, identifying circumstances surrounding an injury can help the physician attain a quick diagnosis and initiate proper treatment.

In adults, sports injuries often cause dislocations as an elbow gives way with a popping sound. Although thicker tendons and ligaments hold the joints of adults more sturdily in place than those of children, tears or ruptures still occur, especially in athletes, such as baseball pitchers, javelin throwers, or tennis champs, who engage in overhead motions at full capacity. Since this intense type of movement involves ligaments around the sensitive ulnar area, pain and swelling may follow with the first treatment usually being the immediate application of ice. If a complete rupture of the ulnar collateral ligament has occurred, corrective surgery may be needed.

Since surgery cannot guarantee success, shock wave therapy offers a nonoperative option for tendinitis and some types of elbow fracture. For these or other conditions, short-term use of a shock wave has been shown effective with long-term results needing more investigation. Other nonoperative options include anti-inflammatory medications, steroid injection, bracing, ultrasound, and laser therapy. None of these seem to provide consistent results, perhaps because of the many variables among patients and insufficient data on how a particular therapy works. With shock wave therapy, for example, some believe that stimulating an area to the point of pain ultimately leads to pain relief as the body kicks in its own analgesia via inflammation and/or hyperstimulation.

Because of the complexities of this active joint, Eric M. Chumbley states that correct diagnosis of an overuse injury "requires an understanding of the anatomy of the elbow, which includes three articulations, two ligament complexes, four muscle groups, and three major nerves." Nevertheless, physical examination of the elbow and surrounding area usually produce a dependable diagnosis with "basic treatment principles . . . described by the acronym 'PRICEMM': protection, rest, ice, compression, elevation, medication, and modalities (physical therapy)."

For many elbow injuries and also conditions of overuse, initial goals focus on reducing inflammation and controlling mobility with therapeutic treatments and exercises added later for strengthening. However, the source of these problems may be the faulty biomechanics leading to osteoarthritis or other degenerative conditions—biomechanics especially weakened in children who decide on a single sport too early, thereby causing repeated stress in one area during their primary growth years. In such cases, young patients may need to be trained to throw a ball correctly or encouraged to add countermovements with other sports using other muscles. Chiropractic or osteopathic maneuvers can also restore elbows of all ages to full function and mobility by releasing nerve entrapment and thus enabling a patient to exercise wide ranges of motion intent on strengthening the joint and preventing future recurrences.

See also DISLOCATED JOINT.

Chumbley, Eric M. "Evaluation of Overuse Elbow Injuries." Available online. URL: http://www.findarticles.com/cf_0/m3225/1_61/59426887/print.jhtml Downloaded on May 27, 2003.

Safran, Marc R. "Valgus Instability of the Elbow Due to Ulnar Collateral Ligament Injury." Available online. URL: http://www.findarticles.com/cf_O/mOKHT/3_5/98314180/print.jhtml Downloaded on May 27, 2003.

Waanders, Nicholas A. "Nursemaid's Elbow: Pulling Out the Diagnosis." Available online. URL: http://www.findarticles.com/cf_0/m0BGH/6_17/63772185/print.jhtml Downloaded on May 27, 2003.

Wang, Ching-Jen. "Shock Wave Therapy for Patients with Lateral Epicondylitis of the Elbow: A One-to-Two-Year Follow-Up Study." Available online. URL: http://www.findarticles.com/cf_O/m0918/3_30/87011593/print.jhtml Downloaded on May 27, 2003.

electromyography This diagnostic test measures the electrical activities of muscles to reveal damage to tissue or neuromuscular junctions between muscles and nerves. An electromyograph (EMG) takes about one to three hours during which time a machine records data supplied through thin needle electrodes inserted into a specific muscle site. As each electrical pulse occurs, tingling or burning briefly results. Apart from small bruises, slight swelling, or just plain feeling jittery during an EMG, the test itself involves very few risks.

electronic muscle stimulator A July–August 2002 release from the U.S. Food and Drug Administration (FDA) reminds readers that electrical muscle stimulators (EMS) fall under their domain due to the Federal Food, Drug, and Cosmetic Act, which allows the FDA to regulate U.S. sales. The FDA, also responsible for fielding complaints of unfounded claims, reports that EMS devices have not been approved as effective methods for weight reduction or for obtaining the rock hard abs as advertised. Indeed, some EMS devices have been shown unsafe as confirmed by shock, burning, bruising, interference with pacemakers, or worse. However, the currently approved devices can be considered useful in toning or firming muscle, but only temporarily, which indicates that time could be better spent in losing weight and exercising regularly. Notable exceptions arise in the medically prescribed use of EMS in treating muscle spasms, preventing muscle atrophy, and reeducating the muscles or increasing a patient's range of motion after a stroke or injury. In such cases, an EMS can help to stimulate, increase, or even restore full muscle function.

U.S. Food and Drug Administration. "Six-Pack Abs Electronically?" Available online. URL: http://www.fda.gov/fdac/features/2002/402_abs.html Downloaded on February 20, 2003.

elevation The opposite of depression, this type of joint movement lifts some part of the body, such as when closing the lower jaw, placing a swollen foot higher than the torso, or otherwise lifting a body part away from the downward pull of gravity.

ergogenics A Gale Group article, "Muscle Madness," in the March–April 2002 *American Fitness*, by the Aerobics and Fitness Association of America, defines ergogenics as sports enhancers "which include everything from steroids to hormones to over-the-counter supplements." Although the goal may be improvement of athletic performance or enhanced muscle function, the real results can be dangerous, with long-term effects yet to be tallied. For example, growth hormones and steroids used for ergogenic purposes can affect the whole body. Unpleasant side effects range from anger to altered hair growth to alterations in growing bones. Because of these and even greater risks, the olympic committees (U.S. and international) and the National Athletic Association banned the use of steroids and growth hormones as athletic enhancements. Still another ergogenic technique, creatine supplementation, has gained some acceptance, but recent studies showed that the body reacts to it by producing formaldehyde—a toxin known to damage cells and muscles.

An earlier report, "Creatine Supplementation," released by the American College of Sports Medicine in June 1998 reported on energy boosts gained with phosphocreatine—the phosphorylated form of creatine—specifically during short-term, intense bouts of exercise but not during aerobics or workouts of longer duration. After a week of creatine supplementation, body mass increased one to three pounds for most individuals, probably because of water retention, which could detrimentally affect those with kidney dysfunction. The report also expressed concerns about the need for studies that test outside the laboratory and that determine the long-term effects of creatine supplementation on children.

Dr. Jordan D. Metzi wrote of similar concerns in his article "Creatine Uses Among Young Athletes," in the August 2001 issue of *Pediatrics.* Since creatine and other nutritional supplements designed to improve athletic performance occur naturally, they are not under the U.S. Food and Drug Administration's (FDA's) watchful eye. Without FDA testing for safety, however, another once-popular product—ephedryl alkaloid—caused disabilities and even deaths of formerly healthy athletes. By 2001, creatine became the popular supplement for giving that extra edge in school sports. However, Dr. Metzi sees the high expectations placed on the performance of children as a "disturbing trend."

Ironically, many people consider nutritional supplements safe because they are "natural," but the final scores are not in. Until studies investigate creatine thoroughly, this amino acid can be naturally produced in the liver and stored in muscles with the help of foods such as milk, red meat, and some fish.

See also EXERCISE; NUTRITION.

Gale Group. "Muscle Madness." Available online. URL: http://www.findarticles.com/cf_0/mo675/2_20/84182809/print.jhtml Downloaded on February 28, 2003.

Kraemer, William J. and Jeff S. Volek. "Creatine Supplementation." Available online. URL: http://www.acsm.org Downloaded on May 28, 2003.

Metzi, Jordan D. "Creatine Uses Among Young Athletes." Available online. URL: http://www.findarticles.com/cf_0/m0950/2_108/77480756/print.jhtml Downloaded on May 28, 2003.

ergonomics The rise of musculoskeletal disorders (MSD) in the workplace has not gone unnoticed. With guidelines provided by the Occupational Safety & Health Administration (OSHA), U.S. companies are being asked to assess the injury and illness records of their employees in an attempt to identify ergonomically incorrect factors at work. Problems with tendinitis, bursitis, carpal tunnel syndrome, sprains, strains, or other pains related to conditions in the workplace will be evaluated, and jobs or departments with a higher percentage of MSD will need closer inspection. To assist in this OSHA challenge, the secretary of labor appointed 15 representatives from academia, industry, labor, medicine, and other professions to the National Advisory Committee on Ergonomics with the January 2003 meeting beginning its two-year charter in hopes of solving ergonomic issues.

The committee is still out on identifying the areas of research needed and the practical strategies to be developed, but some guidelines have been established. In a 2003 press release on office ergonomics, for instance, OSHA advises adjusting a chair and sitting with feet flat, shoulders relaxed, and thighs parallel to the floor. When typing, the keyboard should be at elbow level and wrists straight with the top of the computer screen just below eye level. Additional suggestions include shifting positions frequently, exercising hands and shoulders, and placing often-needed desk items within easy reach.

Meanwhile, in manufacturing, companies have focused on making tools more comfortable, efficient, and safe, according to Steve Spaulding in his article for the November 2001 *Contractor.* A quote included by Professor Richard Marklin, chairman of the American Industrial Hygiene Association's ergonomics committee, says that ergonomics means "designing the work environment around the individual human operator, taking into account his or her strengths and limitations." As Spaulding goes on to point out, "That environment is dependent upon three things: 1) how the task is set up or oriented toward the worker; 2) ambient conditions such as air quality, humidity, temperature; and 3) the physical tools in use."

Spaulding, Steve. "Well in Hand: Manufacturers Are Using the Science of Ergonomics to Make Their Tools More Comfortable, Efficient, and Safe." Available online. URL: http://www.findarticles.comcf_0/m3042/11_48/80682452/print.jhtml Downloaded on May 28, 2003.

estrogen See HORMONE REPLACEMENT THERAPY.

eversion In this joint movement, the arch turns down as the outer side of the foot ascends in a range of motion opposite of inversion.

Ewing's sarcoma Named for the American doctor of pathology who documented this bone tumor in the early 20th century, Ewing's sarcoma affects children and young adults under age 30 with the most frequent occurrences between 10 and 20 years of age. As with other tumors in the Ewing's family, the causes stem from a chromosomal abnormality. Earliest signs of this second most common bone cancer in children (osteosarcoma being the first) include pain and swelling, often in the arms or legs.

Following a study of the prognostic factors in 975 patients, a group of European doctors reported in the September 18, 2000 *Journal of Clinical Oncology* that the key adversity in Ewing's sarcoma comes when the initial diagnosis shows a spread into other regions, especially in bone metastases. However, early detection, the child's age, and better methods of treatment have improved the outlook by 15 percent or more since the mid-1980s—not only of survival but of survival that is relapse free.

In the U.S., the National Cancer Institute (NCI) created a database on the Internet at www.cancer.gov to provide information about clinical trials and new treatments as quickly as possible. Active treatment currently consists of surgical removal of an original tumor, chemotherapy, and radiation therapy. Since a successful outcome involves many medical domains, the NCI recommends "medical centers with a multidisciplinary team including a primary care physician, pediatric surgical sub-specialists, radiation oncologists, pediatric oncologists/hematologists, rehabilitation specialists, pediatric nurse specialists, social workers, and others in order to ensure that children receive treatment, supportive care, and rehabilitation that will achieve optimal survival and quality of life."

Cotterill, S. J., S. Ahrens, et al. "Prognostic Factors in Ewing's Tumor of Bone: Analysis of 975 Patients from the European Intergroup Cooperative Ewing's Sarcoma Study Group." *Journal of Clinical Oncology* 18, no. 17 (September 2000): 3,108–3,114.

exercise Choosing a form of exercising brings a mass of confusing options, such as active, passive, aerobic, anaerobic, calisthenic, dynamic, weight bearing, weight training, physical training, high impact, low impact, warming up, and cooling down. To keep the fun in function, one choice places little merit on competing or excelling but has the goal of good health—a basic concept behind cross training. Instead of selecting one workout regimen for one set of muscles, a person exercises them all. For example, Tuesday's racquetball session leads to Wednesday's ballet class or bike today and play tennis tomorrow—to start with individual interests before developing other skills. Not only does this provide a challenging workout for each group of muscles, cross training avoids overuse injury and stops boredom on the track or treadmill.

After starting with personal interests and aptitude, a well-rounded plan expands for flexibility (stretching exercise), endurance (aerobics to jumping rope), strength (stair-climbing to weight training), and balance (ballet or tai chi). If aims include weight loss, the target requires a higher expense of energy for more calories to ignite and burn. For instance, the Physical Activity Calorie Use Chart from the American Heart Association says jumping rope uses three times more calories than does a leisurely stroll.

To exercise heart muscle, the American College of Sports Medicine offers the following instruction: first find the maximum heart rate by deducting the person's age in years from the number 220. That answer times 0.9 totals the upper limit and times 0.6 the lower limit, with an optimal range somewhere between the two. For a 60-year-old, for example, 220 minus 60 equals 160, times 0.9 makes 144 (the upper limit) and times 0.6 makes 96 (the lower limit), with 120 heartbeats per minute being about right for exercising cardiac muscle—give or take a few beats. The *Merck Manual, Second Home Edition* offers a simpler solution of 20 beats per minute above a person's normal resting rate with precautions, of course, about obtaining prior approval from a doctor then starting slowly for short time periods when beginning any new exercise.

One reason that the heart is the place to start is the resultant rise of oxygen throughout the whole body. Cardiac-strengthening exercise usually means aerobics, too, which heightens activity, burns calories big time, and improves overall endurance. With such a boost, a body can more easily hop into strength training to build bones and muscle mass. Then anaerobic exercises, such as isometrics or weight lifting, can come merrily into play.

The most optimal exercises will be play—unless work needs doing. Say, for example, that one unit of rest lays down the baseline. With that as the scale, washing windows equals about three times one unit of rest. Similarly, painting the house requires about five times the effort of lolling around, and moving a chair probably expends six times the energy of sitting in one. So, why do people lounge around when even moderate exercise of a half hour three to five times a week has been proven to lessen the risks of heart attack, stroke, and other life-threatening diseases? According to the February 15, 2003 "Fitness" column of *Obesity, Fitness and Wellness Week,* some women say they are too busy tending others to take care of themselves. Some felt guilty; some felt unsafe; and some had to fight off dogs when exercising. New immigrants also feared social encounters they could not handle.

Admittedly, housework, yard work, and home maintenance generally solve genuine worries and, well, general excuses. However, jumping rope can be far more fun, especially on a no-pile commercial-type carpet that prevents wearing down cartilage or tearing knee tendons. Besides working muscles and strengthening bones in legs, hips, and thighs, jumping rope firms arms and heats up joints. Coordination improves too unless weak knees and a bad back makes a person need to skip skipping. Otherwise, the National Osteoporosis Society says that just a few minutes each day of skipping—with or without a jump rope—skipping increases hip bone density by 4 percent in little more than a year. If too much jumping at one time seems like too much of a good thing though, 20 jumps five times a day provides enough high-impact activity to strength backbone mass, assuming, of course, a physician says the spine can take it. How much the bones can take and how often is an answer only a physician or orthopedic expert can prescribe. However, all-purpose guidelines almost always recommend starting slowly, warming up, and gently stretching before first beginning to walk. Once a body gets into motion, bike riding, running, and dancing may be only a step away.

For some, exercising that seriously is not possible. Again with a doctor's advice and approval and the supervision of an occupational or physical therapist, strength training provides an option that can help to lessen disability. In fact, one study shows the greatest increase can be seen in those who initially exhibited the least strength with some patients experiencing an average 189 percent increase in knee extension capabilities and 87 percent increase in hip extension strength. Impressively, those numbers translate into better maneuverability in walking or climbing stairs—crucial aspects for self-care. Similarly, strength or resistance training of upper limbs converts into practical abilities, such as pushing up from an armchair, opening a door, or carrying a lightweight bag of groceries. For persons who are elderly, frail, or medically unstable, low-impact exercises can usually be tolerated with a focus on lower extremities particularly helpful for improving mobility. Additional benefits include the reduced risks of falls and increased independence.

One trend on the rise, according to the American Council on Exercise (ACE), places the century-old Pilates method topside of the nation's most popular fitness trends. Designed to strengthen dancers' muscles without adding bulk, "Every Pilates exercise movement requires control of the entire body and focuses on the quality of movement, correct alignment, and proper breathing." Reportedly, this helps posture, flexibility, and body awareness, too, with other sources lauding the latter as being particularly helpful in strengthening stroke victims. Among other predictions, ACE sees "active relaxation" as being on the rise with "Gentler forms of exercise that promote better sleep, longevity, reduced stress, increased energy and an overall sense of well-being."

As people begin to see fitness as a means of building bone density and managing arthritis pain, interests shift from looking good to feeling good, not only in body but in mind. Apparently, more and more physicians and therapists prescribe exercise for their depressed patients, using SMART guidelines in establishing goals for physical activity: Specific, Measurable, Attainable, and Reasonable with Target dates set for success. The results include reducing fatigue, improving sleep patterns, and gaining a sense of accomplishment as a counterweight to self-criticism. However, do positive effects always occur? A study from the University of Missouri–Columbia reported that the immediate effect of 30 minutes of aerobics "was to increase well-being and fatigue but decrease distress relative to baseline measures. Thirty and 60 minutes after exercise, the effect was to increase well-being and decrease fatigue and psychological distress," which means regular exercise is a really SMART thing to do.

When is exercise not so smart? If right after a meal, exercise can divert energy from digestion since the body's efforts will then go into the physical activity rather than into processing food and absorbing nutrients. Prior to mealtimes, though, and especially at the beginning of the day, exercise can help to pump up metabolism, which keeps a person going for hours. One exception, however, comes after a bad night's sleep. If the body already has to work harder to compensate for lack of rest—or for the emotional upheaval that triggered the tossing and turning—exercise just might be too much to handle that day. Similarly, any signs of fever or illness make physical exertion counterproductive, as does a diet heavy in protein. The reason for the latter is that protein has an acidic effect on the body, and so does exercise. Therefore, keeping a healthful acid-alkaline balance does not mean less exercise but possibly less red meat and dairy with more fresh fruits and vegetables. By first conditioning the body's internal environment, the external will be better prepared to exercise all the benefits of good health.

See also NUTRITION.

ACE Media Center. "American Council on Exercise (ACE) Makes Fitness Trend Predictions for 2003." Available online. URL: http://www.acefitness.org/media/media_display.cfm?NewsID=153 Downloaded on February 15, 2003.

American College of Sports Medicine. "Exercise for Health: How Much Exercise is Enough?" Available online. URL: http://www.acsm.org/health%2Bfitness/fit_society.htm Downloaded on February 16, 2003.

Bee, Peta. "Feel the Rope Burn." Available online. URL: http://www.timesonline.co.uk/print/friendly/0,,1-57-633240.00.html Downloaded on April 7, 2003.

Cox, Richard H., et al. "Positive and Negative Affect Associated with an Acute Bout of Aerobic Exercise." *Official Journal of The American Society of Exercise Physiologists (ASEP)* 4, no. 4 (November 2001): 13–20.

Hack, Bradley. "Exercise Valuable for Mental Health." Available online. URL: http://www.acsm.org/health%2Bfitness/fit_society.htm Downloaded on February 16, 2003.

Morter, M. T., Jr. "Fitness vs. Health." Available online. URL: http://www.worldchiropracticalliance.org/tcj/2002/jun/jun2002morter.htm Downloaded on February 13, 2003.

NewsRx. "Why Do Women Exercise Less Often than Men?" Available online. URL: http://www.newsrx.net/welcome_680.cgi Downloaded on February 15, 2003.

Simkin, Barry. "Even Frail Elderly Patients Can Benefit From Exercise." Available online. URL: http://www.geriatrictimes.com/g020831.html Downloaded on February 20, 2003.

Thompson, Dixie L. and David R. Bassett. "Daily Activities Count in Health and Fitness." Available online. URL: http://www.acsm.org/pdf/fitsc202.pdf Downloaded on February 17, 2003.

extension This joint movement, which is the opposite of flexion, increases the angle between bones as the body straightens into an upright stance or anatomical position. If too much stretching occurs—such as when preparing to leap, jump, or throw—the motion then becomes hyperextension with extensor tendon injuries more likely, especially during abrupt or prolonged movements.

See also RANGE OF MOTION; REPETITIVE MOTION DISORDERS.

extensor muscles The fingers stretch. The arm straightens. The extensor muscles extend hinged joints as though opening a door and letting in more length. If bones and muscles reach too far too fast or too often, injuries can occur—as athletes who have overextended themselves occasionally might attest. With the extensor muscles in good working order, however, the body extends to stand up straight and hold out arms in a greeting.

See also FLEXOR MUSCLES.

extracorporeal shock wave therapy A fact sheet from the American College of Foot and Ankle Surgeons explains this noninvasive surgical procedure as directing sound waves to stimulate the body's own healing response. Although the treatment may not be advisable for patients with additional medical concerns, extracorporeal shock wave therapy produces good results for conditions such as heel pain (plantar fascilitis), particularly if six months or so of more conservative treatments have failed. The procedure, which usually requires only local anesthesia, takes about a half hour with light activity recommended for about four to six weeks.

American College of Foot and Ankle Surgeons. "Extracorporeal Shock Wave Therapy." Available online. URL: http://www.acfas.org/brshockwave.html Downloaded on February 15, 2003.

eye Four weeks from a child's conception, eye buds form. By birth, they reveal a glimpse of two grapelike globes filled with clear gel in the back and fluid in the front—a liquid blend of oxygen, glucose, and proteins. On either side of the tough, fibrous whites of the eye (sclera)—but also above, below, and around—six muscles extend in straplike pairs from one end of the optic nerve stem with the other end attaching to the brain. From this central point of view, the small pairs of muscles control eye movement, allowing a view that looks up or down or increases peripheral vision side to side. The muscles also foster facial expressions as eyes roll in amusement or lock into a challenging stare.

When exercising other optical options, ciliary muscles involuntarily contract or expand to accommodate either a faraway view or a closer look while the iris muscles block or let in external light to clarify the picture. Then, when light-sensitive rods and color-sensitive cones have gathered all the information they can process, the optic nerve of each eye relays that data—upside down—to the brain where the visual cortex set the sight aright. Like other muscles in the body, however, eye muscles can experience breakdowns in visual communication or interpretation at various points along the way. If, for example, eye muscles pull the retina too tight, vision becomes myopic (nearsighted). If too slack, hyperopia (farsightedness) occurs. Both conditions can usually be treated with corrective lenses. With strabismus, though, eyes misalign, pulling in or wandering out but, either way, skewing the viewer's perception of what is seen.

With orthoptic treatment, eye muscles can often be trained to work together through strengthening exercises designed for this unique task. Other treatments depend on the particular type of strabismus. For example, muscles that allow vision to cross (esotropia) may require surgery, sometimes not long after a child is born. If muscles let an eye wander (amblyopia), the standard treatment for decades has been to patch the stronger eye in order to strengthen the "lazy eye" with the eye patch or bandage in place for six hours. However, a May 12, 2003 news release from the National Eye Institute of the National Institutes of Health (NIH) says recent studies show two hours of patching have the same positive effect as six, which can make a big difference to—and from—a child's view.

Another option in the March 13, 2002 news release from the NIH's National Eye Institute discusses the use of atropine eyedrops once a day to treat amblyopia instead of an eye patch. Apparently, the drops act on the stronger, unaffected eye by blurring vision, thereby forcing the lazy eye to work harder and, subsequently, strengthen. Although the patch may slightly speed visual improvement, many children do not want to wear one because of skin irritation or, more likely, because of irritating comments from their peers. Since amblyopia will show the most improvement before a child turns seven, consistent treatment is deemed more important than the choice between patch or drops.

To keep all eyes at optimal working conditions, the American Optometric Association suggests regular checkups every two years during childhood and every three during the adult years with annual visits typically beginning after age 60. However, the first eye examination occurs shortly after birth when the medical team looks for congenital disorders, such as strabismus. Drooping muscles of the upper eyelid (ptosis) can also be apparent at birth or later acquired by injury, but surgical repair may not be needed unless the eyelid impedes a person's vision.

Besides muscles, eyes require bone as found in the orbit or bony eye socket that houses each eye. Instead of one continuous bone, seven bones comprise the orbit. They sometimes experience an infection, malformation, or injury. If a fracture should trap an eye muscle and impair the vision, surgical restoration of the involved facial bones may be required.

For many reasons, around 2.4 million Americans have visual impairments with another 1 million categorized as blind according to statistics released March 20, 2002 in the report *The Vision Problems in the U.S.* by the National Eye Institute in partnership with Prevent Blindness America. The study stemmed from an NIH-hosted workshop in 2001 when experts from the U.S. and Europe explored the topic "Craniofacial Muscle Specialization and Disease." With a call for more research of muscle disorders involving the eyes, it will be interesting to see what develops for better addressing the current computer phenomenon of repetitive strain injuries that strain the eyes.

An old adage refers to eyes as the windows of the soul, but physicians may be seeing eyes as windows into a body's well-being. In many disorders, such as rheumatoid arthritis or diseases of connective tissue, joints, and bones, the eyes often reflect early warning signs of an internal condition that needs medical evaluation and attention. Concerning early recognition of musculoskeletal disease, the eyes clearly have it. By looking deeply into a patient's eyes, medical professionals in general might get an inside view of the person's overall health.

American Optometric Association. "Recommendations for Regular Optometric Care." Available online. URL: http://www.aoanet.org/eweb/?webkey=009122e6-9352-4e0c-8379-08d2eb507cdd Downloaded on March 13, 2003.

National Eye Institute. "Eye Drops to Treat Childhood Eye Disorder Work as Well as Patching the Eye." Available online. URL: http://www.nei.nih.gov/news/pressreleases/031302.htm Downloaded on March 13, 2002.

National Eye Institute. "Reduced Daily Eye-Patching Effectively Treats Childhood's Most Common Eye Disorder." Available online. URL: http://www.nei.nih.gov/news/pressreleases/051203.htm Downloaded on May 12, 2003.

National Eye Institute. "The Vision Problems in the U.S." Available online. URL: http://www.nei.nih.gov/news/pressreleases/032002.htm Downloaded on March 20, 2002.

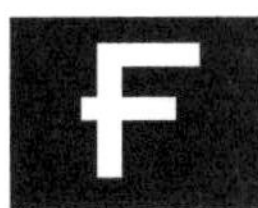

face From forehead to chin, the unique contours and beauty of a person's face depend in large part on the shapes and structures of the underlying bones. Closer to the surface, facial muscles move expressively, communicating a person's reactions even before a word has been said. The forehead wrinkles. An eyebrow lifts. The lips give a grimace or a grin, and at least a glimpse of the person's thoughts have been somewhat revealed.

Anatomically speaking, the face has 14 bones of various shapes, sizes, and thickness, each of which comes with corresponding muscles. Not only does this system nicely sculpt the lines and structure of the face, but facial muscles facilitate function and movement. To provide expression, for example, occipitofrontalis muscles inserted in the occipital bone allow the forehead to crease in surprise or fright, raising eyebrows and widening the eyes. To wrinkle the forehead vertically, perhaps in perplexity or disapproval, corrugator supercilii muscles gather the skin above the frontal bone. Orbicularis oculi muscles outline each eye, enabling the lids to close, and, from the zygomatic bone comes muscle ready for laughter. On either side of the mouth, buccinator muscles attaches to maxillae bone, allowing the curve of a smile or the mouth to round in pursed lips equipped to kiss, whistle, or release the right amount of air to inflate a balloon or to blow a flute in varying degrees of softness.

Besides being such fine instruments of expression, facial bones and muscles provide what is needed to sustain life with water and food. For instance, masseter muscles originating from the zygomatic arch and inserted in the mandible allow the jaw to close. Apparently a closed mouth comes with added meaning and purpose because muscles associated with the temporal bone also close the jaw. Other muscles inserted into the mandible allow teeth to grate and grind in crunching ice, eating, and releasing tension too. With these extraduty tasks to perform, the temporomandibular joint (TMJ) understandably experiences occasional aches, pains, or loss of mobility.

Joint problems aside, the primary disorders attached to the face usually result from some type of trauma—from broken bones to overuse injuries or broken teeth to the facial tics brought on by nerve damage or a bad case of the nerves. If an accident or other trauma involves severe damage to the facial bones, surgical intervention and sometimes a prosthetic device may be required.

One unique aspect of the face is its ability to express the presence of a disorder or a disease. In acromegaly, for instance, the unexpected enlargement of a fully grown adult's jaw and nose and a general coarsening of the facial features often identify this disease of the pituitary gland. Laxity of the facial muscles may indicate a stroke, whereas facial paralysis usually suggests an inflammation, infection, or other damage to the facial nerve with appropriate treatment depending on the cause. In young children especially, a blue face or one that is bluish and swollen indicates a severe respiratory problem requiring emergency medical attention. For all ages, an outbreak of red facial hives accompanied by nausea or difficulty in breathing can signal a life-threatening allergic reaction that also calls for immediate measures to be taken.

When all is well and the body is at rest, facial activities still occur because of the sensory organs located in the face. The nose or mouth inhale and exhale the air needed for life. Even as the body sleeps, eyelids shut out distractions, and the ears between the facial bones and the skull remain alert to danger or the night cries of a child. Once awakened, a face faces a job, the world, and the next day—showing a person's attitudes and determination. However, the face also faces the mirror that speaks of self-acceptance and satisfaction with the person seen. If the image does not compare well with society's or one's own preferences, cosmetic surgery of the face can provide an option when other possibilities seem too flawed. For instance, in a rhytidectomy, loose or wrinkled skin and small pads of fat may be removed from the face or chin in a procedure that medical staff at Johns Hopkins says may take two to four hours. When the bruising and swelling subside in about two weeks, the person usually acquires a more youthful look. Similar results occur with blepharoplasty, which removes excess fat, muscle, and skin from around the eyes in an operation that often takes one to three hours. In rhinoplasty, a plastic surgeon removes bone and cartilage to remodel the nose into a shape that is more pleasing to the patient, with a smaller nose being the typical choice. However, this same type of surgery can also be performed to rescue a damaged nose or to improve nasal passageways when a patient's breathing has been obstructed by an injury or a birth defect.

For children born with craniosynostosis syndrome involving various degrees of facial deformities, a team of medical experts may be called upon to evaluate the severity of the condition and to plan long-range surgical corrections of the eye muscles, teeth, and facial bones with initial surgery sometimes beginning shortly after a child's birth. This midfacial advancement requires coordinated efforts with bone grafts and traditional surgery often taking four to eight years or more, depending on the severity. However, Dr. John W. Polley of the Rush Craniofacial Center at Rush-Presbyterian-St. Luke's Medical Center in Chicago, Illinois, and dentist Alvaro A. Figueroa developed an innovative and much faster technique called rigid external distraction, or RED. Reporting on this for the Associated Press in Washington, D.C., health writer Lauran Neergaard discussed the way that surgery–rigged pulley repairs children's severe facial birth defects in her 2001 article by that name. To correct the misshapen birth defect of a sunken nose and bulging eyes, Dr. Polley separated a child's facial bones and then "attached a pulley-like contraption . . . that her parents tightened each day with a screwdriver, slowly pulling out the sunken bones so they could grow into the right position." With facial bones wired to a halo-shaped device, the child's caretakers could then make twice-daily adjustments with a tiny turn of a screwdriver, providing a daily correction of about one millimeter. Subsequently, as bones move and gaps widen slightly, the body begins to fill the areas by manufacturing new bone, thus avoiding the need for grafts. Long-term investigations of both the success rate and the occurrences of relapse have not yet been established, thus making this procedure still in the experimental stages. Nevertheless, what sounds like torture may have far less traumatic effects on a child than years of surgery, especially since positive results may be seen in only a matter of weeks. For the 5,000 children born with severe craniofacial defects in the U.S. each year, this could be very good news for them and their parents to face.

See also TEMPEROMANDIBULAR JOINT.

Neergaard, Lauran. "Surgery-Rigged Pulley Repairs Children's Severe Facial Birth Defects." Available online. URL: http://www.stopgettingsick.com/templates/print_template.cfm?id=4501 Downloaded on June 2, 2003.

facet joints Another name for the joints in the back portion (posterior) of the spine, the facet joints come in two opposing pairs for each vertebrae with one set facing up and the other down. By effectively coming together as a type of hinged joint, facet joints allow flexion (bending forward) and extension (bending backward) for the spine's normal range of motion. Since these are also synovial joints, a capsule of connective tissue envelopes each and provides synovial fluid for lubrication. This liquid—plus a coating of cartilage around the joint surfaces—enables smooth movement of the spine. If something disrupts this ease of motion, as happens with osteoarthritis, then various stretching exercises, spinal manipulation, and water or hydrotherapy may help the synovial fluids to build up again, thereby reducing pain.

See also JOINT; OSTEOARTHRITIS; VERTEBRA.

falls or falling According to the lengthy document *Health, United States, 2002,* falling accounts for the most frequently cited reason that persons age 45 and older give for visiting a hospital emergency room after an injury. From the National Center for Injury Prevention and Control, the report "Falls Among Older Adults—Summary of Research Findings" warns of the increased risk of falling as a person ages, with more than one-half the falls by people age 65 and older occurring in the home. Unfortunately, an older adult who has fallen once will be two to three times more likely to fall again within the year—an especially troublesome fact since 95 percent of all hip fractures result from falling. The risks increase for stroke victims, persons with more than one chronic disease, and patients with visual, muscular, or balance problems. Thick-soled shoes, alcohol, and medications that cause drowsiness can be factors in falling, too.

While testifying on June 11, 2002 before the U.S. Senate's Subcommittee on Aging (Committee on Health, Education, Labor and Pensions), Dr. David W. Fleming, then acting director of the Centers for Disease Control and Prevention (CDC), called falls "the leading cause of injury death among people 65 years and older," with over 10,000 dying from fall-related injuries in 1999. The following year saw 1.6 million seniors getting emergency treatment for falls, with an estimated 12 million—or one in three—falling each year.

In hopes of reducing those odds, the CDC contributes to the continuing research and development of relevant items, such as hip pads that at-risk people can wear in an attempt to prevent hip fractures or at least lessen their severity. Additionally, the CDC funds ongoing studies to evaluate the causes leading to falls and the areas of intervention that could prevent these occurrences. Recently, for example, CDC research at Vanderbilt University in Nashville, Tennessee, implemented the Tennessee Fall Prevention Program to teach nursing home staff how to identify and reduce hazards regularly encountered in the facilities and also to monitor more closely each patient's use of medicines. As a result of this program, nursing home residents became 20 percent less likely to fall.

Meanwhile, across the country, the CDC has been assisting the California State Health Department in counseling assisted-living and independent seniors about the risks of falls and the sturdier steps that can be taken with home modifications, routine screenings for osteoporosis, regular reviews of medications, visual examinations, and commencement of sensibly chosen exercise programs. Another CDC report, "Preventing Falls Among Seniors," points to inactivity as contributing to the overall body weakness that often precipitates falls. With the recommendations of a doctor or health care professional, exercises can be individually selected to focus on ways to strength muscles while improving balance and coordination. To avoid tripping at home, people may need to evaluate and then remove any potential obstacles, such as clothes or newspapers on the floor and books on the stairs. Nonskid carpet padding or adhesive-backed rugs can also help to lessen a person's likelihood of stumbling. In addition, often-used items can be placed on low shelves so no step stool is required to reach them. Should a stumble begin, a grab bar along each corridor and near the toilet, shower, or bathtub can help people to regain their balance before a full fall occurs. Similarly, stair and porch railings help to prevent falls as do good lighting and thin-soled shoes with nonslip tread.

Practical matters as seemingly insignificant as the length of one's toenails should also be considered. In a lecture given at the inaugural Geriatrics Education Conference and Exposition in New York City, Dr. Helen K. Edelberg, an assistant professor at Mount Sinai School of Medicine, cautioned about long toenails and foot problems, such as bunions, foot deformities, and foot disorders, as being potential sources for falls. Weak ankles and other musculoskeletal conditions, such as cervical spondylosis, arthritis, injury, and tendinitis, can also cause people to lose their balance. As postural instability and increased sway begin to decrease a person's steadiness, normal movements can suddenly become perilous when merely changing body positions or increasing walking speed. In the presence of eye problems or the poor lighting that hinders almost everyone's visual perception, a sudden step-down or that last step on the stairs can be especially hard to see. However, this hazard can easily be corrected with the application of a strip of bright paint or contrast tape. Otherwise, a broken bone or serious head injury can land a person in the hospital where ongoing risk factors may be identified for the first time. Then, a physical therapist (PT) or an occupational therapist (OT) may initiate intervention as part of the rehabilitation process, training the patient in gait and balance, helping to increase range of motion, and providing instructions on safer ways to perform everyday activities at home. If needed, an OT or a PT can evaluate the patient's home environment, making further suggestions for devices that can assist safe ambulation.

Identifying obvious risks, such as a person's refusal to use a cane or a walker while, instead, expecting a wobbly antique table to stop a fall, may be part of an at-home assessment made by an OT or a PT. In a clinical environment, however, the evaluation may consist of gait and balance activities that show how well the patient maintains stability when sitting, rising, standing, and walking. Undoubtedly, the therapist will observe foot drop, too, in hopes of pinpointing physical causes for falling—sometimes with biomechanical measurements of muscle strength and range of motion to define any weaknesses that can potentially lead to another fall. To be on the safe side, though, therapists sometimes show patients how to fall with minimal damage. While a backward fall can lead to more serious injuries of the head, pelvis, and hips, a forward fall usually has less dire consequences and also allows patients to be in the correct position needed to push, pull, or, if need be, drag themselves up again.

Although aging advances the risks of falls for most people, a disability or the recuperative period following surgery can evoke similar concerns. In the first few weeks after hip surgery, for instance, patients may experience increased risks in movements as simple as reaching down to grab an item from the floor. To aid patients in performing this type of daily routine without an assistant, many companies have developed products to help a person reach, grab, dress, or put on shoes. Doorknob extensions and ergonomically designed jar lid openers can also come in handy by relieving hand pressure and, instead, making these leverage tasks be performed by the full movement of the whole arm. For bath time, a sponge on a handle and a soap on a rope can help to prevent falls by keeping needed objects within easy reach. A shower seat prevents the prolonged standing that can cause knees to buckle, thereby allowing the patient to conserve strength for getting out of the bathtub—assisted, of course, by that previously installed bathroom grab bar. With such a varied assortment of devices now available to lessen the risk of falls, falling into the habit of using them when they are not really needed might become the greater risk!

Centers for Disease Control and Prevention (CDC). "Falls Among Older Americans: CDC Prevention Efforts," Available online. URL: http://www.cdc.gov/Washington/testimony/ag061/02.htm Downloaded on February 17, 2003.

Centers for Disease Control and Prevention. "Health, United States, 2002." Available online. URL: http://www.cdc.gov/ nch/products/pubs/pubd/hus/highlits.pdf Downloaded on February 7, 2004.

Centers for Disease Control and Prevention. "Preventing Falls Among Seniors." Available online. URL: http://www.cdc.gov/ncipc/duip/spotlite/falltips.htm Downloaded on February 17, 2003.

Ciocon, Daisy G. and Jerry O. Ciocon. "The Fall Factor." Available online. URL: http://www.rehabpub.com/features/22002/7.asp Downloaded on April 16, 2003.

Knowlton, Leslie. "Preventing Falls, Improving Outcomes," Available online. URL: http://www.geriatrictimes.com/g010920.html Downloaded on June 2, 2003.

National Center for Injury Prevention and Control. "Falls Among Older Adults—Summary of Research Findings." Available online. URL: http://www.cdc.gov/ncipc/duip/SummaryofFalls.htm Downloaded on February 17, 2003.

Staff. "Life Is Hard. Make It Easier with a Helpful Gadget," *Focus on Healthy Aging, Mount Sinai School of Medicine* (June 2003): 4–5.

fascia Whether superficial or deep, this fibrous membrane encompasses the muscles with protective lining and connective tissue. For instance, superficial fascia allows friction-free movement of the skin. In contrast, deep fascia binds the muscles it envelopes, helping to separate one muscle from another while holding each in place. Because this tough connective tissue continuously occurs throughout the body, almost anything that affects the fascia will probably be felt in the areas surrounding the disorder. For example, fasciitis occurs when the fascia beneath the skin becomes inflamed, potentially affecting a large region of the body. With myofascial pain syndrome, pain and tightness of muscles can be sorely felt.

See also FIBROMYALGIA.

fatigue Clinically speaking, muscle fatigue means the lessened production of force in the affected muscle(s). As Dr. Graham Lamb said in his September 2001 talk at La Trobe University, each of the various causes depends on the type of muscle involved as well as the strength and duration of the stimulation it receives. Since a muscle's contraction involves several steps, any interference along the way can hinder its action potential or response. For instance, excess stimuli cause metabolic changes in muscle fiber with variations according to the type—slow-twitch (type I) or fast-twitch (type II). If calcium moves in and out or if glycogen nears depletion, structural damage of muscle fibers could occur and prolong the fatiguing. However, fatigue itself provides the body with a built-in mechanism that prevents muscle cells from dying. If something overrides that system, such as continuing to perform an activity beyond the point of exhaustion, the muscle's contractile apparatus stops working. No more action potential will then be available until the body has had adequate rest and nutrients to reestablish an energetic balance.

With complete muscle fatigue, as described above, the affected muscles cannot function properly. With partial muscle fatigue, though, movement becomes just plain taxing. The body feels weighted down with bags of sand. The legs plod. Feet drag. Empty arms lift tiredly. The usual level of alertness may seem altered, the perception skewed, and the concentration impaired. This type of acute muscle fatigue may occur after a prolonged activity or an intense workout as the body acquires a buildup of natural waste products, such as lactic acid, but ample water and a good night's sleep usually offer some relief.

Like pain, acute and chronic muscle fatigue produce subjective symptoms felt only by the person involved. However, muscle weakness itself can be measured by physical examination and various tests that may help to locate any underlying medical conditions. Chronic muscle fatigue often does indicate a disease or disorder with the possibilities as varied as FIBROMYALGIA, MULTIPLE SCLEROSIS, RHEUMATOID ARTHRITIS, hypothyroidism, chronic fatigue syndrome, tuberculosis, diabetes, anemia, and varicose veins. As a sign of disease or disorder, chronic fatigue goes on and on—even after a reasonable period of rest. With acute muscle fatigue, however, the sudden onset could be symptomatic of a temporary illness, such as mumps or flu, especially if accompanied by a fever.

Assuming no circulatory problem has interfered with the body's vital supplies of oxygen (a problem that indicates a more serious medical condition of the heart or lungs), acute muscle fatigue can often be prevented. Pacing physical activities and exercising regularly (instead of hard or hardly) can help a body maintain its balance. Keeping the muscles fueled with healthful nutrients, such as folic acid and iron, also prevents fatigue.

When all of the above have been ruled out and all of the recently taken medications have been reviewed for side effects, continuing bouts of muscle fatigue could be attributable to emotional factors, such as chronic anxiety, fear, or boredom. Muscle fatigue can also result from a contaminated environment of polluted air, noise pollution, or jolting vibrations that shake the spine and unsettle the nervous system. Lack of sleep can quickly contribute, too, particularly for parents of a newborn or colicky infant. In fact, almost anything that keeps a person awake during regular times of rest will cause fatiguing felt throughout the body. If muscle fatigue seems localized, however, that too can provide a clue in uncovering causative factors ranging from repetitive strain to ill-fitting shoes to eyestrain. Then, new positions in performing a repeated task—or better shoes and a new pair of glasses—can help to quicken steps and equip the person to see more energy in sight.

See also NUTRITION; STRESS.

feet or foot With 26 bones, 33 joints, 19 muscles, and the 107 ligaments and tendons needed to hold each intricate part in place, a foot carries a lot of weight—not by mishap but by design as those who poetically named bones have been swift to see. The tarsus, for example, gets its name from a Greek word for a flat wicker frame but, in the foot's case, a basket weave of bones around the ankle area. Shaped like a little boat, the scaphoid bone has been dubbed the navicular, while the rows of bones in the toes apparently honored the rows of soldiers for whom each phalanx (plural, *phalanges*) was named. Regardless of their names, foot bones need to stay in line or the whole body can host an army of biomechanical problems.

When foot problems become a pain, the most common locations of discomfort seem to be the ball of the foot, around the heel, or in the joints of the toes. Less obvious, however, may be problems with posture, balance, or gait that show up as musculoskeletal conditions, such as a pelvic twist, a misshapen spine, or a misaligned vertebral column, but which actually begin from the ground up. An analogy of the situation might be a picture of solid brick walls placed onto a wobbly, lopsided foundation. The walls might stand for a while, but, eventually, something will give. Similarly, if either or both feet have biomechanical problems in the bones that comprise the arch or the muscles that line the sole of the foot, the entire body will be thrown off balance. As Dr. Mark Charrette explains in his November 2002 article "The Importance of Proper Foot Function," in *The Chiropractic Journal*, "If one or more of the foot's arches is not able to provide the necessary support, or if there has been a breakdown of the plantar fascia, abnormal postural adaptations develop. Additional stress is then placed on all of the joints, ligaments, and muscles involved in helping to maintain upright posture." He concludes by saying, "Posture, as well as balance, coordination, and efficient musculoskeletal function, all depend on the smooth functioning of the foot and ankle complex."

The American College of Foot and Ankle Surgeons concurs, citing common categories of foot and ankle problems as congenital, acquired, traumatic, infectious, neoplastic (involving abnormal tissue growth as occurs in both benign and malignant tumors), and arthritic conditions. Of these, the acquired biomechanical problems may be the most preventable since they often result from physical stress and/or improper footwear. While addressing both of those factors in a fact sheet, "Aerobics and Your Feet," the American Podiatric Medical Association points to poor choice of shoes, hard surfaces, and overuse as primary causes of stress fractures of the foot. If the feet exhibit pronation or the ankles turn inward, orthotic shoes inserts may be needed. Shoes with arches that compensate for expected motions also come recommended with choices depending on the dynamics involved in that particular activity. In aerobic dance, for instance, the impact can be six times the force of gravity, thus necessitating the need for plenty of cushioning. Frequent side-to-side motions in aerobics also require an accommodating arch support with the top of the shoe having sufficient strength to assure the foot's stability. Running shoes, however, do not provide the help needed for aerobics but are instead designed with their unique purpose in mind.

See also BIRTH DEFECTS; FLATFOOT OR FLATFEET; FOOTWEAR.

American College of Foot and Ankle Surgeons. "Surgery of the Foot and Ankle." Available online. URL: http://www.acfas.org/brftankl.htm Downloaded on February 15, 2003.

American Podiatric Medical Association. "Aerobics and Your Feet." Available online. URL: http://www.apma.org/sports/aerobics_printable.html Downloaded on February 26, 2003.

Charrette, Mark. "The Importance of Proper Foot Function." Available online. URL: http://www.worldchiropracticalliance.org/tcj/2002/nov/nov2002charrette.htm Downloaded on February 13, 2003.

female athlete triad A fact sheet from the American Academy of Family Physicians describes this disorder as having three parts affecting 1) eating habits, 2) menstrual periods, and 3) strength of bones. Weight loss, irregular periods, fatigue, and stress fractures can occur as bones begin to thin or osteoporosis develops. To correct this syndrome, a physician may prescribe birth control pills or hormone replacement therapy to help regulate menstrual cycles and stop further bone loss. Natural supplements to replenish any deficiencies of vitamins and minerals will probably be recommended too. However, female athlete triad can usually be prevented by eating regularly, including a wide assortment of nutritious fresh foods in the diet, and choosing moderate exercises instead of sustaining a highly strenuous physical regimen for prolonged amounts of time.

American Academy of Family Physicians. "Sports and Women Athletes: The Female Athlete Triad." Available online. URL: http://familydoctor.org/handouts/599.html Downloaded on February 20, 2003.

femur The longest, strongest bone in the body, this part of the appendicular skeleton goes from hip to knee. Also called the thighbone, the femur fits its rounded head into the hip bone while its smaller distal end articulates with the second largest bone in the body—the tibia of the lower leg. The long bone shape acts like a lever in raising and lowering the leg—and sometimes anything in its way!

In a hard fall, the shaft of the femur can break in a variety of patterns depending on the person's age or other factors. For older people, the head or neck of the femur becomes a commonly fractured site. In young children, growth plate injuries may be more likely to occur. However, for very young children who have not yet begun to walk, a femoral fracture may present evidence of physical abuse, particularly when accompanied by past bone breaks or present bruising. (Unfortunately, the same can be said for suspicious fractures involving nonambulatory residents of nursing homes.)

Of the reported instances of child abuse, 12–29 percent involved femoral fracture with the specific type depending on the type of injury suffered. As one horrible example, a spiral fracture indicates forceful twisting or torsion that is considered highly unlikely for nonambulatory children to do on their own. Retrospective studies that look into case histories over a period of time show high probabilities of physical abuse involving femoral fractures of children less than a year old but dramatically decreasing as the child reaches a second or third birthday. However, parents and other caretakers can themselves become abused by false accusations when dangerous equipment might be to blame. If, for instance, a play center or some similar device allows a nonambulatory child to rotate in one direction with dangerous stops or jolts quickly achievable in the opposite direction, a femoral fracture can conceivably occur. Therefore, to be sure that one potential case of abuse does not lead to another, medical professionals can remain cautious about routinely accepting the conclusions indicated by the statistics. Hence, they should make no assumptions but, rather, probe further, ask detailed questions, and obtain thorough histories in any pediatric trauma.

See also FRACTURES.

Penny Grant. "Femur Fracture in Infants: A Possible Accidental Etiology." Available online. URL: http://www.findarticles.com/cf_O/m0950/4_108/79742698/print.jhtml Downloaded on June 2, 2003.

fiber, muscle In the mouth, bundles of collagen fibers support the teeth and anchor each tooth to bone and/or to adjacent teeth. In the skeleton, fiber creates the spindles that attach each end of a muscle to the corresponding bone, while motor fibers innervate skeletal muscles, thus enabling them to move. How quickly that movement occurs may depend, in part, on variations in the composition of muscle fibers that allow fast-twitch (type II) or the more energy-efficient slow-twitch (type I) responses to transpire. The report "Muscle Fiber Composition and Back Pain," in the July 2002 issue of *The Back Letter,* says that most people have a distinctive mix of both type I and type II muscle fibers. To date, though, no evidence has established that people with chronic lower back pain or other muscle aches have an inadequate or unusual mix of fiber types. Instead, all indications continue to reinforce the overall importance of regular exercise to strengthen muscle fibers and facilitate body movement, albeit fast or slow.

Staff. "Muscle Fiber Composition and Back Pain." Available online. URL: http://www.findarticles.com/cf_0/m0670/7_17/90301364/print.jhtml Downloaded on June 2, 2003.

fibromyalgia Ever since the American College of Rheumatology established the criteria for its diagnostic entry onto the medical scene in the early 1990s, fibromyalgia (FM) has frustrated patients and baffled doctors by its elusiveness. Symptoms of muscular pain, stiffness, and fatigue represent other conditions too, which can make this chronic disorder more recognizable by what it is not. In other words, it is not rheumatoid arthritis nor spinal arthritis nor a number of other possibilities, although it may feel the same and can accompany those or other illnesses. With bouts of anxiety and depression sometimes tossed into the mix of warning signs, fibromyalgia was once seen by skeptics as being all in the head. Yet very real pain resides in muscles and connective tissue at multiple tender points that have been consistently identified in the 3.5 million Americans of all ages who have been affected by this disorder.

In typical instances of fibromyalgia, muscles and soft tissue will often be quite tender to the touch in these specific locations: around the lower vertebrae of the neck, at the insertion of the second rib, around the upper thigh, in the middle of the knee joint, in muscles at the base of the skull, in the neck and upper back muscles, in the midback muscles, on the upper sides of the hips, and on the sides of the elbow. On good days, little or no discomfort may exist. On bad days, the presence of some or all those areas can be felt, especially on rising. In that situation, a hot shower may help to relieve aches or stiffness. Recommended doses of over-the-counter anti-inflammatory medications after meals may also help to calm the inflammation in muscles, joints, and connective tissue.

With disability rates for fibromyalgia estimated as high as 44 percent, the Arthritis Foundation has actively examined numerous possibilities, including behavioral research and the influence of various factors in the environment. In addition, research initiated by the foundation has revealed interesting comparative responses involving the body's normal production of hormones and neuropeptides to convey pain messages from the nerve cells to the spinal cord and brain. These comparative studies show, for example, that FM patients have elevated levels of substance P—the chemical responsible for the body's ability to generate pain signals after an injury. Indeed, some believe an accident or some type of trauma initially activates these signals but then later fails to shut off when healing has begun. Regardless of the causes, studies show the level of serotonin remains consistently low in fibromyalgia patients. This has particular significance since serotonin is the body's naturally produced chemical known to aid sleep and also to restrain the frequency and/or intensity of pain.

In further attempts to locate and document these responses of pain with greater precision, researchers have been putting their brain scans together. While using state-of-the art equipment, fibromyalgia experts scanned and then compared the brain responses of patients with fibromyalgia with those who do not have the disorder. As reported in the May 2002 journal of *Arthritis & Rheumatism*, researcher Richard H. Gracely, Ph.D., and Daniel J. Clauw, M.D., used functional magnetic resonance imaging (fMRI) scans on a group of fibromyalgia patients and a disorder-free group of equal size, subsequently finding some interesting differences. In the non-FM group, increased brain activity occurred only after a pain-inducing pinch but not in response to slight pressure. In contrast the FM patients responded with heightened brain activity in both of those instances.

As of this writing, the National Institutes of Health (NIH) has begun clinical trials on topics as diverse as behavioral insomnia therapy, the efficacy of Reiki, and "Gabapentin in the Treatment of Fibromyalgia" in the hopes of understanding "specific abnormalities that cause and accompany fibromyalgia" and developing better ways to diagnose, treat, and prevent this disorder. From the start, however, the NIH performed groundbreaking studies. By 1999, it had released a fact sheet reporting on those findings, which included abnormally low levels of the hormone cortisol in FM patients.

By 2000 a fact sheet from the American College of Rheumatology (ACR) reported FM as affecting 2 percent of the U.S. population, with seven times more women than men troubled by the disorder, especially women of childbearing age. Suggestions from the ACR included sleep aids, muscle relaxants, heat treatments, occasional applications of cold, massage, occupational therapy, and exercises that incorporate stretching, range of motion, and aerobics to improve the patient's functional performance.

Later investigations have continued to confirm the positive effects of exercise on FM patients. For example, the July 27, 2002 issue of the *British Medical Journal* reported on a study involving 132 FM sufferers who met at a rheumatology clinic in London for one hour twice a week for 12 weeks. Half of the group received relaxation therapy and the other half exercise therapy. At the end of the three-month period, 35 percent of the patients who exercised reported improvements in their condition whereas only about half that number showed similar progress occurring with relaxation training. In a follow-up evaluation a year later, some of the exercise group no longer exhibited symptoms of FM while others in that same group reported noticeable lessening of muscle and joint tenderness.

Meanwhile, a 2002 study by the Touch Research Institutes in Miami, Florida, compared relaxation therapy with massage therapy, with the latter combining several types of massage, each of which used only moderate pressure. After five weeks, both groups reported a reduction of anxiety and depression, but only the group receiving massage therapy experienced lowered levels of the pain-signaling substance P. In addition, FM patients who received twice-weekly massages showed increased levels of serotonin, the chemical that inhibits pain and improves the conditions for sleep. With more restful occasions for the body to heal and to rid itself of toxins as normally occurs during sleep cycles, the study confirms that massage therapy subjects did indeed report less evidence of anxiety and depression with corresponding decreases in measurements of pain.

In addition to massage and more restful patterns of sleep, nutritional support may also be a crucial factor in lessening symptoms. Since malabsorption problems commonly occur in fibromyalgia patients, natural vitamin supplements can be helpful in assuring that the body gets what it needs to maintain energy, strengthen the nerves, and keep muscles, bones, and fibrous tissue in good repair. Similarly, adequate amounts of filtered water, natural fruit or vegetable juices, and mild herbal teas will help to flush out toxins, such as those that accumulate due to poor digestion, pollutants in the environment, food colorings, and the preservatives typically used in packaged foods. White flour, white sugar, and other heavily processed foods should be avoided as should the infamous nightshades (i.e., veggie members of the pepper, tomato, and potato families) that reportedly cause inflammatory responses in arthritis patients. Similarly, foods high in dairy and animal fat can also elicit inflammation as can individually determined foods that cause allergic reactions in FM patients.

Since food allergens vary from one person to the next, keeping a daily journal of the foods and beverages consumed over a four- to six-week period could prove helpful in locating problematic factors in the diet. In addition, daily notations about one's sleep patterns, physical activities, and worries could also prove useful in pinpointing the precise areas that adversely affect a particular individual. By identifying any factors that trigger sleep loss and discomfort, FM patients may then be better equipped to find inventive ways to avoid whatever aggravates their condition. Although this offers no cure, an active role in managing fibromyalgia at least brings hope of relieving fatigue and lessening the pain.

See also NUTRITION.

American College of Rheumatology. "Fibromyalgia." Available online. URL: http://www.rheumatology.org/patients/factsheet/fibromya.html Downloaded on February 17, 2003.

Arthritis Foundation. "Delivering on the Promise in Fibromyalgia." Available online. URL: http://www.arthritis.org/research/research_program/Fibromyalgia/default.asp Downloaded on May 31, 2003.

Balch, James F., M.D., and Phyllis A. Balch. "Fibromyalgia Syndrome." *Prescription for Nutritional Healing, Second Edition.* Garden City, N.Y.: Avery Publishing Group, 1997, pp. 274–277.

DeNoon, Daniel. "Fibromyalgia Pain Is Real." Available online. URL: http://webmd.lycos.com/content/article/48/39261.htm? Downloaded on February 17, 2003.

National Institutes of Health. "Clinical Trials." Available online. URL: http://www.clinicaltrials.gov/ct/gvi/action/Findcondition?ui=D005356+recruiting=true Downloaded on May 31, 2003.

Touch Research Institutes. "Study." Available online. URL: http://www.miami.edu/touch-research Downloaded on February 17, 2003.

Warner, Jennifer. "Exercise Can Ease Fibromyalgia." Available online. URL: http://webmd.lycos.com/content/article/49/40037.htm? Downloaded on February 17, 2003.

fibrosarcoma The American Cancer Society characterizes this cancer of fibrous tissue as most commonly affecting the arms, legs, or torso of patients between age 30 and 55. However, medical staff from the University of Miami School of Medicine report that fibrosarcoma is also the most common soft tissue malignancy found in a child's first year of life, sometimes presenting as a mass at birth with rapid growth during early infancy. Like other sarcomas, the tumor originates in soft tissue, such as the connective tissue of ligaments and tendons, with eradication dependent on prompt detection and treatment. Although fibrosarcomas almost never begin in bone, if left unhindered they spread and may eventually include bone metastasis, which usually involves the appendicular rather than the axial skeleton.

See also BONE CANCER.

University of Miami School of Medicine. "Medical Dictionary." Available online. URL: http://www.med.miami.edu/patients/glossary Downloaded on June 3, 2003.

fibrositis The old term used for fibromyalgia, this chronic disorder presents itself as pain and stiffness in the networking tissue that moves or supports the bones and joints.

See also FIBROMYALGIA.

fibula On the outer part of the lower leg, the fibula articulates with the much thicker, stronger, weight-bearing tibia that resides between the knee and ankle as part of the appendicular skeleton. Also known as the calf bone, the original Latin word places the fibula as the pin or back element that clasps a brooch into place. Since the fibula is indeed quite long and thin, it joins the tibia in being one of the most commonly broken bones in the U.S.—or about 185,000 times each year, according to health information from Johns Hopkins.

See also FRACTURES.

fight-or-flight response The heartbeat quickens. Senses heighten, and hormones ooze forth in the form of corticosteroids freshly manufactured from the adrenal cortex. Beads of perspiration arise on the skin and roll their scent away, eliminating toxins and lowering body temperature. Digestion all but ceases. The liver unloads stores of glucose, providing precious fuel for energy. Blood flow diverts from the skin and internal organs, mustering even more glucose and oxygen for innervating use in the muscles and brain. Now fully charged for action, the body can readily stand its ground and fight or, with amazing speed, flee—not just for the moment but long after the danger has passed.

For many, many thousands of years, this natural response originating from the limbic system—or the primitive part of the brain—controlled instinctive behavior highly appropriate to physical danger, thus helping to preserve the human race. In today's world, however, the circumstances perceived as a peril often come from an unaware boss, a clueless coworker, a distracted spouse, a whining child, a disconcerting computer message, or the distressing headlines in the news—none of which require either fleeing or fighting. Nevertheless, the person who has been affected by such matters immediately acquires an excessive amount of energy to expend with no outlet for doing so. The only thing to conquer may be stress but with a swift bout of exhaustion most likely on the way. Furthermore, if this fight-or-flight response becomes a regular routine at home or work, the body swerves between a heightened state of readiness and debilitating fatigue—an unsettling condition that eventually weakens internal organs, shuts down the immune system, and almost assures the development of ailments ranging from hypertension to chronic musculoskeletal spasms and pain.

Since no one has the power to change anyone but the self, a decision to correct the imbalances can initiate an objective evaluation of any circumstances that frequently lead to a fight-or-flight reaction. For some, the rebalancing efforts may mean making a career change, taking an assertiveness training course, or practicing ways to communicate concerns and feelings with precision and clarity. For almost everyone, though, general recommendations include the addition of sound nutritional support, massage therapy, and relaxing activities, such as praying, playing, painting, singing, or listening to soothing music. As long as a person remains in the throes of heightened mental alertness and physical preparedness, however, just about any immediate and appropriate activity, such as yard work or racquetball, provides a healthy outlet for relieving excess energy. Then, with regular follow-up of individually preferred exercises, the adapting body will adeptly transform the primitive reactions of fight or flight into a fitness choice.

figurative use Literally speaking, muscles overlay skeletal bones of the body, shaping the person's physique or figure. Figuratively speaking, muscles may be motifs for money or power and bones for symbols ranging from death to pet peeves, with no bones about it.

finger or fingers With the wave of a wand or a paintbrush, the five fingers on a person's predominately used hand can perform the magic of art or the orchestration of music. Fingers make things. Fingers fix things. Fingers type, tap, grasp, and beckon for attention while only showing a glimpse of what is really there. Beneath a thin covering of muscle and skin, a total of 14 finger bones (phalanges) extend like magic from the palm of each hand, corresponding to the somewhat shorter 14 bones of the toes on either foot. That makes an amazing 28 bones in the 10 phalanges alone.

In polydactyly, an extra finger exists. However, if the addition consists primarily of soft tissue or skin, it can usually be removed shortly after a child is born. Missing fingers, shortened fingers, and elongated fingers may also emerge at birth, usually because of a genetic disposition but occasionally because of an entrapment or other interference in the womb when the fingers first began to form. In most newborns, though, 10 fingers arrive as expected, ready to reach for food or touch the mother's skin with intricate nerve endings in place to enjoy and record that valuable information.

As children grow, their fingers also develop as devices for exploring and investigating persons, objects, and almost anything else in the surroundings that entice. Then mobility turns to heightened physical activity with fingers getting banged, jammed, dislocated, or broken. Although each type of injury requires relevant treatment, splinting may be needed to correct joint placement and encourage proper growth.

With a mallet finger, a ruptured tendon, or a fractured bone, the tip of the finger may become inclined to bend down and remain in that position. Similarly, inflammation can cause a tendon to become entrapped, such as happens in a trigger finger when the trapped tendon hinders ease of movement. Rheumatoid arthritis, osteoarthritis, and other medical conditions can also cause fingers to become misshapen or deformed. In many such instances, early treatments of either icing or warm-water soaks, anti-inflammatory medications, and exercises that keep the joints flexible can ease pain and improve dexterity in range of motion. If additional treatments become necessary, cortisone injections, splints, or surgery can often restore finger function. Unless nerve damage has occurred, though, fingers continue to feel not only what they touch but what touches them. Although aging sometimes gnarls and claws their beauty, fingers remain sensory instruments. As they reach for reassurance or tactile pleasures, they continue to explore nearby surfaces, sensing, feeling, and recording a caress, a metal railing, a touch of silk.

See also FLEXION CONTRACTURE; TENDINITIS OR TENDONITIS.

first aid According to health information from the Harvard Medical School, the first step in first aid begins with an assessment of the surroundings. In the absence of any immediate dangers, most first aid measures involve direct care—from stopping bleeding to cardiopulmonary resuscitation (CPR).

Although this book's scope does not include such diverse topics as applying the Heimlich maneuver, delivering twins, or pulling a fishhook from a finger, generally accepted recommendations on dealing with potential back, neck, and head injuries or broken bones might be in order, especially when accompanied by manuals from the Harvard Medical School and the U.S. government.

The latter warns in all caps, "If a broken neck or back is suspected, do not move the casualty unless to save his life. Movement may cause permanent paralysis or death." If leg elevation is required to prevent shock, a fractured leg must first be splinted. To do this, *The Official Government First Aid Manual* differentiates a closed fracture as being less apparent than an open one, which breaks the skin, often causing bone to protrude. Then, protecting the wound from further contamination becomes especially vital but without touching, pushing, or otherwise disrupting the exposed bone. With either a closed or an open fracture, however, the injured limb can be immobilized with whatever is at hand—for example, a rolled magazine, a thick newspaper, or a stick. To immobilize an arm, a sling can be made from a belt or piece of cloth with the hand held higher than the elbow.

Medical experts at Harvard also recommend being suspicious of head, neck, and back injuries whenever a person has been in a vehicular collision or has fallen from a height, such as a swimming pool diving board. Care must then be taken not to reposition a victim unless another life-threatening situation, such as an imminent explosion or fire, makes moving the person imperative. Similarly, the helmet of an accident victim should be left on, untouched and in place. If the person remains conscious, a head injury may be indicated by signs of confusion, nausea, poor coordination, or variation in pupil size. For a neck injury, the person may experience stiffness, pain, headache, tingling sensations, or an inability to move. In all of the above cases, however, a call to 911 remains high on the first aid checklist as soon as conditions and a telephone allow. While waiting for medical help to come, most patients should be kept flat, quiet, and warmed by a coat or blanket and a soothing voice to help reduce the likelihood of life-threatening shock.

The Official Government First Aid Manual: A Literary Guide To The Treatment of Illness and Injury. Woodbury, N.Y.: Platinum Press, 2000.

fitness facilities With a trend toward fitness, business travelers and vacationers have seemingly become more interested in the treadmill, pool, or gym facilities at a hotel or motel than the room discounts or other amenities preferred in the past. Now, well-maintained, functioning equipment enables a traveler to keep up with a regular exercise regimen even when away from the home or office. Whether facilities are on the premises—as preferred by most business women—or at a nearby gym, up to 10 percent of business travelers reportedly take advantage of these services.

On the home terrain, Americans currently have over 62,000 personal trainers to choose from in developing individually tailored fitness programs. However, as Charles Stuart Platkin points out in his May 29, 2003 article "Knowledge is Power . . ." for *The Miami Herald,* the personal training industry presently lacks uniform regulation. As long as this situation continues, consumers will need to ask about a trainer's certification as well as his or her particular approach, overall strategy, and requirements for physical evaluations before a fitness training program is designed. Despite the gaps in state and federal requirements, studies show that good indicators of a trainer's expertise include a bachelor's degree in exercise science or accreditation from either the American College of Sports Medicine or the National Strength and Conditioning Association. Both organizations provide local referrals that make awkwardly questioning trainers about their certification no longer necessary. Once fitness training has begun, however, consumers need to evaluate the success of a program continuously, considering, for example, the level of intensity and duration of pain. Although some discomfort can be expected in the beginning, sharp pain should really not be part of the package. If all is well, a fitness program usually takes 10 weeks at the least but with training typically becoming repetitive after six months or so.

One option that often offers variety and accessibility is training at a YMCA. Since its beginnings in

London in 1884, the YMCA has opened fitness facilities now extending around the world. Indeed, the World Alliance of YMCAs presently provides leadership and develops policies for a confederation of 122 national YMCA movements with alliances from Africa to the Caribbean to the Middle East. In addition to physical fitness centers and typically reputable fitness programs in many large towns and cities, the organization also focuses on facilitating spiritual and social fitness. In Orange County, California, for example, a January 25, 2000 article for *PR Newswire* reported on the nonprofit organization's goal of raising funds to be used for financial aid in child care that would go beyond baby-sitting and into strengthening each child's character and body.

More schools may be developing a similar approach. With at least 15 percent of the school-aged children in the U.S. currently assessed as overweight, schools may soon host the next round of fitness facilities. To begin that positive trend, some creative solutions so far include involving children in gardening and in developing environmental awareness while others focus on getting cafeterias to remove soft drink vending machines and offer more tasteful meals based on sound nutritional principles. With hands-on involvement in growing the good foods that fuel energy, most children have what it takes to become active. To further that intent, the U.S. surgeon general called for healthier food choices in schools and daily gym classes. Federal funding for physical education programs also increased by 20 percent in 2003. In addition, some schools have begun to take the initiative in developing programs, depending on what works in the local area. In Downey, California, for example, the West Middle School turned children's interests in popular video games into an opportunity for physical fitness. Participants in the resulting Cyberobics program get a workout on exercise bikes attached to video games. With, for instance, heart rates tabulated by the machines, the children's own level of fitness scores points toward the power awarded video characters. Meanwhile, in a lower-income suburb in Texas, students dance, skate, and paddle kayaks donated by local residents. In Washington, another program combines fitness and science as children perform aerobic exercises and then monitor their own hearts. As people of all ages become more aware of adventuresome and workable possibilities, the most personally designed fitness facilities may soon begin at home.

Collier, Lorna. "Innovative Schools Teach Lifelong Health by Just Saying No to Status Quo." Available online. URL: http://www.miami.com/mld/miamiherald/news/5959871.htm?template=conten-modules Downloaded on June 3, 2003.

Curley, Bob. "The Business of Fitness." *Business Traveler.* (August 2002): 36–39.

Plotkin, Charles Stuart. "Knowledge is Power . . ." Herald. Available online. URL: http://www.miami.com/mld/miamiherald/5957563.htm?template=contentModules Downloaded on June 3, 2003.

PR Newswire. "YMCA of Orange County to Increase Child Care Financial Aid for Local Families in 2000." Available online. URL: http://www.findarticles.com/cf_0/m4PRN/2000_Jan_25/58939955/print.jhtml Downloaded on June 4, 2003.

flatfoot or flatfeet On first appearances, most newborns have flatfeet, but closer inspection usually shows *fat* feet—with a small fatty pad in the arch slowly disappearing as the infant ages. Then, a flexible flatfoot may continue until somewhere around age five with the arch seeming to disappear whenever the child stands. As long as the muscles and joints in the foot and calf of the leg remain functioning and mobile, this painless and normal condition commonly corrects itself without any treatment. However, if foot and leg pain or muscle fatigue begin to occur, the pediatrician or podiatrist will look for indications of a tight heel cord or a rigid flatfoot. One sign, for instance, occurs when the ankle turns inward. If only one foot seems to be involved, the doctor will undoubtedly compare the two feet, evaluating the differences between them and also examining the pattern of wear on the pair of shoes most often worn.

According to a fact sheet from the American College of Foot and Ankle Surgeons, another indicator of painful progressive flatfoot is "too many toes" showing when viewed from the back of the foot. Further evaluations may include moving each foot against resistance and looking for signs of swelling, not necessarily in the arch as much as in the leg's calf muscle. From the back of the knee down the back of the leg, a tendon passes beneath ankle bone before attaching to the arch of the foot. There, the tendon helps to maintain the architectural triumph of the arch while the corresponding muscles enable the heel to lift without dragging as a person walks. If the tendon holds too tightly, though, the foot's range of motion may be hindered, and mild to sharp pain may result. When this type of condition exists, the physician or medical specialist can demonstrate stretching exercises to increase the flexibility of the tendon as well as the foot and leg calf muscles. Shoe inserts may also be recommended as a means of relieving foot pain but with the bonus of making a child's shoes get maximum use until they are outgrown.

In any age group, a fall or injury can cause the arch to drop suddenly, which usually means that a tendon has ruptured. Sharp pains verify this prospect. Then, magnetic resonance imaging (MRI) of the tendon may be needed to locate the extent of damage. However, flatfeet can also occur if foot joints stiffen or if prolonged swelling alters the natural curve of the arch. Regardless of the cause, though, flatfeet need treatment to restore healthful walking conditions and to prevent arthritis from developing. As reported in the American College of Foot and Ankle Surgeons' (ACFAS) February 2003 news release "Correct Flat Feet Before Adolescence," the typical treatment options include shoe modification, orthotic inserts, physical therapy, stretching exercises, and gentle anti-inflammatory medication. Should surgery be needed, a study reported by the same ACFAS news release says that surgical outcomes before adolescence remain high with normal foot functioning generally restored after a four-month recuperative time.

Interestingly, however, many adults do not even know they have flatfeet. According to the American Academy of Orthopaedic Surgeons' (AAOS) October 16, 2002 news release "Ignore Flat Feet and They Might Become Your Archenemy," 75 percent of the people in this country experience foot pain sometime during their lives. Of the 25 percent of North Americans who have flatfeet, many are just not troubled by them. Nevertheless, when left untended, knee pain, tendinitis, and other probabilities can eventually occur. To find out if a foot wears any such risk, the AAOS offers ideas for easy tests that a person can perform at home. An evaluation of often-worn shoes, for example, will show wear on the inside of the sole and the heel area if the wearer has flatfoot. Another test requires that the person spread the fingertips against a wall while standing tiptoe on one foot. (Hint: With a fallen arch, this usually cannot be done.) In addition, as most swimmers know, a wet footprint on dry concrete should show the front or ball of the foot connected to the heel by a much thinner side strip. As those dignified folks at the American Academy of Orthopaedic Surgeons say, a wider side strip means that foot is as flat as a pancake.

See also TENDINITIS OR TENDONITIS.

American Academy of Orthopaedic Surgeons. "Ignore Flat Feet and They Might Become Your Archenemy." Available online. URL: http://orthoinfo.aaos.org Downloaded on February 25, 2003.

American College of Foot and Ankle Surgeons. "Correct Flat Feet Before Adolescence." Available online. URL: http//www.acfas.org/prflatfeet.html Downloaded on February 25, 2003.

American College of Foot and Ankle Surgeons. "Painful Progressive Flatfoot." Available online. URL: http://www.acfas.org/brflatfoot.html Downloaded on February 15, 2003.

flexibility Throughout this book, suggestions continuously occur for exercising range of motion to increase the flexibility of joints. So, what is the big deal about having those flexible connections? Aging naturally causes connective joints to stiffen. However, the number of birthdays does not count as much as inactivity—a primary factor that is usually preventable. Although recent studies show that stretching for flexibility will probably not stop acute muscle injuries from happening, flexing certainly will not be the cause. Instead, five to 10 minutes spent in warm-ups actually does warm muscles, tendons, and ligaments, thereby preparing the body for heightened activity. In sports, such as gymnastics or tennis, that require both strength and agility, gentle stretches before and after a game will relax the muscles and enhance an athlete's overall performance. The key, though, is gently stretching, slowly stretching, and lightly pulling then holding that stretch for a few seconds without the bouncing or overextending that can cause muscle fiber to tear.

When accidents do happen, recovery may be measured by how flexible the person becomes—perhaps not just physically but spiritually and mentally too. People feel better when they can move, which, in turn, inspires more movement. Then, with circulation improved, the body has what it needs to send forth nutrients to form new tissue in new growth and also in the newly remodeled muscles and bones that already exist. Body wastes get transported from the system too, lessening the likelihood of toxic buildup in cells, organs, and muscles. Similarly, the joints receive a better flow of those lubricating fluids that allow for ease of movement. This small lube job is no small matter as it enables persons of all ages to bend, lift, turn, and perform the everyday activities needed for independent living. The resulting flexibility helps people better catch themselves at the first signs of a fall, thus decreasing the likelihood and intensity of those pains that no one wants.

Luebbers, Paul. "Enhancing Your Flexibility." Available online. URL: http://www.acsm.org/pdf/fits202.pdf Downloaded on February 7, 2003.

Staff. "Flex Time." *Sports Illustrated for Women.* (January/February 2001): 30–31.

flexion The opposite of extension, this joint movement decreases the angle between the bones, such as when a hand bends toward the inner wrist, when the head drops toward the chest, or when the toes point downward, away from the leg.

flexion contracture A contracture can occur in any joint. In the elbow, knee, or hip, though, it can often be a subtle indicator of arthritis or another condition that needs to be checked out by a specialist, such as a rheumatologist. Treatment, in such cases, will depend on finding ways to address the underlying cause.

In the hand, a flexion contracture is commonly called *bent finger,* which usually occurs in the middle joint of a finger but may be in a fingertip or knuckle. A fact sheet from the American Association of Hand Surgery says that the affected hand can tighten into a fist, but upon straightening, the bent finger remains "stuck" even if the person presses down on it with the other hand. Spraining, twisting, or jamming a finger may initially cause a contracture. If so, treatment includes relieving the swelling, exercising the finger, and splinting. If the condition remains, a hand surgeon can evaluate the need for surgery.

flexor muscles The opposite of extensors, flexor muscles bring bones closer together, decreasing the space or angle between them as when the arm folds to hold the telephone receiver to an ear and when a hand cups to hold water. In pain, flexor muscles react protectively, curling up the injured part for the whole body to hug and hold.

flexor tendon injury For each thumb and every finger, two flexor tendons attach into the palm, allowing the hand with all its digits to clasp, grasp, bend, extend, or make a fist. If something happens either to pop or to tighten those tendons, movement ceases in that area or occurs only with painstaking motion. Similarly, toes and other moving parts of the body come attached with flexor type tendons, such as the hamstring or the Achilles tendon in the heel—each of which is capable of sustaining damage or scars. Prompt application of ice and anti-inflammatory medications may relieve the pain and swelling. However, if a condition shows no signs of resolving itself, ultrasound treatments or cortisone injections may be needed. A torn or snapped tendon often requires surgical repair as might an older injury with a buildup of scar tissue that hinders the affected joint.

After surgery, the area of repair remains immobile for a while, usually with the help of a splint. A fact sheet from the American Association for Hand Surgery discussing flexor tendon injuries recommends edema control techniques, such as a glove or a wrap worn for light compression. To keep swelling down even more, the hand can be elevated higher than the heart. Although the length of recovery time varies according to each individual, the general expectation is about 10–12 weeks. To assist the healing process, an occupational therapist can provide therapeutic exercises two or three times a week to increase flexibility as the hand begins to mend.

American Association for Hand Surgery, "Flexor Tendon Injuries FAQ." Available online. URL: http://www.handsurgery.org/Flexorinjuries.pdf Downloaded on February 17, 2003.

folic acid The American Society for Nutritional Sciences and The American Society for Clinical Nutrition announced the results of a study in a December 3, 2001 news release entitled "Benefits of Government-Mandated Folic Acid Fortification Greater Than Expected"—which almost says it all. As of January 1998, all enriched cereal grain products, including rice, flour, cornmeal, and pasta, produced in the U.S. had to be fortified with folic acid in an attempt to eradicate certain types of birth defects. With the increased consumption of folate and other B vitamins, however, middle-aged and elderly Americans showed increased benefits too. For instance, the inclusion of folic acid in the diet has had a positive effect in reducing the risks of heart attacks, memory impairment, and strokes. Besides enriched cereal products, fresh food sources include collard and turnip greens, asparagus, broccoli, cantaloupe, beans, peas, and orange juice.

American Society for Clinical Nutrition. "Benefits of Government-Mandated Folic Acid Fortification Greater Than Expected." Available online. URL: http://www.faseb.org/ascn/dec01pr.htm Downloaded on May 5, 2003.

footwear The old saying, "If the shoe fits, wear it," would probably comprise about one-third of the advice from the American Orthopaedic Foot and Ankle Society (AOFAS). As their online health information indicates, a fitting shoe not only fits but is well made and appropriate for the occasion. For instance, AOFAS's "A Guide to Children's Shoes" recommends no shoes for young babies, who need only booties or socks for warmth. Similarly, neither shoes nor socks for toddlers and young children come recommended if indoor surfaces have been deemed safe enough for walking barefoot. Otherwise, shoes fit best by the length, the width, and the depth, with ample toe room to avoid ingrown toenails and other foot problems. Since the feet of young toddlers grow at least a half size every two months and preschoolers about every four months, shoes need to be examined often to make sure they do not press against the toes.

When the time comes for the next pair of shoes, the best choice will be comfortable with no breaking-in required. Although young children do not really need an arch support, a padded insole can feel good to the feet, especially if constructed of natural fibers that allow the foot to breathe. Likewise, the upper part of the shoe should consist of natural leather or cotton canvas with synthetic materials reserved for mesh weaves that also keep feet from sweating or retaining perspiration. For the bottom of the shoe, smooth but nonslippery soles help with traction whereas thick or sticky soles can be awkward, causing the very falls they were meant to prevent. Generally, shoes shaped to look like a foot work best as do flat soles and a snugly fitting heel. For early walkers, high-tops that tie up and stay on well will help to support the ankles and prevent slipping.

The American Podiatric Medical Association (APMA) concurs, adding that both feet should be measured while standing with the size chosen to fit the larger foot. Then, time should be allowed to walk around the store so shoes can be assessed for immediate comfort and even distribution of weight without any signs of pinching. Smooth seams inside a shoe will prevent chafing too. To assure a good fit even further, the shoes should be tried on while wearing the socks or stockings that will be worn with this particular pair of shoes.

These guidelines fit adults nicely, too, with expectations of uniformity within a manufacturer's line and of one's own shoe size never taken for granted. A full-grown foot changes over time as bones shift and body weight increases or decreases. For people of all ages, feet also swell throughout the day, making late afternoon or early evening a good time to get a more accurate assessment of shoe size. According to the APMA, in fact, an average day of walking exerts a force of several hundred tons on the feet of most adults, thus inclining a weakened foot to be injured more than any other part of the body.

If that body happens to be in the military, the addition of shock-absorbing insoles to regulate military regulation boots can help to reduce an otherwise high occurrence of stress fractures. According to a March 2003 news release reporting on this topic for the American College of Sports Medicine, researchers particularly recommend insoles made of a combination of soft and rigid foam with a woven and washable protective covering. Some servicemen and servicewomen seem satisfied with gel inserts too.

In reporting on other safety factors in the January 2000 *Occupational Hazards,* Todd Nighswonger points out the need to consider specific work conditions. For instance, if working hazards include the potential of falling or rolling objects, compression-resistant footwear will be needed—not just a steel-toed shoe but one with a steel cap that covers the toes with full protection. If the possibility of punctures from nails, glass, or sharp metal poses a hazard, the soles should be reinforced with flexible metal—assuming no danger of electrocution exists. If so, soles then need to be made of a nonconductive material, such as rubber, with socks made of fibers that do not conduct electricity. Silk, wool, and nylon will most likely do. Protection against acids and other chemicals may also be required. Rubber soles are a frequent choice but one that does not work well around some environments, such as meat- and poultry-processing plants or oil refineries. Shoe protection from heat and cold need to be considered, too, with specific guidelines available from the Occupational Safety and Health Administration and also from the American National Standards Institute.

When considering protection and long-lasting footwear, the shoe's last offers a last word. In other words, every shoe has a last that is either straight or curved. To discover which is which, draw a full-length, imaginary line down the shoe from the center of the heel through the middle of the toe. A curved last will bulge out, particularly on sports shoes, but this can aggravate or cause foot problems. Additionally, a curved last does not provide adequate support for the muscles and tendons running on the outside edge of the fairly straight-edged foot that most people have. Apparently, some manufacturers of athletic shoes think a curved last adds to stability when the opposite could be true. To know for sure if a design has actually offered support as needed, an inspection of worn shoes may tell all. For instance, if the contour of a shoe becomes misshapen after use, it probably had an inadequate shape from the start. If so, a straighter last—and, possibly, individually designed orthotic inserts prescribed by a foot specialist—can help most feet move in the right direction with a minimum of strain.

See also ORTHOTICS.

American College of Sports Medicine. "Running in Military Boots Could be Made Safer, More Efficient By Adding Insoles." Available online. URL: http://www.acsm.org/publications/newsrelease_030503.htm Downloaded on April 14, 2003.

American Orthopaedic Foot and Ankle Society. "A Guide to Children's Shoes." Available online. URL: http://www.aofas.org/guidekids.asp Downloaded on February 17, 2003.

American Podiatric Medical Association. "Your Podiatric Physician Talks About Footwear." Available online. URL: http://www.apma.org/topics/footwear_printable.htm Downloaded on June 9, 2003.

Nighswonger, Todd. "January 2000." Available online. URL: http://www.findarticles.com/cf_0/m4333/1_62/59557570/prit.jhtml Downloaded on June 9, 2003.

fractures By the year 2050, the American Academy of Orthopaedic Surgeons reportedly expects 650,000 hip fractures annually. At this writing, however, the U.S. government's Agency for Healthcare Research and Quality (AHRQ) says that over 225,000 Americans aged 50 years and older sustain a hip fracture each year. Of these, about 81 percent require hip repair surgery with about 19 percent of those surgeries resulting in complications as reported in the December 2002 AHRQ bulletin, number 268. A 2003 AHRQ bulletin further reports that the greatest risks for postoperative complications arise when patients with abnormal vital signs leave the hospital too soon, even if they go to a rehabilitation or a skilled nursing facility. Despite the discouraging statistics, safety measures can dramatically decrease the above odds since most falls occur at home and most can be prevented.

For many people, however, the problem does not come from falling down but from getting up with spontaneous stress fractures occurring as full body weight goes onto previously weakened bones. For example, osteoporosis can cause compression fractures, which, in turn, increase the rate of morbidity. With early detection and treatment, though, patients with osteoporosis can lessen the risk of fractures by as much as 50 percent. If vertebral compression fractures do occur, treatment traditionally includes bed rest, pain relievers, braces, and physical therapy. Vertebroplasty may also be used to cement bones or kyphoplasty to place inflatable balloonlike devices into the fractured area where they expand to fill spinal voids, thus restoring strength and vertebral height.

Besides the 10 million or more Americans with osteoporosis, another 18 million have low bone mass. Often, this involves metabolic disorders that instigate bone loss with a less-recognized but increasingly frequent cause of low back pain occurring from sacral stress fractures. As with other types of stress fractures, low bone density combined with high activity causes the breakage, but, in this case, vague or dull pain can be easily mistaken for a common backache. After a diagnostic examination has dismissed potential tumors, disk disease, sacroiliitis, or other joint dysfunctions, a magnetic resonance image (MRI) helps to confirm the existence of a sacral fracture. Treatment then involves rest from all weight-bearing activities for about two weeks with nonimpact training in a swimming pool or on a stationary bike for the next six weeks or so.

Additionally, stress fractures can occur as otherwise healthy bones get overloaded during strenuous sports or military maneuvers, especially if the person's footgear is not geared for full support. A February 2000 fact sheet entitled "Stress Fractures" from the American College of Sports Medicine (ACSM) reported that 0.7–15.6 percent of all athletic injuries result in stress fractures, particularly among runners, jumpers, gymnasts, and dancers. Among military personnel, women score the highest percentile in stress fractures with an overall rate of 1–20 percent for new recruits. To avoid the likelihood of stress fractures, the ACSM suggests getting adequate calcium in foods or supplements, gradually increasing the intensity of physical activity, and training on level asphalt that absorbs shock before progressing to grass or uneven terrain. For the long haul, a study reported at an annual meeting of the American Society for Bone and Mineral Research found that women who regularly did back-strengthening exercises for a period of two years were three times less likely to have a spinal fracture.

Besides being named by their location, fractures also have names according to the trauma causing them, such as a stress fracture on a weight-bearing bone or a blowout fracture behind the eye. Additionally, fractures have classifications according to their character. For instance, a spiral leg fracture does indeed have a spiral pattern, whereas a greenstick fracture figuratively compares to the way a green stick breaks—torn and somewhat jagged. A transverse fracture slants crosswise across the bone. An incomplete fracture is just that, while a complete fracture occurs as a full break, just as the name implies. A comminuted fracture results in splintered pieces but may be a closed fracture. In contrast, a compound fracture compounds problems by being a full, open break with bone protruding through the skin, thereby causing concerns about infection.

When a bone breaks, it is important to seek proper FIRST AID and, if needed, call 911. In general, the typical treatment for a fracture includes bone setting by a medical professional followed by non-weight-bearing rest and possibly surgery, depending on the location, severity, and type. Recovery time depends on which bone has broken as well as the person's age. For example, the fractured finger of a five-year-old child may heal in a month while the same injury might take an adult six to eight weeks to heal. Generally, the large bones of the leg take the longest recovery time and, in some instances, may require hospitalization and traction to realign the bone with gentle pulling applied by various devices. For most people, however, a fractured will heal in the body's own time with the bone's own remodeling processes. Nevertheless, prompt medical attention helps healing begin correctly with a minimum of complications.

See also FALLS OR FALLING; FOOTWEAR; SAFETY.

Agency for Healthcare Research and Quality. "Most hip fracture patients do not have medical complications following surgery." Available online. URL: http://www.ahrq.gov/research/jan03/0103RA3.htm Downloaded on March 6, 2004.

American Academy of Foot and Ankle Surgeons. "Stress Fractures." Available online. URL: http://www.aofas.orf/stressfrac.asp Downloaded on February 17, 2003.

Frederickson, Michael, Lara Salamancha, et al. "Sacral Stress Fractures: Tracking Down Nonspecific Pain in Distance Runners." Available online. URL: http://www.physsportsmed.com/issues/2003/0203/fred.htm Posted February 2003.

Linville, Douglas A., II. "Vertebroplasty and Kyphoplasty." *Southern Medical Journal* 95, no. 6 (June 2002): 583–587.

functional neuromuscular stimulation Similar to the therapeutic stimulation used to exercise muscles and avoid atrophy, functional neuromuscular stimulation (FNS) goes a step further by assisting steps, especially when gait training and other conventional forms of therapy have reached a plateau and leveled there. Then, FNS provides an additional boost with treatments the patient can apply at his or her own pace with no assistance usually required. Originally, this was not the case since older systems placed electrodes atop the skin, causing discomfort to some patients and frustration to most because of the time needed to get hooked up to and unhooked from the unit. With improved FNS systems, however, electrodes can be surgically implanted beneath the person's skin and left in place with wires coiled into a small unit kept on the thigh. Not only does this simplify FNS use, but as a patient activates the system, electrical stimulation can reach nerve fibers at a deeper level. The patient subsequently sees visual evidence of muscle contractions and is encouraged to continue activating his or her muscles without the danger of overexertion. Between these therapeutic times, however, the patient can swim or bathe with the small unit left in place, ready for the next round of treatments that can increase muscle strength and help to recover lost mobility.

Daly, Janis J. "The FNS Project." Available online. URL: http://www.rehabpub.com/Features/32003/6.asp Downloaded on April 16, 2003.

G

gait A confident stride, a hesitant step, a firm footfall, a shuffle—the way a person walks can open a gate to revealing attitudes as well as a gait pattern indicative of physical conditions or concerns. From the moment the heel hits the ground, the body's gait cycle carries the foot forward and into a position for the toe to push off as the opposite heel advances. If something interferes with this normal motion, however, something is amiss. To find out what, the pattern of the gait cycle or any other abnormality in walking can offer useful information for a podiatrist or physician when making a diagnosis.

Many of the abnormalities identified when assessing a person's gait have highly descriptive names. For example, a propulsive gait makes a person appear to be charging forth when this positioning may, instead, be a sign of the halting effects of Parkinson's disease or an instance of poisoning, including the highly toxic effects of certain drugs. A scissors gait allows the knees and thighs to thump against each other or to cross in a cutting movement akin to that of a pair of shears. Typically, a trauma to the spinal cord—or, perhaps, cervical spondylosis generating from the upper neck—causes this type of gait as can cerebral palsy. In a spastic gait, however, prolonged muscle contractions on one side of the body can result in foot-dragging, which may be due to a head trauma initiated by an accident, tumor, or stroke. In a steppage gait, a spinal cord trauma or a herniated lumbar disk may cause the toes to point down in foot drop that, in the extreme, can cause the front of a shoe to scrape along the ground. Various diseases, such as poliomyelitis and multiple sclerosis, can also cause steppage and other types of gait problems as can musculoskeletal conditions. A waddling gait, for instance, looks like it sounds with atrophy of the spinal muscles, muscular dystrophy, or congenital hip dysplasia the most common causative factors. Legs of an uneven length, foot problems—from bunions to ingrown toenails—bone fractures, tendinitis, arthritis, and degenerative disk disease also alter the way a person walks, as can ill-fitting shoes.

If a fracture or an injury has occurred, the gait should normalize and improve over time with healing. For chronic conditions, however, treatment will depend on the cause and type of movement. When the very way a person walks increases the risk of falling—as happens with a propulsive gait—a cane or a stabilizing walker may be recommended. In such a circumstance, assistance would be especially essential as the person moves onto an uneven sidewalk or across irregular terrain where getting one's footing is hard. Simply slowing down when walking gives most people the opportunity to assess their surroundings visually or with other sensory tools. Slowing down also gives the body time to adapt physically and rebalance itself. If the legs or feet need bracing and the bones need adjusting to stabilize a gait, spinal manipulation by an osteopath or a chiropractor followed by a prescribed course of physical therapy will generally be helpful in most cases.

Since few people have perfect bodies, many experience at least a slight discrepancy from one leg to another. Eventually, almost all will stub a toe or bang a foot, small matters that, nevertheless, can alter the gait as a person compensates without even being aware of what has happened. The height of heels most often worn can gradually affect the musculoskeletal system, too, as the spine accommodates to subtle changes. The body shifts. The weight rebalances. Ever so slowly, the gait begins to modify, affecting the joints and vertebrae and, perhaps, causing some musculoskeletal problems attributed to other factors, such as bone loss or worn cartilage. If, however, an asymmetrical gait has created an adverse environment that wears away bones and cartilage or otherwise affects the skeletal structure of the body, then correcting the gait could certainly prove useful in treatment.

Another interesting possibility in improving gait relates to motor function, particularly after a stroke or trauma has occurred. At such times, the patient's timing may be off while walking, a problem that can be directly addressed with the inclusion of music in a physical therapy program. As part of the rehabilitation process, a distinctive beat with regular patterns of recurrence can help the person restore a walking cadence, with music to step to and enjoy as the body's motor responses begin to reset themselves.

To find out if gait has caused or is perpetuating a musculoskeletal problem, an evaluation can be made by a physical therapist and/or doctor of osteopathy, chiropractics, or orthopedics. If an incomplete spinal cord injury has affected gait though, innovative treatments may include FUNCTIONAL NEUROMUSCULAR STIMULATION or other types of electrical stimuli to get the muscles moving. At the Miami Project to Cure Paralysis, for example, researcher Dr. Edelle Field-Fote and colleagues have developed a Spinal Cord Injury Functional Ambulation Inventory (SCI-FAI) to assess gait and to record a baseline in order to document a patient's progress with greater precision.

With more biomedical engineering feats in the works, Dr. Field-Fote and others associated with the University of Miami School of Medicine have begun a five-year study funded by the National Institutes of Health to compare the effectiveness of three different combinations of body weight support treadmill techniques for use in gait training. Although no cure presently exists for severed spinal cord injuries, The Miami Project to Cure Paralysis expects successful surgical repairs to be achievable in the future. As Dr. Field-Fote reportedly said, "By determining today what types of rehabilitation interventions lead to the best improvements in function in the shortest period of time, we will be ready for the day when we have the cure."

See also FOOTWEAR; PARALYSIS; REHABILITATION.

Brouman, Sherry. "Walking Off the Pain." Available online. URL: http://www.rehabpub.com/features/1022003/2.asp Downloaded on June 10, 2003.

The Miami Project to Cure Paralysis. "Rehabilitation Studies Gain NIH Funding." Available online. URL: http://www.miamiproject.miami.edu/Library/n102061.htm Downloaded on June 10, 2003.

ganglion cyst In its classic form, this rounded gelatinous growth beneath the skin looks like an extra bone often located opposite the prominent wrist bone. A ganglion cyst may be smaller or larger than the most noticeable bone of the wrist, too. Sometimes arising in other locations, such as behind a fingernail or in the palm at the base of a finger, this fluid-filled sac can feel as hard as bone or as compressible as a rubber ball. Either way, a cyst seldom hurts but can cause discomfort by limiting range of motion in the involved joint. If the cyst has arisen behind a fingernail, the pressure can also bring discomfort but will most likely cause an unsightly nail formation. Since a cyst around a fingernail has often been associated with degenerative arthritis, however, that condition alone would increase the probability of pain and be a cause for further investigation by a rheumatologist.

The reason a cyst arises may not be clear. However, some believe a blow brings one about and, therefore, can take the problem away again. According to one very old but popular home remedy, a ganglion cyst can be burst by being hit with the back side of a Bible. Those who have tried with a hardbound book instead of a leather binding have found that a wrist can be broken by the same means! Some cysts spontaneously resolve themselves with no treatment at all, while others may need to be aspirated by a medical professional who then pulls the fluid through a needle. Should that happen, a fact sheet from the American Association for Hand Surgery says that about 50 percent of the ganglion cysts removed by aspiration will not return. In other instances though, a cyst that causes discomfort may need surgical removal, especially if the location makes aspiration a concern. For example, a ganglion cyst in the palm of the hand places the radial artery in proximity—too close for comfortably aspirating. When surgery offers the best option, it will probably be in an outpatient facility. Then, the procedure usually involves a local anesthetic before removal of the cyst along with a tiny piece of the joint capsule or tendon sheath to which it has become attached. Following surgery, the area may be immobilized for comfort but with therapeutic exercises prescribed shortly thereafter to assist with healing.

American Association for Hand Surgery. "Ganglion Cyst FAQ." Available online. URL: http://www.handsurgery.org/ganglioncyst.pdf Downloaded on February 20, 2003.

gangrene With the original Greek word meaning *an eating sore,* gangrene results in the death of tissue, bone, and sometimes persons. In most cases, the condition begins with a disruption of blood flow to the muscle or bone with causative factors as varied as diabetes, frostbite, arteriosclerosis, and complications following surgery or an injury.

When describing the latter instances, health information from the University of Miami School of Medicine says gas gangrene results from a bacterial infection that destroys muscle tissue, producing pain and pus as the area quickly decays. Because the invading bacteria will likely be anaerobic, it needs little or no or oxygen to penetrate deeply into a wound, where its rapid spreading affects formerly healthy tissue. If the bacteria invades large areas of the body or goes into internal organs before an intravenous-administered antibiotic has had time to work, this gangrenous condition will often be fast and fatal.

In addition to gas gangrene, two primary types of gangrene are classified as wet and dry. A fact sheet from the Mayo Clinic describes dry gangrene as gradually resulting from a reduced flow of blood in the arteries. In contrast, wet gangrene results from a sudden interruption of blood as often happens in an injury, blood clot, frostbite, or severe burn. In its early stages, dry gangrene presents itself as pain with the area turning cold and black if atrophy sets in. In wet gangrene (or moist gangrene, as it is otherwise known), the affected area may initially be hot and red but turn cold and blue with an offensive odor as the condition worsens. Rapid spreading ultimately leading to death can occur with wet gangrene but not usually with dry. In either case, oxygen therapy will probably be needed, although this treatment cannot revive dead tissue. Then, surgical removal or amputation may be required, depending on the location.

Because diabetes often involves loss of sensation or gradual numbing in the outer extremities, those conditions greatly increase the risk of gangrene. Therefore, care must be meticulously taken even in seemingly small matters, such as selecting shoes, trimming nails, moisturizing the skin, and protecting the hands and feet.

All persons, however, need to be aware of the hazardous weather in their own environments and take preventative actions to protect every part of the body. When going out in below-freezing temperatures, wearing capes, coats, gloves, masks, and/or scarves helps to safeguard not only the fingers, toes, and limbs but also the eyes, nose, and lungs.

If frostbite does occur, the extent of damage will depend on how cold the weather is and how long the exposure has continued. Somewhat like the reversal of a sunburn, shallow frostbite may present as whitened skin that peels away after warming, while an area of deeper frostbite will blister and swell. If deep freezing numbs an area, wet gangrene may show itself in gray, soft surfaces that may later require surgical removal. If dry gangrene results, skin surfaces take on a black, leathery look. In any case, immediate warming with a blanket and a hot (not scalding) beverage can help to ward off hypothermia as can immersion in warm water no hotter than 100 to 103 degrees Fahrenheit. Care must be taken, though, not to rub the affected area since this can easily damage tissue in the skin and muscles even more. In addition, blood clots may form in cold-restricted vessels, and rubbing could conceivably dislodge those, adding to the dangers.

According to the second home edition of *The Merck Manual,* yet another risk occurs as tissues thaw, releasing chemicals that can cause irregularities of the heart and toxins in the blood. Additionally, *The Merck Manual* mentions the possibility of reexposure to frigid temperatures with warnings that refreezing the just-thawed tissue will create a greater threat than leaving it frozen. If, for instance, a person has to walk away from the bitter cold on frostbitten feet, the frozen portions of the foot will at least offer some protection to the undamaged tissue. When danger has passed and tissue can be carefully warmed, treatment includes gently washing and applying antibiotic ointment and sterile bandages until professional medical attention can be obtained. Initially large areas of the body may seem to be affected, often appearing to be more severe than the actual damage. Therefore, to save as much of the bone as possible before proceeding with unnecessary amputation, the injured fingers, toes, or limbs may be left intact for several months to give the body ample time to resolve the damage and to heal.

See also DIABETES, EFFECTS ON HANDS AND FEET; FOOTWEAR.

Beers, Mark H., M.D., et al., eds. *The Merck Manual of Medical Information, Second Home Edition.* White House Station, N.J.: Merck Research Laboratories, 2003.

Thomas, Clayton, M.D., et al., eds. *Taber's Cyclopedia Medical Dictionary, Edition 18.* Philadelphia, Pa.: F. A. Davis Company, 1997.

University of Miami School of Medicine. "Glossary-Gangrene." Available online. URL: http://www.med.miami.edu/patients/glossary/art.asp?print=yes&articlekey=14506 Downloaded on June 10, 2003.

genetic factors These basic but ultramicroscopic units of heredity come in pairs, each of which have either dominant or recessive characteristics or a combination of the two. For example, darker colorations of the hair, skin, and eyes will often be dominant over lighter shades. Bone density, body shape and size, and an inclination toward athletics, art, music, poetry, mathematics, or mechanical aptitudes arrive in the gene pool too. In addition, some genes activate the immune system, and some, known as operators, control other genes. As the aptly chosen names imply, modifying genes modify or alter. Inhibiting genes inhibit. Tumor suppressor genes do just that, and sex-linked genes with their X and Y chromosomes determine a person's gender. For the most part, genes generate rather genius maneuvers via genetic codes or guidelines, but sometimes they just do not.

In a genetic disease, for example, some type of abnormality or disorder occurs because of hereditary factors. In the past, people could do little about such matters—nor do they today without genetic counseling. Then, genetic screening or genetic testing, such as occurs with amniocentesis, may be completed to identify specific genetic markers—genes that reveal the inherited traits and dispositions toward disorders or disease. With this microscopically detailed family history and an accurate assessment of the risks, a final decision usually comes down to the potential parents having to decide if they want to proceed with a pregnancy or terminate one that is likely to lead to the genetic disorder for which the previous tests have been made. With genetic engineering, however, alterations can conceivably be initiated in the laboratory with other outcomes in mind.

For example, a March 14, 2003 news release from the Imperial College of Science, Technology, and Medicine in England reported about a new treatment that may have a positive impact on genetic diseases, such as spinal muscular atrophy, which occurs once in every 10,000 births. To keep this from occurring at all, the treatment modifies the manner in which proteins are produced from the genetic code on the deoxyribonucleic acid (DNA). When processing genes into ribonucleic acid (RNA), the genetic information breaks into "islands of information called exons, which need to be stitched together, while the meaningless sequences are removed. If the sequence of an exon is changed, splicing can be disrupted, causing genetic mutations." Conversely, by using short pieces of RNA to put the suitable sequences back into the exon, researchers can then "influence splicing" or manipulate the splicing reaction in order to "restore the proper expression of defective genes."

In the U.S., the National Center for Biotechnology Information (NCBI), which is part of the National Institutes of Health, has made the GenBank database publicly available, listing the DNA and protein sequences of over 105,000 organisms. Although the information usually comes from individual laboratories or larger research projects, NCBI provides GenBank data through their Entrez retrieval system. NCBI also offers daily updates and monthly releases to keep researchers and the general public aware of the latest happenings and findings in genetic research.

With so many changes, possibilities, and controversies involving this topic, any presentation of the facts understandably remains in the genesis stage. Nevertheless, it is already clear that musculoskeletal disorders will indeed be affected by ongoing research and outcomes since a number of diseases caused by defects in genes have already been connected to the formation and function of muscles and connective tissue. For instance, Duchenne muscular dystrophy, originates from a defect in the cytoskeletal protein necessary for maintaining cellular structure, while myotonic dystrophy results from faulty expansion of a muscle protein gene. Brittle bone disease, also called OSTEOGENESIS IMPERFECTA, results from a mutation in the genes that instruct the body about the quality and quantity of collagen to be produced. The common type of DWARFISM, ACHONDROPLASIA, can be inherited by a dominant gene. However, 80 percent of the time, sporadic mutations occur in the fibroblast growth factor within a specific chromosome. In Lou Gehrig's disease, or AMYOTROPHIC LATERAL SCLEROSIS, a genetically coded enzyme reportedly fails to carry out its intended function of converting cellular radicals into safer substances, so this genetic defect ultimately causes cells to die from within. In fibrodysplasia ossificans progressiva—a very rare disease affecting one person in 2 million—the muscles gradually turn into bone. With several genes under investigation at this writing, the evidence may not yet be in. However, even when different genes have been considered, more than one could prove to be a contributing factor. This apparently has been shown to be the case in some instances. For example, current research seems to indicate that more than one gene can be implicated in CHARCOT-MARIE-TOOTH DISEASE, which could explain why the symptoms vary so widely from one person to the next.

Variations bring positive outcomes in genetic coding too, as Dr. Will G. Hopkins of New Zealand points out in his article "Genes and Training for Athletic Performance," published in the April 2001 issue of *Sportscience.* With references made to the published research and findings of Claude and Thomas J. Bouchard, Dr. Hopkins says, "When you compare the physical performance of individuals, heredity is as important as all other influences combined." Furthermore, "If you take a random sample of individuals and train them all the same way, you will not end up with everyone on the same level of performance. Clearly, athletes are individuals who inherit the ability to respond well to training."

As various types of athletic training, the nature versus nurture debate, and issues of ethics encircle the globe, some believe that DNA markers should be used to identify potential athletes, while others think that genetic research should be confined to identifying and rectifying criminals and disease. In a free society, diversity is expected. It should be welcomed with intelligent viewpoints eventually produced on every side, depending, of course, on the knowledge, experience, and educational training of the speakers and, perhaps, on their own very personal combinations of genetic codes.

FSMA. "SMA News Release from the Imperial College of Science Technology and Medicine, England—March 14, 2003: Scientists Discover Possible New Treatment for Genetic Diseases." Available online. URL: http://www.fsma.org/muntoni2003.shtml Downloaded on April 16, 2003.

Hopkins, Will G. "Genes and Training for Athletic Performance." Available online. URL: http://www.sportsci.org/index.html?jour/03/03/htm&1 Downloaded on April 16, 2003.

-genic or -genesis As a suffix, either of these word forms usually denotes a cause or origin. For example, osteogenic conditions originate in bone cells. Additionally, the great bones and well-contoured muscles in a photogenic face just naturally appear attractive in photographs.

gen- or gene- As a prefix, these combinative forms produce words that refer to producing, forming, or originating, such as genesis, which translates as "in the beginning."

gigantism See GENETIC FACTORS; GROWTH HORMONES.

gliding One of the four movements of which joints are capable, gliding depends on one bony surface gliding across another without circular or angular motions. Mandibular gliding, for example, smoothly moves the jaw up and down or back and forth with ease.

gluteus In the buttocks, three paired muscles move the thigh—the gluteus maximus, the gluteus medius, and the gluteus minimus, each of which bear the body in a concerted effort to stand, walk, or stretch the legs. As a person ambles along, motion begins with support resting primarily on the ankles. Then, after the foot has flattened on the ground but before the toes have left again, the gluteus muscles carry the body forward, generating midstance support until the person's weight shifts once again onto the ankles. If, however, the gluteus maximus muscles have received regular workouts resulting in that nicely contoured shape everyone seems to want, the supertight buttocks do not do much for the walk, the stance, or the lower back, except, perhaps, to present a pain.

To loosen up a bit, the American Physical Therapy Association recommends doing a limbering exercise twice a day. To do this, the person lies flat on the back on the floor or a firm mattress with feet flat and knees bent. With the stomach tucked, the right ankle goes atop the left thigh above the knee. Then, while holding that position, both legs come toward the chest and remain for 15–30 seconds. After doing this twice, the stretching exercise repeats with the left ankle on the right leg. Not only does this reportedly stretch the gluteus maximus muscles, the exercise strengthens posture too. If the position seems somewhat tortuous, however, a lighter version of stretching without straining should be tried. For instance, while laying down on a mattress with knees bent and feet flat, the right hand reaches beneath the legs to clasp the left ankle while the left hand similarly grasps the right ankle. While holding that position with the lower legs forming an X, the knees slowly come toward the chest—with no bouncing or hard pulls but with a slight pressure felt on the outer thighs.

When the gluteus needs overall strengthening, hip abduction can also help as the person stands on a level surface (preferably, a low-pile carpet) then opens and closes the legs in a jumping jacks exercise. This assumes, of course, that a physician agrees that the person's spine can handle the jolts. If not, similar results can come with a jumping jack motion by just lying on that carpeted floor (or firm mattress) and moving the arms and legs out then in, out then in. Because the gluteus medius attaches to the pelvis and the top of the thigh, moving the legs out and away from the body requires the assistance of the abductors muscles or the gluteus minimus. Then, as the legs come together again in a straight-leg position, the gluteus medius muscles or adductors of the inner thigh get a workout. This back and forth motion between the adductor muscles and the abductor muscles of the gluteus helps to stabilize the pelvis when standing—or when hopping about from one leg to another.

American Physical Therapy Association. "Don't Be a Tight Ass." Available online. URL: http://www.findarticles.com/cf_0/m1608/4_18/84153416/print.jhtml Downloaded on June 11, 2003.

Anderson, F. C. and M. G. Pandy. "Individual Muscle Contributions to Support in Normal Walking." *Gait Posture* 17, no. 2 (April 2003): 159–169.

golfer's elbow See TENDINITIS OR TENDONITIS.

gout Once called the disease of kings and the king of diseases, this form of arthritis often disables sufferers with chronic pain, fever, and joint tenderness. Although studies eventually revealed gout's connection to inherited factors of metabolism, its tag as the disease of kings most likely fits, too, because of the purine-rich foods associated with the rich. Consuming ale, wine, wild game, red meat, and shellfish—in the past and today—can readily contribute to a buildup of uric acid in the body.

When an excess of uric acid has been reached, gout typically presents pain and redness in the big toe. Evidently, this occurs because of that toe's poorer circulation and lower temperature—two conditions just the opposite of what is needed to circulate and decrease uric acid in the blood. As acid builds in the big toe, crystals begin to form, causing inflammation and pain to settle in the joint. In addition to altering the diet to eliminate any foods high in purine, typical treatments consist of cold compresses, rest, anti-inflammatory medication, and, if needed, a steroid injection into the painful site.

Besides increased production of uric acid in the body, another influence comes from the kidneys as adequate elimination of acids fails to occur. The ingestion of several glasses of filtered water each day may help to stimulate kidney action. However, if a person takes diuretics for another condition, such as hypertension, other approaches may be needed. For instance, the American College of Rheumatology (ACR) suggests directing therapy toward normalizing uric acid levels in the blood, particularly if a patient suffers from frequent gout attacks. With blood tests to assess the levels of uric acid and also the joint fluids examined for an accumulation of crystals, a rheumatologist will consider those results and various other factors to determine whether the problem occurs because of the body's excessive production of uric acid or because of the kidneys' failure to eliminate the uric acid properly. Depending on the outcome, a choice of medications will help the kidneys either to excrete excessive acids or to inhibit production in the first place. Until this normalization occurs, nonsteroidal anti-inflammatory drugs may help to alleviate pain. During an attack, though, products containing aspirin should be avoided.

Of every 100,000 people, 840 have experienced a gout attack, according to the ACR. Those odds increase for those with hypertension, obesity, and diabetes. Although a rheumatologist or primary care physician can provide the assistance needed in managing gout, untreated conditions can eventually result in a misshapen joint that, in turn, brings on more pain. Surgery may then be needed to remove the crystals and repair the damage in the affected joint. Since this may not have highly successful results—and since surgery addresses only one small area of a systemic condition—preventive measures and early management of gout offer the most viable options.

American College of Rheumatology. "Gout." Available online. URL: http://www.rheumatology.org/patients/factsheet/gout.html Downloaded on February 17, 2003.

Johnson, Joyce. "Ask the Doctor Column: Give Gout the Boot." *Retired Officer* (September 2002): 7.

graft or grafting Bone grafts and skin grafts may be the types most commonly known, but grafting can involve any tissue taken from one part of the body—or from the body of another person—to replace other tissue that has been injured or diseased. For this procedure to succeed, replacement tissue not only must be found but must also be compatible with the recipient's system. In bone marrow transplants, for example, complications arise when the donor's T cells (the principal defenders of the body's immune system) see the host site as an invader and, therefore, aggressively begin to attack the tissue of the person receiving the graft. This T cellular confusion can happen right after surgery or at any time during recovery. Either way, graft-versus-host disease (GVHD) usually occurs because of an imperfect match between the donor and the recipient. To prevent GVHD, T cells may be eradicated from the donor's bone marrow before the graft takes place. Additionally, most patients receive immunosuppressive drugs and sometimes steroids to help their own systems accept the graft. As long as the person's immune system remains suppressed, however, visitors need to don disposable masks, gowns, and gloves to avoid exposing the vulnerable patient to bacteria or other contaminants.

Since ideal donors for any type of graft may be hard to come by, researchers continuously investigate the possibilities of various materials. To regenerate trabecular bone, for example, synthetic alternatives included a variety of biodegradable polymer foams, all of which did not necessarily withstand compressive testing. Chemical engineers then decreased the sphere diameter and increased the heating time to enhance the strength with a pore system similar to a reverse template of the trabecular bone's fibrous structure.

In Sydney, Australia, the Orthopaedic Research Laboratories of the University of New South Wales has been testing another potential source of bone grafts—coral. According to a July 2003 release in the *Journal of Orthopaedic Research,* the success of partially converted coral as a material for bone grafts depends on the timing and the completion of a complex sequence of events during bone remodeling and resorption. In other words, if new tissue from the host bone grows into and onto the graft before the graft's porous coralline microstructure breaks down during the resorption process, some promising results could occur.

The body's cycle of breaking down the old and building up the new tissue of bones and tendons provides the continuum into which almost any graft must fit. Since sports play a big role in the number of injuries received, clinical trials, research, and innovative technology often arise from that field. For example, one of the most frequent sports injuries occurs in the anterior cruciate ligament (ACL) of the knee, occasionally necessitating a tendon-bone graft. To complete a successful reconstruction, numerous factors must be considered, such as the technique used to prepare the graft material or the site and also the angle and tension of the graft. With a secure graft fixation, the patient will be able to place weight onto the leg more quickly and with more steadiness or strength. After ACL surgery, however, bone tunnel enlargement can occur, again bringing instability. Several potential causes for this setback exist. Various factors include the reaction of the person's immune system, the toxic effects of substances used to sterilize the grafting material, the amount of cellular loss that occurred during drilling into the bone site, the graft motion or stress on the bone tunnel, and other nonspecific inflammatory responses. Nevertheless, if such problems do arise, they will almost always occur sometime within the first year of receiving the graft.

If an impaired blood supply, rather than an injury, has caused the death of bone tissue, a graft may keep the bone from collapsing, particularly in a weight-bearing area, such as the hip. The trick then comes in collecting tissue from another location in the body but with the very needed blood vessels left intact. As one might expect, such an intricate operation requires several hours with a recuperative time spent on crutches for several months thereafter. When successful, however, the graft not only gives new bone tissue a chance to form, but it also sets up a new source of the blood supply vitally needed to keep the bone alive and mobile.

Laurencin, C. T. "Trabecular Bone Regeneration." *Medical Devices & Surgical Technology Week* (February 16, 2003).

Otsuka, Hironori. "Comparison of Three Techniques of Anterior Cruciate Ligament Reconstruction with Bone-Patellar Tendon-Bone Graft." Available online. URL: http://www.findarticles.com/cf_0/0918/2_31/99292241.jhtml Downloaded on June 12, 2003.

Walsh, W. R., P. J. Chapman-Sheath, et al. "A Resorbable Porous Ceramic Composite Bone Graft Substitute in Rabbit Metaphyseal Defect Model." Available online. URL: http://www.ncbi.nlm.nih.gov/entrez/query.fcgi?cmd=Retrieve&db=PubMed&list Downloaded on June 12, 2003.

Graston technique Since its introduction to chiropractors in November 2001, the Graston technique has found enthusiastic response by offering a workable, innovative approach to treating soft tissue problems. With instruments specifically designed for this method, trained clinicians can reportedly better identify and treat injuries, thus preventing chronic conditions from developing in the joints, lower back, or neck. Many athletic trainers, physical therapists, and occupational therapists have now been trained in the use of the Graston technique too. Regardless of who performs the treatment, six stainless steel instruments do much of the work.

Molded to fit the body's curves, the contoured instruments influence tissue at a deeper level, breaking down old scar tissue in conditions previously considered to be chronic or permanent. To know just where to apply the light pressure or scrapinglike motion, the trained technician uses the specialized instruments in a manner similar to holding a tuning fork or a stethoscope. Instead of listening for adhesions or fascial restrictions though, the chiropractor or therapist can feel resonance that comes through variations in the tissue and respond with greater accuracy than with unaided use of hands.

To see if these benefits lived up to the assertions, researchers from the Schools of Informatics and Allied Health Sciences at Indiana University treated 1,004 patients an average of seven times at various sites around the country over a two-year period. When reporting the results, Dr. Douglas G. Perry summarized five categories of interest in determining the success of the treatments: functionality, pain, numbness, goal achievement, and work status. By the fourth treatment, functionality had improved significantly in the patients' daily activities, work, and recreation. By the end of the therapy sessions, pain had reportedly decreased whereas numbness declined measurably—from 15 down to five on a scale of one to 20. Additionally, 50 percent of the patients said they had reached 90 percent of their therapeutic goals. Likewise, return to full status at work increased from 69 percent at the beginning of the study to 83 percent of the participants going back to work by the time the treatments had ended.

Wilczewski, Karen. "The Graston Technique: Changing the Treatment of Soft Tissue Injuries." *The American Chiropractor* 24, no. 6 (2002): 34.

gravity, effects of Gravity attracts. Gravity holds the Earth in orbit. Gravity guides the structure and function of muscles and bones that succumb to—or resist—gravitational pull. In gravity, the force (*F*) equals the given mass (*m*) of an object and its acceleration (*a*) rate—or so conjectured Sir Isaac Newton (1642–1727) in his famous formula from which the apple fell: $F = m \times a$. When read, this means the force of gravity equals an object's mass times its acceleration. So, what does this formula have to do with muscles and bones? How does gravity affect the musculoskeletal system? Rather, how does a lack of gravity affect muscle and bone? If you take away the force, what will happen?

Space research has looked into such matters since the early days of astronauts when Cosmos flights from Russia showed variations in mammalian bone strength. This instigated numerous studies into muscle atrophy—a phenomenon that occurs not only in the absence of gravity but in the absence of weight-bearing loads on the musculoskeletal system. By understanding the former, better comprehension of the latter may also come to pass. For example, in prolonged space flights, bone mass evidently decreases because a lack of stress decelerates the production of osteoblast cells needed to build new bone cells. To put it another way, less weight on bones means the body kicks back and produces less bone. Therefore, weight-bearing bones, such as in the hips and legs, suffer the greatest effects. On a six-month space mission, this may translate as 1–2 percent bone loss per month. Individuals more inclined to suffer bone loss, however, experienced as much as 20 percent loss of bone mass on longer missions. To be more specific, recent studies showed that up to 1.58 percent bone mineral loss occurred each month from the proximal femur of the thigh during four- to 14-month missions with more than 20 percent loss in knee extensor strength occurring in only 60–80 days.

Since 10 million or more people in the United States alone have problems with bone loss, these findings in space may help countless numbers on Earth. Undoubtedly, the studies will not only help bone mass from diminishing in lumbar vertebrae and legs but may bring light to related problems, such as the subsequent rise of blood calcium levels that increases the risk of kidney problems. Recovery of bone loss also comes into focus as astronauts now have their bone density measured before and after flights with follow-ups a year following their return. Such precisely obtained and documented information allows excellent opportunity for comparative studies, particularly of the axial skeleton, with trabecular and cortical bone measured then compared with individuals who have not set foot in space. Additionally, microscopic changes in muscle filaments and proteins can be examined, focusing on the effects shown in posture, mobility, function, and strength.

Although the consequences of very long space flights to faraway planets have not yet been verified, documentations of short-term bone losses have been confirmed by the National Aeronautics and Space Administration's (NASA's) Skylab program, space shuttle flights, and Russia's Cosmos and space station Mir missions. All parties conclude: reductions in the size and the mass of muscle fiber do occur in space. In the muscles that normally oppose gravitational pull, biochemical changes result as well. Weightlessness affects the release of calcium in bones, and changes occur in muscle protein composition. Why, though, does this lack of gravity matter? What does it have to do with Earth and its gravity-laden musculoskeletal systems?

One hope of space lab research involves a clearer understanding of how muscles function on and around the globe. As researchers investigate the capacity of cells, individual muscle fibers, and groups of muscles, they may be able to establish timelines of typical changes—structurally and functionally—to be expected within each of these units. By seeing exactly what happens and when, scientists can then collect valuable information for better understanding the normal processes of aging. As information from NASA reports, some even hope the factual data and insights gleaned from space research programs will offer solutions to complex medical problems, such as osteoporosis.

Apparently Vanderbilt University Medical Center thinks this will be so since its Center for Space Physiology and Medicine began in 1989. Later it began participating in NASA missions. The center's research now includes such diverse topics as the nervous system, anemia, bone loss, energy balance, and muscle adaptations in conditions relating to weightlessness. Since prolonged bed rest can have similar effects, ongoing studies consider the molecular regulation of bone, the enzymes important in maintaining cellular energy, the mechanical stretch of muscle fiber, and other alterations of the skeletal mass—on both a molecular and a systemic level. To determine the effects of weightlessness on muscle function and fatigue, the center has developed noninvasive methods, such as magnetic resonance spectroscopy, to measure a muscle's state of energy. In yet another research project, investigations of slow- and fast-twitch muscles revealed biochemical changes that may carry weight in addressing muscle atrophy. For example, fast-twitch muscles contract fast to move the body forward. Slow-twitch muscles, however, contract slowly, working against gravity to keep the body upright. Therefore, in space—or in other conditions with effects similar to weightlessness—slow-twitch muscles slowly take on the characteristics of fast-twitch muscles. This means the person returning to Earth, or to an upright position, will have difficulty just standing up and walking around. To prevent such things from happening, exercise and nutrition play a large part in the space program—and here on Earth.

With such microscopic investigations going on today, information will constantly be changing as new findings and new solutions present themselves. Without a doubt, this ongoing research will affect musculoskeletal treatments on Earth, perhaps with some interesting surprises. For instance, in early NASA days, one project took a microscopic look at changes in rats. When caged together, these highly sociable creatures revealed far less altered bone than that experienced by their lonely little counterparts. Furthermore, the rat pack showed faster recovery of bone losses than sole rats left alone in their cages. This strange fact could be significant for people. After all, gravity does attract. Gravity holds the Earth and all its occupants in orbit—together.

Robertson, David and F. Andrew Gaffney. "Investigation." URL: http://www.mc.vanderbilt.edu/gcrc/space/index.html Downloaded on July 6, 1999.

groin pull The leg overstretches. The hips move side to side and then, with a quick stop, change directions. The inner thigh pulls, and within moments, pain and swelling begin. While watching from the bleachers, the fans at a basketball, hockey, or soccer game may applaud the injured player. At home, though, a groin pull gets only a crackling sound when touched. Muscle spasms and loss of leg strength may also occur with ice packs needed for comfort and anti-inflammatory medicine for the pain. Wrapping the thigh with a wide elastic bandage or wearing underwear designed for groin compression may keep the swelling to a minimum during the time it takes to heal. How long that is will depend on the person's age, the level of fitness, the extent of the injury, and the faithfulness with which this conservative treatment has been followed. If not much, further injury and a chronic problem become more likely. If, however, pain develops slowly in the crease of the groin and abdomen with no particular, identifiable injury, health information from the *Runner's World* Web site, www.runnersworld.com, suggests the problem could be a stress fracture in the hip rather than a groin pull. X-rays and other diagnostic tools can verify the latter. However, if an overextension of the adductor muscle has indeed occurred, healing should be apparent when tenderness has left the area. Then the muscles of the inner thighs can be strengthened to avoid future injury. A simple but workable exercise, for example, suggests that the person sits on the floor with the bottoms of the feet clapped lightly together. While maintaining that position, one hand rests on each knee and gently presses down—not hard enough to make a person groan but just until a light tug occurs on the inner thighs.

Staff. "Untitled." Available online. URL: http://205.147.231.44/home/0,1300,1-0-0-417-1-0-P,00.html Downloaded on June 12, 2003.

growing pains An active day of play occupies the minds of most children, but with nightfall, scary shadows and ouches come. For some children, this may be a delay tactic to postpone going to bed. More likely, though, the pains that were not there earlier actually were. The child was just too busy to notice. As with adults who have had an active day, the lack of physical activity at bedtime brings those achy muscles into full focus, making rest difficult or impossible. At such times, the label-recommended dose of ibuprofen or acetaminophen, a light massage, a warm bath, and, perhaps, the application of heat can bring relief. When accompanied by a heavy dose of hugs, comfort measures will generally assuage the pain and assist a child in sleeping. If touch and comfort seem to exacerbate the problem, however, something else could be at work.

Pain not attributable to the day's activity or overuse may indicate an illness, especially if fever, stiffness, redness, swelling, bruising, limping, cramping, or other signs occur. Headaches, joint pain, bone pain, and persistent pain in the muscles or the upper extremities—especially during the daytime—also signal the need for prompt medical evaluation by a pediatrician or rheumatologist. In rare instances, for example, growing pains in a localized area could be part of a process seen in leukemia.

If a child complains of achy legs throughout the day, the problem could be due to an abnormality in the GAIT cycle. Alternatively, the structure and shape of the bones may be the cause. For instance, as the heel touches the ground, an irregular shape would put the foot immediately into an incorrect or awkward position. Another possibility occurs when body weight transfers from the heel onto the arch, at which time the midsection of the foot may flatten out too much, a condition called FLATFOOT OR FLATFEET, thus causing overpronation. Should this occur, the inner side of the midfoot tilts lower than the outside, with pain frequently resulting in the feet, ankles, hips, or thighs.

A fact sheet on this subject from the University of Michigan Health System explains that overpronation comes about because of loose tendons or ligaments attached to the foot bones—a problem that could occur at birth or in an injury. In either case, the child's favorite FOOTWEAR will show revealing patterns of wear that an orthopedic physician or podiatrist will want to examine as well as the child's gait pattern. Should overpronation prove to be the problem, custom-made shoes or orthotics will probably be prescribed. Similar treatments will also be advised for instances of underpronation (supination) where the outside of the foot tilts down and the inside up. After studying various designs used for these orthotic treatments, A. M. Evans, of the University of South Australia, reported on their success in the March–April 2003 *JAPMA, Journal of the American Podiatric Medical Association,* concluding, "These findings may provide the impetus for a more rigorous examination of the possible relationship between pronation and 'growing pains.'"

With debate about whether the latter even exists, children, nevertheless, have inexplicable episodes of leg pain deep in the muscles during the dark of night. Occurrences most commonly begin after age five, although younger children may be affected. One explanation involves the fact that larger areas of cartilage ease a baby's entrance into the world with ossification of bones later occurring as the child grows. Although this natural process will not be noticed by most, children may simply be aware that something feels uncomfortable or different during heightened times of growth. If no other signs of disease or injuries exist but growth spurts do, this may well be a temporary problem that is soon outgrown. Until then, staff from the Texas Children's Hospital remind parents that most instances of growing pains are neither severe nor of long duration, with about 10–15 minutes of pain from the onset to be expected. In the hospital's report for the January–February 2002 issue of *Vibrant Life,* "Relax, It's Just Growing Pains," the medical staff also advises parents or other caretakers to "remain calm, as fear and stress can actually heighten the child's pain."

See also GROWTH AND DEVELOPMENT IN CHILDREN.

American Podiatric Medical Association. "Relationship Between 'Growing Pains' and Foot Posture in Children: Single-Case Experimental Designs in Clinical Practice." *JAPMA, Journal of the American Podiatric Medical Association* 93, no. 2 (March/April 2003): 111–117.

Texas Children's Hospital. "Relax, It's Just Growing Pains." Available online. URL: http://www.findarticles.com/cf_0/m0826/1_18/82605180/print.jhtml Downloaded on June 14, 2003.

growth and development in children At birth, infants can do little more than flail their arms and legs. By 18 months, though, most children have the gross motor skills needed for walking reasonably well and the fine motor skills for scribbling with a fat, nontoxic crayon. By two to two-and-a-half years of age, most children can run and climb the stairs or, perhaps, the furniture. By three, the gait steadies as does a child's ability to draw circles with a now-favored hand, and muscle tone improves as baby fat disappears. By four years of age, children can usually hop up, dress themselves, and then keep on hopping. By five, skipping may be the fun thing to do, and drawings may be identifiable—at least as a suggestion of a person or object. By six, most children can write their names and walk across a low beam or board without falling off, assuming, of course, such feats entice them.

Once children have reached school age, a number of factors cause their growth and development to take a turn toward the personal. The "normal" range allows for tremendous variations in shape, size, motor skills, and physical aptitude. Although most children have major growth spurts just after birth and again during puberty, the rate of growth and the size reached at maturation depend greatly on a unique combination of inherited traits, nutrition, and overall health. As long as a child does well—physically, mentally, and emotionally—comparisons with other children have little value and may serve only to increase an ego or decrease self-esteem. If extreme patterns of growth (i.e., deemed as too much or too little) become a concern, however, comparative growth charts can be a useful tool in signaling problems or medical conditions.

While revising the 1977 growth charts from the National Center for Health Statistics, the Centers for Disease Control and Prevention (CDC) published Growth Charts for the United States, 2000, with laudable considerations made for the wide cultural and racial diversity in this country. Additionally, the new CDC growth charts include assessments of body mass index to evaluate a child's weight in relation to his or her height. While compiling this information, however, the National Health and Nutrition Examination Survey also ascertained a troubling trend showing that the number of overweight children had doubled in the last two decades.

Ironically, concerns also exist regarding underdevelopment of some children at puberty because of poor NUTRITION or eating disorders, such as anorexia. Regarding the latter, studies have often focused on girls trying to be as thin as the lead in a supermodel's appointment book pencil. However, on February 3, 2003, Reuters Health released "Anorexia in Teen Boys Found to Stunt Growth." While studying this phenomenon, Dr. Dalit Modan-Moses of Tel Aviv University and colleagues evaluated a dozen teen boys who had been diagnosed with anorexia nervosa. Growth retardation was shown in 11 of the boys. During treatments, the three boys who again attained normal weight were able to catch up to their anticipated sizes, whereas the teens who remained underweight did not.

Another catch-up situation occurs with young athletes who may restrict growth or delay their maturation because of inadequate nutrients combined with intense physical training. Teens commonly recover such losses between seasons. If training continues for the long term, then developmental delays may also go on. In some cases, lessened stature at full adult height may occur. Regardless, further investigations of the many influences on growth surely warrant a particular focus on the interrelated factors that help children—athletically inclined or not—to reach their full potential.

Daly, Robin M., Shona Bass, et al. "Does Training Affect Growth?" Available online. URL: http://www.physsportsmed.com/issues/2002/10_02/daly.htm Downloaded on February 18, 2003.

Reuters Health Information. "Anorexia in Teen Boys Found to Stunt Growth." Available online. URL: http://www.nlm.nih.gov/medlineplus/news/fullstory_115537.html Downloaded on March 3, 2003.

growth hormones In early life, an overabundance (hypersecretion) of growth hormones causes gigantism of the skeletal system, while an inadequate supply (hyposecretion) causes some types of dwarfism. For middle-aged adults, an overproduction of growth hormones can result in ACROMEGALY. Once an abnormal level of growth hormones at either extreme has been determined by a blood test, timely treatment, such as drug therapy, can help to arrest the condition.

According to a fact sheet from the Human Growth Foundation in Glen Head, New York, human growth hormone deficiency can arise at any time throughout childhood with noticeably slow growth patterns presenting a typical first sign. Causes may be genetic, structural (as in certain types of bone conditions), or due to hormonal disorders attributable to a number of factors. For example, in the rare disorder Cushing's syndrome, the adrenal gland produces too much cortisol hormone, with the results often involving softened bones, muscular atrophy, and general body weakness. Poor nutrition and systemic diseases can contribute to delayed growth, too, with normal growth usually returning once the underlying condition has been successfully treated.

In an editorial for the May 2002 issue of *The Journal of Pediatrics,* Dr. Basil J. Zitelli of the Children's Hospital of Pittsburgh, Pennsylvania, expressed concern about a trend of treating children of short stature with growth hormones. One rationale advocates the need to protect smaller children and teens from being teased or bullied. Another addresses the perceptions that people have—perhaps parents in particular—of tall children being successful children. Although the need for growth hormone therapy for specific conditions certainly has great merit, treating a nondisease of shortness can put a child unnecessarily at risk—physically and emotionally—with little guarantee of achieving the hoped-for results. As Dr. Zitelli suggests, "Perhaps efforts toward increasing the height of normal short children should be redirected toward teaching the acceptance of individual differences and placing value on personal character. The effects of such efforts may extend beyond height to accepting those of us with big noses, cupped ears, or different colored skin."

Human Growth Foundation. "What Are Growth Disorders?" Available online. URL: http://www.hgfound.org/disordersframe.html Downloaded on February 18, 2003.

Zitelli, Basil J. "Editorial." *The Journal of Pediatrics* 40, no. 5 (May 2002): 493–495.

Guillain-Barré syndrome This progressive disorder usually begins in the legs with pain, weakness, and gradual loss of reflexes, such as can be ascertained by tapping the knee. Loss of feeling followed by varying degrees of paralysis occur as the disorder rises up the torso. In severe cases, the person's breathing may be affected within two to three weeks from onset as the disease reaches the most dangerous phase. A ventilator may then be required to assist respiration until the symptoms have subsided, typically in the reverse order from which they first appeared.

In children, misdiagnosis may be common due to similar symptoms of tired leg muscles or growth spurts caused by GROWING PAINS. The lack of a well-established gait pattern with which to compare can also be a source of confusion. Nevertheless, any sign of a limp or a reluctance to walk needs to be investigated by a physician. As an early indicator of Guillain-Barré syndrome (GBS), leg pain, numbness, or tingling may follow a previous illness, such as a virus or tonsillitis. Progressive weakness and lethargy can be symptomatic too. Further along the course of the illness, the child may have some difficulty sitting up. Although less than one child in 100,000 under age 17 acquires GBS, this disease has been classified as the most common cause "of acute general paralysis in developed countries" according to Tjun Tang in the *British Medical Journal.*

Only slightly more adults than children acquire GBS each year with causes often relating to episodes of viral or bacterial infections one to three weeks prior. Immunization shots can also be a triggering factor. In any case, the immune system does not shut off when the instigating source has passed and, subsequently, attacks the myelin sheath that covers the body's peripheral nerves. Should this occur, a lumbar puncture can confirm elevated levels of protein in the cerebrospinal fluid. An electromyography that records muscle activity may also be instructive. Once a diagnosis has been made, treatments depend on the severity of the symptoms. For instance, one possibility includes plasmapheresis to remove the plasma from the patient's blood in hopes of eliminating the antibodies that caused the disease. Intravenous treatments and breathing assistance may also be needed as bed rest surely will. Although 95 percent of the patients recover, GBS can be life threatening, especially if paralysis affects the person's breathing. For this reason alone, hospitalization is needed. However, it is also needed to provide the patient with around-the-clock supervision, frequent repositioning, and passive range of motion exercises to prevent contractures from occurring. Recovery may take two months or more with additional physical therapy or occupational therapy needed for up to two years as the person's strength eventually returns.

Tang, Tjun. "A Painful Hip as a Presentation of Guillain-Barré Syndrome in Children." Available online. URL: http://www.findarticles.com/cf_0/m0999/7279_322/70421588/print.jhtml Downloaded on June 13, 2003.

Worsham, Treesa L. "Easing the Course of Guillain-Barré Syndrome." Available online. URL: http://www.findarticles.com/cf_0/m3235/3_63/60811845/print.jhtml Downloaded on June 13, 2003.

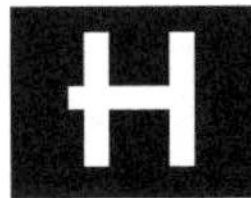

Haglund's deformity Wearers of high heels sometimes call Haglund's deformity a pump bump since this bony prominence usually occurs on the back of the heel when one has often worn dress pumps. A person's inherited foot structure may be the main source of the problem rather than shoe choice, but weight increase, foot stress, and injury can also initiate this painful bump around the area of the Achilles tendon. Then, tight shoes will undoubtedly intensify redness and swelling as bursa become inflamed. Orthotic inserts and open-back shoes can relieve the pressure. Ice packs can reduce swelling and anti-inflammatory medications, such as aspirin or ibuprofen, can lessen pain. Conservative treatments may also include physical therapy, whirlpool baths, ultrasound, and deep massage. If six months or so of nonsurgical care fails to alleviate the problem, surgery may be required to remove superfluous bone and, sometimes, to reattach the Achilles tendon. After surgery, health information from the whymyfoothurts.com Web site suggests foot elevation and ice packs for about 20 minutes every hour or so for a couple of days with weight kept off the foot for three to six weeks, depending on the extent of the Achilles tendon involvement. The podiatrist or orthopedic surgeon will probably suggest toe wiggling and other exercises to help return the corrected foot to normal too.

See also BURSITIS; FOOTWEAR; HEEL.

Staff. "Haglund's Deformity." Available online. URL: http://whymyfoothurts.com/conditions/haglunds deformity.html Downloaded on June 16, 2003.

Hallervorden-Spatz disease With no cure yet for this rare, inherited disease, the National Institute of Neurological Disorders and Stroke (NINDS) of the National Institutes of Health continues to research ways to prevent, treat, and ease this progressively degenerative movement disorder. Health information from NINDS reports that death often occurs within 10 years of the onset of Hallervorden-Spatz disease, but survival may continue for decades. Treatments vary according to each individual's needs. However, they may include occupational therapy, physical therapy, or exercises specifically adapted to alleviate symptoms, such as muscle contractions and spastic movements of the torso, face, and limbs. Overall, therapy typically places an emphasis on providing support and reducing the patient's discomfort in an effort to improve the quality of life.

National Institute of Neurological Disorders and Stroke. "Hallervorden-Spatz Disease Information." Available online. URL: http://accessible.ninds.nih.gov/health_and_medical/disorders/hallervorden.htm Downloaded on June 16, 2003.

hammertoe In most people, most toes lay fairly flat. With hammertoe, however, the profile of a foot may look as though it has one to five little tents since one or more toes bend down in an inverted-V contracture. Women and the lesser digits of the small toes have this condition more often than do big toes and men of every size.

According to a fact sheet from the American Podiatric Medical Association, hammertoes come in two types: flexible and rigid. As one might suspect, a flexible hammertoe still has mobility in the joint and, therefore, can be treated with greater success. Once this developmental stage has passed, however, a rigid hammertoe develops with tight tendons and misaligned or immobile joints.

Sometimes caused by arthritis and sometimes by heredity and other contributing factors, hammertoes in both categories result from abnormalities in the foot that then lead to increased pressure on the tendons and joints. Taping the toes or inserting orthotics may help to correct structural concerns, and using anti-inflammatory medications may decrease the pain. Occasionally, cortisone injections may be prescribed to reduce symptoms too. If rigid hammertoe has occurred, surgery may be needed.

See also FEET OR FOOT; FOOTWEAR; TENDINITIS OR TENDONITIS.

American Podiatric Medical Association. "Your Podiatric Physician Talks About Hammertoes." Available online. URL: http://www.apma.org/topics/hammertoes_printable.htm Downloaded on June 16, 2003.

hamstring In ancient days, "to hamstring" a load-bearing animal or a fast, audacious enemy meant to cripple them. Today's athletes surely hope this will not be a final outcome, especially since the hamstring offers a frequent site for sports injuries. According to health information from Rice University in Houston, Texas, such injuries occur because of poor flexibility in the lower back, abnormal biomechanics, or inadequate stretching exercises and other warm-ups just before beginning a vigorous activity. Sprinting, for example, creates high tension on the hamstring muscles along the back of the thigh, increasing the risk of a sudden tear or other acute injury when starting off too tautly.

When discussing this topic, the American Academy of Orthopaedic Surgeons (AAOS) identifies the hamstring as actually being "a group of three muscles that help to straighten (extend) the leg at the hip and bend (flex) the leg at the knee." Therefore, a "pulled hamstring" consists of "a strain or tear in the muscles or tendons." Since injuries can be prevented easier than they can be cured, the AAOS suggests a stretching exercise that may also help to relieve lower back pain. While sitting on a padded mat or carpet with the left leg extended, the sole of the right foot rests around the left knee as both hands reach toward the upright toes of the left foot. After holding that position—without straining—for about 30 seconds, the legs then reverse their positions for another light stretching toward the toes.

Besides gentle stretches and warm-ups, an understanding of the workings of this muscle group can also help to prevent a hamstring injury. As with other parts of the body, muscles work in sets or pairs, with one muscle contracting while the other relaxes. So, from the back of the thigh, the hamstring muscles contract while, on the front, the quadriceps relax, thus enabling the person to bend that leg. To straighten the leg, the reverse occurs. In either instance, the quadriceps usually have more power, which means the hamstring muscles work harder and/or get fatigued more quickly. This dynamic can make the legs of young athletes especially vulnerable to injury since muscles and bones do not grow at the same rate. During a growth spurt, for instance, the muscles often have not had time to catch up with the lengthening bone, which tightens the hamstrings even more and sets up prime conditions for an injury, especially if a young athlete jumps or abruptly extends a leg. In a serious injury, the muscle pulls away from the bone and can even pull a piece of bone with it. A rupture or tear of this sort will usually leave the person unable to stand up, much less walk or run. Quite likely, surgery will then be needed to reattach the muscle with time out and physical therapy for weeks to come.

For less serious hamstring injuries, treatment generally consists of resting the area and applying compression and also ice packs for 20 minutes every one to two hours or so. As a preventative measure (but one that can also be useful in rehabilitation), the University of Miami School of Medicine recommends good nutrition to keep the body's electrolytes in balance as well as adequate intake of fluids to avoid dehydration, both of which can help to keep muscles from cramping. A well-balanced diet also prevents weight imbalances that can further increase the probability of musculoskeletal injuries.

See also NUTRITION.

American Academy of Orthopaedic Surgeons. "Hamstring Muscle Strain." Available online. URL: http://orthoinfo.

aaos.org/fact/thr_report.cfm?thread_id=137&topcategory=wellness Downloaded on June 16, 2003.
University of Miami School of Medicine. "Hamstring Injuries." Available online. URL: http://www.med.miami.edu/patients/glossary/art.asp?print=yes&articlekey=7079 Downloaded on June 16, 2003.

hand From wrist to fingertips, the hand consists of numerous muscles, tendons, and nerves bound to bones with exotic names like trapezoid, scaphoid, lunate, and triquetrum. A tally of the bones in a single hand includes eight small carpal bones of the wrist and the five metacarpals (body of the hand) with 14 bones packed into the set of five phalanges (fingers including the thumb)—all of which fit together nicely like a small, three-dimensional jigsaw puzzle.

With the ulnar and the median nerves added to this compact but complex system, a half-million hands in the U.S. will undergo surgery each year. Although the reasons for surgical repairs vary greatly, causative factors often include an injury, congenital defect, arthritis, infection, tumor, tendinitis, and nerve compression, such as occurs with carpal tunnel syndrome. Sometimes microsurgery may be required to reattach an amputated part or to reconstruct injured tendons and bone. For the latter, GRAFTING may be needed. Microscopic techniques can also restore damage due to injuries, birth defects, and degenerative disorders, such as osteoarthritis, that sometimes mar the hands and fingers. As examples, the American Academy of Orthopaedic Surgeons (AAOS) says surgery may be needed to remove excess bone growth, to replace a degenerating joint, or to fuse joints together to correct a disfigurement that interferes with range of motion. If, however, a hand has received a deep or gaping wound, a procedure known as flap surgery may be used to take the skin and all of the underlying tissue, including blood vessels, from another part of the body to repair damage on the hand. In severe FRACTURES when a bone breaks through the skin, SURGERY may be needed to align the bones and stabilize the hand, often with wires or other devices to hold fractured bone in place.

Whatever the cause or need for surgical restoration, the AAOS says that therapy may be needed after hand surgery with exercises and activities particularly designed to restore normal function and dexterity. Besides providing post-surgery help, however, an occupational therapist (OT) who specializes in hand care can provide ongoing assistance for a variety of disorders, such as rheumatoid arthritis sprains, tendinitis, and carpal tunnel syndrome. An OT also fosters rehabilitation after a STROKE, AMPUTATION, or INJURY. Typical treatments for the rehabilitation of a hand include splinting and exercise programs to lessen joint stiffness and muscular weakness. If needed, an OT's evaluation of a patient's home or workplace can include a professional assessment that addresses any ongoing sources of strain or pain, thus helping the person to create a safer living environment. The primary goal, however, will ultimately be to restore the patient's hand function to full capacity.

For most people, the handiness of hands often gets taken for granted until an accident or illness suddenly makes it difficult to put on a pair of glasses, lift a glass of water, or ease oneself from a chair. Dexterous and multifunctional, the hands assist in planting a rosebush, peeling an apple, giving directions, and typing a manuscript. Without hands, a person cannot easily open a door or close a window. Hands need holding—by lovers, by parent and children, by the well and the dying. Without hands, the beauty of art, music, and gourmet meals might not be as readily forthcoming. Without the gestures of hands, even the ability to communicate will apparently be diminished.

Some interesting research focuses on the role hands play in communicating to others, yet these current studies show that old assumptions may give only a glimpse of what hand gestures truly do. Waving and gesticulating, for instance, seldom assist the viewer in better understanding what someone has to say but, rather, assist the speaker in the saying. In other words, hands provide other words. Evidently, gesturing can aid the speaker in processing language and identifying, retrieving, or recalling words. Gestures also provide visual cues in a manner similar to imagery by interpreting, illustrating, and, thereby, magnifying a word, phrase, or intention. For example, a welcoming gesture clearly invites someone to come in or come closer, while expanding the hands and arms may indicate a larger embrace or may act as a practical visual aid in demonstrating what happens in a pattern of growth. More than this though, a gesture can assist the speaker in producing words and speech as though physically retrieving something from a shelf.

If gesturing occurs as a person engages in conversation involving the exchange of new information, the hand patterns may themselves become part of the verbal encoding or more thorough assimilation of the new data. Then later, the gesture helps to bring forth that particular word or concept. Therefore, those who use their hands expressively do not lack sufficient words as once thought but have instead found a very effective memory tool for gaining and expanding their vocabularies. According to these present findings, people with high verbal skills gesture more than those with less command of their native language.

As further studies confirm this interesting turn of the hand, the results could conceivably affect education with new insights and innovative approaches. For example, children might no longer be cautioned to sit still and learn but, rather, be encouraged to gesture, gather, and greedily grab onto new language, thus better equipping them to sort through and handpick each apt word to use.

American Academy of Orthopaedic Surgeons. "Hand Surgery." Available online. URL: http://orthoinfo.aaos.org/brochure/thr_report.cfm?Thread_ID=48&topcategory=Hand Downloaded on June 16, 2003.

Frick-Horbury, Donna. "The Effects of Hand Gestures on Verbal Recall as a Function of High- and Low-Verbal-Skill Levels." Available online. URL: http://www.findarticles.com/cf_0/m2405/2_129/901079/print.jhtml Downloaded on June 16, 2003.

hand, inflammation of the joints Many years ago, a scrappy teenager might shove a fist toward someone's face with the challenge, "Want a knuckle sandwich?" Assuming either survived into old age, today's answer might be, "Yes!" A gripping ability to make a fist means the hinged knuckle joints of the fingers still have what it takes to perform tasks, such as guiding a pencil, holding a fork, typing at a keyboard, buttoning a shirt, or making a for-real sandwich. If arthritis has set into the knuckle joints, however, pain and deformity can hinder fine motor skills of the hand, making daily activities difficult if not impossible.

Although an injury, such as happened in that fistfight, can cause arthritis in a hand, arthritic conditions elsewhere in the body could be the source of trouble. Other causative factors may indicate an underlying medical condition or damage done through overuse as the ligaments loosen, allowing the knuckle joints to slip. Knowing the reasons may seem to be a moot point but can be helpful in directing a course of treatment, for example, in locating and changing any activities that contribute to the joint dysfunction. Typically, treatments include pain relievers or anti-inflammatory medication with joint aspiration or corticosteroid injections sometimes needed. If these efforts fail to bring relief and increased range of motion, a fact sheet on metacarpophalangeal joint (MP) arthritis from the American Society for Surgery of the Hand says, "Some advanced cases of MP joint disease may need surgery. Two types of surgery are commonly performed. The first is generally done in less severe cases and is called synovectomy or soft-tissue replacement. If the tendons have slipped out of place, they are put back into place over the knuckle joint. If the small muscles of the fingers are causing the fingers to lean toward the small fingers, the muscles are operated on to stop the fingers from being pulled toward the little finger. The second type of surgery is joint replacement and is generally used on more severe cases of MP joint diseases. The diseased metacarpophalangeal joint is replaced with an artificial joint." The risks include acquiring an infection after surgery, and, over time, breakdown of the replacement joint can occur. Barring complications, the hand will usually be immobilized for several days and then a course of therapy begun for four to six weeks. Splinting may continue if needed to assure pain relief and to assist in limiting movement until full range of motion has been restored to the fingers and the knuckle joints.

See also JOINT ASPIRATION/INJECTION.

head Here is a riddle: a bone is a bone is a bone, but when is a bone a head? Answer: the larger end of a bone is a head, and the first toe bone over a finish line can be ahead too. As relating to the upper part of the body though, a head is a house—not only housing the sensory organs of sight, sound, smell, and taste but housing a storehouse of information in the brain. If that brain happens to be quite large, the head might also house an ego.

Assuming, however, that trauma, birth defects, and disease have caused no disruptive disorder to the head, this extraordinary structure consists of 29 bones articulating through suture joints and the hinged joint of the jaw. With eight cranial bones, 14 facial bones, six tiny bones (ossicles) in the ears, and that little detached hyoid bone at the base of the tongue, the head gets a heads up for holding the body's good sense—and the sensory instruments of the senses—in well-rounded balance.

To complete this architectural feat, the two major portions of the head can be categorized as the facial mass and the cranial mass. The former sits on the front section, facing ahead, and the cranial mass rounds out the back part. This assumes, of course, that naturally rounded heads have been well-received by the owner's culture, which, even today, may not necessarily be the case. Even a century or so ago, people thought the practice of intentional head molding had ceased around the world, relegating these deformations of structural character from the Neolithic and Bronze Ages to museum collections or archeological digs. Presumably gone were the straps, pads, and other light pressures once used to bind an infant's head, ancient practices that often signified the person's eventual adult status within a community. However, modern-day research has confirmed that head molding does indeed continue, globally, into the 21st century.

In a study of child care practices carefully guided by anthropological protocol and by the federal regulations relating to studies of human subjects, researchers from the University of Illinois at Chicago discovered that women of varied cultural backgrounds shape their babies' heads from birth to around age three, when the fontanels have usually closed. What begins as hand molding the heads of newborns gradually evolves into the use of constricting caps, tight headbands, or firmly bound blankets on older infants and young toddlers, thus completing the desired effect as passed on by one's elders. Interestingly, this culturally diverse study showed that all of the women knew how to accomplish these procedures, whereas the men did not. Additionally, all of the participants said they molded their babies' heads to assist the development of their child's beauty, intelligence, or health. For example, some women wanted their children to have the dimpled cheeks deemed beautiful by so many. To achieve this effect, they rubbed the child's zygomatic bones with upward circular motions and light pressure. Simultaneously, women from other cultures manually molded and rounded a child head in hopes of assisting intelligence. Although this study brought no evidence of the opposite effect occurring, the feasibility of accidental damage to the brain or sensory organs could exist.

Pediatricians and other physicians who have been made aware of head-molding practices will surely need to handle their inquiries in a highly sensitive manner to avoid giving cultural offense. However, a far more frequent occurrence may be the positional molding of an infant's head, which usually happens by accident or, perhaps, by ignorance. Either way, about one of every 100 infants exhibits this once-rare condition that typically presents as asymmetrical flattening on the back of a child's head and a corresponding misalignment of the ears or facial features. This seems to come about more frequently and unavoidably in multiple births when babies experience womb crowding or when low birth weight necessitates prolonged hospitalization. In general though, positional molding began to increase dramatically after the 1993 recommendation from the American Academy of Pediatrics encouraged parents and caretakers to place infants on their backs rather than on their stomachs to prevent Sudden Infant Death Syndrome (SIDS). Although this procedure successfully contributed to a decline of SIDS, instances of positional molding subsequently arose. In addition to this causative factor, chronically busy parents or other caretakers seem to be more inclined to leave an infant in a car seat or a baby carrier for longer periods of time. Therefore, to correct the problem or to avoid altogether flattening the back of the baby's skull, caretakers may be advised to pick up a restless child, gently rub the head, reposition the baby with care, and keep a watchful eye. If this does not help, a pediatrician may prescribe a medical device, such as a dynamic orthotic cranioplasty band.

See also CRANIUM; FACE; HEADACHE; HEAD INJURY; TORTICOLLIS.

FitzSimmons, Ellen, et al. "Infant Head Molding: A Cultural Practice." *Archives of Family Medicine* 7 (January/February 1998): 88–90.

Littlefield, Tim. "Directing Symmetrical Cranial Growth: Positional Head Molding in Multiples." *Twins* (July/August 1999): 24.

headache Sometime within the year, 90 percent of the men in this country and 95 percent of the women will have at least one headache. With those and other interesting facts to offer, the American Council for Headache Education (aptly initialed ACHE) categorizes headaches as two main types: primary and secondary, with 90 percent of occurrences in the first category. That is especially good to know since a primary headache seldom signals an underlying medical condition or disease but, rather, results from tension, sinus pressure, or other factors that are seldom life threatening. Secondary headaches, however, can result from an infection or some type of pressure within the skull, such as happens with a tumor. If a tumorous growth has begun, pain progressively worsens with accompanying signs, such as nausea, visual disturbance, or a disruption of speech, gait, or coordination.

Fortunately though, a tumor-induced headache is a rare occurrence. Much more likely causes of secondary headaches involve arthritis, where the pain often intensifies on movement, or with a fever, which causes the blood vessels in the head to swell. In either instance, a rheumatologist or primary care physician will prescribe appropriate treatment. For the resulting headaches, anti-inflammatory medication may help to relieve the pain. If headaches arise from a structural problem, such as TMJ (TEMPOROMANDIBULAR JOINT), that can also be addressed by a primary care physician, dental specialist, or a chiropractor. CHIROPRACTIC adjustments of the vertebrae, particularly in the neck and upper back, can be especially helpful when the spine has gotten out of alignment, causing the head to throb.

Similarly, cervicogenic headaches can arise because of an accident, aging, or a structural irregularity in the nerves and muscles of the head or neck with pain often activated by movements as simple as turning the head in conversation or holding a phone. In such instances, abnormal tenderness, restricted range of motion, and changes in muscle contour present confirming signs with treatment likely to involve some type of physical rehabilitation. For example, trigger point therapy may be used to break up fibrous tissue by way of a needle. For headache-producing abnormalities that involve connective tissue, muscles, or joint dysfunctions, manual therapy provided by a chiropractor or an osteopath can usually be performed safely with good results. Cervical traction that stretches the neck muscles and ligaments can also provide relief, assuming there is no instability of the cervical vertebrae. To evaluate this and other possibilities, a thorough physical examination will include an assessment of the person's posture and any musculoskeletal involvement. In addition to physical rehabilitation, treatment may include medication, relaxation therapy, injections, biofeedback, or surgery, depending on the diagnosis and the severity of the condition.

Health information from the National Institute of Neurological Disorders and Strokes advises that underlying disorders other than musculoskeletal conditions may present as headaches accompanied by pain in the eyes or the ears. When headaches persist, especially in children or in adults with no prior history of head pain, a physician may order a blood test or X-rays to rule out conditions as varied as thyroid disease, blood clots, or anemia. Severe headaches after a HEAD INJURY usually bear closer scrutiny with a computed tomography (CT or CAT) scan and/or magnetic resonance imaging (MRI). An eye exam may also be ordered to assess any signs of weakened eye muscles or pupils of unequal size.

Locating the precise point of pain can be complicated by the network of nerves extending over the scalp and into the face and throat. Muscles around the head and face can also be sensitive to pain, but the brain and the skull bones themselves do not hurt since they have no pain-sensitive nerve fibers. Therefore, pain will usually be referred from somewhere else. In addition, sinus pressure can cause the eyes and head to ache but, so can a migraine. To differentiate between those two common sources of headache, the report "Sinus Headaches Versus Migraine" by the National Headache Foundation (NHF) says that true sinusitis presents not only a headache but also postnasal drainage or congestion often accompanied by facial pressure or tenderness when touching the cheeks or forehead. A cough, fatigue, or pressure in the ears may accompany a sinus headache, too. Chronic conditions of sinusitis can be medically confirmed by X-rays. When self-diagnosing, though, the triggering factors for a headache may provide false clues. For instance, weather changes can produce a sinus headache, but weather can also trigger a migraine.

According to statistics provided by the NHF, one migraine sufferer resides in every four homes, with about 28 million people or 13 percent of the population affected in the U.S. Only a relatively small number, however, experience an aura or that flash and shimmer of light with which the migraine has come to be identified. More likely, symptoms will include sensitivity to light and sound, sometimes accompanied by nausea or queasiness. Although preventative medications may be prescribed for those who have regular migraines each month, other medicines provide acute therapy after an attack begins. To hold migraines to a minimum, patients may be advised to keep a journal to help identify any triggering factors, especially since these vary from person to person. Some common instigators, for instance, include environmental triggers, such as exposure to smoke or bright lights, emotional stress, hormonal fluctuations, lack of sleep, and lack of exercise.

According to a 2003 online survey conducted by the NHF, 41–43 percent of those who responded said that exercise lessened the severity and the frequency of their headaches. With admonitions about consulting a primary health care advisor prior to beginning a new exercise program, the NHF further suggests warm-ups and adequate hydration before and after physical activity. Concern should be shown for the diet, too, by not skipping meals but avoiding foods that previous journal keeping has implicated as triggering an attack.

See also NUTRITION.

National Headache Foundation. "Sinus Headaches Versus Migraine." Available online. URL: http://www.headaches.org/professional/presskit/FinalMigraineFacts4-5.html Downloaded on April 7, 2003.

National Institute of Neurological Disorders and Stroke. "Headache Information." Available online. URL: http://accessible.nind.nih.gov/health_and_medical/disorders/headache.htm Downloaded on June 19, 2003.

Zasler, Nathan D. "Physical Treatment of Cervicogenic Headache." Available online. URL: http://www.achenet.org/articles/70.php Downloaded on April 7, 2004.

head injury According to a July 2001 report from the National Institute of Neurological Disorders and Stroke (NINDS), "Shaken baby syndrome is a severe form of head injury that occurs when a baby is shaken forcibly enough to cause the baby's brain to rebound (bounce) against his or her skull." A graphic and rather gruesome analogy would be to consider the three-second effects of a blender. Should the child happen to survive such abusive treatment, the symptoms range from lethargy to loss of consciousness with the added prospects of vomiting, convulsions, dislocated bones, and crippling injuries to the neck or spine. Yet, ironically, the NINDS reports, "There usually are no outward physical signs of trauma."

According to data from the American Academy of Pediatrics (AAP), 15–38 percent of the infant mortality rate in the United States relates to shaken baby syndrome. If a pediatrician or other physician has cause to suspect this form of child abuse, verification can usually be made by computed tomography (CT or CAT) scan with magnetic resonance imaging (MRI) following those results. To guide doctors in handling and reporting such matters in a timely but sensitive manner, the AAP issued a report from their Committee on Child

Abuse and Neglect in the July 2001 issue of *Pediatrics*.

For preschoolers, older children, and adults, severe head injuries usually occur by accident. According to a fact sheet from the Centers for Disease Control and Prevention (CDC), bicycle-related head injuries alone account for about 153,000 emergency visits and 17,000 hospitalizations in the U.S. each year, with the highest rate of injury and the highest instances of death among children under 15 years of age. With the use of a sturdy helmet, however, CDC estimates that at least one life could be saved each day in this country and one head injury prevented every four minutes.

When a head injury does occur, immediate concern arises about bleeding inside the skull, especially worrisome since this can be delayed from 24 to 72 hours and still present no conclusive signs. To help people know what to look for, the University of Maine Cooperative Extension offers online health information. "First Aid for Head Injuries" lists such telling symptoms as loss of memory, visual problems, bleeding or other fluids draining from the ears or sinus cavities, nausea, and irregular breathing. If a bump erupts on the head, however, the size does not necessarily correspond with the extent of an INJURY.

Until emergency treatment and appropriate medical tests can be obtained, ice compresses can help to lessen the swelling. This reduction could be crucial in keeping pressure from building within the skull if blood vessels or protective tissue have been compromised. The most likely occasions for that to happen will be during a vehicular accident, physical abuse, or a fall from a great height. Thanks, however, to the hardness of the skull and the protective layers of tissue and fluids that cushion the brain, most head injuries will not be severe but will, nevertheless, be scary due to the profuse bleeding that is likely because of the many blood vessels around the scalp. In such cases, the first response of aid should be to stop the bleeding by applying firm pressure to the area for five minutes or so with a clean, dry cloth or towel to avoid further contaminating the wound. If this does not check blood flow or if a deep puncture has occurred, stitches may be needed to close the wound and a tetanus shot administered. After the person has been treated by a medical professional, the recommended dose of acetaminophen may be given for pain but not aspirin since its blood-thinning action may cause a wound to start bleeding again.

See also SAFETY; SKULL.

Chatfield, Joanne E. "Clinical Briefs: AAP Report on Shaken Baby Syndrome." Available online. URL: http://www.aafp.org/afp/20020101/clinical.html Downloaded on June 17, 2003.

National Ag Safety Database. "First Aid for Head Injuries." Available online. URL: http://www.cdc.gov/nasd/docs/d000801_d000900/d000815/d000815.html Downloaded on May 15, 2003.

National Bicycle Safety Network. "The Problem." Available online. URL: http://www.cdc.gov/ncipc/bike/problem.htm Downloaded on May 15, 2003.

National Institute of Neurological Disorders and Stroke. "Shaken Baby Information Page." Available online. URL: http://www.nind.nih.gov/health_and_medical/disorders.shakenbaby.htm?Format=printable Downloaded on June 17, 2003.

heart attack If this life-threatening situation occurs, a call to 911 should immediately be followed by aspirin, preferably chewed, whether it is the chewable kind or not since this helps the body more quickly absorb aspirin's blood-thinning action. If the person is in cardiac arrest—i.e., unconscious, no pulse, and not breathing—cardiopulmonary resuscitation (CPR) must begin at once to get life-flowing blood and oxygen circulating again. To do this, the person's throat passage must first be cleared so puffs of breathe can be given, mouth-to-mouth twice for every 15 chest compressions. With both hands on the victim's chest, 80 to 100 compressions each minute applies the force most often needed to keep an adult alive until medical help arrives. Since every minute matters, that 911 call brings trained staff and equipment onto the scene so no time will be lost unnecessarily in an emergency waiting room. State-of-the-art equipment used later can sometimes bring a person back from cardiac arrest, but a mere four to six minutes of not breathing will usually result in brain damage.

However, the American Heart Association reports that the survival rate for victims of cardiac arrest can increase from 5 percent to up to 74 percent if treatment begins within those first five critical minutes.

On January 29, 2003, the National Institutes of Health (NIH) released a study that showed MRI provides a faster, more accurate way to diagnose heart attacks. According to the study, only about 40 percent of heart attacks can be diagnosed in emergency departments that still use standard tests and procedures, but magnetic resonance imaging (MRI) provides a more accurate and much faster diagnosis. Not only does this technology show a medical team how well the heart muscle is functioning and how well the blood is flowing, an MRI reveals the location and intensity of any heart damage that has occurred. Since an MRI takes only about 40 minutes or so, appropriate and timely treatment can begin right away without additional, potentially damaging delays.

Also according to the American Heart Association, about 7.6 million adults in this country do survive a heart attack each year. With this vital organ continuing to beat to its own rhythm, the heart functions as a life-propelling device that pumps nutrient-rich and oxygenated blood to all organs and muscles of the body. Like other muscles in motion, those in the CARDIAC MUSCLE actively alternate cycles of contracting and relaxing. Unlike other muscles, though, the uniquely structured cardiac muscle fibers produce a person's heartbeat. Also unlike most other muscles, heart muscle operates involuntarily. No one has to remember to get a heart up and moving, but choices about EXERCISE and NUTRITION can be made to enable this vital organ to function in better health.

When the heart does not operate well, numerous factors can lead to an attack that may or may not result in cardiac arrest. For instance, malformations in the heart can occur at birth. Heredity, aging, obesity, physical inactivity, or disorders, such as hypertension and diabetes, can increase the risks of problems developing later. Damage can also occur in the heart tissue, perhaps because of other seemingly unrelated medical conditions that eventually affect the heart or because of the sudden onset of a virus, a high fever, or a severe electrical shock. At other times, the arteries constrict or become blocked by fats or mineral deposits that slowly accumulate, like sediment, during the body's regular cycling processes. Regardless of what causes an obstacle in one or more of the arteries, blood begins to pool around the constricted area, allowing a clot to form. If that blood clot dislodges and interrupts the heart's involuntary cycle, the diminished flow of blood and oxygen will soon cause the person to experience symptoms, such as shortness of breath, light-headedness, and, perhaps, a cold sweat. Then cardiac muscle may tightly contract, creating a sensation of heavy pressure, weight, or pain in the center of the chest and often radiating down the arms or into other parts of the body.

To prevent these precarious life-and-death situations, the American Heart Association recommends regular physical examinations to detect and treat problems that put the person at a greater risk for having a heart attack. In addition, the association advises people in general to watch their weight, avoid excesses in lifestyle, eat nutritious low-fat foods, and exercise regularly. If a heart attack or a cardiac event has already occurred, the same advice holds true with modifications made by the cardiologist or a primary care physician, depending on the individual's needs. For instance, some cardiac patients may require total bed rest, but many can begin walking for a few minutes each day while still in the hospital, gradually increasing the time of a daily walk to a half hour or so. If the doctor advises monitoring during a new treatment of exercise, a cardiac rehabilitation setting provides such a facility. There, patients can use stationary bikes, rowing machines, and treadmills, with the latter being a particular favorite. In addition to the emphasis on physical fitness and nutrition, a cardiac rehabilitation center may also include counseling on relevant subjects such as anger management, lifestyle changes, or social interactions aimed to help the cardiac patient find ways of managing and reducing STRESS.

heart muscle See CARDIAC MUSCLE.

heat therapy Almost since the beginning of time, people have known the healing comfort of a warm sun massaging an achy back or felt the therapeutic effects of bathing in a hot sulfur spring. Hot water, hot moist cloths, hot paraffin, or hot mud have all had medicinal value in various times and cultures. With most of those treatments still in use today for musculoskeletal conditions, newer therapies include modern versions of heat packs, warm whirlpool baths, ultrasound, and a hydrocollator. This last item is immersed into hot water and then removed and wrapped in a terry cloth holder designed to keep moist heat around the area of the neck collar for about a half hour. Similar devices can be purchased and warmed in a microwave for one to one-and-a-half minutes and then applied locally. To make a heat pack at home, uncooked rice poured into a cotton tube sock then tied in a knot at the open end can provide an effective source of dry heat once microwaved.

Although some patients seem to thrive with the dry heat found in heat lamps and heating pads, moist heat generally works best for most people, assuming, of course, that sensitive skin can take it or that desensitized skin will not be adversely affected. Either extreme warrants exceptional care be taken in using heat therapy on an infant, elderly stroke victim, or anyone else with impairments of circulation or sensations in the skin. In most instances though, the warmth of moist heat feels more comfortable than dry and, therefore, can be more comforting. Since the dampness allows heat to reach deeper into the body, this can be particularly therapeutic when a person has reached the rehabilitative phase of an injury.

To keep the heat itself from injuring a patient, health information provided by the Ohio State University Medical Center recommends that 140 to 160 degrees Fahrenheit be used for moist heat packs with six to eight layers of toweling to avoid burning the skin. After applying for 15 to 20 minutes, the redness may continue for up to six hours with the heat continuing to have some effect during that time. For whirlpool baths, the recommended temperatures range from 98 degrees to 104 degrees Fahrenheit for about 20 minutes as the soothing water swirls around the person, improving overall circulation. Since this has been known to increase blood pressure too, a physician's advice should be sought, especially in the presence of pregnancy or hypertension, or similar conditions. Care should also be taken to protect the skin, regulate the temperature settings, and avoid falling asleep during heat therapy, particularly if it is unsupervised. Otherwise, the idea is to relax and let the heat increase blood flow throughout the body, soothing the muscles and joints.

Because heat therapy helps to enlarge blood veins and vessels, the enhanced circulatory effects brings nutrients to the outer extremities and carries away body wastes—conditions that often prove optimal for healing. Only recently, however, has warming therapy become available for the treatment of chronic wounds. For example, Dr. Luther C. Kloth, a professor of physical therapy at Marquette University in Milwaukee, Wisconsin, and his colleagues worked with the local Zablocki Veterans Affairs Medical Center to complete a clinical trial on the effectiveness of a warming therapy device in treating pressure ulcers. Although the study was randomized, patients had to meet certain criteria to assure that healing might be possible, thus eliminating those with a terminal illness or with less treatable conditions, such as uncontrolled diabetes. With 43 wounds and 40 patients from 42 to 101 years of age, the study began. For half of the patients, a warming therapy device was used with a foam cover for protection and a plastic window for inspection as researchers inserted an infrared heating element to deliver warmth to wounds of various sizes. After 12 weeks, the results showed that the wounds treated with warming therapy healed more than 50 percent faster than those who had been given the standard treatments. As clinical research continues, new standards for treating older wounds and injuries may be set in this warming therapeutic trend.

National Institutes of Health (NIH). "NIH Study Shows MRI Provides Faster, More Accurate Way to Diagnose Heart Attacks." Available online. URL: http://www.nih.gov/news/pr/jan2003/nhlibi-29.htm Downloaded on February 14, 2003.

Wolski, C. A. "Wounds and Warmth." Available online. URL: http://www.rehabpub.com/Features/42002/9.asp Downloaded on June 20, 2003.

heel The heel (calcaneus bone) encompasses the foot's rounded posterior behind the ankle, where all sorts of indignities may occur from the heel puncture used to draw a blood sample in a newborn baby to the heel spurs that occasionally arise as people age. Additionally, inflammation around the Achilles tendon sometimes signifies an underlying medical condition, such as arthritis or ankylosing spondylitis. If a disease affects the body's musculoskeletal system, most likely the heel will show some proof. For instance, a thickening of the tendon may reveal a case of gouty arthritis, while a bone abnormality may confirm a structural flaw in the foot's biomechanics.

In the fact sheet "Heel Disorders and Treatments," the American College of Foot and Ankle Surgeons (ACFAS) suggests self-care treatment at the onset of heel pain, assuming, of course, that no accident or injury necessitates an immediate medical evaluation. For nonemergency use, the ACFAS recommendations include a regimen of ibuprofen or aspirin taken according to label directions for several days to reduce inflammation of the tissue. To alleviate tenderness and swelling in the heel even further, the foot can be placed in an adequately sized container that is then filled with tap water to the ankle level and with ice cubes added every five or six minutes for a chilling 30-minute soak three times a day. This icy footbath can especially provide relief right after an activity that cannot be postponed or curtailed, but cold therapy is not at all recommended for patients with a circulatory problem of the extremities, such as occur with diabetes. For patients in general, other suggestions include wearing comfortable FOOTWEAR with soft or rubbery soles, stretching the calf muscles daily, and avoiding vigorous activities until the heel has completely healed. If substantial healing does not occur within a week or so, a professional medical evaluation will certainly be needed.

The ACFAS Clinical Practice Guideline Heel Pain Panel made a report to develop a standard and a comprehensive medical strategy. It is entitled "The Diagnosis and Treatment of Heel Pain" and says, "As a rule, the longer the duration of heel pain symptoms, the longer the period to final resolution of the condition." Having first identified mechanical factors as the most common instigator of heel pain, the panel then acknowledged other causatives as being "traumatic, neurologic, arthritic, infectious, neoplastic, autoimmune, and other systemic conditions," with diagnostic testing and correct treatment directed at the source of the problem. Since the panel recognized that patients will usually try various self-remedies before seeking medical advice, suggestions begin with the importance of obtaining a careful history, "including time(s) of day when pain occurs, current shoe wear, activity level both at work and at leisure, and history of trauma." With that information available to adapt a personalized course of treatment, the panel further suggests, "An appropriate physical examination of the lower extremity includes range of motion of the ankle with special attention to decreased range of motion of dorsiflexion of the ankle, palpation of the inferior medial aspect of the heel, palpation of the medical aspect of the heel, the occurrence of bilateral symptoms, and angle and base of GAIT evaluation." A physical evaluation may also include the most appropriate type of radiograph as needed.

Depending on the patient's needs, treatment of the heel may include nonsteroidal anti-inflammatory drugs (NSAIDs), padding or strapping the foot, injecting the site with corticosteroids, and continuing the self-care tactics outlined above as, of course, deemed appropriate by the physician. If improvement can be noticed within six weeks, therapy will probably continue until a good outcome has been obtained. Otherwise, a referral may be made to a podiatric foot and ankle surgeon. Then, "The second phase of treatment for the referred patient includes continuation of the initial treatment options with considerations for additional therapy: the use of custom orthotic devices, especially in the biomechanically malaligned patient, the use of night splints to maintain an extended length of the plantar fascia during sleep, a limited number of corticosteroids injections, and cast immobilization for 4–6 weeks or the use of a fixed ankle walker-type device to immobilize the foot during activity." If a weight increase has caused damage or added to heel stress, a weight-loss program will also be recommended. Surgery may also be advised if a bone spur remains or if the heel suffers a pathological condition, such as an inflamed bursa or a diseased tendon. Regardless of the particular set of circumstances or the individualized course of treatment, the ACFAS panel reports that symptoms in 90–95 percent of the patients will be resolved within a year.

See also NUTRITION.

American College of Foot and Ankle Surgeons. "Heel Disorders and Treatments." Available online. URL: http://www.acfas.org/brheelds.html Downloaded on February 15, 2003.

Clinical Practice Guideline Heel Pain Panel. "The Diagnosis and Treatment of Heel Pain." *The Journal of Foot and Ankle Surgery* 40, no. 5 (September/October 2001): 329–340.

herbs for muscles and bones As with any effective treatment for the musculoskeletal system, an optimal choice of herbs depends on a person's symptoms and condition, not on the motivation of whoever happens to be pushing a particular product. As to be expected, most television and print advertisements, for example, will laud the herbs they package and sell as though the herbs are ideal for everyone. Although one product cannot possibly fit all, the herbs and herbal combinations themselves may be fine. Less expected perhaps, but far more insidious is the "expert" advice of a store clerk who wants to sound quite knowledgeable but just is not. Therefore, locally fresh-grown herbs, tasty herb teas, and culinary herbs—spices found in the grocery story—will usually be the safest ones to try for general usage. As a counterpart to that rule of thumb from the kitchen, the bitter herbs, or ones that taste really yucky, will rarely (if ever) be good choices when consumed frequently or in larger quantities. In a pinch, a pinch may be exactly right for therapeutic purposes, especially if the well-recommended herb will be consumed for only a short period of time followed by an equal number of days off. Before playing with a potentially strong herb, however, a good guideline may be to follow the advice of herbal handbooks compiled by reputable authors and publishers—not just one book, but three or more respected sources who consistently report that the same herb should be used for the same reasons. Even then, a person's individual responses to foods must also be a major consideration.

For example, most reliable sources agree that black walnut has been shown to reduce the toxic effects of artificial ingredients, preservatives, food coloring, bacteria, pesticides, and other pollutants that can accumulate, especially if a person has not ingested enough filtered water to wash them away. Instead of ridding everybody's body of poison, though, black walnut can itself produce a dangerously poisonous effect in those who have allergies to nuts. Therefore, even a completely natural herb is not universally safe. Herb use and herbal therapy require not only common sense but a sense of one's own person.

With these disclaimers and the personal adjustments needed, herbs can provide supportive help in an overall healthy diet. For example, the regular use of alfalfa in a salad can provide the chlorophyll and numerous other nutrients considered particularly helpful for circulation throughout the body. The often-lauded *Ginkgo biloba* can do the same but may evoke headaches. Besides, ginkgo is just not something that people usually sit around munching.

Assuming they are relevant to a condition, culinary herbs can usually be consumed with greater safety and, often, to good effect—perhaps with gourmet meals occurring in the process. For instance, oregano has been said to ease neuralgia and bruised muscles, while cherries and strawberries have long been considered a home treatment for arthritic conditions, such as gout. For rheumatism, herbs such as basil and oregano or vegetables such as asparagus may alleviate aches and pains. Depending on the type and cause of a headache, herbs like basil, marjoram, and rosemary may come just in time with thyme also considered healing for headaches and a number of other painful events. In addition, thyme taken off the spice rack can provide a local antiseptic salve or paste to treat a cut or wound. If sore muscles and painful joints occur, herbs can be used externally in hot plasters made of mustard or wet, warm compresses that apply ginger or hot onions to the site. However, just as the ingestion of herbs can cause problems for those with a food allergy, the external application of an herbal treatment can evoke unsightly skin eruptions and other irritations for those with sensitive skin.

Other factors to consider when choosing herbs include any counterproductive effects on medications, which will usually be caused either by overlapping purposes or by hindering a drug's effect. Therefore, it is crucial to ask a physician or a pharmacist about any contraindications and also to read carefully the information that comes packaged with each medical product. More importantly, the primary care physician and all specialists will need a list of the herb capsules taken (even if infrequently) before they can safely prescribe pharmaceutical treatment. As a general rule, however, no herb should be taken for the same symptoms or for the particular condition that a prescribed or an over-the-counter medicine will treat. For instance, most herbalists agree that devil's claw reduces inflammation in muscles and joints, but this herb should not accompany use of aspirin, ibuprofen, or other NSAIDs (nonsteroidal anti-inflammatory drugs) having similar effects. Likewise, an herb known to relax the muscles, such as passionflower, chamomile, or valerian (the organic source of valium), should not be combined with either a prescribed or an over-the-counter muscle relaxant.

As another precaution, a person should begin with one new herb only, whether as a spice, a tea, or an herb capsule, giving it a week or so before trying the next relevant herb that comes highly recommended by several reliable sources. This means, of course, that a combination herb capsule should not be tried at all until the safe use of each ingredient has been previously ascertained. For infants, young children, and pregnant and nursing women, even greater precautions must be taken when investigating the use of individual herbs. Likewise, various medical conditions come with particular concerns. For instance, the *PDR for Herbal Medicines, First Edition* cautions about the use of echinacea in treating an infection or an inflammation in people with autoimmune disorders, "Because of a conceivable activation of autoimmune aggressions and other over-reactive immune responses."

For almost everyone, harsh or medicinal herbs, such as goldenseal *(Hydrastis canadensis)*, must be used in the aforementioned few days on and equal days off pattern to avoid an accumulative effect that can result in a toxic overdose. Should this happen anyway, treatment usually consists of ingesting activated charcoal or very burned toast. However, to lessen the possibility of any adverse effects, a full glass of filtered water should be drunk when taking an herb capsule or the stronger liquid forms of herbs found in a homeopathic remedy or tincture. With simple precautions, a sensible consideration of one's own body, and the time allowed for a much slower but natural course of treatment to begin, a well-chosen herb can bring healthful support to the body's inborn response toward healing.

See also NUTRITION.

Fleming, Thomas R., et al., eds. *PDR for Herbal Medicines.* Montvale, N.J.: Medical Economics Company, Inc., 1998.

herniated disk Whether a physician or specialist refers to this condition of the vertebral disk as ruptured, prolapsed, or slipped, the outcome remains the same—pain or numbness in the neck or limbs—either of which has usually been caused by pressure on the spinal nerves. The common term of *slipped disk* can be misleading though as to what actually transpires. Between the bones of the spinal column, the disks provide a cushiony effect that protects the vertebrae from receiving an ongoing shock as a person runs, walks, or merely stands. The outer ring of each DISK (annulus) supplies strength and structure by the means of a complexly woven, tough, fibrous, gristlelike cartilage, while the center or nucleus of the disk adds a rubbery springiness felt throughout the spine. If rupturing occurs, the gelatinous center oozes, giving a radiographic picture that erroneously appears to show a slippage of one or more disks.

A fact sheet from the American Academy of Orthopaedic Surgeons (AAOS) offers some reasons this condition develops, one of which has to do with age. As people get older, water content generally decreases in their muscles, bones, and disks, allowing the latter to shrink and, subsequently, narrowing the space between the vertebrae. This narrowing then results in a loss of flexibility.

Normal wear and tear consequently causes painful disruptions of the disk, while added body weight can compress them even more. Poor posture or poor positioning during a physical chore that requires lifting can also have an adverse effect as can sudden jolts and pressures on the spine. Since four out of five people in this country occasionally experience lower back pain, that symptom alone does not indicate the presence of a herniated disk unless, perhaps, pain or numbness began with an injury, such as a blow to the back or a fall. Otherwise, a more telling sign may be sciatic pressure with weakness, tingling, numbness, or a sensation of burning shooting down the hips and into the lower limbs. Although some patients may demand X-rays or magnetic resonance imaging (MRI), such tests may not be clinically significant in confirming a herniated disk that will be treated conservatively anyway. At least in the beginning, a conventional course of treatment will probably include bed rest and over-the-counter or prescription-filled pain relievers. Cold compresses can also be applied for 20 minutes several times throughout the day or evening. If muscle spasms begin, though, heat therapy may prove to be more useful. Short walks and therapeutic exercises to strengthen the back or abdominal muscles may also be advised.

According to the AAOS, these measures may bring the desired relief. If not, the physician may suggest epidural injections of cortisone to soothe the spinal nerves and enable the patient to complete a course of physical therapy. Sometimes, the doctor may use enzyme injections to dissolve enough of the prolapsed disk to remove pressure from the affected nerve. If pain continues, an MRI or computed tomography (CT or CAT) scan can then be useful in revealing any damage a ruptured disk has caused to the nearby nerves or muscles around the spine. For instance, a fragment of a disk could be lodged in the spinal canal, pressing on a nerve and causing loss of function. If so, a laminectomy is traditionally performed. This type of SURGERY requires overnight hospitalization and a general anesthesia to remove the disk or part of the vertebrae. However, newer surgical techniques may require only a local anesthetic in an outpatient setting.

In the May 2001 issue of *The Back Letter*, an article entitled "Do Uncontained Disc Herniations Resolve within Weeks? Should Surgery Be Delayed?" reports that a study from Japan indicates surgical delays can give a disk time to resolve itself in several weeks as "the body's defense system attacks and absorbs uncontained disc herniations, leading to early radiographic and clinical resolution." With exceptions made for those having severe conditions, this protocol reduced by almost 50 percent the discectomies that the researchers would normally have performed within a year. In this country, few spine specialists advocate early surgery except as warranted by injury or other circumstances requiring extreme measures to be taken with speed. As the article points out, however, the decision to proceed with surgery often reflects the patient's ability to cope with symptoms or to tolerate the indefinite delay a disability could bring. With no easy solution in any case, researchers may bring more light to the subject by establishing precise baselines and comprehensive methodologies for confirming the extent of a disk herniation and then treating subsequent conditions with a closer look at the unique individual who ultimately lives with the uncontained disk.

American Academy of Orthopaedic Surgeons. "Herniated Disk." Available online. URL: http://orthoinfo.aaos.org/fact/thr_report.cfm?thread_id=185&topcategory=spine Downloaded on March 6, 2003.

Staff. "Do Uncontained Disc Herniations Resolve within Weeks? Should Surgery be Delayed?" Available online. URL: http://www.findarticles.com/cf_0/m06670/5_16/75607517/print.jhtml Downloaded on May 17, 2003.

hiccup or hiccough In this poetic instance of onomatopoeia imitating sound, a hiccup by any spelling is actually singultus—the involuntary contraction of muscles in the diaphragm accompanied by the well-orchestrated closing of muscles in the larynx. Often occurring after an abrupt intake of air, classical hiccups may begin with a rhythmic sound adding audio to the annoyance. With occasional intermissions possible, an acute case of hiccups may last up to 48 hours, while persistent hiccups go on and on. If more than two months of hiccuping continues, the problem may be classified as intractable with treatment depending on one of about 100 potential causes. The most common cause involves a gastrointestinal problem of some type. H. S. Smith and A. Busracamwongs stated, "Causes may be natural or drug induced, and the same agents that are used to treat hiccups may also induce them," a problem that can be particularly troublesome when it affects the remaining quality of life in an elderly or a terminally ill patient.

Some successful home remedies generally focus on raising the level of carbon dioxide in the blood, which initially got out of balance as the person hyperventilated or breathed too rapidly. To counteract this inequity, the person holds his or her breath or breathes into a paper bag, not plastic. Another old remedy invigorates the vagus nerve that runs from the brain to the stomach. To follow this suggestion, the person drinks water quickly and rhythmically or swallows crushed ice. However, an amusing remedy mentioned by *The Merck Manual* has the person gently pull the tongue and rub the eyeballs. If done simultaneously, that feat would surely be worth witnessing, whether the hiccups go away or not!

Beers, Mark H., M.D., et al., eds. *The Merck Manual of Medical Information, Second Home Edition.* Whitehouse Station, N.J.: Merck Research Laboratories, 2003, 545.

Smith, H. S. and A. Busracamwongs. "Management of Hiccups in the Palliative Care Population." *American Journal of Hospital Palliative Care* 20, no. 2 (March/April 2003): 149–154.

hinge joint Similar to the hinged lid of a box, a hinged joint opens (extends and straightens) or closes (flexes and bends.) These joints encompass synovial fluid to keep the knees, elbows, fingers, and toes moving smoothly, back and forth.

See also JOINT.

hip As muscles and ligaments wrap around the hip bones and hollows like so many rubber bands and fan belts, the pelvis and thigh come together in a BALL-AND-SOCKET JOINT that forms the pelvic girdle. Around this complex system, cushionlike fatty pads of varying thickness provide additional protection to the hips. Supportive muscles in the abdomen, groin, and buttocks also add protective value and assist in providing the stability needed to bear the body's weight. These adjacent muscles help to decrease sway and increase a person's mobility too. As the head of the femur (thighbone) snugly cradles into the deep socket of the pelvis's acetabulum, the resulting structure permits remarkable range of motion rivaled only by the shoulder joint. To assure smooth movement even further, the synovial lining of the joint supplies small amounts of lubrication that keep the hips shifting and swinging—hopefully, friction free.

For most people, this structural network works exceptionally well. The pelvic girdle adapts to stresses that occur during the active growth spurts of puberty and the sudden weight gains or additional strains of pregnancy. Heightened physical activity and impact sports can affect hips, too, with signs of damage often showing up as groin pain or loss of motion in the joint. If, however, stiffness or general pain regularly arrives when getting up or bending down, this may signal the advent of an underlying condition, such as arthritis or osteoarthritis, which requires a medical evaluation by a rheumatologist or a primary care physician. With so much potential movement in the hips, dislocations can also occur, sometimes as early as in the womb where crowding or BIRTH DEFECTS can cause disruptions of the bones. If the hip becomes dislocated or otherwise damaged, the effects will surely be felt up and down the appendicular skeleton to which the pelvic girdle belongs.

Because of the close proximity to the body's abdominal region, a hip disorder may first seem to be related to the digestive tract. When discussing this diagnostic problem in the November 2002 *Focus, Journal of the American Chiropractic Association* (ACA), an article quotes Dr. Leo Bronson—the vice president of the ACA Council on Orthopedics at that time—as saying, "The one sign that really gives you a clear indication of hip pathology is pain with range of motion in the hip, particularly extreme abduction or internal rotation." If a hip disorder has occurred or a biomechanical problem has been ascertained, chiropractic or osteopathic therapy may include manipulation of the joints, release of the constricted muscles, electrical stimulation, ultrasound, and myofascial stretches, which also address the muscular involvement in the lower back and spine as well as the pelvic region. If the person's gait has been affected, that too will need to be assessed with follow-up exercises and orthotics frequently prescribed for a continuation of the therapy at home.

Besides the more typical biomechanical problems, hips also suffer from overuse injuries as occurs when a leg overstretches or when improper equipment has been worn. In addition, repetitive motion can affect the pelvic girdle—again with poor shoes, tools, and other equipment often lacking the protective support needed. Less likely may be an infection in or around a hip joint. However, evidence will often be given through localized redness, swelling, and/or a fever that generally affects the whole body. Similarly, other underlying medical conditions evoke signs elsewhere. For instance, the presence of osteoarthritis or bone degeneration may show up in blood tests or bone mineral density tests. X-rays alone, however, might not provide a clear picture because of the hip's many angles and contours. Therefore, magnetic resonance imaging (MRI) may be required to diagnosis what is happening.

A lot does happen to the hips, especially as people get older, heavier, and/or more sedentary. According to statistics mentioned in a January 2003 release from the Agency for Healthcare Research and Quality (AHRQ), approximately 350,000 hip fractures occur in the United States each year. For those FRACTURES involving hospitalization, a study by AHRQ says that early release places the patients at a greater risk. If other abnormal vital signs exist at the time of discharge, the person has a 60 percent greater chance of readmission within a couple of months and an overwhelming 360 percent greater likelihood of dying than those who remain under hospital care until the condition stabilizes. To identify the risks even better, Dr. Ethan A. Halm, M.P.H., of the Mount Sinai School of Medicine, developed a list of dangerous problems that need to be resolved before discharging a patient with a hip fracture. These include a fever over 101 degrees Fahrenheit, either a high or low extreme in blood pressure, extremes in heart rate, a high rate of breathing, poor oxygenation of the blood, the inability to eat, a wound infection, acute chest pain, shortness of breath, or a mental status at variance with the person's level of alertness prior to the occurrence of the fracture.

A February 2003 release from the American Academy of Orthopaedic Surgeons (AAOS) says that 90 percent of hip fractures result from a FALL. With baby boomers from the post–World War II days now entering retirement age, a rise in hip problems has been predicted with the possibility of 650,000 hip fractures occurring by 2050. That translates to 1,800 hip fractures per day in the U.S. alone. As AAOS further reports, the Hospital for Joint Diseases Research Group recently studied patients over age 65 in good mental and physical health. It found that, after a hip fracture, only 41 percent regained their former levels of mobility with 59 percent incurring decreased mobility or lessened independence when performing their daily chores.

Because so much depends on the hips and hip joints in adequately bearing and moving the body's weight, Dr. Robert D'Ambrosia—noted author, surgeon, and former president of AAOS—says, "If you can prevent one of these fractures from occurring, it's a lot better than trying to fix it afterward." While aiming toward that goal, Dr. D'Ambrosia expects the orthopedic community to evaluate hip protectors. Though no manufacturer guarantees complete success in preventing hip fractures, these innovative products offer a promising solution, particularly for high-risk patients with osteoporosis or other types of degenerative bone disease. When discussing this topic in "Elderly Can Benefit from Hip Shields, Study Says," published in the November 23, 2000 *Detroit Free Press* health news, Associated Press writer Janet McConnaughey reports that a two-year study in Finland involved 653 at-risk participants. Of the 13 patients who broke their hips during this time, nine were not wearing hip shields.

Almost everyone agrees that falls hasten the occurrences of hip fracture, yet many at-risk persons reportedly do not like the inconvenience or the bulkiness of wearing a hip shield. Additionally, most do not admit to needing a walking aid even though such devices can help to prevent falls from happening. A physician, occupational therapist, or physical therapist can prescribe the optimal choice for an individual among the numerous devices available. For those who decide for themselves that a cane might be useful, the American Physical Therapy Association (APTA) offers some important suggestions for people with hip problems. For instance, to get the right height, a cane needs to be almost straight when held upright as the person stands. Another valuable tip in the APTA 1998 publication "Taking Care of Your HIP" says that the person can relieve stress on a damaged hip by using the cane on the *opposite* side rather than the same side, as often assumed.

The APTA further recommends exercises for people with hip problems to promote flexibility and to strengthen the pelvic girdle. To do the later, the guide offers a "Standing Hip Strengthener" exercise where the person stands up straight while holding onto the back of a nonwobbly upright chair and then slowly extends one leg out to the side—about 12 inches. When that position has been maintained for 10 seconds or so, the leg slowly returns to the starting point, and the opposite leg repeats the movement. Alternating repetitions then continue for about 10 times or until the side of either hip has begun to tire.

To strengthen the buttocks, abdomen, and hamstring muscles that help to support hip movement, the APTA guide further suggests that the person lies on a floor (although a firm mattress or other padded surface might be sensible for some) with the knees bent and feet flat. As the person focuses on tightening the abdominal muscles, the pelvis tilts upward slightly, creating a straight line with the knees. After holding that position for 15–20 seconds, the person relaxes a moment and then repeats the EXERCISE eight to 12 times. For this or any other exercise done while lying down, however, special care should be taken to support the curve of the neck with a small pillow or a rolled hand towel to avoid straining the upper vertebrae.

In their January 2001 health release, the National Institute of Arthritis and Musculoskeletal and Skin Diseases (NIAMS)—part of the National Institutes of Health—says an exercise program that strengthens the pelvic girdle can also improve the positioning of the hips and, subsequently, relieve pain. If inflammation continues though, NIAMS suggests using nonsteroidal anti-inflammatory drugs (NSAIDs) in either over-the-counter strength or a stronger prescription provided by a doctor. To a lesser extent, some physicians may prescribe the use of corticosteroids to reduce joint inflammation, such as occurs with rheumatoid arthritis. Since this medication may cause further damage to the joint and, possibly, adverse side effects, such as weight gain and a lowered resistance to infection, corticosteroid treatments will need to be monitored by a rheumatologist or a primary care physician. Care should also be taken when discontinuing this treatment due to its effects on the body's natural production of hormones.

If the use of medications, exercise, physical therapy, and walking aids, such as a cane or walker, does not succeed in lessening pain and increasing joint function, NIAMS says the joint damage should be detectable by X-rays before a doctor recommends other options, such as HIP REPLACEMENT SURGERY. The most likely reasons for that surgery may be osteoarthritis, rheumatoid arthritis, injury, bone tumors, or avascular necrosis—the latter of which results when an inadequate blood supply to a hip eventually causes loss of bone. Before replacing the hip, however, NIAMS suggests an osteotomy as another option to be considered if at all viable. In that procedure, the surgeon will remove the damaged bone and tissue and then will reposition the hip joint, allowing the body to resume its correct position. Although recovery may take up to a year, an osteotomy can alleviate hip pain and eliminate the risks unique to a hip replacement. To establish the likelihood of its long-term effectiveness though, a patient's age, overall health, and quality of bone would be important factors to take into account before making a decision.

See also CALCIUM; NUTRITION.

Agency for Healthcare Research and Quality. "Patients with Hip Fractures Who Leave the Hospital Too Soon Are at Risk." Available online. URL: http://www.newswise.com/articles/2003/1/HIPFRCT2.AHC.html Downloaded on February 14, 2003.

American Academy of Orthopaedic Surgeons. "One in Every Three Seniors Will Fall." Available online. URL: http://www.newswise.com/articles/2003/2/AGING.OSR.html Downloaded on February 14, 2003.

American Physical Therapy Association. "Taking Care of Your HIP." Alexandria, Va.: American Physical Therapy Association, 1998.

McConnaughey, Janet. "Elderly Can Benefit from Hip Shields, Study Says." Available online. URL: http://www.freep.com/news/health/hip23_20001123.htm Downloaded on March 1, 2003.

National Institute of Arthritis and Musculoskeletal and Skin Diseases. "Publication No. 01-4907." Available online. URL: http://www.niams.nih.gov. Downloaded on February 19, 2003.

Staff. "Untitled." *Focus, Journal of the American Chiropractic Association*. Available online. URL: http://www.merchiro.org/publications.couldshowthatwith Downloaded on July 30, 2004.

hip replacement surgery All surgery carries some risks, but orthopedic surgeons Richard Rothman and William Hozack of the Rothman Institute at Thomas Jefferson University Hospital in Philadelphia, Pennsylvania, have been working to lessen the perils by means of a limited-incision hip replacement. A report in the February 16, 2003 *Medical Devices & Surgical Technology Week* says this less invasive surgical procedure makes a four- to six-inch incision and takes only about 35–45 minutes, as demonstrated on the Internet during a January 15 Web cast from the operating room. Although the variables in any recovery depend on the individual patient and the surgeon's experience or skill, a limited-incision hip replacement technique usually results in less blood loss, less postoperative pain, and less time in the hospital. Ease in rehabilitation can, reportedly, be expected too.

Perhaps more typically, hip replacement surgery generally lasts about two to three hours during which time the surgeon eliminates the damaged bone tissue and cartilage from the hip joint. After taking numerous measurements prior to selecting the best PROSTHESIS, the surgeon then pushes the femur (thighbone) from the socket and inserts one or more parts into the site. Again, a surgeon has a variety of choices available—metal alloys, plastics, polymeric materials, and ceramic on ceramic—each of which has either a similar or a greater strength than the healthy version of the original bone. When selecting the right combination and also when deciding other matters, such as whether to use cement, the doctor considers the stability of the surrounding bone, the extent of the replacement, and the person's age. If, for instance, only part of a joint shows damage or disease, the surgeon may perform a partial hip placement, which frequently leaves the acetabulum intact but replaces the head of the thighbone. If a total hip replacement proves necessary, decisions have to be made about using a cementless procedure or using various types of cement to create an immediate bond, thus allowing the prompt mobility that is particularly vital for an elderly patient. With age a primary consideration, younger patients (typically under 50) may receive a cementless hip replacement with materials selected to encourage bone ingrowth during the body's natural bone-remodeling process.

Regardless of the material used, the American Academy of Orthopaedic Surgeons (AAOS) says each substance will have certain characteristics in common. They are all biocompatible with the body to avoid either a local or a systemic rejection response. They all resist corrosion and wear, thus lessening the need for replacement of the replacement and, most importantly, preventing the further destruction of bone. Each choice of material has high standards of fabrication, and all have mechanical properties meant to duplicate the bone structures that they will replace.

In a total hip replacement, health information from the AAOS describes the implant process as having three parts. The replacement stem fits into the femur (thighbone) for stability. The artificial ball replaces the head of the femur. Additionally, the artificial cup replaces the hip socket. Some designs allow a custom fit of each individual part, while others come in a single unit. When added together, the components weigh about 14–18 ounces, depending on the measurements and the person's needs. For patients weighing over 165 pounds, the success rate reportedly lessens. For 80 percent of the patients, though, a hip replacement can be expected to last about 20 years.

From the Agency for Healthcare Research and Quality (AHRQ), the report "Researchers Compare Strategies for Treating Elderly Patients Who Have an Infected Hip Prosthesis" says that 1 percent of the patients will incur an infection of the hip prosthesis. One option then repeats the costly surgery in hopes of improvement. Yet another approach involves surgically cleaning and removing the infected tissue in a procedure known as debridement. Although another infection could possibly occur, debridement may be a better option for a frail and elderly patient, who, according to the AHRQ research, will gain "2.2 to 2.6 more months in quality-adjusted life expectancy than replacement of the prosthesis."

When all goes well with a hip replacement, as usually does occur, the time needed for recovery will depend on whether the surgeon has used cement to hold the prosthesis in place to get a patient up and moving again with the greatest speed. For the cementless hip surgery often preferred for younger patients, recuperation will necessarily be slower since the body needs ample time for bone remodeling to transpire, thus incorporating the material and stabilizing the joint. Despite this delay, however, the cementless option has the advantage of lasting longer and encouraging natural bone growth. In either case, physical and/or occupational therapy will be needed when the hip can bear weight again.

A tip sheet from the American Occupational Therapy Association offers some safe and comfortable ways to ease into daily activities as patients become more mobile. Just sitting, for example, works best when using a raised chair or another elevated surface to help the patient avoid bending forward or crossing the ankles or the knees. Getting dressed may require a dressing stick to assist in putting on underwear or slacks, again without bending down. Similarly, a sock aid and a shoehorn can help patients evade bending from the waist. To carry a hot liquid, container covers come well-advised. To prevent tripping, loose rugs should be removed from every room the patient enters. When working at a counter, a high stool will help as will various devices used almost anywhere to help recovering patients safely reach, carry, and lift objects until they are completed healed and hip again.

See also JOINT REPLACEMENT.

Agency for Healthcare Research and Quality. "Researchers Compare Strategies for Treating Elderly Patients Who Have an Infected Hip Prosthesis." Available online. URL: http://www.ahrq.gov/research/May01/501ra9.htm Downloaded on June 26, 2003.

American Occupational Therapy Associations. "Daily Activities After Hip Surgery." Available online. URL: http://www.aota.org/Featured/area6/links/link02r.asp Downloaded on June 26, 2003.

Staff. "Surgeons Demonstrate How Limited Incision Hip Replacement Reduces Risk." *Medical Devices and Surgical Technology Week* (February 16, 2003): 38.

homeopathy See MEDICAL ALTERNATIVES.

hormone replacement therapy In the last half century or so, hormonal replacement therapy (HRT) became the "in" treatment, perhaps not too coincidentally beginning with the women's liberation movement. At that time, HRT appropriately began to address the symptoms of menopause naturally arising as the female body loses estrogen. By replacing this loss, HRT subsequently lessened other concerns regarding bone mass, osteoporosis, and bone fracturing that frequently occur as women age. Although many questions remain as to whether HRT reduces bone fractures as some believe, numerous unbiased studies have shown that restoring a woman's estrogen supply to its premenopausal state does indeed prevent bone loss and actually causes bone mineral density to increase. With the potential of these healthful benefits though, widespread use of HRT developed into a sort of panacea or general all-purpose treatment for postmenopausal women.

In an insightful editorial published in the *Southern Medical Journal,* Editor Ronald C. Hamdy, M.D., F.R.C.P., F.A.C.P., offered this challenging statement, "Clinicians, however, need to ask themselves what exactly are they trying to achieve while treating the particular patient sitting across from their desk. They then need to refer to the evidence-based data concerning the best available medication to treat that condition. If they are trying to relieve postmenopausal symptoms, estrogen is probably the best medication available. If, on the other hand, they are trying to treat hypercholesterolemia or osteoporosis, then maybe they should consider other medications which have been shown to be effective in the management of these particular conditions."

As Dr. Hamdy pointed out earlier in his editorial, HRT entered the medical scene prior to the rigorous testing later required by the Federal Drug Administration and other regulatory agencies to assure product use and safety. Now, under the auspices of the National Institutes of Health, thorough research has begun, conducted by the Women's Health Initiative (WHI) study. The results are expected in 2005. Until then, definitive answers about HRT may not be forthcoming, but controversies continuously abound. For example, one WHI trial ceased in July 2002 when evidence pointed to HRT as increasing the risk of stroke, heart attack, and breast cancer. Then, the May 28, 2003 issue of *JAMA, The Journal of the American Medical Association,* reported on the "Effect of Estrogen Plus Progestin on Stroke in Postmenopausal Women." The article concluded, "Estrogen plus progestin increases the risk of ischemic stroke in generally healthy postmenopausal women. Excess risk for all strokes attributed to estrogen plus progestin appears present in all subgroups of women examined." The May 27, 2003 *FDA Talk Paper,* published by the U.S. Food and Drug Administration (FDA), offered its conclusions on the WHI findings, saying, "The combination estrogen and progestin increased the risk of dementia in women 65 and older and failed to prevent mild cognitive impairment (memory loss.)" FDA approval had never been given for the use of HRT in preventing cognitive disorders, and the administration's official word continues to be cautionary. In similar manner, the "FDA continues to advise women to talk to their doctors, and if they decide that estrogen and progestin containing products are appropriate, they should use the lowest dose for the shortest duration to reach treatment goals, although it is not known at what dose there may be less risk of serious side effects."

See also EXERCISE; NUTRITION.

Hamdy, Ronald C., M.D. "Hormonal Replacement Therapy: Fact or Fiction." *Southern Medical Journal* 94, no. 12 (December 2001): 11,141–11,142.

U.S. Food and Drug Administration. "WHIMS Study on Estrogen/Progestin." Available online. URL: http://www.fda.gov/bbs/topics/ANSWERS/2003/ANSO1226.html Downloaded on June 28, 2003.

Women's Health Initiative. "Effect of Estrogen Plus Progestin on Stroke in Postmenopausal Women." Available online. URL: http://jama.ama-assn.org/cgi/content/abstract/289/20/2673 Downloaded on June 28, 2003.

Huntington's disease Inherited, progressive, and ultimately fatal, this devastating brain disorder reveals early symptoms of muscular clumsiness and involuntary twitching that eventually deteriorate into an inability to walk, speak, or swallow. Although the initial signs typically appear in midlife, onset may begin as early as age two or as late as 90 with children of Huntington's disease (HD) victims having a 50-50 chance of inheriting the disease, or, rather, the fatal gene that has been isolated as the causative factor.

With the disease first described by Dr. George Huntington in 1872, researchers discovered over 100 years later (in 1983) the mutant gene responsible for HD—a protein comprised of amino acids appropriately dubbed huntingtin. In its normal state, huntingtin occurs in the cytoplasm of most cells in the body where, as studies suggest, the gene helps to develop and sustain brain function—unless something goes wrong and the opposite occurs. Since cells "can survive in a dysfunctional state for some time, . . . it appears that turning off the mutant gene can result in reversal of neurodegeneration," according to Anne B. Young in *The Journal of Clinical Investigation.*

The fall 2002 issue of *Toward A Cure,* published by the Huntington's Disease Society of America, reports on the studies of J. Timothy Greenamyre, Ph.D., and colleagues at Emory University in Atlanta, Georgia. They concluded that the "mutant huntingtin protein has direct, harmful effects on mitochondria"—those tiny power plants that energize all cell function. Therefore, the team believes that understanding how the mutant gene harms the mitochondria may offer solutions in protecting nerve cells and slowing—or stopping—the progression of HD.

Until this promising research develops into practical application, the treatments for HD progress with each advancing stage. A characteristic approach usually involves memory tools, walking aids, physical therapy to aid mobility, and occupational therapy to help patients perform daily chores, such as dressing and feeding themselves. Massage for muscle spasms or contractures may also be beneficial. As the disease advances, HD patients often require highly attentive supervision, especially when eating or sipping fluids to help prevent them from aspirating those substances. In general though, treatments continue to focus on making the individual as independent and as comfortable as possible to maintain his or her quality of life.

Greenamyre, J. Timothy. "In Focus: Study Helps Researchers to Understand Role of Mitochondria in HD." Available online. URL: http://www.hdsa.org/edu/PDF/TAC_Fall_2002.pdf Downloaded on July 20, 2004.

Young, Anne B. "Huntingtin in Health and Disease." *The Journal of Clinical Investigation* 111, no. 3 (February 2003): 299–302.

hydration Water, water everywhere, but not enough people will drink—or so implies a survey by the Cornell Medical Center and the International Bottled Water Association. Of the 3,003 Americans responding, only one in five met the minimum of the eight eight-ounce glasses of water per day recommended by most sources. For active people, nine to 10 glasses of eight ounces each come closer to compensating for the daily losses that occur even during sleep. In times of heat, stress, fatigue, fever, or illness, the need for water increases even more, especially for infants, young children, athletes, or the elderly, who seem more prone to dehydration. Fresh fruit, milk, and natural juices add toward daily water intake. However, caffeine-rich drinks, such as coffee and sodas (and to a somewhat lesser degree, tea) do not count. These liquids act as a diuretic and increase dehydration. If the day's intake of water does not meet a body's demand, natural functions diminish in a relatively short time. Dry skin, grogginess, and fatigue often present as the first symptoms of thirst. By the time a person notices, "I'm thirsty," dehydration has already begun. This presents a real danger simply because water accounts for 60–70 percent of the solid tissue in the body, including muscle mass and vital organs. Nothing can substitute water's vital function in distributing nutrients, ejecting toxins, protecting joints, carrying oxygen, generating energy, and balancing electrolytes, such as sodium, potassium, and chlorides (salts), needed for bone and muscle health.

A study entitled "Dehydration and Muscle Metabolism" by the Division U.S. Army Research Institute of Environmental Medicine investigated the effects that loss of water has on muscles. It finds that muscle strength is generally not compromised, yet muscle endurance diminishes by 15 percent and aerobic endurance lessens, too. Such findings remain consistent with other studies that frequently focus on the effects of hydration in sports or athletic performances.

Michael F. Bergeron, Ph.D., F.A.C.S.M., reports on this subject in "Playing Tennis in the Heat: Can Young Players Handle It?" in the August 2002 *Current Comment* by the American College of Sports Medicine. He says, "One of the best ways a tennis player can better tolerate competing in the heat is to maintain adequate hydration." Otherwise, performance problems range from being "off" to muscle cramps and heat exhaustion. Dr. Bergeron further notes, "Many tennis players *begin* play or training dehydrated. The more dehydrated a player is at the beginning of a match, the more body temperature will likely rise during play—especially if the match goes long." Additionally, players lose sodium and chloride, which then need to be replaced before rehydration can occur. If an imbalance continues, however, the problem becomes potentially life threatening. To avoid this, Dr. Bergeron recommends 24 ounces of fluid be drunk for each pound lost during a game—a general rule that might, likewise, be important when engaging in other activities.

Somewhat less expectedly perhaps, one activity in which dehydration greatly affects the body occurs in the labor room. In the article "Hydration Reduces Prolonged Labor," published in the April 1, 2000 *Family Practice News,* Kate Johnson reports on a study by Dr. Thomas Garite, chairman of obstetrics and gynecology at the University of California, Irvine. Dr. Garite is quoted as saying, "Laboring women, especially after prolonged labor, often appear dehydrated." In this country, however, the fluid intake has commonly been well monitored and yet intentionally limited in the labor room. To challenge this ongoing practice, Dr. Garite studied 195 randomly selected women and found that 26 percent of the low-hydration group experienced labor that lasted over 12 hours, whereas only half that number in the high-hydration group endured prolonged labor. Although more studies will be needed to ascertain the range of optimal fluid levels that can be safely suggested and administered, Dr. Garite reportedly said, "Laboring women may not require as much fluid as distance runners, but our suspicion was that they may be closer to runners than resting patients." Undoubtedly, most new mothers would agree.

Bergeron, Michael F. "Playing Tennis in the Heat: Can Young Players Handle It?" Available online. URL: http://www.acsm.org/health+fitness/pdf/current comments/healhydr.pdf Downloaded on February 9, 2004.

Cornell University Medical Center Nutrition Information Center. "New Survey Shows Most Americans May Suffer From Dehydration." Available online. URL: http://www.bottledwater.org/public/BWFactsHome_main.htm Downloaded on April 14, 1998.

Johnson, Kate. "Hydration Reduces Prolonged Labor." Available online. URL: http://www.findarticles.com.cf_0/m0BJI/7_30/62050612/print.jhtml Downloaded on June 27, 2003.

Montain, Scott J., Sinclair A. Smith, et al. "Dehydration and Muscle Metabolism." Available online. URL: http://www.usarie.army.mil Downloaded on June 27, 2003.

hydrotherapy Therapeutic use of water, ice, and steam has treated musculoskeletal injuries and diseases for many centuries among many peoples. Whether by sweat lodge, sauna, steam baths, cold compresses, whirlpools, or swimming pools, numerous physical therapy clinics and hospitals use hydrotherapy to treat a variety of conditions, such as bone pain, muscle pain, inflammation, rheumatoid arthritis, spinal trauma, headaches, muscle disorders, and swollen ankles or feet. Although many of the treatments can continue at home or in a fitness center, some require medical supervision—for example, the whirlpool baths that stimulate circulation in paralyzed limbs or the hyperthermia baths that immerse a patient in hot water to generate a fever when an ill body has failed to produce one on its own. Frail patients, children, or those with limited body awareness will also require full supervision.

When selecting between HEAT THERAPY and COLD THERAPY, the best choice depends on the symptoms or goals intended. For instance, heat typically calms the body, whereas cold stimulates and invigorates. Therefore, tired muscles and general fatigue might warrant a warm soaking, while fevered feet might ache for a cooling footbath. In a home, hospital, or other therapeutic setting, a combination of well-regulated hot and cold treatments often proves useful too. For instance, to relieve pain, swelling, congestion, and infections affecting the muscles and bones, sitz baths that alternate hot and cold water can bring effective relief. In most cases, however, specific guidance for regulating procedures will be needed from a doctor or other medical specialist to assure safe, optimal settings of the time and temperatures needed to produce the desired effect.

Fact sheets on water therapy from www.spine-health.com suggest an aquatic medium as being ideal for patients whose land-based options have become limited, especially since water offers both buoyancy and resistance when performing exercise. Although children and patients with a limited range of motion will need very careful supervision, water reduces the risks of injury from a fall while providing the support needed for friction-free movements. The latter is especially helpful in many musculoskeletal conditions, such as arthritis, where joints often remain painfully inflamed. For example, in the presence of low back pain that has worsened during walking, pool exercises provide options that range from simple routines in the shallow water to treadmills submerged in the deeper water. Often, an otherwise healthy patient can independently manage beneficial exercises by just hanging onto the side of a swimming pool in water slightly above the waist, bringing the outer knee toward the chin, holding that posture for a moment, and then reversing the position. Similarly, leg-raising exercises can be eased with the water's support, whereas the water offers strengthening resistance when merely walking in a pool near the shallow end.

In general, hydrotherapy eases gravitational pull, proving useful, therefore, in diverse situations where gravity produces strain. This includes, for instance, childbirth, when women often find that the buoyancy of water helps to relieve labor pains and ease the baby's birth. At the opposite end of life, hydrotherapy can ease the pain, stress, and discomfort of terminally ill patients. Although precautions must be taken to assure sanitary conditions free of troublesome bacteria and to adjust the temperature settings carefully for safe use, a program of hydrotherapy can bring effective treatment in helping the body to readjust its own temperature settings.

Staff. "Water Therapy Exercise Program." Available online. URL: http://www.spine-health.com/topics/conserv/water/water001.html Downloaded on June 28, 2003.

Staff. "Water Therapy Exercises." Available online. URL: http://www.spine-health.com/topics/conserv/water/water002.html Downloaded on June 28, 2003.

hyper- The addition of this prefix places the word above and beyond an established standard but does not necessarily mean a positive effect. For example, hyperactivity denotes excessive mobility and restless movements that can be difficult to handle in young children or in patients whose cognitive levels show signs of impairment. Hyperthermia results in extreme body temperature that can be threatening in the case of heat stroke, a condition that may occur during excessive weather or during sports activities. However, hyperthermia can be useful when well regulated by a trained physician or a therapist in treating various types of pain and musculoskeletal conditions.

See also HYPO-.

hypermobility syndrome See JOINT HYPERMOBILITY SYNDROME.

hypertrophy The opposite of this condition—or atrophy—means a muscle gets put to little or no use. In contrast, hypertrophy results from overuse or a continuation of strenuous exercise. A fact sheet from the Muscle Physiology Laboratory at the University of California–San Diego, explains this as beginning with "an increase in the neural drive stimulating muscle contraction." As greater demands on a muscle continue, "the message filters down to alter the pattern of protein expression" in the body, with hypertrophy occurring up to two months later. "The additional contractile proteins appear to be incorporated into existing myofibrils (the chains of sarcomeres within a muscle cell). There appears to be some limit to how large a myofibril can become: at some point, they split. These events appear to occur *within* each muscle fiber. That is, hypertrophy results primarily from the growth of each muscle cell, rather than an increase in the number of cells."

Hypertrophy can occur in body areas as varied as the adenoids, prostate, and heart muscle, but the disorder often results from a corresponding imbalance. For example, in the article "Benign Asymmetric Hypertrophy of the Masticator Muscles," published in the December 2000 *Ear, Nose and Throat Journal,* Enrique Palacios of the Louisiana State University Health Science Center discusses common instances of facial asymmetry. Assuming that clinical investigations with radiographs have eliminated other possibilities, the hypertrophy very likely has been caused by bruxism—the teeth grinding that occurs during sleep or jaw clenching during times of tension.

Some people, however, acquire hypertrophy on purpose. For instance, an individual trying to build massive muscles may have hypertrophic effects in mind. The training methods will vary from one source to the next, but the general idea entails mechanically loading the muscles to induce hypertrophy, with or without the assistance of creatine and/or other supplements. Another principle includes the frequent application of a stimulus with progressive increases in muscle loading until muscular growth has ceased. Then, the person lessens the conditioning effort and later picks up again, increasing the load until the desired effects—or the maximum level of strength—have been obtained, either of which varies from person to person and from age to age.

In investigating the later, the American College of Sports Medicine (ACSM) discusses "The Physiology of Aging" in the February 2001 *Current Comment* with these interesting comments, "Aging is not just the passage of time, but rather an accumulation of biological events that occur over a span of time. If we define aging as the loss of one's ability to adapt to a changing environment, then biological or functional age becomes a measure of one's success for adaptation." With the loss of muscle mass a concern most people experience after age 50, researchers note characteristic losses first occurring in the forearms and lower legs. Although one's age does affect muscle mass and function, the ACSM says, "Recent studies all seem to agree that elderly skeletal muscle is able to adapt to short term (12 weeks) training programs by increasing strength through muscle hypertrophy . . . and improved functional performance." One two-year study, for example, provided a training program of two sessions per week for 42 weeks followed by a 10-week time-out for testing and resting. Then another 42-week session began with three sets of exercise having 10–12 repetitions. Reportedly, strength continued to improve among men and women with no prolonged plateaus for either group. Therefore, the ACSM states, "Age should not be a limiting factor for beginning an exercise program (but that medical approval should be obtained), and that the exercises should be progressive in nature, individualized, and involve all the major muscle groups." Such training can be especially useful in maintaining posture, retaining balance, building strength, and assuring the muscular function needed for mobility and an independent life. As an added bonus, the increased circulation that comes with exercise often lessens pain.

See also ERGOGENICS; EXERCISE.

Bemben, Michael G. "The Physiology of Aging." Available online. URL: http://www.acsm.org/health+fitness/pdf/currentcomments/physio.pdf Downloaded on February 9, 2004.

Palacios, Enrique. "Benign Assymetric Hypertrophy of the Masticator Muscles." Available online. URL: http://www.findarticles.com/cf_0/m0BUM/12_79/68924385/print.jhtml Downloaded on June 27, 2003.

University of California–San Diego. "Hypertrophy." Available online. URL: http://muscle.ucsd.edu/musinfo/Hypertrophy.shtml Downloaded on January 24, 2003.

hypo- The opposite of hyper-, this prefix means that one thing is less than, under, or beneath something else, usually a particular standard. For example, hypocalcemia signifies the presence of less calcium than the body needs to maintain healthy muscles, heart tissue, and bones, whereas hypoproteinemia results from too little of the protein needed to build cells and body tissue. In hypothermia, a person's body temperature drops below normal—from 98.6 to around 95 degrees Fahrenheit, thus cooling the body to a level dangerously close to shutting down the circulatory and respiratory systems. In some cases though, highly regulated hypothermia can be used effectively in lessening blood flow during surgery or in performing specific types of musculoskeletal therapy.

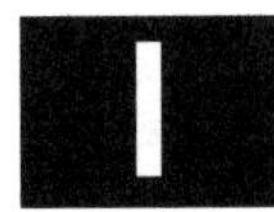

idiopathic juvenile osteoporosis Unlike its more common counterpart of juvenile osteoporosis, idiopathic juvenile osteoporosis (IJO) has no known association with any other medical condition. Nevertheless, the results of primary and secondary juvenile osteoporosis may be the same as the body resorbs more bone than the remodeling process can produce. In fact, this rare form of bone disease may not be apparent until IJO causes spontaneous fracturing in the long bones of previously healthy children, a phenomenon that generally occurs between the ages of eight and 14. Within two to four years of onset—or after the rapid growth of puberty has ceased—this disorder may go into remission as suddenly and mysteriously as it began. With the first signs usually presented in lower back pain or aching hips and feet, a pediatrician or medical team will rule out other causes that appear more likely. Once IJO has been diagnosed, however, the basic strategy—according to the National Institutes of Health Osteoporosis and Related Bone Diseases National Resource Center—will be to protect the spine and other bones from vertebral compression fractures or other types of breakage until remission occurs as, fortunately, often happens. Until then, typically protective treatments include crutches, medication, physical therapy, and other means of alleviating stress from the weight-bearing bones. Otherwise, spinal impairment or collapse of the rib cage can occur, causing permanent disability. Therefore, the sooner the detection, the better the likelihood of providing the supportive care needed.

Although a child's growth will often halt during the active presence of IJO, his or her normal growth pattern usually resumes when the disease remits. Since this does not always happen though, the National Institute of Child Health and Human Development has completed a recent study of the use of alendronate (Fosamax)—a drug that stops bone resorption—with reportedly good results. A June 4, 2003 update on the clinical trial says, "Researchers believe that children treated with alendronate will improve bone strength and decrease the amount of fractures caused by osteoporosis." This could prove to be of consequence as the child enters the later adults years, particularly in light of other studies from the National Institute of Child Health and Human Development. One says, "Even mild childhood osteoporosis may have long-term consequences since individuals who achieve a less than normal bone composition (peak bone mass) during the first 20–30 years of life may be at an increased risk for osteoporosis as adults."

See also BONE LOSS; BONE MASS; JUVENILE OSTEOPOROSIS; OSTEOGENESIS IMPERFECTA; OSTEOPOROSIS.

National Institute of Child Health and Human Development. "Treatment of Childhood Osteoporosis with Alendronate (Fosamax)." Available online. URL: http://clinicaltrials.gov/ct/gvi/show/NCT00001720?order=1 Downloaded on June 4, 2003.

iliotibial band The iliotibial band plays well on the outside of the thigh, providing the leg and knee with the stabilization needed to climb stairs, get in and out of a vehicle, or race in a marathon. If, however, a runner consistently practices on only one side of the road near the shoulder, the outside foot will always be lower, causing inflammation of the IT band. This normally tough group of fibers can also be stressed by various biomechanical abnormalities, such as an extreme pronation of the foot, discrepancy in the leg lengths, pelvic tilt, or legs that bow. When a workout focuses on strengthening quadriceps muscles, the IT band may tighten too much for comfortable flexibility. If biomechanics, overuse, or repetitive motion have strained the IT band, health information from Rice University recommends first correcting any biomechanical flaws and/or training errors and then resting the area for a while. Ice packs, massage, and gentle stretches can help to relieve the pain and restore leg function. A variety of leg-swinging and hip-rotating exercises that work each of the muscles in the legs, hips, and thighs can strength the entire region, too, and help to prevent future imbalances.

immobilization Characteristically, the human body requires not only energy but synergy, with all parts functioning well in synchronized accord. If one part suffers, all parts feel it and respond accordingly. For instance, an injury or surgery in one area can have traumatic effects elsewhere, especially since connective tissue connects one part to the next. Therefore, recovery does not depend only on the skill and promptness used in treatment but on the body's ability to remobilize again. For this reason, a primary goal in most musculoskeletal disorders will be to get a patient up and moving as quickly as possible. If that is impossible, the adverse effects of immobility will likely include edema, swelling, stiffness, and pain as the circulation slows and body fluids pool. If immobility continues unchecked, degradation of the soft tissue can lead to progressive weakening of the muscles and bones, eventually destroying cartilage or bone and causing muscles to atrophy. In addition, prolonged immobilization can lead to the haphazard healing of tissue rather than the normally parallel pattern, thus complicating matters more in a condition known as cross-linking. As these random configurations of growth cause adhesions of the soft tissue, more stiffness results in joint dysfunction or lessened range of motion. To avoid this complex sequence of events, immobility can be addressed in most cases by physical therapy and an individualized course of exercise. If not, medical options include both manual and mechanical means of providing continuous passive motion, particularly when the weight-bearing bones, such as the legs or hips, have sustained some type of damage. Should active exercise prove too painful, controlled passive motion can help to alleviate the discomfort in a slower but safer manner, thereby overcoming immobility and the multitude of problems that inactivity often brings.

See also ACTIVITY; EXERCISE.

Hammersfahr, Rick and Mark T. Serafino. "Early Motion Gets the Worm." Available online. URL: http://www.rehabpub.com/Features/32002/2.asp Downloaded on April 16, 2003.

impingement syndrome A thesaurus might offer verbs like *encroach, intrude,* or *impose* as substitutes for *impinge,* and that is what happens within the human body as one thing gets into another's space. This may occur, for instance, in the mouth when a tooth forcibly erupts through bone and tissue or when vertebrae narrow in stenosis, pressing uncomfortably against the spinal cord. Repetitive motions in an occupation or sports activity can also cause an impingement syndrome to occur in active joints. Like TENDINITIS, impingement may involve painful inflammation of the bursa sacs, called BURSITIS. If this happens to be located in a shoulder, the subsequent swelling may pinch the surrounding structure, squeezing the *rotator cuff* in a painful impingement. Besides this more common example, an impingement syndrome can also occur in the shoulder's coracoid process.

In the report "Coracoid Impingement" in the January 2000 *American Journal of Sports Medicine,* Dr. Michael F. Ferrick of the Department of Orthopaedic Surgery, Darnall Army Hospital, Fort Hood, Texas, says, "Patients with this disorder usually have localized pain anteriorly, especially with forward elevation, internal rotation, and cross arm adduction. . . . Initial treatment is non-operative and based on activity modification and physical therapy, but operative decompression may be required if conservative measures fail." In addition to analgesic pain relievers and anti-inflammatory medications, Dr. Ferrick recommends, "The first line of treatment for coracoid impingement should be a program of activity modification, with avoidance of provocative positions, and physical therapy to strengthen the rotator cuff muscles and stabilize the scapula."

Ferrick, Michael F. "Coracoid Impingement." Available online. URL: http://www.findarticles.com/cf_0/m0918/1_28/61826878/print.jhtml Downloaded on June 30, 2003.

infantile paralysis See POST-POLIO SYNDROME.

infant massage From the first arrival of an infant's wail, a nurturing parent responds by gently holding, cradling, and stroking skin so silken that one touch encourages further contact. These tactile responses aid both parent and child in establishing a bond and acquiring instant means of comfort, communication, and relief from stress. On the other hand, if a premature infant arrives with an extremely low birth weight (ELBW) of 2.2 pounds or less, the most nurturing mother may not have opportunity to provide loving contact since the baby may be whisked into neonatal care. Usually, parents will visit as soon as safely possible, yet they may feel awkward—or even terrified—when handling a tiny infant. If the parents happen to be inexperienced, their lack of confidence may further exasperate the new relationship and the more relaxed environment that are optimal for their and their child's well-being.

In addition to these immediate concerns, studies by the Agency for Healthcare Research and Quality indicate a higher prevalence of poor physical growth of ELBW babies throughout childhood and into the teen years where more catch-up growth and less health problems may finally occur. With developmental delays likely until then, however, half of the ELBW adolescents experienced functional limitations, while one-third showed less ability to participate in normal or extracurricular activities at school. Therefore, the most effective treatments might begin right after birth before further conditions have occasion to arise, thus making massage a good option to consider.

For many centuries in many countries, infant massage has been used to stimulate health and launch a close bond between parent and child. Research, though, has only recently focused on these time-proven benefits. According to experiments by the Touch Research Institutes at the University of Miami School of Medicine and the Nova Southeastern University, massaging touch can promote physiological changes, such as improved circulation and strengthened muscles in infants and children of all sizes.

In the article "Premature Infant Massage in the NICU," in the May–June 2003 issue of the *Neonatal Network*, J. M. Beachy of the Children's Hospital Newborn Special Care Unit at Doctors West, Columbus, Ohio, reports that, in the past, nurses hesitated to use this ancient and economical treatment for fear of overstimulating an infant. Indeed, if not done correctly on a frail infant or one with respiratory distress, massage could have contrary and potentially dangerous effects. With proper training and timely application, however, safe results can benefit even the tiniest newborn. For instance, recent studies show that massage therapy assists infants in gaining weight, improving their development scores, bonding with their caregivers, and receiving earlier hospital release.

Although infants with wounds or injuries should rarely be given a massage and, even then, only with high levels of medical training, parents of premature or delicate babies can be taught safe techniques by a licensed therapist who specializes in infant care. For parents in general who want an infant to experience the benefits of massage, www.infantmassage.com offers helpful tips, such as beginning with a timely moment. This automatically excludes bath time for babies under five months since bathing repeats the stimulatory effects of massage, while massaging at bedtime would be counterproductive. Otherwise, watching the baby's response matters more than clock-watching. With legs as a starting point, a massage will get off to a less-intrusive start, mainly because most infants have become accustomed to having their legs handled during a diaper change. Conversely, an unexpected attempt to massage the chest might be met with a wail of protest.

To avoid friction on a baby's sensitive skin, a pure-quality, cold-pressed vegetable cooking oil, such as sesame, safflower, or the very lightest grade of clear olive oil, can lubricate the massager's fingers and minimize chafing. Unlike mineral oil or petroleum-based products, vegetable oil can absorb well into the baby's pores for an added healthful effect, whereas perfumed lotion will irritate sensitive skin. Once the adult's trained hands have been lightly lubricated, a series of long, gentle strokes will apply minimal pressure appropriately but without being feathery or ticklish since those touches usually annoy an infant as much as they do an adult. If the baby cries, flails his or her arms in and out, or otherwise expresses displeasure, the massage should cease and another time attempted. For instance, when cradling and comforting a healthy infant, the head and spine may be lightly massaged with gentle circular motions but, again, with a keen eye on the baby's response and the positive feedback that is needed to continue.

Beachy, J. M. "Premature Infant Massage in the NICU." *Neonatal Network* 22, no. 3 (May/June 2003): 39–45.

Staff. "Infant Massage." Available online. URL: http://www.infantmassage.com.au/tips/ Downloaded on June 30, 2003.

infections of spine A microorganism, such as a virus, bacterium, or fungus, can enter the spine through an injury—or, more rarely, a surgical incision—then rapidly multiply into a primary bone infection. If the invader enters elsewhere—say, staphylococcus through a finger cut or streptococcus via a strep throat—a secondary bone infection could occur, although this would be unusual. However, primary bone infections seldom happen too.

In the report "Infections of the Spine" for www.spineuniverse.com, doctors Michael J. Young and Richard T. Holt of Spine Surgery, Louisville, Kentucky, say, "True infections are uncommon, particularly in the industrialized countries of the world. The estimated annual frequency is 0.037 for disc space infection, 0.037 for bacterial vertebral osteomyelitis and 0.037 epidural abscesses. Post-operative wound infections range from 1% after a simple discectomy to 6-8% after attempted fusion with hardware." Because of the rarity and the inconclusive symptoms, such as unrelenting back pain that could point to more likely problems, diagnostic delays can occur, especially in the absence of fever. Once a magnetic resonance imaging (MRI) scan confirms an infection, the treatment usually includes a long-term course of antibiotics, often given intravenously at first and, later, orally. If an infection results from a postoperative wound, aggressive treatment includes debridement (surgical wound cleaning), suction, or irrigation of the area as well as antibiotic therapy.

In a scientific paper, "Complex Spinal Deformities in Severe Spinal Infection," presented to the international organization for spinal surgeons, Groupe International Cotrel Dubousset, Doctors Southern, Hammerberg, and DeWald of the Spinal Surgery Section, Department of Orthopedic Surgery, Rush-Presbyterian-St. Luke's Medical Center in Chicago, Illinois, reported on their study of 57 cases and concluded, "Although most primary spinal infections can be treated non-operatively, there are situations where operative treatment becomes necessary. Our indications for surgery are neurologic compromise, intractable pain, structural instability or failure of nonoperative management to prevent progressive bony destruction." Successful management also depends on the patient's own immune system. When properly addressing a problem, though, tissue samples provide important data for identifying the organism responsible for the infection. Then debridement and bone grafting may be needed to treat a severely ill patient or surgery to correct any spinal deformities that have resulted from the infection.

See also BONE INFECTION.

Southern, Edward P., Kim W. Hammerberg, et al. "Complex Spinal Deformities in Severe Spinal Infection." Available online. URL: http://www.gicd.org/p4_96Complex.html Downloaded on June 30, 2003.

Young, Michael J. and Richard T. Holt. "Infections of the Spine." Available online. URL: http://www.spineuniverse.com/displayarticle.php/article235.html Downloaded on February 19, 2003.

inflammation In the presence of an injury, illness, infection, or allergen, the body defends the area under attack by applying pressure and putting on the heat. This response characteristically evokes redness, pain, and fever, symptoms that can be useful to a point by burning out a problem. For instance, the body's protective response to an invasion of microorganisms may include releasing natural chemicals into the area to dispose of the trespassers along with any dead tissue left in the wake of the assault. This defense system also clears the way for new growth and repair. If, however, outside help arrives too soon, the very medication intended to reduce pain or fever can suppress the body's active effort to restore itself. If a fever reducer arrives too late though, the situation can flare into a life-threatening encounter, especially for young children, frail patients, or those having a weakened immune system. Then, ice compresses or cool baths can help to keep the body temperature from rising further while sponge baths of icy water—on the pulse points only and never on the chest—can often bring a fever down with greater haste.

Because these remedial procedures require a highly watchful eye and excellent timing, they bring to mind the maxim: medicine is not a science only, but an art. Indeed, both aspects come together in detecting and treating the cause of localized inflammation, especially if a rheumatologist or a primary care physician also has reason to suspect an infectious etiology. If some type of infectious disease does exist, the standard treatment for inflammation may be exactly what is needed to cause an infection to grow! Therefore, the presence of an inexplicable inflammation—or an inflammatory response to a potential allergen or illness—may require heavy-duty surveillance by a medical professional.

For many people, inflammation of the joints can be attributed to ARTHRITIS, with the treatment depending on which of over 100 forms has been detected. Rheumatoid arthritis, for example, requires treatment as an autoimmune disease, making inflammation of the joints symptomatic, rather than the primary problem. In some types of arthritis, swelling and inflammation may indicate an accumulation of fluids in the joint, thus necessitating joint aspiration. The specific location of an inflamed area can be an important factor, too. In ankylosing spondylitis, for instance, inflammation will most likely attack the spine or large joints of the body with the accompaniment of pain and stiffness. As a representative of reactive arthritis, Reiter's syndrome presents joint inflammation as a reaction to an infection elsewhere, such as the urinary or intestinal tract, with other symptoms occurring in the eyes or skin. This means the entire situation needs medical evaluation, not just the inflamed joints. Muscles can also become inflamed, perhaps indicating viral infection or the onset of muscle disease. With such diverse possibilities for inflammatory responses in the muscles and bones, each requires medical evaluation and treatment.

See also HAND; INFLAMMATION; INFLAMMATORY MUSCLE DISEASE.

inflammatory muscle disease According to education information from the National Neuroscience Institute (NNI), inflammatory muscles disease often results "when the patient's immune system damages the body's own muscle tissues." Although children may be affected, such conditions occur more often in adults. Treatments possibly include medicines that suppress the immune system. The typical movement reported by the NNI says, "Patients with these diseases develop progressive weakness of the hip and shoulder muscles over a few weeks or months, sometimes with difficulty in swallowing."

To stimulate new research "on this uncommon and understudied family of diseases," the National Institute of Arthritis and Musculoskeletal and Skin Diseases (NIAMS) conducted a "Workshop on Inflammatory Myopathy" on April 5–6, 2000. The workshop first summarized what is presently known and then emphasized what is still unknown in an effort to marshal cooperative forces in finding more solutions. For example, attention was drawn to the role of T cells in inflammatory myopathy, the use of prednisone in easing inflammation (but with cautions of side effects), and the use of magnetic resonance imaging (MRI) in providing evidence of the biochemical state of a muscle. Focus then turned to fostering collaborative clinical trials, "perhaps through the establishment of a consortium involving both neurologists and rheumatologists, the two major medical specialties caring for myositis patients." After various presentations,

NIAMS challenged the workshop participants toward support in "(1) Better understanding of basic muscle responses to the mechanisms of injury and repair. (2) Dissection of the processes by which muscle cells are damaged and repaired in the inflammatory myopathies. (3) Deeper exploration of the role of inflammation in dystrophies and possible other muscle diseases. (4) Establishment of a collaborative clinical group."

Indeed, similar interests extend around the world. From Edinburgh, *ANCR, Advances in Clinical Neuroscience and Rehabilitation* published "Inflammatory Muscle Disease" by Gillian Hall. It discussed diagnostic concerns that include assessing the patient's age, the presence of skin rash, the condition of the autoimmune system, the location of specific muscle involvement, muscular weakness, and symmetrical versus asymmetrical presentation in muscular shape and strength. Blood analysis and radiological screening may also be deemed appropriate, while "muscle biopsy provides histological confirmation of disease." However, previous treatments may need to be reevaluated too. For instance, "Patients who fail to respond completely to long-term steroid therapy may be developing a steroid myopathy," which would, "of course, only be exacerbated by the further use of steroids." Since the early 1900s, some reports have suggested the involvement or the increased risk of cancer. "Therefore, particularly in older patients, a search for an underlying malignancy is warranted."

When reporting on this matter, a 2001 "Summaries for Patients" by the American College of Physicians—American Society of Internal Medicines states, "People with idiopathic muscle disease, such as dermatomyositis or polymyositis, are clearly at increased risk for cancer." While defining inflammatory muscle diseases, the report also offers a clarifying overview, "The muscles of the body sometimes become inflamed, resulting in symmetrical weakness of the legs and arms. When the cause of inflammation is not known, it is referred to as idiopathic. This weakness is unrelated to exercise and may be accompanied by muscle aching or tenderness. The two main types of idiopathic muscle inflammation are known as polymyositis and dermatomyositis." To investigate the reports of the additional risks of cancer, researchers examined the files from a central pathology service in Australia and then evaluated the records of 537 patients diagnosed as having idiopathic muscle inflammation. "Compared with the general population, people with dermatomyositis had a sixfold higher risk for cancer, and people with polymyositis had a twofold higher risk."

Buchbinder, R., A. Forbes, et al. "Incidence of Malignant Disease in Biopsy-Proven Inflammatory Myopathy. A Population-Based Cohort Study." *Annals of Internal Medicine* 134, (June 19, 2001): 1,087–1,095.

Hall, Gillian. "Inflammatory Muscle Disease." *ANCR, Advances in Clinical Neuroscience and Rehabilitation* 2, no. 2 (May/June 2002): 2,002–2,003.

National Institute of Arthritis and Musculoskeletal and Skin Diseases. "Workshop on Inflammatory Myopathy." Available online. URL: http://www.niams.nih.gov/ne/reports/sci_wrk/2000/myoreportsummary.htm Downloaded on July 1, 2003.

inheritance See BIRTH DEFECTS; GENETIC FACTORS.

injury When an initial injury receives improper care, secondary injury can result. If given adequate time and treatment though, a healing response typically begins in the tissue as inflammation prepares the way for body repairing and remodeling. At first, the damaged areas seems to hug around itself, sealing off with vasoconstriction to conserve blood pressure and blood clotting to guard blood flow. This is followed by a release of innate chemicals primitively ready to duke it out with whatever gets in the way. Redness around the site occurs as histamine collects, and hemorrhaging causes swelling. The temperature may rise, and irritated nerve endings send pain signals in case the mind forgets—all of which restrict joint mobility and muscle activity as warning signs to stay put. Eventually though, damage control ceases, and repairs begin as countless cells and substances remove dead tissue and then reorganize the body's effort into reconstructing muscle and remodeling bone.

Depending on the severity of an injury, the often-recommended RICE method of Rest, Ice, Compression, and Elevation assists the recuperative period by calming down the body and alleviating discomfort. In "What to Do for Simple Athletic Injuries," the Yale Sports Medicine Center page recommends RICE for at least 48–72 hours with "under no circumstances" warnings regarding heat of any kind during this time, including hot baths and showers that can increase swelling and inflammation. Regarding rest, Yale has this word of caution, "Stop the activity, immediately! To prolong stopping could cause further damage to the injured part." Ice, too, should be applied as soon as possible for 20–30 minutes every hour or so to control swelling and decrease muscle spasms. During and between ice treatments, compression of the injured area helps to minimize swelling with an elastic bandage or tape wrapped firmly—but not tightly enough to hinder circulation or cause tingling and numbness. Prior to rest or sleep, the wrap can be loosened a bit more with the injured part elevated above heart level to drain surfeit fluids from the site and further reduce the swelling.

Because the musculoskeletal system has so many moving parts, injuries can come through overuse or overextension as athletes, office workers, and equipment operators will attest. For example, a baseball player who practices and plays a game with the same throwing arm may become aware of the drawbacks of repetitive motion as compression occurs on the outside of the elbow and tension on the inside. If an overextended throw contributes to the problem, ligaments may stretch, and, over time, bone spurs may erupt at the damaged site. In addition to RICE treatment, severe cases may require surgery to reconstruct a joint or tighten the pulled area. Alternatively, if the shoulder or rotator cuff has an impingement, this too may require surgery with physical therapy needed to get back into the game and keep a player playing.

Through use, wear and tear, or the normal processes of aging, the body's many joints, ligaments, tendons, muscles, and bones often experience injury. Accidents also occur with spinal vertebrae receiving the jolt of a whiplash or bones breaking. In the wintertime, for instance, snow skiing accidents top the list with 278,730 injuries in 2001, according to the U.S. Consumer Product Safety Commission. Snowboarders tallied 164,261 injuries and ice hockey players scored 41,438 injuries that same year. Although most of the damage resulted in sprains and strains, dislocated joints and fractured bones sometimes required long-term medical care. To avoid such problems, the American Academy of Orthopaedic Surgeons joined forces with the Prevent Injuries America! program, urging people of all ages to follow five basic guidelines. Know and abide by the rules of the sport. Wear appropriate gear for protection. Check equipment and know how to use it. Warm up before playing. When feeling tired or in pain, avoid participating in a sport or any other activity that requires heightened alertness and agility.

Accidents and injuries do not just happen during play, though. In the guest editorial "Injury Prevention: Blurring the Distinctions Between Home and Work" published in *IP Online, Injury Prevention,* Dr. G. S. Smith of the Liberty Mutual Research Institute for Safety writes, "In today's global business environment, with its increasing number of self-employed, contractual, and home-based workers, many workplaces are not covered by regulatory agencies, such as the Occupational Safety Health Administration. The rapid growth of telecommuting, for example, presents some unique health and safety challenges. Given the changing nature of the workplace, a new, comprehensive community approach to injury prevention is needed, one which takes into account the blurring of the lines between work and non-work environments that is increasingly prevalent in society."

See also ERGONOMICS; FRACTURES; REPETITIVE MOTION DISORDERS; SAFETY; WHIPLASH.

Smith, G. S. "Injury Prevention: Blurring the Distinctions Between Home and Work." Available online. URL: http://ip.bmjjournals.com/cgi/content/Full/9/1/3. Downloaded on June 6, 2003.

intoeing When seeing feet point toward each other, some have dubbed this condition as *pigeon* *toes*—a common occurrence in young children that may, or may not, be outgrown. Either way, a primary problem can be in getting shoes to fit, although some children also experience twisting of the tibia (leg bone) or femur (thighbone), which could present a cause for surgery. For most children, however, braces, special shoes, or orthotics will correct this usually painless problem. Therapeutic foot stretches may also help when given according to the pediatrician's or podiatrist's instructions. According to the American Academy of Family Physicians, a cast may also be required, but most children present straighter feet and legs by age six to eight. If not, the American Orthopaedic Foot and Ankle Society recommends surgery only if the child is eight to 10 with a persistent problem causing significant concerns in walking.

See also FEET OR FOOT; FOOTWEAR; GAIT.

intradiskal electrothermal therapy (IDET) Healthcare information from Emory University calls intradiskal electrothermal therapy IDET "a novel, minimally invasive procedure to relieve back pain caused by degeneration to the disks in the low back." From the University of Chicago Spine Center, doctors F. Todd Wetzel and Thomas A. McNally reported on the "Treatment of Chronic Discogenic Low Back Pain with Intradiskal Electrothermal Therapy" in the *Journal of the American Academy of Orthopaedic Surgeons,* saying, "Chronic discogenic low back pain is difficult to treat. Nonsurgical care is the rule for most patients. When this fails, IDET may offer an alternative between the extremes of continued nonsurgical therapy and lumbar spinal fusion. Preliminary data are encouraging, with reported therapeutic success rates of 60% to 80%. Given the limitations of study design in reports to date, however, additional clinical data continue to be collected."

Wetzel, F. Todd and Thomas A. McNally. "Treatment of Chronic Discogenic Low Back Pain with Intradiskal Electrothermal Therapy." *Journal of the American Academy of Orthopaedic Surgeons* 11, no. 1 (January/February 2003): 6–11.

intramuscular hematoma Following a blow or injury, bleeding can occur within the muscle but usually reabsorbs into the body within five to 42 days, disappearing entirely within three to five months. In an acute or a chronic hematoma, however, the clinical task will be to rule out a tumor of the soft tissue, assuming blood coagulation time has been shown to be normal.

See also MUSCLE CONTUSION.

inversion The opposite of eversion, this joint movement points the big toe up and away from the body.

See also EVERSION; RANGE OF MOTION.

iron Some people with musculoskeletal problems pump iron to build strength, while others need to consume iron. Some, however, may be consuming too much. For example, a group of doctors from the Departments of Environmental Health, Neurology, and Epidemiology and also the University of Washington School of Medicine in Seattle, Washington, presented a paper in the June 10, 2003 *Neurology,* warning of the particular risks to Parkinson's disease patients from ingesting high levels of iron with high manganese intake. Previously, the February 22, 2001 release from the Public Information Committee for the American Society for Nutritional Sciences and the American Society for Clinical Nutrition said iron deficiency may be "common among non-elderly persons throughout the world, but many elderly Americans have too much—rather than not enough—iron in their body," with men being twice as likely as women. Although the Public Information Committee said further investigation would be needed to show which specific foods often elevate levels of iron, the study showed that one-fifth of the total daily iron intake came from iron-fortified cereals consumed by participants whose ages ranged from 67 to 96.

Age can be an important factor in having too much iron or too little, as most often happens with women of childbearing age. With heavy monthly periods, women can lose considerably more iron since two-thirds of this essential mineral resides in the hemoglobin of the blood. Besides excessive blood loss, iron deficiency anemia can result from low dietary intake, inadequate absorption, and lack of supportive vitamins, such as vitamin A, which helps to activate iron, or vitamin C, which helps the body to absorb iron. If an iron deficiency does occur, the presenting signs may include fatigue, weakness, inability to concentrate, fluctuations in body temperature, and lowered resistance in the immune system. However, an underlying medical problem of the musculoskeletal system may also be at work, for instance in a chronic inflammatory disorder. In such cases, management of the condition by a rheumatologist or other specialist will be essential in getting the anemia under control, particularly since dietary iron and supplements do not address the causative factor.

For most people, the biggest issues in absorbing dietary iron relate to what type of iron has been consumed, how much the body has already stored, and whether anything interferes with its absorption. For instance, the body usually absorbs heme iron quickly from dietary sources, such as meat, fish, and poultry. Less absorption, though, generally occurs of the nonheme iron found in lentils, beans, cereals, and grains. Moreover, sources such as calcium, soybeans, and the tannins in tea can further reduce the body's utilization of nonheme iron. Therefore, reading product labels and noting the recommended dietary allowance (RDA) guides to the daily intake of iron and other nutrients remain highly significant. However, an optimal guide might include consuming a daily assortment of fresh foods with the variety changing from one day to the next to assure a balanced diet.

See also NUTRITION.

Powers, K. M., T. Smith-Weller, et al. "Parkinson's Disease Risks Associated with Dietary Iron, Manganes and Other Nutrient Intakes." Available online. URL: http://www.ncbi.nlm.nih.gov/entrez/query.fcgi?cmd=Retrieve&db=PubMed&list_uids=127 Downloaded on July 1, 2003.

Wood, Richard J. "For Many Elderly Americans Who Have Excess Iron in their Body, Taking Iron Supplements is Unnecessary and May be Dangerous." Available online. URL: http://www.faseb.org/ascn.march01pr.htm Downloaded on May 5, 2003.

isometric exercise This type of exercise works toward toning muscle and strengthening bone density but without any joint movement, an important consideration for those with arthritis or other painful disorders affecting the joints. One isometric example might be tightening the buttocks, holding that position for five to six seconds, releasing the tension, and repeating five to 10 times. An isometric exercise might also be pushing against a wall or walking through the resistance of waist-high water in a swimming pool. However, in the article "Isometric Exercise Introduced," on www.fitnesszone.co.za, Dr. Jeremy Sims of the U.K. cautions, "If you suffer from heart disease or raised blood pressure, you should stay clear of isometric training. During muscular contractions in this form of exercise, blood pressure can rise quite profoundly."

Sims, Jeremy. "Isometric Exercise Introduced." Available online. URL: http://www.fitnesszone.co.za/strength3.htm Downloaded on July 1, 2003.

isotonic exercise Unlike isometrics, an isotonic exercise utilizes joint movement with corresponding muscles contracting, such as occurs in doing push-ups or lifting weights. The primary caution here involves developing one set of muscles at the expense of others.

See also EXERCISE.

isthmic spondylolisthesis See DEGENERATIVE DISK DISEASE; HERNIATED DISK.

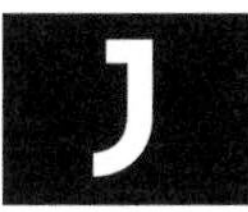

jaw The upper jawbone of the maxilla, which extends from the top teeth to the eyes, normally provides an excellent partner for the lower mandible—the largest, strongest, and only movable bone in the face. For most people, the jaw shows strength, character, and, sometimes, a set purpose, including a stage for grinding one's teeth, reciting a poem, singing, or speaking out persuasively. However, a malformation can disrupt these structural effects as well as the jaw's function. In an early embryonic state, for example, the right and left sides of the mandible may fail to fuse, resulting in a cleft jaw that's both unsightly and troubling to one's health.

According to the American Association of Oral and Maxillofacial Surgeons, over 10 million people suffer from various degrees of jaw deformity. A severe case, for instance, may involve a lack of bone formation, as happened with a boy missing half his jaw at birth. In "The Rib Bone that Transformed into a Jaw Bone: An Amazing Miracle in Jaw Surgery!" the September 12, 2000 *PR Newswire* reported of the condition, telling of a four-inch section of rib removed from the child's own body and then sculpted, grafted into place, and secured with titanium pins. Since the procedure did not require wiring, the boy could speak and eat within the week. A 10-year follow-up later assured the innovative surgeon, Dr. Mansoor Madani of Temple University in Philadelphia, Pennsylvania, that the boy's face had remained symmetrical with the rib-jaw replacement growing at the same rate as the opposite side, thus allowing normal function of the TEMPOROMANDIBULAR JOINT (TMJ).

At the opposite extreme, even slight TMJ dysfunction may cause different levels of discomfort, dental problems, and/or headaches. A distracting jaw click can make speaking be problematic, too. Depending on the severity of the condition, a course of treatment with chiropractic adjustment or acupuncture may help. However, an uncorrected jaw dysfunction generally means the person will have some degree of difficulty in eating, sipping fluids, or swallowing. An improper bite also affects a patient's oral health to such an extent that the American Association of Oral and Maxillofacial Surgeons (AAOMS) reports that around 24 million adults in this country completely lack teeth. This may, of course, be due to poor nutrition and/or poor hygiene of teeth and gums, but jaw irregularities can perpetuate problems until, over time, even a new set of dentures may be unable to provide a comfortable fit. If a severe shrinkage of the jawbone has occurred—as may eventually happen after the teeth have been removed—grafting may be required to establish a stable foundation for denture wear. Replacement of bone may also be needed to provide a secure structure for imbedding dental implants or for attaching a partial denture or a dental bridge. With the continuation of an irregular bite, however, eating may become less and less appealing.

In addition to these health concerns, a person may be displeased with the way a jaw irregularity affects the facial alignment. For example, a vertical imbalance may give the appearance of a toothless smile, while a horizontal imbalance may cause the chin to project in a pugilistic look or, conversely, recede into a weak chin. When discussing the surgical options for these conditions, a fact sheet entitled "Cosmetic Orthognathic Surgery (Alteration of the Jaws)" by the Mayo Clinic in Rochester, New York, states, with the parentheses theirs, "The goal of treatment is to shorten or lengthen the horizontal, vertical, or transverse dimensions of the jaw so that the facial soft tissue, teeth, and other facial structures are in proper functional and aesthetic balance. Other surgical and medical evaluations also may be required to assess associated cosmetic (skin, nose, and neck) and functional (speech, airway, sleep) problems."

An immediate cosmetic concern may draw a person into considering corrective surgery, but a long-range bonus comes in orthodontic treatments that usually accompany reconstruction of the jaw. Correcting such problems earlier in life will undoubtedly help a person to avoid the malnutrition that sometimes comes with aging. Moreover, correcting a jaw abnormality can have a positive outcome on one's sleep. This does not, however, always mean a need for surgery. In reporting on this topic as studied by J. Pancer, S. Al-Faifi, M. Al-Faifi, and V. Hoffstein of the University of Toronto, the article "How Effective Are Oral Appliances for Managing Snoring and Sleep Apnea?" appeared in the May 2000 issue of *Journal of Respiratory Diseases.* When the 75 patients in the control group used a mandibular advancement appliance as a nonsurgical means of repositioning the jaw, the sleep "apnea/hypopnea index fell from 44 to 12 events per hour, and the arousal index fell from 37 to 16 events per hour," thereby exhibiting an improvement in sleep conditions. Apparently, the participants' mates experienced these benefits too, as the formerly frequent loud snoring of their partners dropped from 96 percent to only 2 percent.

Without such mechanical devices to assist its forward positioning, the lower jaw typically recedes during sleep and, likewise, during times of trauma, such as when an unconscious victim is on the scene. Then, an adjustment similar to mandibular advancement may be manually required through jaw thrust, a maneuver that glides the jaw forward to open the airway, thus enabling the unconscious person to breathe or to receive cardiopulmonary resuscitation (CPR) should that be needed.

With most victims usually awake to notice, an accident or injury to the face will more likely damage, break, or dislocate a jaw. If a break occurs on one side of the mandible, quite likely the opposite side will show breakage, too, according to the National Institutes of Health (NIH.) However, if damage takes place in the maxilla (upper jaw), the injury may be severe enough to affect other areas of the face, neck, or brain. Breathing may also be distressed, further necessitating a 911 call and prompt treatment by a trained medical professional. If the victim has to be transported, the broken or dislocated jaw should be immobilized by cradling in the hands or securing with a wide elastic bandage, a towel, or other nearby workable source of fabric slipped beneath the jaw and tied atop the head.

Damage can come about because of a motor accident, industrial accident, assault, sports injury, or other mishap, but the NIH reports the most common cause of a broken or dislocated jaw occurs through a traumatic blow to the face. Then, restorative surgery may be required to reconstruct facial structures. If the reconstructive process includes a jaw implant, for example, that specific aspect of the restoration process may take one to two hours of surgery, during which time the surgeon creates pockets inside the mouth by making incisions near the lower part of the bottom lip. According to "Facial Implants," from the American Society of Plastic Surgeons, risks of that particular procedure include bleeding, infection, and, possibly, the eventual shifting of the implant. In most types of cosmetic and reconstructive surgery, however, some temporary swelling and bruising can be expected as can difficulty in smiling, talking, and eating for a while. For instance, a soft or liquid diet may be needed for four to six weeks with restricted movement of the lower jaw. Shortly thereafter, orthodontic treatments may begin with the length of time depending on the work needed to assure jaw stability and function. In the process, overall health conditions usually improve too.

See also BIRTH DEFECTS; CLEFT LIP AND PALATE; DISLOCATED JOINT; FRACTURES.

American Association of Oral and Maxillofacial Surgeons. "What Is Oral and Maxillofacial Surgery?" Available online. URL: http://www.aaoms.org/public/Pamphlets/whatisoms.pdf Downloaded on July 18, 2003.

American Society of Plastic Surgeons. "Facial Implants." Available online. URL: http://www.plasticsurgery.org/public_education/procedures/index.cfm Downloaded on July 2, 2003.

Mayo Clinic. "Alterations of the Jaws (Cosmetic Orthognathic Surgery)." Available online. URL: http://www.mayoclinic.org/orthognathicsurgery-rst/index.html Downloaded on February 9, 2004.

National Institutes of Health. "Medical Encyclopedia: Jaw—Broken or Dislocated." Available online. URL: http://www.nim.nih.gov/medlineplus/ency/article/000019.htm Downloaded on July 2, 2003.

Pancer, J., S. Al-Faifi, et al. "How Effective Are Oral Appliances for Managing Snoring and Sleep Apnea?" Available online. URL: http://www.findarticles.com/cf_0/m0BS0/5_21/63768253/print.jhtml Downloaded on July 2, 2003.

PR Newswire. "The Rib Bone that Transformed into a Jaw Bone: An Amazing Miracle in Jaw Surgery." Available online. URL: http://www.findarticles.com/cf_0/m4PRN/2000_Sept_12/65149866/print.jhtml Downloaded on July 2, 2003.

joint As the 206 bones of the body come together at various angles and junctions, each articulation creates a joint that is either movable or is not. Those capable of movement can accomplish one (or more) of four possible actions: (1) a gliding motion, (2) an angular motion, (3) circumduction, or (4) rotation. In a gliding motion, for example, one bone slides along another in ideally a smooth movement, such as occurs in the jaw when the tongue feels for an achy tooth or the lower lip juts into a pout. In the angular motion that occurs between the long bones of the arms or legs, the joint angle increases or decreases with flexion and extension—for instance, as a person lifts an object overhead or kicks a soccer ball. In circumduction, a long bone circumscribes a circle, such as when shoulder movement allows an arm to wind up for a baseball pitch. In the action of rotation, joint movement occurs inward and outward, such as happens with the elbow when swatting the birdie in a badminton game or waving good-bye in a windshield wiper motion.

These four little moves make a tremendous variety of activities possible. However, to make possible the moves themselves requires three of the body's four kinds of joints. That fourth or remaining type of joint belongs to the immovable category, such as the fixed joints that occur in the little vertebrae naturally fused together in the lower part of the spine. Also, the sutures of the skull articulate as fixed joints, absorbing shock but permitting almost no movement once a baby's fontanels have ossified at around 18–24 months of age. Otherwise, the movable joints throughout the body move descriptively as a hinge joint, a pivot joint, or a ball-and-socket joint, depending on the size and shape of bone involved and the movement needed.

With structure and function working cooperatively for most people most of the time, the body's largest, heaviest hinge joint comes together in each knee, either of which, expectedly, encounters the most common occurrences of injuries. Elbows also have their damaging moments, especially since two types of junctions occur in a hinge joint and a pivot joint that meet in that small space, synchronizing the effort toward activity. The highly versatile ball-and-socket joint, however, can outperform every other joint in the body, with the shoulder capable of the most complete range of motion. With slightly less possibility of movement than found in a mobile shoulder, the hip's ball-and-socket joint carries full body weight, which also makes it a strong candidate for damage.

Fortunately, the body has protective devices to shield and stabilize each joint during times of heightened activity. For instance, the bones themselves may come capped with tough cartilage. To protect the movable joints further—also known as the synovial joints—a lining of synovial membrane covers the inside of each joint capsule, which fills with a lubricative synovial fluid. For added support and protection, sturdy ligaments steady the joints and keep them in alignment. Tendons attach the muscles needed for action, muscles that also pad the bones protectively should a fall occur. As if these efforts were not enough, the body also supplies sacs filled with more lubricating fluids and then places those bursas among the muscles, tendons, and bones near the joints in a joint effort similar to packaging a person's moving parts in a unique form of bubble wrap.

See also BURSITIS; RANGE OF MOTION.

joint aspiration/injection Each of these endeavors involves the therapeutic insertion of a needle into a joint, often with the same goal of reducing pain, but, nevertheless, with a reversal of procedures. Aspiration (also known as arthrocentesis) draws fluid from a joint, either to relieve pressure or to obtain a sample for testing the conditions that may be causing a joint to swell. Conversely, an injection has the opposite action of inserting some type of liquid into the joint for medicinal purposes. In an August 2001 fact sheet discussing both instances, the American College of Rheumatology (ACR) explains, with the parentheses their own, "Fluid obtained from a joint aspiration can be sent for laboratory analysis, which may include a cell count (the number of white or red blood cells), crystal analysis (so as to confirm the presence of gout or pseudogout), and/or culture (to determine if an infection is present inside the joint.) Drainage of a large joint effusion can provide pain relief and improved mobility. Injection of a drug in the joint may yield complete or short-term relief of symptoms."

With the most likely joints either being weight bearing or the small joints in the hands, joint injections usually insert an anti-inflammatory medication or a corticosteroid directly into the site to treat painful conditions, such as rheumatoid arthritis. In a degenerative disease, such as osteoarthritis, an injection may be used to lubricate a joint inflamed due to the friction often caused by dryness. Regardless of whether a test or a treatment consists of injections or joint aspiration, the most common side effects include an allergic reaction to anything from the skin cleanser used to prepare the site to the typically small amount of bandaging tape applied afterward to the medication itself. Other risks involve "post-injection flare," which presents "joint swelling and pain several hours after the corticosteroid injections," a side effect the ACR says "occurs in one out of 50 patients and usually subsides within several days." Whether long-term joint damage will result from the frequent use of corticosteroid injections remains to be proven, but another risk includes inadvertently rupturing the tendon near the injection site. However, an infection seldom arises after a joint injection, according to statistics from the ACR, with about one in 15,000 patients experiencing this risk.

American College of Rheumatology. "Joint Aspiration." Available online. URL: http://www.rheumatology.org/patients/Factsheet/injection.html Downloaded on February 17, 2003.

joint hypermobility syndrome As a characteristic feature of this hereditary condition, a joint readily moves beyond its expected RANGE OF MOTION. Sometimes the excessive movement indicates the presence of an underlying disorder, such as MARFAN SYNDROME or Ehlers-Danlos syndrome, the latter of which affects elastic connective tissue throughout the body as primarily exhibited through the skin. In investigating still another possibility, researchers at Johns Hopkins Medical Institutions reported their findings in the September 6, 2002 release entitled "Flexible Joints Associated with Chronic Fatigue Syndrome" (CFS). According to this medical report, children and teens with CFS are 3.5 times more likely than their peers to have hyperflexible joints. However, the lead researcher, Dr. Peter C. Rowe, professor of pediatrics at the Johns Hopkins Children's Center, also says, "We know that about 20 percent of healthy adolescents have joint hypermobility, but clearly most do not go on to develop CFS" More likely, perhaps, may be the development of talents that use this extraordinary flexibility to a positive effect, such as in the heightened performance of a dancer, tennis player, acrobat, pianist, or other virtuoso.

A fact sheet, "Hypermobility Syndrome," prepared for the University of Miami School of Medicine by William C. Shiel Jr., M.D., F.A.C.P., F.A.C.R., says, "Signs of the syndrome are the ability to place the palms of the hands on the floor with the knees fully extended, hyperextension of the knee or elbow beyond 10 degrees, and the ability to touch the thumb to the forearm." Although such feats may seem enviable to those who experience the opposite condition of joint immobility, hypermobility can also result in pain as joints overextend. Higher instances of scoliosis can occur as can as injuries, such as a dislocation or a sprain, resulting from the extra movement of a joint. Dr. Shiel goes on to say, however, that joint hypermobility syndrome will sometimes improve as a child enters the adult years.

Information from the Hypermobility Syndrome Association in Bristol, England, explains that the differences in the formation of connective tissue proteins, such as collagen, give hypermobile joints greater laxity in movement, which, correspondingly, makes them more susceptible to injury. Additionally, the stretchy ligaments often cause the muscles to work harder to keep joints properly aligned, thus evoking pain and muscle spasms or causing the person to experience recurrent falls.

In his article "Pain and the Hypermobility Syndrome," for The Hypermobility Syndrome Association's Web site, Dr. Rodney Grahame, emeritus professor of rheumatology at University College Hospital in London, says, "A little known fact is that hypermobility occurs in many individuals in a few joints only. It does not necessarily have to affect all of one's joints." This, too, can present problems, of course, because of the excessive wear and tear that gives a person the propensity toward arthritic conditions. However, Dr. Grahame further suggests that persons with joint hypermobility syndrome "in addition to their proneness to injury, dislocation, and osteoarthritis, may also have a fault in the way their pain signals are picked up for onward transmission to the brain, where they reach consciousness." Since a possible correlation between the brain and pathways of pain has been noted elsewhere, researchers have apparently begun to focus on this potential aspect of joint hypermobility syndrome(s) with more clinical studies of the complex issues hopefully forthcoming.

Grahame, Rodney. "Pain and the Hypermobility Syndrome." Available online. URL: http://www.hypermobility.org/painandhms.php Downloaded on June 28, 2003.

Johns Hopkins Medical Institutions. "Flexible Joints Associated With Chronic Fatigue Syndrome." Available online. URL: http://www.hopkinsmedicine.org/press/2002/September/020906A.htm Downloaded on July 3, 2003.

Shiel, William C. "Hypermobility Syndrome." Available online. URL: http://med.miami.edu/patients/glossary/art.asp?print=yes+articlekey=390 Downloaded on June 28, 2003.

joint movement See RANGE OF MOTION.

joint replacement Accidents, birth defects, degenerative joint disease, and general wear and tear make joint replacement surgery a viable option in reconstructing a joint, restoring function, and removing pain. Also known as arthroplasty, the success of joint replacement surgery may depend on more than the surgeon's skill and experience. For example, a wrist joint replacement typically eliminates pain and increases mobility but does not necessarily return full range of motion, especially if the procedure includes fusion. New prosthetic designs, however, have begun to address these concerns as researchers develop cementless wrist implants capable of improving both mobility and strength in the hand.

In a February 2003 press briefing, the American Academy of Orthopaedic Surgeons discussed advancements in minimally invasive surgery (MIS) for use in repairing hips, knees, and shoulders. Orthopedic surgeon Kristaps J. Keggi, who developed an MIS technique used with more than 6,000 patients over 10 years, was quoted as saying, "Minimally invasive surgery for total hip arthroplasty has reliably shown in thousands of patients to lead to smaller incisions, less blood loss, fewer complications, and an earlier rehabilitation than traditional total hip arthroplasty."

As arthritis or other conditions bear down on the weight-bearing joints, the instances of pain will increase, breaking into sleep cycles but, less noticeably perhaps, breaking down bone until a joint becomes progressively more restricted or misshapen. Then, a timely question may be asked, as happens in the article "Is It Time for Joint Replacement?" in *Focus on Healthy Aging* published by the Mount Sinai School of Medicine. To help people to know for themselves whether the time has come for arthroplasty, Dr. Marvin Gilbert, Clinical Professor of Orthopedic Surgery at the Mount Sinai School of Medicine, responds, "It is an operation meant to relieve pain and improve the quality of your life. The only indication for it is your decision that the arthritis is interfering enough so that you can't do the things you want to do—that it interferes with your quality of life." Although this varies according to each person's age, level of pain, the severity of the condition, and other circumstances, such as income, independence, and job responsibilities, Dr. Gilbert offers another decisive word, "It's possible to delay surgery, but in most cases it's more advantageous to have the procedure before the bone ends have begun to break down or the joint has begun to become deformed. In other words, it's better if you can still walk on your own in the surgeon's office for an evaluation."

American Academy of Orthopaedic Surgeons. "Minimally Invasive Surgery May Improve Outcomes for Patients Undergoing Joint Repair." Available online. URL: http://www. Newswise.com/articles/2003/2/MINEVAS.OSR.htm Downloaded on February 14, 2003.

School of Medicine, Mount Sinai. "Is It Time for Joint Replacement?" *Focus on Healthy Aging* 6, no. 4 (April 2003): 1–2.

jumper's knee See TENDINITIS OR TENDONITIS.

juvenile arthritis Across America, 300,000 children live with some type of arthritis or rheumatic disease. Either condition profoundly affects young lives by limiting a child's abilities to perform simple tasks. By age 18–44, however, those numbers rise—one boy or girl at a time—to 8.4 million arthritis sufferers, according to the Arthritis Foundation, with millions more at risk for its development. How can this happen? With causes generally unknown, researchers have noticed certain genetic markers appearing more commonly in childhood arthritis. However, the condition offers no indications of being inherited and rarely occurs more than once in a family. Juvenile arthritis may also challenge detection because of symptoms similar to the normal GROWING PAINS. For instance, a child may experience stiffness upon awakening or a reluctance to use a limb. Pain, fever, and fatigue may occur with lessened mobility. If left untreated, a progressively worsening condition can cause joint deformity or stunted growth.

According to a fact sheet, "What Is Juvenile Arthritis?" from the American College of Rheumatology, "A number of other conditions can mimic juvenile arthritis, such as infections, childhood malignancies, musculoskeletal conditions, or other less common rheumatic disease." Treatment can be tricky too because some medications used for adult arthritis have not been approved for children by the U.S. Food and Drug Administration (FDA), while other drugs can have adverse effects on normal growth. The type of medicines and therapies chosen for each individual, however, will depend on the type of arthritis exhibited. To alleviate overall symptoms and strengthen young muscles and bones, a program of nutrition, exercise, and physical or occupational therapy can help to prevent disability. Although devices, such as splints, may be needed, regular participation in school events whenever possible will help to give a child valuable opportunities for normal activities, the development of social skills, and a means of building self-confidence. Regardless of the treatment deemed best for a particular child, the cooperative efforts of parents and a pediatric team specializing in rheumatology can work toward remission but with ongoing considerations of each specific individual. To assist further, some state agencies and vocational rehabilitation programs can provide resources for a family who needs help in managing the costs and the very best treatments available for their child.

See also JUVENILE RHEUMATOID ARTHRITIS; NUTRITION.

American College of Rheumatology. "What Is Juvenile Arthritis?" Available online. URL: http://www.rheumatology.org/patients/factsheet/jra.html Downloaded on February 17, 2003.

juvenile osteoporosis When this rare condition occurs among children and adolescents, another underlying medical condition usually proves to be the causing factor. According to a fact sheet on this topic by the National Institutes of Health

Osteoporosis and Related Bone Diseases National Resource Center, some common medical disorders that affect bone health in children may include JUVENILE ARTHRITIS, diabetes mellitus, OSTEOGENESIS IMPERFECTA (more often known as brittle bone disease), hyperthyroidism, hyperparathyroidism, Cushing's syndrome, malabsorption syndromes, anorexia nervosa, or kidney disease. Since the symptoms and treatments vary according to the primary cause, a rheumatologist and a team of pediatric specialists will provide an individual course of action. Besides juvenile osteoporosis—or secondary osteoporosis, as it may also be known—the primary condition of IDIOPATHIC JUVENILE OSTEOPOROSIS has no known disease as the underlying source of bone problems.

See also ANOREXIA AND BONE LOSS.

Osteoporosis and Related Bone Diseases National Resource Center. "Juvenile Osteoporosis." Available online. URL: http://www.osteo.org/newfile.asp?doc=r609I&doctitle=Juvenile+Osteoporosis Downloaded on June 28, 2003.

juvenile rheumatoid arthritis The most common form of arthritis in children, juvenile rheumatoid arthritis (JRA) may present only mild symptoms yet incur some serious complications, such as inflammatory eye disease that can lead to blindness. As the fact sheet "Juvenile Rheumatoid Arthritis" by the Arthritis Foundation elucidates, including the parentheses, four major changes may develop in a joint, with characteristic features of JRA being "joint inflammation, joint contracture (stiff, bent joint), joint damage and/or alteration or change in growth. Other symptoms include joint stiffness following rest or decreased activity level (also referred to as morning stiffness or gelling), and weakness in muscles and other soft tissues around the involved joints." Each child, of course, will experience symptoms in varying degrees with one day dissimilar to the next. When other diseases have been ruled out, however, a diagnosis can usually be made if arthritis has persisted in one or more joint for a minimum of six weeks. Questions then turn to which type of arthritis the child has encountered and what kind of treatment will prove most effective in relieving the pain and encouraging normal childhood growth and activities.

To clarify the situation, a fact sheet, "What Is Juvenile Arthritis?" from the American College of Rheumatology (ACR) says, "Juvenile arthritis is a chronic condition that causes inflammation in one or more joints and begins before the age of 16. . . . Though all have joint inflammation in common, they behave very differently, may require different treatment approaches, and have different outcomes." Of the different patterns involved, ACR also says, "*Systemic onset type* begins with very high fevers, frequently has a skin rash and shows evidence of inflammation in many internal organ systems as well as the joints. About 10 percent of children with arthritis will have this type. *Pauciarticular onset disease* affects fewer than five joints. About half of all children with arthritis are in this category. Some of these are very young, from infancy to about age five, and have a risk of developing inflammatory eye problems. Regular eye exams are essential. Others are older and may evolve into one of the adult forms of arthritis. *Polyarticular disease* has more than five joints affected (often many more) and can begin at any age. Some of these children have adult type rheumatoid arthritis that begins at an earlier age than usual."

Formerly, JRA presented no clear diagnostic tools nor clear course of action. However, after collaborating with physicians from 14 countries over a three-year period, the American College of Rheumatology recently approved criteria for the ACR Pediatric 30—the standard by which those who treat JRA can now measure the improvements in each child. It is hoped these valuable guidelines will help to manage the disease and provide a baseline for evaluating what works and what does not in developing an individualized course of treatment.

American College of Rheumatology. "What is Juvenile Arthritis?" Available online. URL: http://www.rheumatology.org/patients/factsheet/jra.html Downloaded on February 17, 2003.

Arthritis Foundation. "Juvenile Rheumatoid Arthritis." Available online. URL: http://www.arthritis.org/conditions/DiseaseCenter/jra.asp Downloaded on July 4, 2003.

juvenile spondyloarthropathy syndromes In these related syndromes affecting nine- to 11-year-old boys more often than girls of similar age, joint swelling typically occurs in the lower extremities, such as the hips. Although blood tests may help to rule out other types of diseases, they do nothing to identify members of juvenile spondyloarthropathy syndromes, which include juvenile forms of ANKYLOSING SPONDYLITIS, REITER'S SYNDROME, and other types of ARTHRITIS, many of which have been addressed under separate entries.

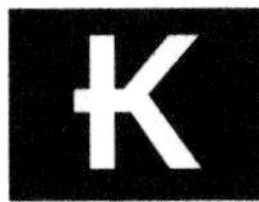

knee The pressure to be groovy could well describe the knee. Every time the leg bends or stretches, the patella (kneecap) slides along a groove at the lower end of the femur (thighbone.) Then, as the knee rests, the patella floats in a bed of quadriceps muscles in the thigh. This means the leg muscles need to maintain a reasonably good balance to hold the patella in place. Also, the femur's smooth groove and the cartilage that lines the kneecap need to retain an even texture, shape, and the right amount of thickness to keep the knee on track. This well-coordinated structure helps the patella to align properly and go back and forth between floating and gliding. Otherwise, the kneecap can get stuck in a groove or shift off center and dislodge. The shove of an outside impact or a sudden twisting movement can push the patella aside too, thwarting full leg function.

To keep this from happening, the body has several well-placed devices that offer stability. Below the kneecap, for instance, the large patellar tendon attaches to the front of the tibia (shinbone.) Meanwhile, on either side of each knee, the medial collateral ligaments and the lateral collateral ligaments provide support while the anterior and the posterior cruciate ligaments make an X across the center of the patella, adding even more steadiness. To secure the knee further, the anterior cruciate ligament (ACL) connects the front of the shinbone to the back of the femur, thus keeping the thighbone from sliding forward. This upfront positioning, however, makes the ACL prone to injuries, as can happen through a direct blow to the knee in a contact sport or in a fall that forces the leg into an odd angle or abnormal position.

Normally, the knee has a reasonable range of motion, from zero degrees at a standstill to a kicking 135 degrees. To make this range possible, however, requires the longest, strongest bone in the body—the thighbone (femur)—to be coupled with the shinbone (tibia) at the main joint of the knee. Between those two bones lies the thick, fibrous, wedge-shaped cartilage pad of the meniscus that acts both as a protecting device and as a gliding surface for the joint. This is not the knee's only joint, though. A medial joint forms within the inner and outer compartment of the adjacent bones. The patella then creates a third joint with the femur, articulating as the patellofemoral joint. To cap things off more, a joint capsule with fluid-filled sacs of bursas encompasses the full joint system. Then, to supply ongoing nourishment to the area, blood vessels keep nutrients flowing and circulation going in the popliteal space behind the knee and also in the large upper and lower leg muscles that activate the knee complex. How active this complex system becomes will depend on the person, of course. Regardless, the knee has a lot riding on it. As the largest weight-bearing joint in the body, a knee may need a little help in staying groovy and in keeping a body upright and mobile.

Not surprisingly though, the knee has the distinction of being the body's most commonly injured joint. Despite all of the above built-in precautions, the connective ligaments in the knee can stretch out of shape. Cartilage can wear out. Bursas can burst. Fluids can spill. Tendons can rupture, and menisci can ski downhill over time or in a fall. In addition, degenerative bone conditions, such as osteoarthritis, can affect the knee as can excess body weight and an ongoing choice of poorly designed or ill-fitting shoes. As long as damage remains minimal, ice packs, immobilization, and elevation will usually be able to reduce the swelling and minimize pain.

To relieve stress on the knee even further, an elastic bandage, a brace, or a splint can immobilize the joint while giving the body ample time to heal. Even with these therapeutic efforts though, swelling may continue, thereby necessitating a need for anti-inflammatory medication. In some cases, such as TENDINITIS, a cortisone injection may also be required. Exercise in general will encourage circulation throughout the body and also promote healing, but exercises designed to strengthen the crucial quadriceps and other muscles in the legs will especially support the knee. In addition, a variety of physical activities, such as bicycling with a knee brace, swimming, and walking in hip-high water, may also come recommended. If knee damage has been caused by a chronic medical condition, such as osteoarthritis or another degenerative disease, however, a primary care physician or a rheumatologist can work with a physical therapist, occupational therapist, chiropractor, or sports trainer in treating the complex issues involved in stabilizing the knee and restoring mobility.

See also ARTHRITIS; BURSITIS; JOINT REPLACEMENT; KNEE SURGERY; PATELLOFEMORAL SYNDROME.

knee surgery Some surprising results in knee surgery can be found in the article "A Controlled Trial of Arthroscopic Surgery for Osteoarthritis of the Knee," published in *The New England Journal of Medicine*. Lead by author, researcher, and surgeon Dr. J. Bruce Moseley, a two-year study conducted by the Department of Veterans Affairs and the Baylor College of Medicine investigated the outcomes of certain types of arthroscopic surgery on patients whose knees had been damaged by osteoarthritis. To see if common procedures proved to be effective and, thus, warranted, Dr. Moseley and his staff divided 180 patients into three randomized groups, each of which underwent surgeries that took about an hour. One group received arthroscopic debridement to remove dead or damaged tissue in the knee. Another group received arthroscopic lavage to flush loose particles from the joint. The third group received nothing but a tiny incision. During the 24-month follow-up, all three groups reported some relief in pain and some improvement in joint function, but the actual surgeries showed neither superior nor inferior results to those obtained by patients receiving the placebo treatment. None of the surgeries, however, attempted to replace an osteoarthritic knee.

Since the topic of OSTEOARTHRITIS is discussed elsewhere, the nonsurgical options will not be addressed here. However, a May 2002 release from the Agency for Healthcare Research and Quality (AHRQ) reported the positive results of total knee replacement surgeries among a group of osteoarthritic patients. After taking into account the person's overall health and the increased risks that older patients have of developing serious complications, the AHRQ study revealed, "After 4 years, nearly 90 percent of patients had a good to excellent outcome. After 5 years, 75 percent had no pain. 20 percent had mild pain. 3.7 percent had moderate pain. Only 1.3 percent had severe pain." In addition, an illustrative chart provided by AHRQ showed that 14 percent of the participants could climb stairs before knee replacement surgery while 77.4 percent could maneuver those same steps afterward. To detail the results even more, another AHRQ chart showed that 7.5 percent of the individuals age 65–69 could walk 10 blocks before surgery whereas 50.7 percent could do so after they had a knee replacement. Interestingly, 8.7 percent of those 85 and older could walk the same distance prior to surgery whereas only 34.0 percent could walk 10 blocks afterward—an improved outcome but one, nevertheless, that demonstrates the significance of a patient's age. As a further consideration of age factors, the AHRQ study showed that patients 80 and older were three times as likely as the younger age group of 50–59 to experience major postoperative complications, such as pulmonary edema, heart attack, or death.

Although every surgery comes with certain risks, such as the development of a blood clot or an infection, less invasive procedures generally minimize the dangers. With that in mind no doubt, orthopedic surgeon Richard Hallock of Hershey, Pennsylvania, and engineer Barry Fells designed the UniSpacer knee system that fills the space formerly occupied by cartilage, thereby allowing patients to avoid or postpone total replacement of the knee—perhaps for another 10 years, assuming the UniSpacer has been inserted at an optimal time. Besides this option, another slightly older procedure developed elsewhere uses an allograft to replace a damaged meniscus in hopes of stopping further degradation of the joint. To do that arthroscopic procedure—usually in an outpatient setting—the surgeon performs a meniscus transplantation by grafting the donor's healthier cartilage tissue of similar shape and size into the site and then affixing the allograft with bone anchors and sutures. Although weight bearing on the repaired joint will not usually be advisable for six weeks or so, a range of passive exercises typically begins right away to assist flexibility and motion, with about 90 percent of the patients experiencing immediate relief of knee pain.

In addition to these procedures, the continuous improvement of techniques offers some innovative options for grafts or other reconstructive efforts in very specific sites of the knee, such as the anterior (ACL) and posterior (PCL) cruciate ligaments. The success of such efforts will then depend on "a number of variables, such as graft material, tunnel placement, number of bundles reconstructed. . . . [M]ethod of fixation and position of the knee at the time of fixation may affect these surgical outcomes. Although it is generally agreed that an ACL replacement graft should be tensioned and fixed with the knee at or near full extension, the appropriate knee flexion angle at the time of graft fixation for PCL reconstruction remains a subject for debate," according to Dr. Christopher D. Harner of the Musculoskeletal Research Center, Department of Orthopaedic Surgery, University of Pittsburgh, Pennsylvania. In further investigating the topic of knee angle or knee positioning during surgery, Dr. Harner explained, "As there exists no standard procedure for graft fixation during a PCL reconstruction, the objective of this study was to assess the effect of knee flexion angle and an anterior tibial load at the time of graft fixation." After studying these effects, Dr. Harner concluded, "These data suggest that fixing the graft at full extension results in increased graft forces and restricted knee motion. Clinically this would be referred to as an overconstrained knee, potentially leading to early graft failure or loss of motion." Therefore, to counter those effects, the "graft fixation with the knee flexed best restores intact knee biomechanics for this reconstruction," an outcome consistent with data from other studies.

For patients who have suffered an injury or sustained damage through a chronic condition, such as progressive arthritis or severe osteoarthritis of the knee joint, total knee replacement surgery may prove to be the best choice, especially for those weighing less than 200 pounds. To assure even further the most successful outcomes, the advancements in technological research and designs have taken the complexity of the knee's structure into account by replicating natural motion, thus restoring greater function. Artificial materials used to replace a diseased joint have also improved, with the variables depending on an individual's unique needs. For instance, some may require the replacement of as many as three bone surfaces.

Typically, a total knee replacement will involve surgical removal of the end of the femur (thighbone) with a metal shell inserted in its place. Then, a plastic device replaces the end portion of the tibia's lower leg bone, while another plastic piece or button goes under the back surface of the kneecap. If a ligament needs replacing, a polyethylene post may be chosen to do the job. However, the fact sheet "Knee Implants," published online by the American Academy of Orthopaedic Surgeons, says, "Components are designed so that metal always articulates against plastic, which provides smooth movement and results in minimal wear." With titanium or cobalt/chromium-based alloys used for the metal and ultra-high-density polyethylene for the plastic, the total weight of the components usually ranges between 15 and 20 ounces. Despite the excellence of these materials, however, deterioration can eventually transpire with a prosthetic joint, just as with a natural one. Therefore, longevity or hard wear may require additional surgery at some future time. Meanwhile, the assistance of physical therapy and a lifestyle designed to include helpful exercises, such as swimming or golf, can increase the mobility of most patients, perhaps for years to come.

See also ANTERIOR CRUCIATE LIGAMENT INJURY; EXERCISE; KNEE; JOINT REPLACEMENT.

American Academy of Orthopaedic Surgeons. "Knee Implants." Available online. URL: http://orthoinfo.aaos.org/fact/thr_report.cfm?Thread_ID=279+topcategory=Knee Downloaded on July 5, 2003.

Harner, Christopher D. "The Effect of Knee Flexion Angle and Application of an Anterior Tibial Load at the Time of Graft Fixation on the Biomechanics of a Posterior Cruciate Ligament-Reconstructed Knee." Available online. URL: http://www.findarticles.com/cf_0/m0918/4_28/63985249/print.jhtml Downloaded on April 18, 2003.

Moseley, J. Bruce. "A Controlled Trial of Anthroscopic Surgery for Osteoarthritis of the Knee." *The New England Journal of Medicine* 347, no. 2 (July 11, 2002): 81–88.

WGAL Channel. "Device Less Invasive Than Replacing Knee: Unispacer Recipient is Doing Well." Available online. URL: http://thewgalchannel.com/health/1356297/detail.html?type=print Downloaded on April 4, 2002.

knock-knees According to the press release "Your Child's Foot Care: Every Step Counts," published by the American College of Foot and Ankle Surgeons (ACFAS), the condition of "Knock knees is normal for 3–7 year olds and usually correct by adulthood." If the possibility of a gait problem exists, however, the ACFAS recommends checking for signs of abnormal wear or other irregularities in the pair of shoes a child most often uses. Nighttime leg cramps need additional investigation, too, to help determine if medical treatment will be needed.

More serious instances of knock-knees can arise in adult years as a sign of spinal misalignment often emanating from the pelvic bones. This can occur, for example, in women with wider hips who become active in sports. As the ankles shift away from the body's midpoint and the knees come closer together, the person's legs turn inward, generating undue stress, tension, and pain around the kneecaps. Assuming the condition results from overuse rather than degenerating joints in the hips or knees, chiropractic adjustments may be able to realign the bones whereas physical therapy and exercise could help to hold them in place. An evaluation by an orthopedic specialist may also be advised.

See also FEET OR FOOT; FOOTWEAR.

American College of Foot and Ankle Surgeons. "Your Child's Foot Care: Every Step Counts." Available online. URL: http://www.acfas.org/prchild_foot.htm Downloaded on July 4, 2003.

kyphosis In growing children, DISKITIS can tilt the spine, causing kyphosis as an abnormal curvature develops. According to the National Institutes of Health, poor posture, trauma, infection, developmental problems, connective tissue disorders, disk degeneration, or other underlying medical conditions can also result in kyphosis at any age. Symptoms ranging from mild backaches and fatigue to difficulty in breathing. In the latter case, for instance, respiration may be constricted as the chest becomes progressively more concave and the upper back more rounded until a hunchback effect has been achieved.

Before any treatment begins, all potential disorders or underlying diseases, such as OSTEOPOROSIS, must either be ruled out or become the primary emphasis in a medical course of action. If poor posture proves to be the singular cause of kyphosis, therapeutic treatments may consist of adjustments aimed to realign or correct the bones with individualized exercises aimed to strengthen the back muscles supporting the spine. Again, this would be done assuming no degeneration of joints and vertebral bones exists nor any potentially perilous contraindications, such as a vertebral fracture. If more serious causatives have been implicated, early detection, appropriate therapeutic treatment, and a corrective course in retraining the body to stand up straight may help to avoid an eventual need for surgery.

To help patients straighten a spinal curvature without surgical intervention, the December 2000 fact sheet "Kyphosis (Curvature of the Spine)" published online by the American Academy of Orthopaedic Surgeons (AAOS) recommends exercise, particularly to strength the abdomen and stretch the hamstrings, and then adds this encouraging word, "As posture improves, the kyphosis naturally diminishes." Although the AAOS reports, "Any curvature over 50 degrees is considered abnormal," the criteria for surgery is "if the curve is greater than 75 degrees." Should that occur, the surgical goal then aims to reduce the "curvature by straightening and fusing the spinal segments together."

See also BACKACHE; BONE DEVELOPMENT; CALCIUM; EXERCISE; OSTEOPOROSIS; SCOLIOSIS.

American Academy of Orthopaedic Surgeons. "Kyphosis (Curvature of the Spine)." Available online. URL: http://orthoinfo.aaos.org/fact/thr_report.cfm?Thread_ID=247&topcategory=spine Downloaded on July 4, 2003.

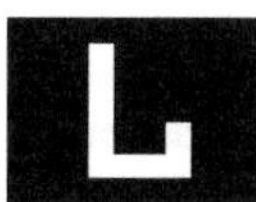

laminectomy This surgical procedure removes part of the upper portion of the vertebral arch (lamina) where spinal nerves pass through vertebrae. As a means of relieving pain or numbness caused by neural impingement, a laminectomy may involve one or more vertebrae, depending on how many instances of bony overgrowth have compressed the spine or pinched the nerves. Such conditions may occur, for example, in degenerative arthritis or spinal stenosis. Also, bone spurs and calcium deposits can form in or around a vertebra, causing undue pressure on other areas of the spine. When conservative treatments of at least three months have failed, health information from the National Institute of Arthritis and Musculoskeletal and Skin Diseases (NIAMS) suggests considering this surgical options, especially if numbness has interfered with walking or proper functioning of the bowels and bladder. Then, a decompressive laminectomy can expand the interior vertebral space, alleviating pressure on the affected nerves. If lumbar spinal stenosis has been the primary causative, a laminectomy may also include fusing vertebrae to stabilize those segments of the spine. As with any surgery, risks include the potential of a blood clot or an infection. With a laminectomy, though, such possibilities as the inadvertent tearing of spinal membrane must also be considered. In addition, NIAMS points out that the degenerative or chronic condition leading to a need for surgery will likely recur in five years or so. Until then, however, successful removal of the bony overgrowth and corresponding release of spinal pressure will give most laminectomy patients some relief in pain as well as improved ambulation.

NIAMS Health Topics. "Questions and Answers About Spinal Stenosis." Available online. URL: http://www.niams.nih.gov/hi/topics/spinalstenosis/spinal_sten.htm #spine_i Downloaded on October 1999.

larynx Commonly called the voice box, the larynx lies between the pharynx (muscular tube of the throat) and the trachea (airway to the lungs), banding cartilage and ligaments protectively around the vocal cords. At the front of the throat, a laryngeal prominence, known as the Adam's apple, becomes even more prominent during puberty when it has a say in deepening the voice—in girls as well as in boys. Meanwhile, at the rear of the throat near the entrance of the voice box, the epiglottis tilts back as the larynx rises, allowing safe passage of food into the esophagus while keeping food from entering the forbidden zone of the trachea. Without that little leaf-shaped epiglottis though, a person could choke on the most appealing food in the garden.

A more likely problem with the larynx occurs in laryngitis—a singer's nightmare with symptoms of a sore throat, dry cough, hoarseness, and sometimes even difficulty in breathing as inflammation of the mucous membrane of the larynx causes the throat to swell. This condition may be attributable to irritants in the air or to an infection brought on by a bacteria or a virus. Occasionally, hoarseness in the larynx may be due to an underlying medical condition, such as inflammatory arthritis, affecting the arytenoid cartilage. In the case of that vocalist or a public speaker, though, overuse could be the cause. Appropriate treatment will depend on the causative factor, but relief may come with rest and avoidance of the potential irritant. The inhalation of moist air will usually help too. However, young children with laryngitis may occasionally experience spasmodic episodes in their throat muscles, which may be soothed with the application of moist heat.

Although unrelated to that particular complication of laryngitis, similar spasms may occur in any age group. However, individuals between 30 and 50 are most likely to be affected by the voice disorder known as spasmodic dysphonia or laryngeal dystonia. As the muscles around the larynx suddenly move involuntarily, a person may have difficulty saying more than a word or two before experiencing a break in the voice or speaking in a strangled or constricted manner. According to the fact sheet "Spasmodic Dysphonia," by the National Institute on Deafness and Other Communication Disorders (NIDCD), the three types of spasmodic dysphonia include abductor spasmodic dysphonia, adductor spasmodic dysphonia, and mixed spasmodic dysphonia. Those complicated-sounding names basically mean that the voice box opens or closes inappropriately. With the adductor muscles closing, the voice shuts off, making the speech sound choppy or as if the person had developed a stutter. With the abductor muscles opening, too much air escapes from the lungs, so the breathy voice sounds weak or hushed. If the voice box alternates between opening and closing, the mixing includes both sound effects with many plausible variations.

Since the origins of spasmodic dysphonia continue to be unclear, numerous ideas have been voiced—from psychogenic to neurogenic—while causes may simply vary yet increase under stress. For instance, the same causative factors that lead to laryngitis have been implicated, but spasmodic dysphonia can also coincide with various movement disorders, such as blepharospasm (uncontrolled blinking or closing of the eyes). Muscle twitches or tremors and involuntary movements of the face, torso, or limbs may also accompany spasmodic dystonia of the larynx. According to NIDCD, a diagnosis will usually be made by "identifying the way the symptoms developed as well as by careful examination of the individual." Typically, that examination may include an ear-nose-throat specialist (otolaryngologist) to examine the vocal folds to see if other causes for a voice disorder, such as a tumor, exist. A speech-language pathologist may evaluate the patient's voice and voice quality, while a neurologist may look for signs of other muscle movement disorders. In milder cases, voice therapy may be prescribed. If the condition impedes the person's speech enough to make communication difficult, psychological counseling may be helpful. In any case, the NIDCD says, "Currently the most promising treatment for reducing the symptoms of spasmodic dysphonia is injections of very small amounts of botulinum toxin (botox) directly in the affected muscles of the larynx." As NIDCD goes on to confirm, this same substance may be injected into facial muscles to give the appearance of younger, smoother skin. Again, this same bacterium—as found in improperly canned foods—can give a person food poisoning. To convert this potential poison into a medicinal effect, "The toxin weakens muscles by blocking the nerve impulse to the muscle. The botox injections generally improve the voice for a period of three to four months after which the voice symptoms gradually return."

To see if other options could replace the botulinum toxin type A (BTXA) used as a fairly standard course of treatment for dysphonia, a medical team from Thomas Jefferson University in Philadelphia, Pennsylvania, presented their findings in "Botulinum Toxin Type B for Treatment of Spasmodic Dysphonia: A Case Report" in the *Journal of Voice.* According to the study, the BTX neurotoxin offers one of seven possibilities, from A to G. As the report further stated, "However, some patients develop resistance to botulinum toxin type A after initially responding well to the therapeutic injections then gradually becoming less responsive to increasing doses of BTXA." Therefore, the study focused on the use of botulinum toxin type B with the medical team summarizing "that BTXB may be safe and effective for the treatment of laryngeal dystonia," especially in patients resistant to BTXA. The research team then concluded with this word of caution, "Additional studies investigating the dose-response relationship of BTXB in the larynx, development of resistance to BTXB, and the long-term safety of BTXB injections are warranted."

National Institute on Deafness and Other Communication Disorders. "Spasmodic Dysphonia." Available online. URL: http://www.nidcd.nih.gov/health/voice/spas Downloaded on July 7, 2003.

Thomas Jefferson University. "Botulinum Toxin Type B for Treatment of Spasmodic Dysphonia: A Case Report," *Journal of Voice* 16, no. 3 (December 18, 2001): 422–424.

leg Attached to the pelvis above, the feet below, and the knees near its midpoint, the articulations of the leg express an impressive range of motion. Backward, forward, around and around, or out to the side and in—the long bones of the leg move the whole body with the assistance of powerful muscles in the hip, calf, and thigh. Indeed, various medical drawings, stripped of skin, illustrate the long bones of the legs embedded deeply within protective layers of muscles. These layered straps of muscles go up, down, and diagonally, strapping together the femur, the patella, the tibia, and the fibula. Once descriptive, those Latin names translate respectively into the thighbone, the small pan of the kneecap, the larger shinbone in the leg's lower front, and the clasping pin of the long, thin bone toward the back of the leg calf. The muscles, too, have Latin names like soleus—the flat bands in the lower calf that insert at the upper shaft of the fibula and extend down to the feet, allowing a foot to flex—or the popliteus that originates in the femur, permitting flexion in the leg. Each of the joints, ligaments, tendons, nerves, arteries, and veins in the legs also have names—as happens all through the body—to bring precise forms of identification into place when medical treatment may be needed.

In the legs, the most likely injuries occur with bumps and bruises, common to all kinds and ages of people, but usually treated with cold cloths or ice and rest. More serious but also fairly common damages can occur as a bone breaks. Often, fracturing in a leg disrupts one of the cylindrically shaped long bones whose hollow channel is filled with yellow marrow, bone matrix, and other matter concerning the nerves or circulation of blood in the bone's interior. If breakage occurs anywhere along the bone, everything in its path may suffer until the fracture mends, usually with the help of a cast or, perhaps, with traction to assure the bone's correct alignment. When that does not help—or when a severe break appears—a rod, a metal pin, or a bone graft may be surgically implanted to hold the bone together.

In an injury, over time, or because of excess weight, the protective cartilage pads between the bones may also wear down, ultimately causing friction and inflammation as the hard surfaces rub together and degenerate into other problems, such as osteoarthritis. Because the legs support the upright and mobile body, however, muscles will eventually react to the deteriorating conditions in the bones. For instance, they may cramp, ache, go into spasms, or atrophy with leg disuse. Muscles, too, can be damaged as fibers overstretch beyond elasticity or as tendons pull or as circulation slows. At such times, the sedentary conditions that often result may become a breeding ground for blood clots, which, when triggered from the legs, can shoot off a blood bullet toward the heart. Illnesses, diseases, or other unknown causes can get a body down too. As long as the legs get the feet moving again, the person will usually be able to get going in whatever direction a mobile, independent life may lead.

See also ARTHRITIS; EXERCISE; FALLS OR FALLING; FOOTWEAR; GAIT.

Legg-Calvé-Perthes disease When something disrupts the normal flow of blood to a bone, deterioration will eventually occur, sometimes in as little as one to three weeks, assuming that nothing quickly corrects or alleviates the contributing factor. If the location of the insufficient blood supply happens to be in the hip of a child age four to 10, the result may be Legg-Calvé-Perthes disease (LCPD)—an occurrence more likely among boys than girls, according to a 2003 fact sheet from the National Institutes of Health (NIH). In addition, recent research indicates the potential of some type of blood-clotting disorder as a source of LCPD. Regardless of the causatives, NIH says the cessation of a blood supply usually affects the head of the femur (thighbone) in one leg, although both legs could conceivably experience deterioration. Initial symptoms may include pain in the knee, thigh, or groin with possible atrophy of the muscles in the upper thigh and a noticeably restricted movement in the hip. Besides investigating and treating an underlying disorder, the general medical aim will be to protect the hip joint from more stress and injury until bed rest or immobilization of the affected area has allowed normal bone growth to resume. That hoped-for outcome usually results with prompt treatment, thus giving a young body time to heal without a permanent deformity.

National Library of Medicine. "Medical Encyclopedia: Legg-Calvé-Perthes Disease." Available online. URL: http://www.nlm.nih.gov/medlineplus/print/ency/article/001264.htm Downloaded on July 7, 2003.

leukemia As a major type of malignancy, leukemia emanates from abnormal marrow in the bone where rapid overgrowth of white blood cells (leukocytes) affects every part of the body. Some cases may be acute, which means the normal bone marrow cells remain undeveloped, thus failing to function properly as abnormal cancer cells proliferate into maturity and replace or crowd out the healthy cells. Conversely, other cases of leukemia may be chronic, with slower development of the abnormal cells giving the healthy cells a little more time to mature and carry out their normal functions.

Besides these two main groups of acute and chronic, the many forms of leukemia further divide into distinctive classifications made by the specific type of white blood cells involved. According to the fact sheet "Questions and Answers About Leukemia," jointly provided by the American Cancer Society and the National Cancer Institute, "The most common types of leukemia are acute lymphocytic leukemia, acute myeloid leukemia, chronic lymphocytic leukemia, and chronic myeloid leukemia. In children, leukemia is the most common cancer, and acute lymphocytic leukemia is the most common type of leukemia. In adults, acute myeloid leukemia is the most commonly occurring type, followed by chronic lymphocytic leukemia."

Whether fast or slow, the progress of most types of leukemia results in severely lowered or weakened red blood cells with symptoms of anemia, fatigue, weakness, and frequent infections. Early signs may also include fever, chills, and other flu-like signs with progressive weight loss and increasing pain developing in the bones and joints. A complete medical history will assist a diagnosis as will blood tests and imaging tests to evaluate the condition of the bones. Biopsies of bone marrow or lymph nodes may also be ordered, depending on the specific type of leukemia that is suspected. Again, according to the precise type, treatments may include a course of antibiotics to support the immune system, blood transfusions to reestablish the red blood cells, and, in some cases, surgery to remove the patient's spleen. In most cases though, chemotherapy will almost always be used to eradicate the cancer-causing microorganisms chemically. That treatment may be used alone or in conjunction with other therapies. Regardless, the chemo itself may cause additional problems by increasing the frequency of nausea, the suppression of bone marrow, and the loss of hair.

Ironically, exposure to high doses of radiation may be one of the many possible causes of acute lymphocytic leukemia (ALL)—the most common type in children under age 15, with 3,800 new cases arising in the U.S. each year. As reported in a fact sheet by the Leukemia and Lymphoma Society, this type of leukemia is unlike all others since ALL occurs at different rates in different global locations with higher incidences reported in more highly developed countries. Subtypes exist too, often presenting signs of bleeding, paled complexions, or pin-sized red spots beneath the skin.

Skin rashes also appear in another type known as juvenile myelomonocytic leukemia (JML), where brown spots on the skin and enlarged lymph nodes may occur. In JML, the liver and the spleen usually enlarge so that an infant fails to thrive and children become lethargic as fevers persist and infections occur. In chronic myelomonocytic leukemia (CMML), however, patients will typically be over 50. About 75 percent of the cases diagnosed after age 60, according to the Leukemia and Lymphoma Society, who goes on to say, "Weakness, infection, or exaggerated bleeding may bring patients to medical attention. Enlargement of the liver and spleen occur in about half the patients." Reporting on this in the society's fact sheet "FS-17—The Chronic Myelomonocytic Leukemias," a suggestion similar to an earlier one for parents states, "Since current treatment for CMML rarely leads to durable remissions, it is important for newly diagnosed patients to discuss clinical trial options with their health care team." With the society reporting a survival range of 10–60 months, CMML patients may also want to consider stem cell or BONE MARROW transplantations. With that choice of treatment, the best match between a patient and a donor will generally come from the marrow of blood-related bones.

At any age, any type of leukemia brings traumatic consequences for each patient and also for each family. To look into these often devastating effects, researcher S. Phipps from the Division of Behavior Medicine, St. Jude Children's Research Hospital in Memphis, Tennessee, studied the "Reduction of Distress Associated with Paediatric Bone Marrow Transplant: Complementary Health Promotion Interventions." In the article by that title in *Pediatric Rehabilitation,* Phipps investigated the potential benefits of various techniques in alleviating mood disturbances and other distresses that commonly arise during lengthy and, sometimes painful, treatments. The complementary medical treatments included in that study included relaxation therapy, imagery, and expressive therapy as attempts to reduce stress. In terms of each person's perception of helpfulness, however, the two most promising treatments that emerged—for patients and parents, too—were massage therapy and humor therapy. Perhaps, that winning combination of nonthreatening touch and a touch of laughter will soon be clinically shown to be the most likely therapies for all gravity-laden people.

American Cancer Society and the National Cancer Institute. "Questions and Answers About Leukemia." Available online. URL: http://www.cdc.gov/NCEH/radiation/phase2/mleukemi.pdf Downloaded on February 9, 2004.

Leukemia and Lymphoma Society. "FS_15_Long_Term and Late Effects of Treatment for Blood-Related Cancers." Available online. URL: http://www.leukemialymphoma.org/all_mat_toc.adp?cat_id=&item_id=9965&viewmode Downloaded on July 9, 2003.

Leukemia and Lymphoma Society. "FS_17—The Chronic Myelomonocytic Leukemias." Available online. URL: http://www.leukemia-lymphoma.org/all_mat_toc.adp?cat_id=&item_id=69974&viewmode Downloaded on July 9, 2003.

Phipps, S. "Reduction of Distress Associated with Paediatric Bone Marrow Transplant: Complementary Health Promotion Interventions." *Pediatric Rehabilitation* (October/November 2002): 223–234.

lifting Improper lifting can cause all sorts of ills, from a hernia in the groin to a herniated disk. Yet many people simply forget there is a correct way to lift and a way almost guaranteed to cause a musculoskeletal problem. The March 2000 fact sheet "Preventing Back Pain at Work and at Home," published online by the American Academy of Orthopaedic Surgeons (AAOS), offers these helpful suggestions on lifting. Plan ahead; get in a position close to the object; separate the feet about a shoulder width to provide a base of support; bend at the knees—not the back; tighten the stomach muscles; and let the legs do the lifting. For picking up light objects, an optimal lift-off position places the body across the item with one knee slightly bent and the other behind as the person leans and reaches with one hand while placing the other hand on a sturdy surface, such as a table or upright chair, for protective support and balance. To lift a cumbersome or heavy object, however, the AAOS wisely advises, "Get help."

The American Academy of Family Physicians (AAFP) concurs. In their fact sheet "Lifting Safety: Tips to Help Prevent Back Injuries," updated online in 2001, the AAFP suggests testing every load by pushing the object with the hands or feet to see how easily it moves—an important caution, too, in assessing those small little packages that could well be loaded with lead. If an object can be lifted without strain, however, getting a grip may keep the item from slipping. Vertebral disks can slip, of course, especially if the back arches as the person lifts an item overhead. A back belt will probably do nothing to improve the situation or to protect the back. More likely, strong muscles in the arms, back, and legs will provide the most protection and give strong bones the best leverage in hustling and muscling whatever needs a lift.

Besides the obvious need to build strength prior to lifting, the Spine & Sport Foundation reported on the "Contribution of Aerobic Fitness and Back Strength to Lift Capacity." As published on the www.spineandsport.com Web site, the investigations of Matheson, Mooney, Legget, Schneider, and Mayer broke new ground in studying the relationships among spinal strength, aerobic capacity, and lift capacity. With the help of 45 healthy female participants, the research team concluded, "It may be inappropriate to use lift capacity as an indicator of the severity of spinal impairment in a disability determination system without taking into account the individual's aerobic capacity." Therefore, treatments intended to improve the lift capacity of patients having a spinal impairment might also assess how much oxygen the persons can safely lift in their lungs.

American Academy of Family Physicians. "Lifting Safety: Tips to Help Prevent Back Injuries." Available online. URL: http://orthonifo.aaos.org/fact/thr_report.cfm?thread_ID Downloaded on March 6, 2003.

American Academy of Orthopaedic Surgeons. "Preventing Back Pain at Work and at Home." Available online. URL: http://orthoinfo.aaos.org/fact/thr_report.cfm?thread_id=130&topcategory=spine Downloaded on March 6, 2003.

Spine and Sport Foundation. "Contribution of Aerobic Fitness and Back Strength to Lift Capacity." Available online. URL: http://www.spineandsport.com/foundation/research/aerobic.asp Downloaded on July 8, 2003.

ligament These tough, shiny bands of fibrous tissue bind the ends of bones together in the joints and connect cartilage, but not too rigidly. Although tendons attach the muscles to their corresponding bones, ligaments lend support to nearby muscles in the region. A ligament can either assist or limit a joint's range of motion, too. Therefore, its versatility can make it susceptible to injury if a person exceeds normal movement. Over time, the ligaments can stretch with use or become unstable in the presence of an inflammatory condition, such as rheumatoid arthritis. Then, even a normal motion, such as a hearty cough or an exuberant stretch or an extra round of bowling, could cause a joint to strike a new position with no more stretch to spare.

limb-girdle muscular dystrophy Health information in the March 2000 "Facts About Limb-Girdle Muscular Dystrophy LGMD," from the Muscular Dystrophy Association (MDA), says, "Limb-girdle muscular dystrophy (LGMD) isn't really one disease. It's a group of disorders affecting voluntary muscles, mainly those around the hips and shoulders—the pelvic and shoulder girdles, also known as the limb girdles." LGMD often starts in childhood or adolescence, though sometimes later. Girls and boys are equally affected by one of a dozen or more forms, each of which has been classified by the genetic flaws that seems to be the primary causatives. In any case, LGMD will not itself be fatal but may adversely affect vital organs of the heart or lungs as the disease progresses. According to the MDA, first signs may present a "waddling" gait, which often develops because of weakened muscles in the legs and hips. Weakness in the shoulders may make the arms heavy so that activities, such as combing hair or pulling on a T-shirt, become more difficult. Fine motor skills, such as holding a fork or picking up tiny objects, may be progressively harder to control, too. Eventually, the person may need a wheelchair or scooter to avoid frequent falls as skeletal muscles decline in strength and voluntary muscles fail to cooperate. An LGMD patient, however, will retain full mental capacity and full use of his or her senses.

Because LGMD primarily affects the musculoskeletal system, treatments for all forms of the disease focus on supportive devices to aid mobility. Should complications arise in the heart or lungs, monitoring becomes vital. For most people with LGMD, occupational therapy and physical therapy will be prescribed. Although opinions may vary about the most helpful types of exercise, intense exercise could actually hasten muscle damage. Physical therapy in general, however, will encourage greater mobility and range of motion in the joints, hopefully preventing contractures and problems with spinal curvature. For instance, water exercises or swimming in the accompaniment of other people can help to tone muscles without adding to the muscular stress. Likewise, occupational therapy may focus on keeping the hands flexible, perhaps with the therapist prescribing devices, such as arm supports, to make everyday tasks more workable at home, in the classroom, or in the workplace.

Muscular Dystrophy Association. "Facts about Limb-Girdle Muscular Dystrophy." Available online. URL: http://www.mdausa.org/publications/fa-lgmd-qa.html Downloaded on February 17, 2003.

limping With numerous possibilities to consider, such as an injury, a birth defect, or legs of unequal length, the sudden development of a limp in a child may be caused by something as simple as an undetected pebble or a sandspur in the shoe. The 2003 fact sheet "Pediatrics: Limp and Joint Pain," by doctors Heidi Koch and Mark A. Graber of the Department of Pediatrics, Family Medicine, and Emergency Medicine, University of Iowa College of Medicine, says a common cause of limping is transient tenosynovitis or the "irritable hip" that sometimes follows a streptococcal infection. With rest and ibuprofen, this temporary condition may resolve in a day or two. However, the possibility of other dangers make close follow-up vital. For example, the rapid onset of a septic hip joint can present the need for emergency treatment and even surgical intervention. In such cases, however, the patient will generally show clear signs of being ill.

When a limp seems to come on gradually or subtly, some possibilities of an underlying medical conditions include LEGG-CALVÉ-PERTHES DISEASE, OSGOOD-SCHLATTER DISEASE, DISKITIS, and JUVENILE RHEUMATOID ARTHRITIS, each of which requires thorough medical investigation. Muscle strains and sprains can also happen to people of all ages, especially during times of increased activity. In younger children, a slight twist can occur in an active playtime with no particular incident to point to, but often, the RICE method of Rest, Ice, Compression, and Elevation can ease a minor limp mysteriously acquired within the day. If limping persists or is accompanied by other symptoms, such as a fever or unremitting pain, a doctor's evaluation will be needed.

See also FOOTWEAR; GAIT.

Koch, Heidi and Mark A. Graber. "Pediatrics: Limp and Joint Pain." Available online. URL: http://www.vh. org/pediatric/provider/pediatrics/familypracticehandbook/limpandjointpain.html Downloaded on March 6, 2003.

load tolerance Everyone alive has some kind of load to carry that may or may not seem tolerable. In relation to the musculoskeletal system, however, load tolerance refers to the various types of physical stresses that act on body structures, such as motion (kinetic stress), force, vibration, and temperature. Those stresses load the body, while the body's physiological responses indicate the level of tolerance involved. In other words, the biomechanical question may be how much can this body take? For instance, how much moving around can be endured without collapsing? How much force or vibration can be withstood? How cold is too cold, how hot is too hot? Are these load tolerances ones that industries and governments can safely address with solutions tolerable by all?

As load tolerance affects various people in various ways, lower backs often carry the weight, but what really weighs too heavily? A team of doctors and researchers from the Biodynamics Laboratory and School of Public Health, Ohio State University, Columbus, reported findings from the study "The Influence of Psychosocial Stress, Gender, and Personality on Mechanical Loading of the Lumbar Spine" in *SPINE*. With "anxiety inventories" and blood pressure readings to gauge the reactions of 25 participants, the researchers found, "Psychosocial stress increased spine compression and lateral shear, but not in all subjects. Differences in muscle coactivation accounted for these stress reactions. Gender also influenced spine loading: Women's anterior-posterior shear forces increased in response to stress, whereas men's decrease." Since numerous studies have focused on such factors as ergonomics in the workplace or influences of repetitive motion on low back disorders (LBD), this group of researchers expressed surprise at the associations found between spine loading and personality types. They concluded, "This study has shown, for the first time, that there is a potential biomechanical pathway associated with psychosocial stress. In addition, individual factors, such as gender and personality traits, dictate how psychosocial stress manifests itself—with increases in muscle coactivity and spine loading. Collectively, these results suggest that one should consider these factors' effects on the human system when attempting to evaluate causality of LBD in the workplace."

Marras, William S., Kermit G. Davis, et al. "The Influence of Psychosocial Stress, Gender, and Personality on Mechanical Loading of the Lumbar Spine." *SPINE* 25, no. 23 (2000): 3,045–3,054.

locomotor training In an attempt to retrain reflexes after sustaining damage to the spinal cord, a patient practices stepping with the help of a therapist. Even if the treadmill movement affects no change in a state of paralysis, locomotor training assists circulation and enables the patient to experience a decrease in infections while generally gaining and maintaining a more positive outlook.

See also GAIT; PARALYSIS.

lordosis See SWAYBACKED OR SWAYBACK.

lumbago Muscle strain, arthritis, a ruptured disk, poor circulation, and bad posture can cause the small of the back to ache, but the dull lumbar pain of lumbago can also occur for no particular reason. According to Dr. Jeffrey N. Katz, the codirector of the Center for Spinal Disorders at Brigham and Women's Hospital in Boston, Massachusetts, over 80 percent of the adults in this country will have lumbago at least once. However, 90 percent of those cases resolve in three months, with about 1 percent developing into recurrent pain in the lower back or lumbar region. With the causes of lumbago often unclear, so too is the treatment. In reporting on "Lumbago Strikes Many, Usually Resolves Quickly" in the June 1, 2000 *Family Practice News,* author Mitchel L. Zoler summarized Dr. Katz's address at a conference sponsored by Primary Medicine Today and the Harvard Medical School, saying, "Patients should be encouraged to continue their full, routine activity as soon as possible, including work. Bed rest should be discouraged." Although nonsteroidal anti-inflammatory drugs (NSAIDs) may be used for pain relief, muscle relaxants will primarily help to ease muscle spasms or disrupted sleep. Chiropractic adjustments and exercises to strengthen the lower back may also be helpful in preventing future episodes of lumbago. To differentiate between a case of lumbago or sciatica, however, Dr. Katz reportedly recommended that medical professionals check to see if a patient can elevate and extend each leg—a quick test that 80 percent of the sciatica suffers will not pass.

See also SCIATICA.

Zoler, Mitchel L. "Lumbago Strikes Many, Usually Resolves Quickly." Available online. URL: http://www.findarticles.com/cf_0/m0BJI/11_30/63690775/print.jhtml Downloaded on July 7, 2003.

lumbar or lumbo- As either a combinative form or a word that stands alone, this refers to the area around the backside, between the pelvic region, and the lower ribs of the thorax. When combined with other word forms, the reference usually locates a precise spot. For example, lumbosacral points to the lumbar region nearest the sacrum—the posterior of the pelvis located on the backside of the hips—while the lumbocostal area pertains to the loins and ribs. When the word stands alone, however, it means the area often referred to as the small of the back. However, the Latin *lumbar* translates as "the loin." Because of the biblical expression to "gird up the loins" in times of trouble, people usually think the loin refers to the front of the thighs or the area most likely to be covered by a loincloth. To be anatomically correct though, the region extends from the curve of the back and includes the sides of the waist, the ideal location for packing one's pockets or loading down drawstring bags with possessions and then cinching on a belt before taking off in a run. Since the five lumbar bones of the lower vertebrae come with five pairs of nerves rising from the spinal cord, today's aches and pains in the lumbar region could be from frequent loading to gird up and go.

See also BACK; FIGHT-OR-FLIGHT RESPONSE; VERTEBRA.

lumbar puncture Commonly called a spinal tap, a lumbar puncture (LP) withdraws a sample of cerebrospinal fluid through the insertion of a needle into the small of the back located in the spine's lumbar region. Often, the procedure has a diagnostic or life-saving purpose, for instance in confirming a suspected case of encephalitis, meningitis, brain tumor, or another disease. In rare instances, spinal fluid may also be removed in an attempt to decrease the pressure of spinal fluid. More commonly, however, an LP may be used to treat a disease as the medical professional inserts an antibiotic, cancer drug, or other medication into the spinal canal.

lupus As an autoimmune disease, lupus attacks the person's own body, including cells, tissue, organs, skin, and joints. Many types exist. However, according to a fact sheet from the National Institutes of Health Osteoporosis and Related Bone Diseases National Resource Center, systemic lupus erythematosus remains the most common type and the one generally referred to as lupus. Often, symptoms may go away during remission. When they flare up again, inflamed joints frequently become painful or swollen, making a person less inclined to continue the physical activities most needed to assure bone health and mobility. Depending on the involvement of major organs, an appropriate choice of medications and therapeutic agents can usually help to control flares and keep a person active. Otherwise, a sedentary patient may become at a higher risk than normal for the development of OSTEOPOROSIS, particularly since women comprise 90 percent of the patients who have been diagnosed with lupus. Therefore, helpful maintenance of the musculoskeletal system may parallel the preventatives suggested for osteoporosis.

Osteoporosis and Related Bone Diseases National Resource Center. "What People with Lupus Need to Know About Osteoporosis." Available online. URL: http://www.osteo.org/newfile.asp?doc=r801 Downloaded on February 19, 2003.

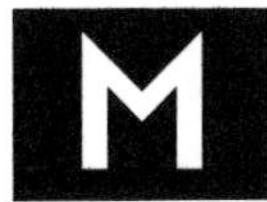

magnetic resonance imaging Unlike X-rays and a COMPUTED TOMOGRAPHY scan (CT or CAT scan), magnetic resonance imaging (MRI) employs radio waves and magnet strength to obtain detailed pictures for diagnostic purposes. For instance, an MRI can help a physician locate the source of pain, bleeding, swelling, or degeneration in a bone or joint as imaging reveals tiny tearing in a muscle, ligament, or tendon. To describe this process, the January 2002 "MR Imaging (MRI)—Musculoskeletal" fact sheet by the Radiological Society of North America, explained, "Radio waves are directed at protons, the nuclei of hydrogen atoms, in a strong magnetic field. The protons are first 'excited' and then 'relaxed,' emitting radio signals, which can be computer-processed to form an image. In the body, protons are most abundant in the hydrogen atoms of water—the 'H' of H_2O—so that an MRI image shows differences in the water content and distribution in various body tissues. Even different types of tissue within the same organ, such as the gray and white matter of the brain, can easily be distinguished."

Although a conventional X-ray may better show bone and a CT may work best in the presence of certain conditions, such as bleeding, other limitations of an MRI mainly focus on metal since this can heat up during the procedure. Therefore, an MRI technologist will usually ask about surgical plates, pins, or screws and other implants, such as a heart pacemaker, intrauterine device, or hearing aid. Questions about any recent exposure to metal shavings may also come up, and removal of all metals, from braces to bracelets, will be required. Since some eyeliners and other beauty products contain metallic iron oxide, makeup may need to come off, but tattoos could be a problem. For many, the claustrophobic feeling of being inserted into a giant tube can be problematic, too, but new designs may help, as may a sedative. The latter can be particularly helpful since the procedure may take from 15 to 45 minutes with patients required to remain completely still for a few seconds or a few minutes at a time. Pregnant patients, however, must wait until after the baby comes.

Besides the usefulness of an MRI in obtaining a diagnosis, "Functional MRI refers to imaging not only the anatomy of a tissue but also the extent to which the tissue is involved in performing some task." In their article, "Functional Magnetic Resonance Imaging of Muscle," published in *Exercise and Sport Sciences Reviews,* doctors Ronald A. Meyer and Barry M. Prior of the Departments of Physiology and Radiology, Michigan State University, East Lansing, Michigan, reported, "A characteristic of many neuromuscular diseases (e.g., amyotrophic lateral sclerosis, postpolio syndrome, diabetic neuropathy) and of advancing age is the gradual loss of motor neurons." The doctors then concluded, "In sum, muscle functional MRI is well-suited for examining normal and abnormal patterns of muscle recruitment within individuals during exercise and may prove useful for diagnosing and monitoring the progression of motor neuron disease."

Apparently, the National Aeronautics and Space Administration (NASA) would agree. The informational report "MRI-Compatible Spinal Compression Harness," prepared by Dr. Alan R. Hargens for the NASA Ames Research Center in California, discusses the limitations of an MRI in detecting certain types of spinal problems or abnormalities that appear during exercising, laboring, or just lolling around in an upright position. As patients typically recline during an MRI, they literally take a load off, which, therefore, offers no indication of the changes that occur—for example, in spinal curvature—when the person experiences normal loading conditions. However, a NASA-developed harness corrects that problem in "a safe, comfortable system to allow such diagnoses by applying forces to the spine during non-invasive imaging. This system was derived from the need to alleviate back pain in astronauts during spaceflight."

See also GRAVITY, EFFECTS OF.

Meyer, Ronald A. and Barry M. Prior. "Functional Magnetic Resonance Imaging of Muscle." *Exercise and Sport Sciences Reviews* 28, no. 2 (April 2000): 89–92.

National Aeronautics and Space Administration. "MRI-Compatible Spinal Compression Harness." Available online. URL: http://spacephysiology.arc.nasa.gov/projects/mri.html Downloaded on June 13, 2003.

Radiological Society of North America. "MR Imaging (MRI)-Musculoskeletal." Available online. URL: http://www.radiologyinfo.org Downloaded on June 13, 2003.

magnet therapy With claims going back at least to the lodestone Cleopatra placed in her bed as an antiaging device, modern-day advocates hail the magnet as a means of improving circulation, relieving pain or muscle soreness, and promoting the healing of fractured bones. Some say magnet therapy can assist sufferers of arthritis, fibromyalgia, rheumatoid arthritis, back pain, and fatigue with magnetic energy supposedly able to increase the wearer's energy or detect the lack thereof, thus making magnets allegedly useful in diagnosing a disease. Skeptics often scorn these unconfirmed ideas with their choice of emotionally charged adjectives, such as *preposterous, insane, and ridiculous.* Interestingly though, both promagnet and antimagnet activists strongly warn people not ever to wear a magnet in conjunction with an electrically charged, battery-operated pacemaker or when undergoing magnetic resonance imaging (MRI).

If magnetic pull had a set value proportionate to its strength with no other considerations, that might help to clarify the issue and more readily gauge or validate research findings. However, the present form of measurement can be confusing or even misleading. Logically, the magnetic strength calibrated in gauss would be expected to have a greater pull with an increase in numerical units. Indeed, manufacturers of magnet products often advertise to this effect, lauding magnetic strength—from mattresses to wristband magnets—as 300–3,000 gauss and up. Yet other factors come into play, such as the proximity of a magnet to the area under treatment, the static or pulsating quality of the magnet, and its degree of involvement with water or other types of molecules, such as fat. Therefore, magnet strength may not always be as it first seems. As an illustration of the confusion that abounds, who would expect a refrigerator magnet to measure about 10 gauss while only 0.5 gauss reportedly gauges the magnetic field of the whole world?

With opinions toward magnet use still poles apart, individuals often convey their personal experiences as a decisively positive or negative charge. For instance, in her article "Winning Secret to Pain Free Training," published in the October 2002 *Natural Muscle,* professional fitness competitor and model Kim Hartt said, "We are constantly searching for medications, devices, etc., which will reduce or mask the pain, so we can push our bodies even further to achieve the optimum look." Having tried muscle relaxants, ultrasound, pain medications, and ointments, Hartt liked the idea of magnet therapy as "non-invasive with no side effects." After making reference to the positive and negative charges found in electricity, Hartt went on to say, "Direct current comes from natural sources. This is why we feel better when we are outdoors—this energy flows through our bodies connecting us with our own natural energy field. Alternating current comes from artificial energy fields that supply our TVs, computers, lights, hairdryers. . . . By using the magnets on our body, this will form a protective barrier (a shell of sorts) which will protect the body from these constant bombardments of alternating current."

While magnetic celebrities and sports figures continue to extol magnet therapy, researchers have been pulled into debates using an early study conducted by Dr. Carlos Vallbona at Baylor's Institute for Rehabilitation Research in Houston, Texas. In his report "Response of Pain to Static

Magnetic Fields in Postpolio Patients: A Double-Blind Pilot Study," coauthored by C. F. Hazlewood and G. Jurida and published in *Archives of Physical Medicine and Rehabilitation*, the stated objective was "to determine if the chronic pain frequently presented by postpolio patients can be relieved by application of magnetic fields applied directly over an identified pain trigger point." With the help of 50 patients diagnosed with post-polio syndrome, the study focused on relieving muscular or arthriticlike pain with an "Application of active or placebo 300 to 500 Gauss magnetic devices to the affected area for 45 minutes." The intensity of that static magnetic field ranged at the low end of commercially produced magnets commonly used for home therapy. However, as Dr. Vallbona and associates explained, "The intensity of the applied magnetic fields was rather low in relation to that applied in other studies, and we did not attempt to assess a dose-response effect. It is likely that the level of penetration of the magnetic field is related not only to the magnet's intensity, but also to the distance between the superficial area to which the device is applied and the site of the trigger point that lies on the fascial plane of a muscle, tendon, or joint." Because of this interest in obtaining close contact between the magnet and the source of pain, the study did not include obese patients. Otherwise, "The results of this randomized pilot clinical trial show that static magnetic fields of an intensity of 300 to 500 Gauss are effective in the control of pain in patients with the postpolio syndrome. Whether the pain was of a myofascial or arthritic nature, it seemed to respond equally well to the static magnetic field and the effect was noticed within 45 minutes from the onset of the application." More specifically, the patients who received the actual magnet device experienced 76 percent reduction in pain as compared with the placebo group, who had a 19 percent pain decrease. In conclusion, the Baylor team identified other areas warranting further investigation, "(1) Dose-response to pain relief; (2) duration of the effect after applying a static permanent magnetic field; (3) identification of the local and central effects of magnetic fields on the same pain area; (4) effect of the simultaneous application of magnets on several pain trigger areas; (5) possible difference of effect of various sizes and shapes of a magnetized device; and (6) cost effectiveness of pain management with magnetic fields versus traditional pharmacologic or physical therapy modalities."

In a December 6, 2002 update, "Magnet Therapy," the Harvard Medical School reported, "Scientific evidence suggests that pulsed electromagnetic fields may help repair bone fractures that have not adequately healed after several weeks." The report also indicates that the use of nonpulsing magnets, such as the static magnets commonly found in commercial products, have not been clinically proven to provide consistent—or any—particular pain relief. Questions continue, too, regarding the many premises associated with magnet therapy, such as improving circulation, alkalinizing body fluids, relaxing blood vessels, or altering nerve impulses. Nevertheless, the magnetic field has drawn researchers from universities, businesses, and government into unbiased evaluation and ongoing clinical trials in hopes of captivating the magnet's therapeutic value or quieting its allure. Until then, one can only consider how much medicinal force a static refrigerator magnet might have.

Hartt, Kim. "Winning Secret to Pain Free Training." *Natural Muscle* (October 2002): 56.

Harvard Medical School. "Magnet Therapy." Available online. URL: http://www.intelihealth.com/IH/ihtPrint/WSIHWOOD/8513/34968/358833.html?d=dmtCon... Downloaded on July 10, 2003.

Vallbona, Carlos, C. F. Hazlewood, et al. "Response of Pain to Static Magnetic Fields in Postpolio Patients: A Double-Blind Pilot Study." *Archives of Physical Medicine and Rehabilitation* 78 (1997): 1,200–1,203.

mandible This horseshoe-shaped bone of the lower jaw anchors the bottom set of teeth and provides a place for the attachment of facial muscles and the facial artery. The slight protuberance from the front locates the chin (mentum). When viewed in profile, a small column of bone tops in a process that fits into the temporal bones of the skull, creating the TEMPOROMANDIBULAR JOINT.

See also JAW.

Marfan syndrome The National Marfan Foundation reports 200,000 people in the U.S. with this inherited disorder or other related disorders of the connective tissues that can affect the cardiovascular system, the eyes, and the skeletal system. Although no cure presently exists, medical management by specialists in cardiology, ophthalmology, and orthopedics can improve the prognosis and lengthen the person's life, making early detection and treatment crucial. As relates to muscle and bone, the foundation describes typical symptoms as spinal curvature, an abnormally shaped chest, loose joints, and disproportionate growth frequently resulting in tall stature.

According to the October 2001 health information from the National Institute of Arthritis and Musculoskeletal and Skin Diseases (NIAMS), "A person with Marfan syndrome often has a long, narrow face, and the roof of the mouth may be arched, causing the teeth to be crowded. Other skeletal abnormalities include a sternum (breastbone) that is either protruding or indented, curvature of the spine (scoliosis), and flat feet." Because connective tissue is meant "to hold the body together and provide a framework for growth and development," defective tissue can adversely affect most of the systems of the body. NIAMS then added, "However, a range of treatment options can minimize and sometimes prevent complications." In order to protect the skeletal system, "Annual evaluations are important to detect any changes in the spine or sternum. This is particularly important in times of rapid growth, such as adolescence. A serious deformity can not only be disfiguring but can also prevent the heart and lungs from functioning properly. In some cases, an orthopedic brace or surgery may be recommended to limit damage and disfigurement."

Questions and Answers About Marfan Syndrome, Publication 02-5000. Bethesda, Md.: The National Marfan Foundation, 2001.

massage therapy With the trained use of hands—or other parts of the body, such as the elbows—the American Massage Therapy Association (AMTA) defines massage as "manual soft tissue manipulation, and includes holding, causing movement, applying pressure to the body" with the overall purpose of "a series of actions aimed at achieving or increasing health and wellness." To apply this therapeutic pressure, licensed massage therapists use a variety of strokes, depending on their training and the patient's particular needs. For example, AMTA says the commonly known Swedish massage uses "a system of long strokes, kneading, and friction techniques on the superficial layers of the muscles, combined with active and passive movements of the joints." Other types of massage focus on releasing tension in specific areas. For example, therapists cup their hands, fingers, or the edge of their hands and then apply short taps during a procedure known as tapotement. In the bodywork form of massage, myofascial release utilizes long, stretching strokes to relieve tension in the fascia. In contrast, trigger point therapy concentrates finger pressure on specific sites of irritation with a goal of breaking muscle spasms and pain.

In the 2001 fact sheet "Massage Therapy Facts for Physicians," the AMTA reported, "An increasing number of research studies show massage reduces heart rate, lowers blood pressure, increases blood circulation and lymph flow, relaxes muscles, improves range of motion. . . . Although therapeutic massage does not increase muscle strength, it can stimulate weak, inactive muscles." This can be particularly helpful in offering therapeutic relief to patients with arthritis, carpal tunnel syndrome, fibromyalgia, tension headaches, muscle fatigue, and reduced range of motion. Indeed, after conducting a randomized study of 262 patients age 20–70, the Agency for Healthcare Research and Quality (AHRQ) released their findings in the report "Massage May Be an Effective Alternative to Conventional Medical Care for Persistent Back Pain." According to this AHRQ study, "After 10 weeks, massage patients had less severe symptoms than self-care patients (3.41 vs. 4.71) and less dysfunction than self-care (5.88 vs. 8.92) and acupuncture (5.89 vs. 8.25) patients." In qualifying these results, however, AHRQ went on to say, "Because many acupuncturists felt constrained by protocols that prohibited them from using herbs and Chinese massage, it is unclear whether a less constrained approach would have been more effective. It also is unclear which aspect of massage therapy makes it effective."

Although this study showed the benefits of massage on the lower back, and, indeed, other studies have validated the positive effects on conditions such as muscle tension and fibromyalgia, massage therapy could produce adverse effects in some types of illness or disorders. For instance, the same massage that therapeutically invigorates the circulatory response in most people could, conceivably, disperse an otherwise localized infection, say, in a boil, or could foster the spread of cancer cells formerly self-contained in a malignant lump or tumor perhaps close to the skin surface. Likewise, a blood clot could inadvertently be dislodged in certain patients or conditions, too. For those with brittle bone disease or OSTEOGENESIS IMPERFECTA, massage could be dangerous as it would be in patients with burns, skin eruptions, or the decreased skin sensitivity that often accompanies severe cases of diabetes. For those with osteoporosis or rheumatoid arthritis, a deep massage or joint manipulation could very well exacerbate the condition.

With those precautions in mind, however, another AHRQ report presented an interesting turn of events that may offer solutions, especially in providing therapeutic massage and other forms of manual therapy to relieve pain in high-risk or unusually fragile patients. A report on the AHRQ-sponsored research conducted by Timothy S. Carey, M.D., M.P.H., of the University of North Carolina, summarized the findings in the AHRQ document "Training Primary Care Physicians in Manual Therapy Gives Them Another Way to Treat Back Pain Patients." It said, in part, "Apparently, limited training in manual therapy offers only modest benefit compared with high-quality conventional care for acute low back pain. However, in an exploratory analysis, patients who received more intense manual therapy (four or more maneuvers) from their PCPs [primary care physicians] recovered normal functioning more quickly than those who received less intense therapy." Less measurable results, perhaps, include the assistance of a primary care physician in fostering an environment conducive to healing and improving quality of life.

Along somewhat similar lines, Kathy Dion, of the Springfield Hospital Alternative Therapy Center in Springfield, Vermont, discusses the benefits of medical massage in her article "Massage Therapy—What Is It?" in the March 19, 2001 issue of *Healthcare Review.* She says, "Medical massage can be used to prevent muscular atrophy in cases of broken bones, to reduce inflammation in strains and sprains, to reduce inflammation of sciatica and lumbago, to increase circulation of varicose ulcers, to stimulate normal bowel movements, and more." After acknowledging that massage may not always be indicated in some patients or conditions, Dion points out the importance of being well-informed as to the contraindications. Indeed, with the American Medical Association reporting that over half the visits to a doctor apparently relate to stress, therapeutic massage techniques sometimes belong primarily in a primary care physician's hands.

See also INFANT MASSAGE.

Agency for Healthcare Research and Quality. "Massage May Be an Effective Alternative to Conventional Medical Care for Persistent Back Pain." Available online. URL: http://www.ahrq.gov/research/jul01/701ra3.htm Downloaded on June 30, 2003.

Agency for Healthcare Research and Quality. "Training Primary Care Physicians in Manual Therapy Gives Them Another Way to Treat Back Pain Patients." Available online. URL: http://www.ahrq.gov/research/apr01/401ra11.htm Downloaded on July 11, 2003.

American Massage Therapy Association. "Massage." Available online. URL: http://www.amtamassage.org/about/definition.html Downloaded on February 25, 2003.

American Massage Therapy Association. "Massage Therapy Facts for Physicians." Available online. URL: http://www.amtamassage.org/about/physicians/htm Downloaded on February 25, 2003.

Dion, Kathy. "Massage Therapy—What Is It?" Available online. URL: http://www.findarticles.com/cf_0/m0HSV/3_14/79788217/print.jhtml Downloaded on July 11, 2003.

mastoid process Apparently, those who descriptively named body parts in early times thought the rounded protrusion of the mastoid bone behind each ear resembled a Greek *mastos* or breast. As an extension of the temporal bone, the mastoid process offers a shapely spot for attaching the various muscles of the face and jaw. Before the advent of antibiotics, however, the mastoid offered the dangerous site for mastoiditis, once a leading cause of death in children.

According to information from the National Institutes of Health describing that still worrisome condition, "Mastoiditis is usually a consequence of a middle ear infection (acute otitis media). The infection may spread from the ear to the mastoid bone of the skull. The mastoid bone fills with infected materials and its honeycomb-like bone structure may deteriorate." Although that deterioration may require surgery to remove part of the bone and drain the mastoid, the need for surgical intervention in a mastoidectomy does not usually happen without warning. Typical symptoms often present as ear pain, ear drainage, fever, and local redness with a protrusion of the affected ear becoming more noticeable as mastoiditis worsens. Prompt treatment with antibiotics, including antibiotic injections into the site, may help to bring the condition under control.

The tendency to treat all ear problems in children with a course of antibiotics has been somewhat curtailed in recent years—not only because overuse eventually renders a medication ineffective but also because of the complications that frequently occur in the digestive tract. In other words, an antibiotic does not necessarily discriminate between "good" and "bad" microorganisms. Thus frequent or prolonged use will quickly disturb the body's ability to process food effectively. Therefore, almost any use of an antibiotic—in children or in adults—means that the addition of cultured foods, such as yogurt or buttermilk, and supplements of acidophilus can be particularly helpful in offsetting the side effects of weakened digestion or intestinal disturbance.

In the Netherlands, "Guidelines from the Dutch College of General Practitioners advise antibiotics only for children with a complicated course of AOM (acute otitis media) or for those at greater risk of complications." While discussing this current practice in "Small Rise in Mastoiditis During Watchful Waiting," published in the June 1, 2001 *Family Practice News,* Miriam E. Tucker reported that the higher rise of mastoiditis among Dutch children "adds up to only about two extra cases of acute mastoiditis per 100,000 per year." Although families and the medical community would certainly prefer to have no extra cases, "The advantages of watchful waiting include fewer antibiotic-associated costs, side effects, and resistance rates." Reportedly, 1995 statistics showed that 27.5 percent of the children in the United States had become resistant to penicillin whereas antibiotic treatments had lost their effect on only 1.1 percent of the children in the Netherlands. This may seem insignificant but could matter greatly in cases of mastoiditis when the body's prompt receptivity to antibiotic treatment can be vitally needed.

National Library of Medicine. "Medical Encyclopedia: Mastoiditis." Available online. URL: http://www.nlm.nih.gov/medlineplus/print/ency/article/001034.htm Downloaded on July 11, 2003.

Tucker, Miriam E. "Small Rise in Mastoiditis During Watchful Waiting." Available online. URL: http://www.findarticles.com/cf_0/m0BJI/11_31/76333437/print.jhtml Downloaded on July 11, 2003.

medical alternatives A 2002 study supported in part by the Agency for Healthcare Research and Quality (AHRQ) reported that up to one-half of the patients who visit complementary and alternative medical providers also see a conventional physician. Researchers collected data on more than 1,800 visits with a minimum of 99 practitioners in each complementary medical field and found that chiropractors and massage therapists primarily see musculoskeletal problems while acupuncturists and naturopathic physicians often treat a wider range of conditions. Interestingly, the median duration of basic training for an acupuncturist is three years, whereas chiropractors and naturopathic physicians require four years of specialized training. A traditional doctor of allopathic medicine also spends four years in medical school but with three years of additional supervision in a typical residency training program.

To offer a more thorough account of the AHRQ study, the research team headed by Daniel C. Cherkin, Ph.D., presented the paper "Characteristics of Visits to Licensed Acupuncturists, Chiropractors, Massage Therapists, and Naturopathic Physicians" in *The Journal of the American Board of Family Practice*. Dr. Cherkin found that "about 75% of visits to acupuncturists and naturopathic physicians were for chronic conditions, 20% for acute problems, and 5% for care not related to illness (including preventive and wellness care)." About half of the visits to massage therapists concerned chronic problems, while wellness visits comprised about 30 percent. Trips to a chiropractor showed fairly even distribution, with chronic care accounting for 45 percent of the visits, acute care 40 percent, and 12 percent not related to an illness. Similarly, "Visits to conventional physicians were also evenly split between acute and chronic problems (37% of each), and they provided care not related to illness (preventive) for 18% of the visits." The remaining percentages generally related to injury or preoperative and postoperative follow-ups.

See also ACUPRESSURE; ACUPUNCTURE; CHIROPRACTICS; HERBS FOR MUSCLES AND BONES; MASSAGE THERAPY; NUTRITION.

Agency for Healthcare Research and Quality. "Up to One-Half of Patients Seeing Complementary and Alternative Medicine Providers Are Also Seeing Conventional Physicians." Available online. URL: http://www.ahrq.gov/research/mar03/0303ra18.htm Downloaded on June 30, 2003.

Cherkin, Daniel C. "Characteristics of Visits to Licensed Acupuncturists, Chiropractors, Massage Therapists, and Naturopathic Physicians." *The Journal of the American Board of Family Practice* 15, no. 6 (November/December 2002): 463–472.

meniscus See KNEE.

metacarpals See FINGER OR FINGERS.

metatarsals See TOES.

minerals See NUTRITION.

mouth Although the opening to almost any cavity can be referred to as a mouth, the one located in the lower facial cavity occurs between the cheeks and contains the teeth and tongue. In times of illness, the mouth of the face can appear to be dry, coated, strawberry-colored, patchy, spotted, or dotted with a suspicious rash, making it a convenient opening for a physician to peer into and get a better idea of what is going on inside the body.

movement disorders An intercepted pass in a sport, such as football or soccer, tosses out only a rough analogy of what happens in a movement disorder. A person thinks about moving from here to there, but the brain does not pass on the message properly. Something in the spinal cord may hinder the information from reaching the musculoskeletal system, thus intercepting the body's ability to respond with appropriate action. To define the situation more precisely, the fact sheet "Movement Disorders," prepared by staff at the Kennedy Krieger Institute in Baltimore, Maryland, states, "Movement disorders describe a group of neurological conditions characterized by abnormalities in the quality and quantity of spontaneous movements. While the clinical presentation ranges from an almost inability to move to severe constant and excessive movement, they are usually divided into groups primarily with excessive movement (hyperkinetic movement disorders) and those with diminished movements (bradykinetic movement disorders). These disorders affect the speed, quality and ease of movement, and do not lead to weakness or paralysis." In adults, the more commonly known movement disorders include Parkinson's disease and Huntington's disease. In children, though, "Specific diseases are less commonly identified, and the disorders are often described by the type of movement observed."

To discuss the classification and definitions of those movements, Dr. David J. Burns, consultant and senior lecturer in neurology at the Regional Neuroscience Centre in Newcastle, Scotland, presented his "Approach to the Patient with a Movement Disorder" in *Advances in Clinical Neuroscience and Rehabilitation,* published in Edinburgh. As Dr. Burn stated, "The key to success in diagnosing and managing patients is to establish the phenomenology of their movement disorder. Although the broad division of patients into those who move too much (hyperkinetic disorder) or move too little (hypokinetic or akinetic-rigid disorder) is simple enough, to the inexperienced physician, differentiating jerky dystonia from tremor or tics for chorea, for example, may not always be straightforward. There may also be a mixed movement disorder present, such as myoclonic dystonia." Therefore, "When approaching the patient with a movement disorder, the value of a careful history and examination can never be under-stated, even if the diagnosis may seem obvious from the moment the patient first walks into the consultation room." In addition, Dr. Burn advises careful consideration of the use of "drugs, both past and present, as a potential cause for the movement disorder." To assist diagnosis further and, thus, determine the appropriate treatment, suggestions include evaluating the patient's specific actions, the speed and frequency of a movement, and the rhythm, for instance, whether intermittent or ongoing. An assessment of the person's posture may also provide valuable information as can the analyses of blood tests, genetic tests, tissue biopsies, and cerebrospinal fluid. Although a choice of medications and therapies will depend on the specific type of movement disorder, the level of depression exhibited may also be a crucial factor in a course of treatment. If the disorder proves to be hereditary, genetic counseling will usually be advisable, too.

Burns, David J. "Approach to the Patient with a Movement Disorder." *Advances in Clinical Neuroscience and Rehabilitation* 3, no. 2 (May/June 2003): 27–28.

Staff. "Movement Disorders." Available online. URL: http://www.kennedykrieger.org/kki_print_inside.jsp?pid=1095 Downloaded on July 11, 2003.

MRI See MAGNETIC RESONANCE IMAGING.

multiple myeloma Within the soft, spongy marrow of the bone, cells come forth in an orderly manner and then systematically release themselves into the body at the right moment for their particular type and task. Of these many cells, one kind of white blood cell develops into a plasma cell that is meant to stand guard, ready to produce whatever type of antibody may be needed to fight any invading microorganisms that bring infection or disease. When cancer cells interfere with this action, however, the structures and designs of the plasma cells change. They can no longer develop—on call—into the uniquely varied types of antibodies needed to protect the immune system. Instead, they become exactly alike. They become abnormal, profuse, and no longer plasma cells but, instead, myeloma cells that return to the bone marrow or attach to the hard outer shell of bone. There they form a mass or a tumor. If only one bone has been involved, plasmacytoma occurs. If, however, myeloma cells locate more and more sites in or around the bones to build other malignant masses, then multiple myeloma results.

The 2002 updated booklet *What You Need To Know About Multiple Myeloma* from the National Cancer Institute further explains that bone cancer begins in bone, but multiple myeloma starts in the cells of the very immune system the plasma cells were meant to protect. This distinction has significance because the diagnosis and treatment differs from that of BONE CANCER. Both will often require chemotherapy and, sometimes, radiation. However, patients with multiple myeloma or plasmacytoma may need additional treatments or medications to eradicate the myeloma cells. Supportive care may also be required to brace and support the damaged bones, while exercise therapy may be useful in strengthening bones typically weakened by a loss of calcium. As bones continue to release too much calcium into the blood, hypercalcemia eventually affects the kidneys, sometimes necessitating dialysis. A treatment of plasmapheresis may become necessary, too, to flush out excess antibodies produced by the myeloma cells. Because multiple myeloma weakens the immune system, a patient will also need to take special care in avoiding any infections and infectious diseases. Other family members or those who have been exposed to certain chemicals or radiation do well to have regular medical checkups, especially since multiple myeloma can often be detected in a routine physical exam even before the appearance of characteristic symptoms, such as anemia, weight loss, frequent infections, kidney problems, and weakness of limbs.

As with other types of cancer, early detection may prove crucial in actively managing this disease. Because the challenges of multiple myeloma can be difficult to control, the National Cancer Institute says, "Many researchers are looking for more effective treatments. They also are looking for treatments that have fewer side effects and for better ways to care for patients who have complications caused by this disease. When laboratory research shows that a new method has promise, doctors use it to treat cancer patients in clinical trials. These trials are designed to find out whether the new approach is both safe and effective and to answer scientific questions. Patients who take part in clinical trials may have the first chance to benefit from improved treatment methods, and they make an important contribution to medical science." To assist in this process, the National Cancer Institute Information Resources can be found on the Internet at www.cancer.gov or by calling the toll-free number (800) 4-CANCER.

National Cancer Institute. "What You Need to Know About Multiple Myeloma." Available online. URL: http://www.cancer.gov Downloaded on September 16, 2002.

multiple sclerosis In any given week, about 200 people in the U.S. will be diagnosed with multiple sclerosis (MS). According to the National Multiple Sclerosis Society (NMSS), approximately 400,000 Americans presently acknowledge having MS, and about 2.5 million people in the world may be chronically affected. Most often, this neurological disease affects young adults between the ages of 20 and 50, with twice as many cases reported in women than in men. However, the numbers present only an estimate since the symptoms vary widely from one person to the next and often within each individual.

As the January 8, 2003 NMSS update, "Just The Facts," explains, "One person may experience abnormal fatigue, while another might have severe vision problems. A person with MS could have loss of balance and muscle coordination making walking difficult; another person with MS could have slurred speech, tremors, stiffness, and bladder problems. Even severe symptoms may disappear completely, and the person will regain lost functions. In severe MS, people have partial or complete paralysis on a permanent basis." Why do such unpredictable symptoms occur with so much variation? An understanding of the disease may help to clarify.

Again, the NMSS explains, "MS symptoms result when inflammation and breakdown affect myelin, the protective insulation surrounding nerve fibers of the central nervous system (the brain and spinal cord). Myelin is destroyed and replaced by scars of hardened 'sclerotic' tissue. These are called plaques, and they appear in multiple places within the central nervous system. Myelin is often compared to insulating material around an electrical wire; loss of myelin interferes with the transmission of nerve signals. Some underlying nerve fibers are permanently severed in association with the loss of myelin." Despite this deterioration and the body's ineffectual attempts to rebuild myelin tissue, two-thirds of the MS patients will remain mobile, although a walker or wheelchair may be needed during flare-ups when balance becomes a problem and muscles fatigue.

These random flare-ups occur in about 75 percent of the instances of MS, making the category of relapsing-remitting MS the most common. Another 15 percent experience primary-progressive MS, which involves "a slow but nearly continuous worsening of their disease from the onset, with no distinct relapses or remissions. However, there are variations in rates of progression over time, occasional plateaus, and temporary minor improvements." The NMSS refers to the remaining instances as secondary-progressive, which combines the other categories of MS. Therefore, early treatment with U.S. Food and Drug Administration-approved "disease-modifying" drug can "help to lessen the frequency and severity of MS attacks, reduce the accumulation of lesions (areas of damage) in the brain, and slow the progression of disability." In addition, a number of therapies can alleviate common symptoms, such as muscle spasticity, pain, fatigue, and weakness, thus helping the doctor and patient better manage MS and increase the likelihood of a productive life with normal life expectancy.

National Multiple Sclerosis Society. "Just The Facts." Available online. URL: http://www.nationalmssociety.org/pdf/brochures/JustFacts.pdf Downloaded January 8, 2003.

multiple system atrophy A rare, neurodegenerative disease of unknown causes, multiple system atrophy (MSA) develops gradually with most of the instances diagnosed in men over 60, according to information from the National Institutes of Health. As neurological damage occurs, multiple systems of the body become affected with symptoms varying so widely that subcategories have been formed to include Shy-Drager syndrome, Neurologic orthostatic hypotension, Shy-McGee-Drager syndrome, and Parkinson's plus syndrome. Indeed, most MSA patients develop the shuffling gait and tremulous movements associated with PARKINSON'S DISEASE. Symptoms also may include dizziness, visual changes, unstable posture, muscle tremors, muscle rigidity, and difficulties in movement. The latter may involve movement of facial muscles needed for expression, speech, and eating. When mobility has been affected, frequent FALLS may occur. With no cure for MSA and no present means of slowing its progression, treatments will generally focus on controlling blood pressure, regulating the heart rate, and alleviating symptoms.

muscle In each skeletal muscle, the simplest function begins with alternating filaments of protein—actin and myosin—interacting to make a single myofibril. Then hundreds—sometimes thousands—of those minuscule myofibrils pack tightly together into one tiny fiber of muscle with microscopic dabs of slowly energizing fat to lubricate the layers.

Although little more than an elongated cell, each muscle fiber develops distinctive characteristics in structure, function, and biochemical make-up. Sometimes a slow-twitch (type I) fiber emerges. Sometimes a fast-twitch (type II) fiber does. Either way, this very excitable tissue individually reacts to all sorts of stimuli, from body mechanics and body chemicals to an electrical production of conduction as ions travel across the cellular membrane, instigating the changes needed to generate ACTION POTENTIAL.

If left by itself, a muscle fiber would be only a long, lonely, little cell where things keep hopping and nothing much happens. However, by bonding with other fibers of muscles, nerves, and tendons, the resulting bundles or fascicles enable the muscle to contract. How fast or how slow that contraction will be depends on the fiber type. For instance, if fast-twitch fibers dominate, more speed and force can occur. If slow-twitch fibers prevail, so can endurance. Either type would only produce a lot of movement going nowhere, though, if not for each fiber's connection to a tendon or a bone.

As muscle tissue attaches to the body's frame, the origin of a striated (striped) skeletal muscle typically begins in a more stationary part of the bone and then crosses a joint (sometimes two) before inserting into a more mobile section. Often, these skeletal muscles come in counterbalanced pairs that produce the body's outer movements as each responsive fiber contracts or relaxes to mobilize that particular joint. Throughout the musculoskeletal system, such movements usually happen voluntarily—unlike involuntary contractions in the heart and in the internal organs. Yet involuntary responses can also occur in the skeletal system—for instance, when muscles activate spontaneously to protect the body in an accident or FALL.

In general, the strength of a movement depends on the strength of the muscle. This is determined not only by the number of fibers but also by the motor unit (sarcomere), which results as a motor nerve innervates each set of myofibrils. Since one motor unit may have 50 times the power of another, all fibers do not have the same capacity, but then, that is not needed anyway. For example, the small stapedius muscle of the ear just does not need the strength of the erector spinae group of muscles on each side of the VERTEBRAE that, with the help of deep back muscles, keep the spine upright and mobile. Nor do the muscles that roll the eyes need to be as large as those used to roll a stalled car onto the side of a road. If that vehicle happens to stall on a cold wintry day, muscles also help to regulate and maintain body temperature by generating heat as they contract. In fact, information downloaded April 28, 2003 from the www.training.seer.cancer.gov Web site of the National Cancer Institute's SEER Program—Surveillance, Epidemiology and End Results—stated, "Nearly 85 percent of the heat produced in the body is the result of muscle contraction."

With over 600 skeletal muscles occurring in the body, cooperative groups form by the location and/or characteristics held in common. For instance, the vastus muscles have the vastest size, whereas maximus refers to large muscles, minimus to small, longus to long, and brevis to short. When categorized by form, deltoid muscles have a triangular shape, and rhomboid muscles develop parallel sides of equal length, showing the silhouette of a rhombus. Other shapes, as well as the directions of a muscle fiber, provide ways of grouping too, with rectus meaning straight, transverse across, oblique diagonal, and orbicularis circular. Then, there is the matter of location, such as the PECTORAL muscles of the chest, the GLUTEUS muscles in the buttocks, and the brachii in the ARMS.

In addition, a muscle's point of origin provides a category for identification. For example, the sternocleidomastoid originates in the STERNUM and CLAVICLE and then inserts into the MASTOID PROCESS. Yet another category arises at that point of origin but this time depending on how many heads one muscle needs. If stability and strength require more than one connection, those two heads make a BICEPS, while three heads occur in TRICEPS and four in QUADRICEPS. Besides these categories, other groups arise from the muscle's action such as ABDUCTOR, ADDUCTOR, FLEXOR, EXTENSOR, levator (leverage or lifting), or masseter (chewing). Muscles may also be grouped by general body regions, such as the facial muscles, pelvic muscles, or whatever muscle it takes to keep a body moving along in the activities of life.

National Cancer Institute. "SEER Program-Surveillance, Epidemiology and End Results." Available online. URL: http://www.training.seer.cancer.gov Downloaded on April 28, 2003.

muscle contusion Better known as a bruise, a contusion occurs when a damaged blood vessel leaks into the surrounding tissue, such as commonly happens with a bump or bang. A lack of vitamin C, aging, and the presence of medications, such as a blood thinner, can cause bruising to occur more readily. However, the pattern predictably includes a red spot on the site followed by a blue or purple coloration that, within a week or so, will change to yellowish brown before disappearing altogether. If a contusion remains after a couple of weeks, health information from the University of Miami Web site says, "A second and much less common problem occurs when the body deposits calcium, the material that makes up the majority of bone, in the area of injury. The area becomes tender and firm. This process is called heterotopic ossification or myositis ossificans."

In writing "Evaluating and Managing Muscle Contusions and Myositis Ossificans" for *The Physician and Sportsmedicine,* doctors Larson, Almekinders, Karas, and Garret recommended a "three-step management for myositis ossificans," which includes pain control, restoration of mobility, and functional rehabilitation. "If the disorder persists but remains asymptomatic, as is most common, no additional treatment is needed. If the mass is symptomatic with continued muscle atrophy, limited joint motion, and pain after conservative treatment, we recommend excision after bone scans confirm that the lesion is mature (usually 6 to 12 months)." Whether surgical removal of a lesion becomes a rare necessity or not, myositis ossificans—as well as common instances of muscle bruising—require a cold compress to minimize blood flow to the area, thus keeping the contusion to a minimum. Elevating the area above the heart and wearing an elastic or compression-type bandage may also help to keep down swelling and pain.

Larson, Christopher M., Louis C. Almekinders, et al. "Evaluating and Managing Muscle Contusions and

Myositis Ossificans." Available online. URL: http://www.physsportsmed.com/issues/2002/02_02/feb02.htm Downloaded on February 10, 2004.

University of Miami School of Medicine. "Bumps and Bruises (Contusions and Ecchymoses)." Available online. URL: http://www.med.miami.edu/patients/glossary/asrt.asp?print=yes&articlekey=302 Downloaded on July 14, 2003.

muscle cramp Sometimes referred to as a charley horse or a stitch, muscle cramping can be brought on by exercise, odd positions of a leg or foot, overuse, fluid imbalance, injury, alcohol, diuretics, and some medications. According to a 2002 fact sheet, "Muscle Cramps," from The National Parkinson Foundation (NPF), a muscle cramp can be identified as "a strong, painful contraction or tightening of a muscle that comes on suddenly, lasting from a few seconds to several minutes. It often occurs in the calf and foot while lying in bed at night or while exercising. Soreness in the muscle may last for hours after the hard, tense cramp has stopped." NPF says that muscle cramps can result from exposure to toxins, such as a bacterial infection or a spider bite. However, a diseased organ or another underlying medical condition—for instance, a neuromuscular disease, such as multiple sclerosis—can also be the primary causative. In PARKINSON'S DISEASE, for example, the NPF says the most common cause of leg cramps results from "a relative lack of medication," with cramps usually occurring "at night when medication levels are low." The foundation further distinguishes between cramps and peripheral vascular disease, which "is hardening and narrowing of the arteries (atherosclerosis) that supply blood to the arms, legs, and other parts of the body," thereby resulting in a reduced blood flow. "The main symptom of peripheral vascular disease in the legs is a tight or squeezing pain in the calf, foot, thigh, or buttocks that occurs during exercise (such as walking up a hill or a flight of stairs, running, or simply walking a few steps). This pain is called intermittent claudication. It usually occurs after a certain amount of exercise and is relieved by rest. As the condition gets worse, leg pain may occur after only minimal activity or even when at rest."

For most muscle cramping, however, home treatments may suffice. To discuss those options, a fact sheet from the Department of Human Services, Victoria, Australia, recommends treatments that "lengthen the cramping muscle using a gentle, sustained stretch then lightly massage the area until the cramp subsides. . . . In cases of severe cramp, an icepack applied for a few minutes may help the muscle to relax." To prevent cramps from occurring in the first place though, suggestions typically include a regular routine of gentle stretches, warm-up and cooldown during times of heightened activity, well-fitted shoes, massage, healthful nutrition, and drinking lots of filtered water.

National Parkinson's Foundation. "Muscle Cramps." Available online. URL: http://www.parkinson.org/muscramps.htm Downloaded on February 26, 2003.

muscle disease According to patient education information from the U.S. government's National Neuroscience Institute (NNI), "Muscle diseases occur in all age groups and can cause serious physical disability. Their impact is especially severe when children and young adults are affected. The needs of these patients are numerous and complicated, and frequently not adequately met. Some muscle diseases respond well to medical treatment, while many of the physical disabilities can be improved or prevented." Because muscle diseases have different causes and take different forms, treatments also differ. As a general guideline, however, the NNI stated, "For simplicity, we can divide muscle diseases into two major categories—those that are genetic, i.e., related to a gene disorder, and those that are not." Genetic diseases include congenital myopathies and various forms of muscular dystrophies. Nongenetic instances include autoimmune disorders, hormonal disorders, and drug-induced conditions. In most cases, primary symptoms present as progressive muscle weakness, occasionally resulting in atrophy. As the NNI aptly concluded, "We strongly believe that the patient with muscle disease must be treated with awareness of the range of problems associated with the disease—medical, physical, genetic, psychological, and social. The first step is always an accurate and specific diagnosis, because specific medical treatment and genetic counseling can only be given with an accurate diagnosis. Physiotherapy and physical aids may be required to help extend physical independence and prevent complications, such as joint contractures."

National Neuroscience Institute. "Muscle Diseases." Available online. URL: http://www.nni.com/sg/muscular.htm Downloaded on February 28, 2003.

muscle loss As people get older, muscle fibers in general decrease in size and number, but fast-twitch fibers in particular show a slower rate of production and lower level of strength. Since muscles do not contract as quickly as they once did, muscle force may diminish too. More than this, though, the loss of skeletal muscle mass also occurs in a process currently referred to as sarcopenia—a term coined from *sarco-*, which refers to flesh or muscle, and *-penia*, which means a loss or deficiency.

In discussing the topic in "The Physiology of Aging: What You Can Do to Slow or Stop the Loss of Muscle Mass," published in the May–June 2002 issue of *American Fitness*, Dr. Michael G. Bemben stated, "Researchers often agree that sarcopenia is not caused by a single factor but is primarily due to a complex interaction of muscle (myopathic) and nerve (neuropathic) alterations, in addition to a declining stimulus to these two physiological systems from decreased physical activity." Among these complex factors, changes in the endocrine system and nutritional deficiencies may also contribute to muscle loss. However, the article "Encouraging News on Muscle Loss and Aging" in the October 2001 issue of *The Back Letter* reported on findings that cast doubt on the popular hypothesis of poor protein synthesis causing muscles to break down faster than they rebuild. Since the first findings on this in the innovative Volpi study—published in the American Medical Association's *JAMA*—focused on older men in fit condition, additional research will be needed to study women and also men who have become sedentary or overweight. Nevertheless, preliminary investigations show that muscle protein production may not be affecting muscles as much as expected. If not, PHYSICAL THERAPY and adequate EXERCISE may be as important in avoiding the loss of muscle as that combination can be in preventing BONE LOSS.

In official statements by the American College of Sports Medicine, the July 2000 *Current Comment* on "Exercise and the Older Adult" said, "Strength/resistance training will help offset the loss in muscle mass and strength typically associated with aging, thereby improving functional capacity." To clarify and make the point even stronger, the statement continued,

> The consequences of sarcopenia can be extensive; individuals are more susceptible to falls and fractures, impaired in ability to regulate body temperature, slower in metabolism, possibly deficient in glucose regulation and may suffer an overall loss in the ability to perform everyday tasks. Muscle atrophy appears to result from a gradual loss of both muscle fiber size and number. A gradual loss in muscle cross-sectional area is consistently found with advancing age; by age 50, about ten percent of muscle area is gone. After 50 years of age, the rate accelerates significantly. Muscle strength declines by approximately 15 percent per decade in the sixties and seventies and by about 30 percent thereafter. . . . Because sarcopenia and muscle weakness are so prevalent in the aging population, it is important to devise strategies for preserving or increasing muscle mass in the older adult. With increased muscle strength come increased levels of spontaneous activity in both healthy, independent older adults and very old and frail men and women. Strength training, in addition to its possible effects on insulin action, bone density, energy metabolism, and functional status, is also an important way to increase levels of physical activity in the older adult.

With those thoughts in mind, the April 2001 *Current Comment* focused on "Resistance Training in the Older Adult." Speaking on behalf of the American College of Sports Medicine, the author of the report, Dr. Darryn S. Willoughby, offered suggestions for developing a training program, beginning, of course, with the crucial need to get prior approval from one's physician. Then a workable plan includes a weekly regimen of two to four sessions lasting a maximum of 20–45 minutes with 48 hours between to avoid muscle overuse and fatigue. Regarding the type of movement needed, Dr. Willoughby said, "Exercise may be categorized as either multi-joint, meaning more than one joint is dynamically involved to perform the exercise (e.g., bench press, shoulder press, leg press), or uni-joint, meaning only one joint is dynamically involved (e.g., bicep curls, triceps extensions, leg extensions). In the older adult, the resistance-training program should focus primarily on multi-joint exercises." With one set of each exercise progressing to a maximum of three sets, "an average of two sets of each exercise would be beneficial for most individuals. To avoid excess fatigue, a two-to-three minute rest period between sets and exercises is recommended." In addition, "research has also shown intensities ranging from 65–75% of maximum to significantly increase muscle strength. Therefore, in order to increase strength while simultaneously decreasing the risk of musculoskeletal injury that often accompanies higher intensities of resistance training, a low-intensity to moderate-intensity range of 65%–75% is recommended." This means that an older person capable of lifting 100 pounds should not exceed lifting 75 in a resistance-training program. As Dr. Willoughby also said, "There is an inverse relationship between intensity and repetitions, indicating that as the intensity increases, the repetitions should decrease. Based on previous research, a rep continuum has been established that demonstrates the number of repetitions possible at a given relative intensity. For example, an intensity of 60% relates to 16–20 reps, 65% = 14–15 reps, 70% = 12–13 reps," with "100% = 1 rep." To maintain variety and progressively build strength, Dr. Willoughby offered this advice, "In terms of the rate of progression, one should consider attempting to progress their resistance-training program on a monthly basis. However, it should be noted that increasing the intensity in some older adults may be contraindicated due to orthopedic and/or other medical limitations. As a result, making adjustments in other training variables would be recommended."

American College of Sports Medicine. "Exercise and the Older Adult." Available online. URL: http://www.acsm.org/health%2Bfitness/pdf/current+comments/EOA.pdf Downloaded on February 10, 2004.

Bemben, Michael G. "The Physiology of Aging: What You Can Do to Slow or Stop the Loss of Muscle Mass." Available online. URL: http://www.findarticles.com/cf_0/m0675/3_20/86230658/print.jhtml Downloaded on July 15, 2003.

Staff. "Encouraging News on Muscle Loss and Aging." Available online. URL: http://www.findarticles.com/cf_0/m0670/10_16/80299512/print.jhtml Downloaded on February 28, 2003.

Willoughby, Darryn S. "Resistance Training in the Older Adult." Available online. URL: http://www.acsm.org/health%2Bfitness/pdf/currentcomments/EOA.pdf Downloaded on February 10, 2004.

muscle relaxant To reduce muscle pain, tightness, and spasms, these prescription drugs usually act on the central nervous system, easing cramps and tension caused by an injury, overuse, or a chronic condition, such as FIBROMYALGIA. Some types of muscle relaxants work by making muscle fibers contract less. Others interfere with calcium release or another action, such as the nerve impulses that travel to the muscles. Regardless of the type, most muscle relaxants make a person feel light-headed or at least somewhat less alert. Therefore, these medications work best when accompanied by rest and relaxation. Conversely, the addition of alcohol and other medications can often heighten or hinder the intended results, increasing the side effects. Because this could create a dangerous situation, the primary care physician needs to be aware of all other prescriptions and over-the-counter drugs a patient takes, including herbs. In addition to these precautions, the risk of an adverse reaction to any new medication remains a possibility, especially in the presence of medical conditions, such as a heart problem or diabetes. A more subtle risk occurs, however, as a muscle relaxant relieves pain and discomfort, thereby enabling a person to feel perfectly capable of using an injured muscle, which, subsequently, could increase damage. With rest, PHYSICAL THERAPY, and other medically advised treatments, a muscle relaxant can offer an effective tool for helping the body relax into healing.

muscular dystrophy Not a disease but a group of genetic diseases, muscular dystrophy (MD) causes progressive degeneration of the skeletal muscles controlling voluntary movement. However, the heart or other involuntary muscles may be affected as well. According to the MD information page provided by the National Institute of Neurological Disorders and Stroke, "Duchenne is the most common form of MD affecting children, and myotonic MD is the most common form affecting adults. MD can affect people of all ages. Although some forms first become apparent in infancy or childhood, others may not appear until middle age or later." With no specific treatment existing for any of the many forms of MD, medications and therapies will depend on the particular type. For example, myotonic MD may require a pacemaker to regulate the heart. In other forms of MD, orthopedic surgery may be required to reposition painful joints or correct abnormalities of the skeletal system. In most patients though, orthopedic devices can help to support the musculoskeletal system, while physical therapy can help to prevent contractures.

Information updated September 5, 2002 by the National Center on Physical Activity and Disability at the University of Illinois–Chicago gives guidelines for exercise while cautioning of the need to obtain prior consent from a primary physician and a cardiologist. Care should also be taken to remain aware of respiratory problems and muscle fatigue with reasonable goals established before exercise begins. Otherwise, muscle weakness may increase rather than muscle strength. Should this occur, passive exercise and stretches can be performed by a therapist to keep the muscles toned until MD patients can initiate active movement on their own. Then, the potential benefits of exercise include "maintenance and improvement in muscular strength for performing activities of daily living such as stair climbing." In addition, an exercise program can "slow the rate of increased weakness or contracture development," thus enabling the person to prolong ambulation and maintain respiratory capacity. By strengthening the skeletal muscles that assist posture, MD patients can often slow scoliosis, too.

National Center on Physical Activity and Disability. "Fact Sheet on Muscular Dystrophy and Exercise, from NCPAD." Available online. URL: http://www.ncpad.org/Factshthtml/muscualrdystrophy.htm Downloaded on February 20, 2003.

National Institute of Neurological Diseases and Stroke (NINDS). "NINDS Muscular Dystrophy (MD) Information Page." Available online. URL: http://www.ninds.nih.gov/health_and_medical/disorders/md.htm?Format=printable Downloaded on July 12, 2003.

musculoskeletal disorder This wide range of disorders involving the nerves, tendons, muscles, and bones can range from mild backaches to debilitating conditions, such as numbness and joint dysfunction. Because musculoskeletal disorders have frequently been caused in the workplace, governmental studies have often focused on such topics as ergonomics, repetitive motion injuries, and the safety risks involved in performing a job.

To assist diagnoses of acute disorders lasting longer than six weeks, the American College of Rheumatology (ACR) published "The Guidelines for the Initial Evaluation of the Adult Patient with Acute Musculoskeletal Symptoms" in *Arthritis & Rheumatism,* the official journal of the ACR. The article stated, "A systematic approach starts with a careful history and physical examination. . . . Diagnostic testing to reassure patients is generally unnecessary and test results may be abnormal in the absence of rheumatic disease," which could further confound the issue. For example, in discussing "Some Statin-Induced Muscle Problems May Not Be Detected by Standard Blood Tests," the September 20, 2002 *AMA Science News Media Briefings* from the American Medical Association explained, "Creatine kinase is released when muscle damage occurs from any cause. Measuring the blood levels of this enzyme can indicate if there is destruction of muscle. Some muscle disorders, however, weaken muscle without damaging muscle membranes. These disorders do not cause the release of creatine kinase."

A continuation of the earlier ACR guidelines said, "Musculoskeletal emergencies may present with acute symptoms. These conditions include infection (for example, septic arthritis, subacute bacterial endocarditis and sepsis, osteomyelitis, necrotizing fasciitis), systemic vasculitis, acute myelopathy or spinal cord compression, fracture, deep vein thrombosis, and anterior compartment syndrome or tumor," each of which will usually be suggested by red flag signs. These red flags that require "urgent evaluation and management of the patient with musculoskeletal symptoms" include a trauma involving soft tissue injury or fracture; hot, swollen joints indicating systemic rheumatic disease or gout; constitutional signs, such as fever or weight loss, implying infection, sepsis, or systemic rheumatic disease; weakness pointing to the entrapment of a nerve or to a motor neuron disease; and diffuse symptoms signaling such possibilities as myositis, metabolic myopathy, the presence of a toxin, or a degenerative neuromuscular disorder. If pain originates from a joint, treatment may focus on resting the area and avoiding weight-bearing activities. When pain appears to be general or vaguely related to a joint, a bone lesion could be the source of the problem. If a systemic rheumatic disease, such as rheumatoid arthritis or lupus, causes the musculoskeletal condition, however, prolonged morning stiffness may occur with general malaise, fever, fatigue, or other signs of multisystem involvement. Regardless of the cause or type of musculoskeletal disorder, a doctor's evaluation will be crucial both in diagnosing and in managing the condition.

See also CARPAL TUNNEL SYNDROME; EXERCISE; LIFTING; TENDINITIS OR TENDONITIS.

American College of Rheumatology. "The Guidelines for the Initial Evaluation of the Adult Patient with Acute Musculoskeletal Symptoms." Available online. URL: http://www.rheumatology.org/research/guidelines/musc/musc-dis.html Downloaded on February 15, 2003.

American Medical Association. "Some Statin-Induced Muscle Problems May Not Be Detected by Standard Blood Tests." Available online. URL: http://www.ama-assn.org/ama/pub/print/article/4197-6750.html Downloaded on November 5, 2002.

myasthenia gravis When something chronically disrupts the normal transmission of nerve impulses to the muscles, a neuromuscular disease will eventually result. If that something happens to be the antibodies meant to protect the immune system, the autoimmune disease that develops will likely be myasthenia gravis. According to the April 21, 2003 fact sheet from the National Institute of Neurological Disorders and Stroke (NINDS), the disease can occur in anyone at any age but most commonly affects women under age 40 or men over 60. The first symptoms include weakness of the eye muscles, difficulty in swallowing, and slurred speech. In addition, NINDS reports, "Symptoms, which vary in type and severity, may include a drooping of one or both eyelids (ptosis); blurred or double vision (diplopia) due to weakness of the muscles that control eye movements; unstable or waddling gait; weakness in arms, hands, fingers, legs, and neck; a change in facial expression; difficulty in swallowing and shortness of breath; and impaired speech (dysarthria)." If the respiratory muscles become affected—as can happen in weakened patients during times of infection or fever—the resultant medical emergency may require a respirator to aid breathing. More often, however, myasthenia gravis can be controlled through medications that suppress production of abnormal antibodies and through therapies that reduce muscle weakness. Because the thymus gland, located in the upper chest beneath the breastbone, may be involved in imbalances of the immune system, a thymectomy—or surgical removal of the gland—will improve symptoms about 50 percent of the time. If the thymus proves to be the source of the immune dysfunction that causes the ongoing miscommunication between nerves and muscles, the thymectomy itself may present a cure.

National Institute of Neurological Disorders and Stroke. "Myasthenia Gravis Fact Sheet." Available online. URL: http://www.ninds.nih.gov/health_and_medical/pubs/myasthenia_gravis.htm Downloaded on April 21, 2003.

myofascial pain syndrome This chronic musculoskeletal disorder can be difficult to detect because referred pain often burns, stabs, or nags its way into an area other than the point of origin. Besides this dilemma, one muscle may be involved or a whole muscle group. According to a fact sheet from Beth Israel Medical Center, Department of Pain Medicine and Palliative Care, in New York City, "The pathophysiology of myofascial pain remains somewhat of a mystery due to limited clinical research; however, based on case reports and medical observation, investigators think it may develop from a muscle lesion or excessive strain on a particular muscle or muscle group, ligament, or tendon. It is thought that the lesion or the strain prompts the development of a 'trigger point' that, in turn, causes pain." These trigger points can be identified as a physician or other medical person trained in anatomy presses specific areas with the fingers and thumb in an attempt to locate active points in the tender skeletal muscle associated with local or regional pain. A latent trigger point, however, may subsequently activate. Alternatively, a secondary trigger point may become hyperirritable because of an overload emanating from another muscle. Instead, a satellite myofascial point may react to a trigger point located somewhere in the general region. Therefore, locating the specific spot may be a challenge, especially important if an injection of botulinum toxin or a corticosteroid is needed to rest the area and alleviate the pain. Otherwise, physical therapy, gentle stretching exercises, and massage therapy come highly recommended by Beth Israel Medical Center, the first in the country to combine pain medicine and palliative care.

Department of Pain Medicine and Palliative Care. "Myofacial Pain." Available online. URL: http://www.stoppain.org Downloaded on February 25, 2003.

myogram See ELECTROMYOGRAPHY.

myopathies Muscle weakness, muscle tension, muscle pain—such discomforts can affect even the healthiest individual at one time or another as can joint pain and swelling. When these symptoms do not pass, however, or when they are accompanied by a fever, rash, or difficulty in breathing and swallowing, a myopathy may be at work. If so, the causes may remain unknown. Often, though, an environmental factor or genetic predisposition can be the instigating source of trouble, according to a 2000 fact sheet from the American College of Rheumatology (ACR.) To detect a myopathy, a rheumatologist will usually assess "a history and physical exam, certain laboratory tests, muscle biopsy, and electromyography (the study of the electrical activity of muscle). Other diseases or conditions, such as hypothyroidism, toxin exposure, drug reactions, and genetic disorders may also affect muscles and need to be ruled out." Because myopathies typically affect a person's autoimmune system, the ACR explained, "These complex diseases can involve many body organs and, while not curable, many of the symptoms can be treated effectively with patient education, physical and occupational therapy, and medications."

American College of Rheumatology. "Myopathies." Available online. URL: http://www.rheumatology.org/patients/factsheet/myopathi.html Downloaded on February 17, 2003.

my- or myo- Not to be confused with the *myc-* or *myco-* referring to fungi, either of these prefixes identifies a word with muscles in some way. For example, myalgia refers to the vague, widespread muscle tenderness accompanying rheumatism or other conditions, such as fibromyalgia. Myocardial concerns heart muscle. Myoma is a benign muscle tumor. Myoclonus relates to muscle spasms and myodynia to muscle pain. Myofibril describes a filament that makes up muscle fiber, while myonecrosis depicts the death of muscle fiber and myatrophy the wasting of muscle. Myochorditis involves inflammation of the vocal chords, and myatonia means a lack of muscle tone, just like it sounds.

myositis *Myo-* refers to muscle, and *-itis* means inflammation. So a temporary case of myositis can result from an infection, injury, or overuse of the muscles involved. As a chronic condition, however, a fact sheet from the Myositis Association defines myositis "in the medical terms of dermatomyositis (DM), polymyositis (PM), inclusion-body myositis (IBM), and juvenile forms of myositis (JM or JPM)." According to the association, early signs include, "Trouble rising from a chair, climbing stairs, or lifting arms; Tired feeling after standing or walking; Trouble swallowing or breathing."

In the May 1, 2002 "Myositis" fact sheet from the University of Washington Orthopaedics & Sports Medicine, Dr. Frederick A. Matsen III stated, "All forms of myositis involve chronic, or persistent, muscle inflammation. This muscle inflammation almost always results in weakness, and less often in heat, swelling, and pain of the muscles. Myositis can affect many parts of the body. Sometimes the joints, heart, lungs, intestines, and skin can become inflamed." About five to 10 people out of every million are affected in the U.S., and women usually experience the disease more often than men. However, children between age five and 15 may also be affected. In all age groups, myositis will likely result in abnormalities in the immune system, too. Therefore, Dr. Matsen goes on to say, "A person with myositis will need to manage the condition and to adjust to the changes it brings. This may involve continuing to take medicine and seeing a doctor regularly. It may also require changing some activities, especially during periods of increased pain and weakness. For most people with myositis, however, treatment . . . is satisfactory, and they can lead productive lives. Myositis is more serious if it affects the breathing muscles, the heart, is combined with a tumor, or if certain auto-antibodies are present. People with these complications will need to be monitored even more closely by their doctors."

Matsen, Frederick A. "Myositis." Available online. URL: http://www.orthop.washington.edu/arthritis/types/myositis/01 Downloaded on February 28, 2003.

The Myositis Association. "About Myositis." Available online. URL: http://www.myositis.org/about_myositis.org/about_myositis/index.html Downloaded on July 12, 2003.

myositis ossificans See MUSCLE CONTUSION.

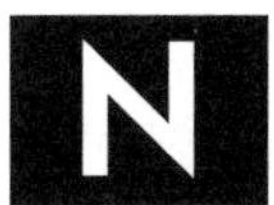

nasal bone See NOSE.

naturopathy With American roots going about 200 years deep, this branch of medicine traditionally believes in strengthening an individual rather than in curing a specific disease. According to the Coalition for Natural Health, most naturopaths typically focus on a person's wellness. "Whether they emphasized the use of hydrotherapy, nutrition, manipulation, herbs, or homeopathy, the goal for all practitioners of natural healing was to stimulate the body to heal itself."

Until the late 1800s, medical colleges routinely taught homeopathic, herbal, and nutritional principles in addition to surgery as a standard course of study. However, as Suzanne C. Lawton, N.D., explained, "Gradually, the pharmaceutical direction to isolate components of the herbs created more potent, but potentially more toxic drugs." With the tremendous technological and medical advances of the 20th century, however, naturopathic medicine fell from use until recent years when people seeking alternatives rediscovered three foundational concepts of naturopathy: (1) the healing power of nature, (2) gentle, noninvasive treatments, and (3) the determination to diagnose and treat the cause of an illness or a disorder rather than its symptoms.

When used as a preventative measure or a means of health maintenance for the musculoskeletal system, naturopathic concepts can be especially effective. Interestingly, the old practices of HYDROTHERAPY, NUTRITION, and SPINAL MANIPULATION have been taken up today in CHIROPRACTICS, OSTEOPATHY, OCCUPATIONAL THERAPY, and PHYSICAL THERAPY to treat certain types of ARTHRITIS, INJURY, or other perplexing conditions of the muscles and bones.

See also MEDICAL ALTERNATIVES.

Lawton, Suzanne C. "Naturopathic Medicine." Available online. URL: http://www.naturopathyonline.com Downloaded on July 22, 2003.

Natural Health. "The History of Traditional Naturopathy." Available online. URL: http://www.naturalhealth.org Downloaded on August 12, 2003.

neck People often speak of superb individuals as being head and shoulders above the crowd, but the relatively small area between the two can sometimes be overlooked. Although an average neck does not carry the weight of the world as the SHOULDERS seem to do, this cervical part of the spinal column carts around 10 or more hefty pounds of HEAD. Besides that ongoing task, the neck plays a large part in turning the EYES and EARS toward opportunities, whether by changing focus and perspective or by performing acts and acrobatics in the form of pivoting the head into the next position. Such feats of function have been made possible by design. As happens throughout the spinal column, the cervical spine contains individual bones—in the neck's case, seven—separated from one another by cushiony intervertebral DISKS. Not only do these disks provide the spinal structure needed for mobility, they act as shock absorbers as movement occurs.

Without this neck action, a body would appear owl-like or as wooden as a mannequin. Without the normal S curve of the neck, however, the head would arise straight from the shoulders as on a stiff pole. Indeed, some peoples' heads seem to do so after, for instance, a WHIPLASH injury. In those unfortunate cases, a rigid cervical area will seldom be the only problem, though, as the loss of a normal neck curve can affect the spinal cord and even one's ability to think. Such complications occur because an arch of bone at the back of each VERTEBRA provides the series of hoops through which the spinal cord must travel from the brain toward the tailbone. So, if an accident—or poor POSTURE or another causative, such as TORTICOLLIS—straightens that normal curve, the subsequent change of position in those bones may cause pressure on the spinal nerves. Although pain relievers may help somewhat to pacify the compressed nerve endings, medication cannot usually address the stiffness or rigidity, but SPINAL MANIPULATION often can. For instance, a chiropractor or osteopath may be able to restore the S curve gradually over a course of weeks with the number of visits varying according to the seriousness of the condition.

Severe injuries and those involving BONE LOSS or damage to the tendons may require immediate referral to a surgeon. For minor misalignments, though, self-adjustments can often be made by lying on the floor with a hand towel rolled into the curve of the neck. With the knees at a 90-degree angle and the lower legs over a chair seat or sofa, the person remains in this "seated" position while on the back for about 20 minutes once a day. Carpet or a padded mat may keep this maintenance exercise from being perceived as a form of torture. However, if the positioning provokes discomfort, two 10-minute sessions may be more effective, assuming any pain or ache begins to dwindle rather than intensify.

Aside from a neck trauma, the daily balancing act most people do can also cause a loss of S curvature as GRAVITY shifts the body forward, adding to the cervical neck pull. Bending studiously over a book, for example, can make a 10-pound head generate up to 30 pounds of pull, lessening the neck curvature, causing neck pain, and even affecting the blood supply to the brain, thus making it difficult to concentrate or focus. If a person's balance also becomes affected, FALLS can occur more readily. If neck pressure and swelling restrict the nerves in the spine, the ARMS and HANDS can go numb. Application of cold compresses can help to reduce swelling, while doing exercises suggested by a doctor or therapist can strengthen the neck muscles and increase flexibility. To assist the neck in maintaining the S curvature regained by spinal adjustments, gentle massages—performed by oneself or a licensed therapist—can help the neck retain its litheness in keeping the head balanced above the shoulders moving through the crowded schedule of a day.

necrosis With its Greek origins referring to a state of death, necrosis involves the loss of living bone cells or muscle tissue. Often, this occurs because of the lack of blood flow to an affected area. However, external factors, such as a trauma, radiation, a chemical agent, or some medications, can cause necrosis too. In addition, various types of necrosis exist, with names usually based on the causative or form of presentation. For example, anemic necrosis can result from a disturbance in the circulatory system, while avascular necrosis interrupts blood supply to a bone. Dry necrosis presents a dry form of GANGRENE, with moist necrosis having the opposite effect.

See also OSTEONECROSIS.

neuromuscular disorders Although some may liken these disorders of the nerves and muscles to an electrical malfunction, others may speak of a failure to communicate. For example, nerves can release chemical messengers or neurotransmitters that never arrive, such as happens when a disconnected wire fails to conduct electricity. In other instances, a chemical substance known as acetylcholine gets to the muscle just fine, but the motor end plate attached to that muscle's membrane either does not receive or does not relay a moving message. With little or no instruction passing from the nerves to the muscle at the neuromuscular junction, the muscle has no reason to respond with a contraction.

When a malfunction exists in the neuromuscular junction, a disorder, such as MYASTHENIA GRAVIS, may be at work, whereas damage to the nerves themselves may result in CHARCOT-MARIE-TOOTH DISEASE or SPINAL MUSCULAR ATROPHY. Other types of neuromuscular disorders can arise because of an encounter with botulism, nerve gas, a black widow spider bite, or certain types of drugs, insecticides, and plant extracts. In the latter case, the results may be intentional. For instance, a surgical procedure may require the use of a curare (a plant extract previously used for poisoning arrow tips) to paralyze an area temporarily in order to prevent twitching in the surrounding muscles during an operation. Conversely, other neuromuscular disorders can result from overactive nerves that repeatedly transmit signals, causing a chaotic response as affected muscles become overstimulated, sometimes to the point of stiffness. In those instances, a physician may prescribe a sedative or an anticonvulsant, depending on the patient's need as determined by the symptoms, case history, and appropriate tests.

Although a traumatic ACCIDENT or INJURY can mess with anybody's nerves, subtle factors, such as body temperature, can contribute too. In the article "A Test of Nerves," authors Dr. Michael E. Powers and student Geoffrey C. Dover of the University of Florida stated, "One of the physiological effects of cooling or heating involves peripheral nerve function, as changes in tissue temperature have been shown to alter nerve conduction. . . . Because of this, it is possible that cold may potentially impair neuromuscular function if the delivery of the afferent signal from the periphery or motor response has been slowed. In contrast, heating may actually improve neuromuscular function." The article made reference to previous neuromuscular research where measurements, such as muscle strength and balance, were taken to examine the changes brought about by varying degrees of heat or cold but with no single conclusion made from those findings. "Thus, although nerve function appears to be impaired by tissue cooling, this does not necessarily mean that joint and muscle function will be impaired. Likewise, it does not necessarily mean that neuromuscular function will improve when heating the tissue. It would be of benefit for the clinician to observe and possibly test the effects of these treatments on each individual patient. In this way, safe and effective protocols for rehabilitation can be established and administered."

Powers, Michael E. and Geoffrey C. Dover. "A Test of Nerves." Available online. URL: http://www.rehabpub.com/features/42003/3.asp Downloaded on April 2003.

neutral position Not unlike the neutral gear of a car, a neutral position in the body places each joint motionless and at rest. For the neck, wrists, and ankles, this means a straight extension with no twisting, bending, stiffening, or tension holding. The elbow and knee joints can also maintain a neutral position at a 90-degree angle, such as when sitting or when holding an upright body on the knees. While praying for neutrality can certainly be effective, a more physical application generally helps to correct one's stance. For example, a neutral position in standing will place the feet about a shoulder's width apart with the toes pointed forward, the knees flexed slightly, the arms hanging loosely at the sides, and the spine erect and lengthened without either arching or compressing the vertebral bones. In this position, breathing naturally occurs from the abdomen. When seated in a chair—purchased, of course, for correct ERGONOMICS—a neutral position places both feet flat on the floor with toes aimed forward and the knees at a 90-degree angle directly over a corresponding pair of uncrossed ankles. Again, breathing comes from the abdomen with the spine neither arched nor compressed but upright, the head nicely balanced, and the chin level. By making the appropriate adjustments in the chair's tilt, height, and placement and the even eye level of a computer monitor or TV screen, the musculoskeletal system can remain unstressed and neutral without having to accommodate to unyielding equipment or twisted positions that can get almost anybody's body bent out of shape.

node As a type of knot or protuberance, nodes normally occur in the lymphatic system and also in the sinoatrial or sinus node of the heart, the latter of which acts as a built-in pacemaker. In the musculoskeletal system, however, a node usually means trouble. A syphilitic node, for example, indicates congenital syphilis, which results in sensitive and painful inflammation at the end of the long bones. In patients with RHEUMATOID ARTHRITIS or OSTEOARTHRITIS, Bouchard's nodes present themselves as the bony enlargement of the finger joints closest (proximal) to the body, whereas Heberden's nodes occur in the last phalanges of the fingers farther away or distal to the body's center. In addition to these instances, which often result in deformities of the hands, Haygarth's nodes present with joint swelling, again because of rheumatoid arthritis. Treatment depends on the causative, but in most cases, a sign of nodes sends signals to see a rheumatologist.

nonsteroidal anti-inflammatory drug (NSAID) According to the American Academy of Orthopaedic Surgeons, "Nonsteroidal anti-inflammatory drugs, or NSAIDs (pronounced en-said) are the most prescribed medications for treating conditions such as arthritis." Besides pain relief, NSAIDs help to reduce fever and also inflammation in the muscles and joints, mainly by blocking the action of two protein enzymes: COX-1, which normally protects the stomach lining, and COX-2, which the body instinctively produces as first aid when joints become damaged or inflamed. Therefore, the NSAIDs known as aspirin, ibuprofen, and other generic names cause systemic irritations, such as disruptions in the stomach or the kidneys, especially when taken in large doses and on a regular or prolonged basis. In addition, most NSAIDs increase the likelihood of bruising or bleeding. Nevertheless, physicians often prescribe a daily dose of 81 mg of any good brand of aspirin to reduce life-threatening blood clots that lead to a stroke or heart attack, even if an episode of the latter has already begun. Although a doctor does not have to prescribe any over-the-counter medicine, any NSAID should be taken regularly only with a physician's recommendation. Then, with a minimal dosage and a buffered variety, aspirin will be less likely to irritate the stomach than higher doses, which may not be needed anyway.

Acetaminophen also does not upset the stomach since it acts on the liver, rather than the digestive tract, but overuse or a body's poor response to this nonprescription drug can potentially cause liver damage. Since it lacks anti-inflammatory properties and antirheumatic effects, acetaminophen cannot, technically, be classified as a nonsteroidal anti-inflammatory drug but can be used as a substitute for one when an NSAID-sensitive patient needs only an analgesic or pain reliever.

Several updates on acetaminophen by the online *Science Daily* discuss its use. For example, findings from a study at Baylor College of Medicine stated that toxicity from acetaminophen overdose results in the primary reason patients in the United States become hospitalized for liver failure. As the article explained, "When a person takes acetaminophen, the liver produces small amounts of a potentially harmful compound called NAPQI (N-acetyl-p-benzoquinone imine). Normally, the liver uses another chemical called glutathione to quickly neutralize NAPQI." If that antidote comes in short supply though, toxicity results. Therefore, the treatment for overdose typically focuses on restoring glutathione in the liver, which can be effective, assuming there is adequate time for this to work. However, the Baylor study revealed that a more efficient approach may be to block the toxic response from happening, which, to date, has been done in mice, not people.

To put the poisoning into perspective, an update on the same Web site stated, "Acetaminophen is quite safe when taken accordingly to package recommendations. Eighty-three percent of our patients who developed acute liver failure had exceeded the daily maximum recommended dose of four grams." Dr. William M. Lee, the principal investigator for the study conducted by the University of Texas Southwestern Medical Center at Dallas, commented that 73 percent of those affected were women. Whether male or female, though, "68 percent of patients with acute liver failure related to acetaminophen overdose recovered with supportive care and 6 percent required transplantation." Another approach, of course, would be to avoid overmedicating in the first place or to take activated charcoal tablets at the first sign of toxicity. In extreme circumstances, such as the lack of tablets or of a nearby medical facility, the venomous effects will often subside—hopefully below the danger zone—with the ingestion of very burned toast.

Since the potentiality for toxicity exists with any medication, patients need to be aware of their own bodily responses and also the reaction of one medicine to another. Although a toxic effect may not occur in most cases, counterproductive effects often will. For example, findings from the University of Pennsylvania Medical Center indicated "Ibuprofen Blocks Aspirin's Ability to Protect Against Heart Attacks; Common Arthritis Drugs Can Stop Aspirin from Thinning the Blood." Yet another release warned, "Researchers Show COX-2 Inhibitors Interfere with Bone Growth, Healing." This update of a study from Stanford University Medical Center "found that selective COX-2 inhibitors—a class of medications widely prescribed for painful inflammatory conditions, such as osteoarthritis and rheumatoid arthritis—interferes with the healing process after a bone fracture or cementless joint implant surgery," an effect that other studies have shown as occurring with NSAID use, too. However, Dr. Stuart Goodman, lead author of the Stanford study, now circumvents this concern by advising patients to avoid using NSAIDs and other COX-2 inhibitors for six weeks after a fracture or surgery to allow time for new bone growth to occur without suppression.

Patients with intestinal problems might also be well advised to consider a time out from the use of NSAIDs. A 2003 article entitled "Camera Pill Reveals Damage from Anti-inflammatory Drugs" stated, "Non-steroidal anti-inflammatory drugs (NSAIDs) may damage more of the intestine than previously thought, according to images taken by a swallowable, capsule-size camera pill used in a Baylor College of Medicine study." With endoscopy, "the tool detected small bowel erosions in 62 percent of NSAID users compared to 5 percent of non-NSAID users." Severe damage did not occur in the latter group but did in 23 percent of the patients using NSAIDs, particularly those ingesting "high doses of indomethacin, naproxen, oxyprozocin and ibuprofen."

In the article "NSAIDS and Musculoskeletal Treatment," Doctors Steven D. Stovitz and Robert J. Johnson said, "Because NSAIDs have profound side effects, they should not automatically be the first choice for treating musculoskeletal injuries." With other options, such as rehabilitation and activity modification, offering good aids for recovery, NSAIDs play a "useful, but limited" role—for example, in treating RHEUMATOID ARTHRITIS or BURSITIS but not SPRAIN, STRAIN, and overuse injuries. This is mainly because their effectiveness has not been adequately investigated or justified in light of the side effects. Nevertheless, the anti-inflammatory properties of NSAIDs usually place them in a top spot on the therapeutic list. As doctors Stovitz and Johnson said, "The problem with this viewpoint is that, in addition to being a sign of injury, inflammation is a necessary component of the healing process." With NSAIDs among the most widely used drugs in this country, it may be time to find out if their use proves counterproductive to long-term healing.

See also COLD THERAPY; EXERCISE; HEAT THERAPY; NUTRITION; PAIN MANAGEMENT.

American Academy of Orthopaedic Surgeons. "What are NSAIDs?" Available online. URL: http://orthoinfo.asos.org/fact Downloaded on August 13, 2003.

The Physician and Sports Medicine. "NSAIDS and Musculoskeletal Treatment." Available online. URL: http://www.physsportsmed.com Downloaded on August 14, 2003.

Science Daily. "Camera Pill Reveals Damage from Anti-Inflammatory Drugs." Available online. URL: http://www.sciencedaily.com/releases/2003/05/030522083447.htm Downloaded on August 14, 2003.

Science Daily. "Ibuprofen Blocks Aspirin's Ability to Protect Against Heart Attacks; Common Arthritis Can Stop Aspirin from Thinning the Blood." Available online. URL: http://www.sciencedaily.com/print.htm Downloaded on August 14, 2003.

Science Daily. "Understanding Acetaminophen Poisoning." Available online. URL: http://www.sciencedaily.com/print.htm Downloaded on October 14, 2002.

Science Daily. "UT Southwestern Researchers Say Overdoses of Acetaminophen Cause Most Cases of Acute Liver Failure." Available online. URL: http://www.sciencedaily.com/releases/2002/12/021217072713.htm Downloaded on December 17, 2002.

nose Somewhere around the center of the face, this prominent triangle presents the dual passageways of the nostrils, which house the sensory organ of smell as well as respiratory aids for the body, such as an air-warming device or air-filtering system of minuscule hair. At the bridge of the nose where sunglasses sit, a miniature version of the larger triangle occurs in tiny nasal bones shaped in an upward-pointing V, while the remainder of the projection consists mostly of cartilage. More cartilage and bone occur behind the dividing line of the nasal septum. This septum forms the two passages of the nasal cavity, a behind-the-scenes space comprising mucous membrane, blood vessels, and hair filters made of cilia.

Being on the front lines of the face, a nose constantly wars with adverse conditions, such as frigid air, air pollution, airborne germs, allergens, foul odors, and physical assault. As some parents have unfortunately found, children have been known to hide small objects, including fingers, in nasal passageways. Eventually, any or all of the above cases of nose abuse can result in disorders ranging from nosebleeds to broken noses, with those occasional sneezes meant to clear the sinuses the way a cough can clear the lungs. More serious may be a nasal obstruction, such as happens with a deviated septum, nasal polyps, tumor, or an infection that spreads into facial sinuses, all of which need to be thoroughly checked out by a physician. If left unchecked, a broken nose may mend in a misshapen manner, but a nosebleed can become life threatening and require packing and, perhaps, cauterization or surgery, particularly when located deep within the nasal cavity. For most nosebleeds though, a patient should not lie down but sit or stand with the head level, not tilted, while pinching the nose with the thumb and index finger for about five or 10 minutes until the bleeding stops. However, pinching a nose to make it slimmer or turned up, will not work—not even with a clothespin—as this author and other schoolgirls of the 1950s will certainly attest.

notochord In an embryonic state, large cells cram into a sheath of firm connective tissue, creating the rodlike notochord. As development of the spine continues, individual VERTEBRAE emerge, gradually forming the vertebral column.

numbness Unlike a dozing limb that awakens one's senses with tingling, numbness presents nothingness. No pain, no tingling, but a feeling of dead weight accompanies this lack of sensation, which may be partial or complete. Usually located in one or more body extremities, numbness can occur from poor circulation, such as in advanced conditions of diabetes, hypothermia, or frostbite. Besides diminished blood flow to an area, numbness can be caused by numerous factors, such as a toxic response to drugs, alcohol, tobacco, or lead; a vitamin B_{12} deficiency; hypothyroidism; a REPETITIVE MOTION DISORDER, such as CARPAL TUNNEL SYNDROME; long-term radiation; or a neurological condition, such as MULTIPLE SCLEROSIS or the onset of a stroke. Eating pufferfish can cause numbness, too. More common causatives may be HERNIATED DISK, bone tumor, and MUSCULOSKELETAL DISORDERS, such as ARTHRITIS and SPINAL STENOSIS, which can place undue pressure on the nerves, or an INJURY, which can damage or sever them. Questions about the precise location of numbness, the duration or length of occurrence, the surrounding circumstances, and other accompanying symptoms will provide the primary care physician with a case history that determines the best tests and treatment. However, until the main cause has been detected and resolved, special care must be taken to avoid bumping, banging, or further injuring a numb area.

nutrition Despite the remarkable diversities among human beings, everybody's body requires certain vital (life-giving) substances, known as nutrients. A study of these nutrients, their chemical principles, and their physical effects on each molecular membrane, each minuscule cell, and each microfiber of muscle and bone would take volumes of discussion to give an adequate account of what well-balanced nutrition does for energy, health maintenance, normal growth, and repair. To highlight the headlines, however, takes five stars: proteins, carbohydrates, vitamins, minerals, and fat—with no escaping the latter unless a person wants to dry up skin, bones, and hormones.

Since fat seems to weigh heavily on people's minds, dietary fats can be a good starting point to consider in nutrition, depending on the type as well as frequency of consumption. Insoluble in water, these lipids help the body oxidize carbon dioxide and water, thus producing heat conducted as energy. Although usually absorbed through the intestines, the emulsified fats, such as cream or butter, are acted on in the stomach where they give a person a greater sense of being full or, in the extreme, being uncomfortably bloated. Conversely, a fat-free or almost lipid-free diet may make a person want to gnaw something. Therefore, researchers at Brigham and Women's Hospital and the Harvard School of Public Health investigated feelings of fullness and the taste enhancements that fattier foods bring, proclaiming the "Mediterranean Diet Found to be More Effective than Strict Low-Fat Option." "A moderate fat diet based on the diets of southern Europe and the Mediterranean allows for a greater variety of foods that are considered very appetizing compared with a strict, bland, low-fat diet. The main dietary fats in a typical Mediterranean diet are unsaturated. Unsaturated fat, or 'healthy fat,' has been associated with lowering cholesterol."

Indeed, olive and canola oils provide healthy substitutes for the saturated fats in meat, butter, coconut, cocoa butter, or palm oil and also for those hydrogenated fats in margarine and most commercially baked products. While saturated fats saturate a body with cholesterol by pumping up the liver's production of cholesterol, the polyunsaturated fats in safflower, sunflower, soybean, corn, and most other liquid vegetable oils apparently do not inflate artery-clogging levels of cholesterol in the bloodstream. Meanwhile, healthier monounsaturated fats, such as the olive and canola oils in most Mediterranean meals, seem to have no effect at all on cholesterol in the blood but, like their fatty friends, add calories. The trick, then, is to add enough monounsaturated fats to transport hormones, regulate transmissions of nerve impulses, and keep the cells, bones, and muscle fibers of the body well lubricated. If, however, a body succumbs to saturated fats that lodge in the intestines or overdoses on other fats that keep making the rounds through the digestive tract and bloodstream, an increase of fiber-rich foods can break this lipid chain. Soluble fibers, such as those in beans, oat bran, and apples, help to lower cholesterol levels. Insoluble fibers, such as those found in wheat bran, provide that sense of fullness that enables a person to eat less and still feel satisfied. Too much fiber, however, can bind fats, vitamins, and minerals, making those nutrients leave the body before their healthy properties have been put to good use. With processed foods far from a natural state though, too little fiber has proven more likely in this country, resulting in an influx of obesity, colon cancer, and other diseases of the digestive tract.

As nature would have it, carbohydrates come to the rescue by providing tasty sources of fiber and offering energy for all body functions, particularly empowering the brain, central nervous system, and skeletal muscles. With carbon (C), hydrogen (H), and oxygen (O) comprising carbohydrates, their low-calorie calories become readily available for energy production. Furthermore, these compact CHO packages help to regulate the body's use of protein and fats—for instance, as the latter requires carbohydrates to break down lipids in the liver. With the exception of milk, carbohydrates come in virtually every plant known and grown so, barring flood or drought, they will usually be available everywhere.

Proteins, too, appear almost everywhere food exists. Although complete proteins come in meat, eggs, soy, and dairy products, incomplete ones can be put into a whole as easily as slapping together a peanut butter and jelly sandwich on whole wheat bread. It is all in the mathematics: a body requires a couple dozen amino acids to function well, but only nine of these must be supplied by foods. Complete proteins have all of the sources found in food, whereas incomplete proteins have varying assortments and levels that need to come together to compute as a complete protein. One might memorize and measure each of the amino acids. Basically, though, a combination of almost any kind of grain with almost any kind of bean adds up nicely. For example, combining red beans and rice or refried beans in a grain tortilla or corn and lima beans in a dish of succotash produces a complete protein. That small effort can be crucial since the building blocks of protein—amino acids—appear in the body more often than any other substance, except water.

A scarcity of clean, filtered water has devastating effects on muscles and bones. The total lack of water brings on dehydration resulting in death. Less dire, of course, is a lack of protein. Nevertheless, this has consequences, such as the loss of energy, loss of hair, higher susceptibility to infection, swollen joints, and weakened muscles. Therefore, it helps to know when protein consumption falls too low. As a loose guideline on page 232 of the book *Food and Healing,* author Annemarie Colbin said, "a craving for sweets, especially when accompanied by a craving for fats, often signals a minimal protein deficiency." Indeed, food cravings in general may signal an imbalance in body chemistry between alkaline and acid as determined by a simple litmus test, available from most pharmacies. Conversely, too much protein can cause imbalances in body fluids and make bones lose precious minerals, such as CALCIUM. For instance, a high-protein diet (or one high in sugar) creates higher acidity in the blood, thus dissolving calcium from the very bones that store and need it.

Besides that important mineral, others include potassium, phosphorus, sodium, magnesium, sulfur, and chlorine, which appear in body tissue in relatively high levels. Lesser amounts occur in trace minerals. Regardless of the quantity needed, all have been proven essential in the physiological processes that strengthen nerves and bones. For instance, minerals help a body maintain the right amount of water, keeping fluids from becoming either too alkaline or acidic. Minerals also help a body produce hormones and other chemicals required for digestion, metabolism, reproduction, and tissue repair. Like vitamins, minerals act as catalysts that assist the nerves in transmitting messages to the muscles, thus causing contractions and movement.

Occasionally, though, minerals and vitamins get in each other's way—for example, as calcium interferes with the body's absorption of iron. More often, vitamins assist the effectiveness of minerals—for example, the ability of vitamin C (ASCORBIC ACID) to increase the body's use of iron. Some of the B vitamins (crucial for healthy nerves) can be absorbed in the body only with the aid of phosphorus, while vitamin D assists in calcium absorption. This teamwork can work the other way around, too—for instance, as the mineral zinc helps the liver to convert beta-carotene into vitamin A.

With so much body work going on between vitamins and minerals, most people cannot begin to know it all, much less remember. Therefore, persons interested in good health maintenance practices may be inclined to pop vitamin pills or take supplements of the major and trace minerals. Although this may seem to be the easiest route to covering all the bases, it seldom is. Knowing how much of each vitamin and supplement to take requires someone to measure and mathematically calculate the unique needs of each person—and the needs of each individual change from day to day. In addition—or, perhaps, subtraction—a problem even with all-purpose pills is they are pretty much dead matter. Although taking vitamins and/or minerals can be effective and expedient in replenishing nutrients known to be lacking, those supplements contain none of the enzymatic action found in real foods. Fresh, uncooked fruits and vegetables—particularly pineapple and papaya as well as soy and soured products, such as yogurt, sour cream, or buttermilk—come packed with enzymes that increase energy production, detoxify the body, keep down body weight, build resistance to infection or disease, and bring welcome relief to musculoskeletal aches and pains.

An easy menu might include a mixture of fresh fruit at breakfast with whole-grain cereal or toast and a fresh vegetable salad for lunch or dinner with small strips of skinned, unmarbled meat. However, a blast of dressing can ruin the effort. Obviously, a low-fat, low-calorie salad dressing will be preferable in keeping down fat consumption, but less apparent may be the need for a preservative-free choice. Since most bottled dressings on the grocer's shelf contain various types of preservatives, those ingredients also preserve enzymes from breaking down and spoiling, which means the enzymatic action ceases in foods, too, making a salad almost as nutrient poor as fast food, except the salad will still have fiber. Therefore, a better choice will be a homemade olive oil and vinegar dressing or a squeeze of lemon or a premixed dressing located on a refrigerated shelf to inhibit spoilage while keeping the enzymes intact. For the greatest nutritional punch, in-season foods grown locally will provide the maximum amounts of vitamins and minerals.

If, however, there is any cause for concern about a lack of nutrients, signs can usually be noticed. According to Dr. Howard F. Loomis, "the cardinal signs presented by a body that needs supplemental enzymes are the symptoms of indigestion, fever, redness, swelling, pain, and abnormal joint movement." Unfortunately, a typical response will often be to medicate those symptoms without getting to the source of a problem. If left uncorrected, "Quite simply, the body can tear down its own tissues to get protein, carbohydrates (as glucose), and lipids when they are needed. All three food substrates are necessary to maintain health, but protein clearly is the most important among equals." When protein stores dip low, early signs of deficiency include edema of the hands and feet, increased secretions from the sinuses, lessened circulation, and muscle cramps. When carbohydrate deficiency occurs, those conditions reverse somewhat, with muscle weakness and a dry mouth, throat, or sinuses. The person may also find it difficult to concentrate yet become easily startled. Similarly, if a body lacks adequate fat, the loss of lipids results in dry skin and bones or muscle tremors.

As long as a wide variety of foods remains available and affordable, however, an unbalanced diet need not become a problem. When fresh fruit and veggies are eaten in abundance with whole-grain breads and cereals at most meals, the diet will become nicely balanced with the twice-daily addition of a complete protein and mere dabs of tasty fat at the tiny tips of the scale.

Loomis, Howard F. "Recognizing Diet-Related Symptoms." Available online. URL: http://www.worldchiropracticalliance.org Downloaded on February 13, 2003.

Peanut Institute. "Mediterranean Diet Found to be More Effective than Strict Low-Fat Option." Available online. URL: http://www.peanut-institute.org Downloaded on February 21, 2003.

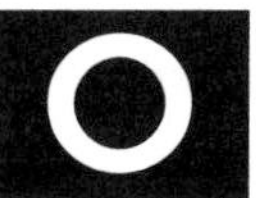

obesity See WEIGHT, EFFECTS OF.

occupational therapist (OT) These skilled professionals come equipped with at least a bachelor's degree, clinical internship, and successful completion of examinations taken on a national and, usually, a state level, too. This process assures that an OT will provide quality assistance while helping an individual recover independence. Quite often, an OT focuses on regaining use or improving control of the musculoskeletal system, for instance after an ACCIDENT, AMPUTATION, BIRTH INJURY, REPETITIVE MOTION DISORDER, SURGERY, or STROKE. In addition, an OT may assist patients in finding ways to increase mobility, muscle tone, strength, or balance in the presence of ARTHRITIS, MULTIPLE SCLEROSIS, and other chronic conditions.

According to the article "Information for Consumers," downloaded on February 25, 2003 from www.aota.org, the Web site of the American Occupational Therapy Association, "Services typically include: customized treatment programs aimed at improving abilities to carry out the activities of daily living; comprehensive evaluation of home and job environments and recommendations on necessary adaptation; assessments and treatment for performance skills; recommendations and training in the use of adaptive equipment; guidance to family members and caregivers."

See also FIBROMYALGIA; HIP REPLACEMENT SURGERY; JUVENILE ARTHRITIS.

American Occupational Therapy Association. "Information for Consumers." Available online. URL: http:// www.aota.org Downloaded on July 21, 2004.

orthopedic biomechanics This branch of research into the musculoskeletal system aims to carry microscopic questions from the laboratory into sizable answers for people's lives. By concentrating in areas such as bone architecture, joint kinematics, muscle forces, microdamage, and reconstruction, various teams of scientists and engineers work toward designing preventatives or developing more effective surgical methods, therapeutic treatments, and ORTHOTICS. To do this requires the technology of ultrasound, motion analysis equipment, and computerized models to consider questions like the following. How much weight can one bone carry? How far can a ligament bend without breaking? What effects does flooring material or a golf swing or bone loss have on the musculoskeletal system, and what can be done to halt degenerative processes?

See also RESEARCH.

orthopedics When people think of bones, they usually think of an orthopedic specialist. Indeed, this medical science addresses prevention and professional treatment of the many disorders or injuries that disturb the musculoskeletal system and its supportive structures, such as cartilage or ligaments. Such treatment may simply involve the prescription of a particular type of ORTHOTIC. Because concerns with muscles and bones often affect the entire body, however, an orthopedic physician may be called upon to coordinate the diagnostic tests, surgery, and therapeutic treatment provided by a cooperative team of other physicians and therapists.

orthopedic trauma ACCIDENTS, INJURY, and various types of bone FRACTURES obviously evoke orthopedic trauma, but recent studies have focused on what happens to a person after bones heal and muscles regain elasticity. The American Academy of Orthopaedic Surgeons reported, "Any illness or psychological disturbance that has a substantial negative impact on outcome after trauma cannot be ignored. In some cases, post-traumatic psychological illness may have a stronger effect on outcome than the severity of the injury itself." To study the ongoing impact of an orthopedic trauma, Dr. Adam J. Starr's research followed up the conditions of 330 patients who, within an average of 14 months, had suffered injuries ranging from motorcycle collisions to horseback riding accidents to gunshot wounds. Although not expected, the more time that had elapsed since the initial injury, the greater the risk of symptoms typically associated with the type of post-traumatic stress disorder (PTSD) first defined by combat veterans. Such symptoms include recurrent recollection of the incident, avoidance of associated places or activities, emotional outbursts or mood swings, sleeplessness, and hypervigilance. In Dr. Starr's study of orthopedic trauma patients, 52 percent exhibited PTSD, indicating the need for therapeutic treatment of the whole person—and not just the obvious wounds—following any traumatic event.

American Academy of Orthopaedic Surgeons. "PTSD Found in 52% of Patients Who Experience Orthopaedic Trauma." Available online. URL: http://www.newswise.com Downloaded on February 5, 2003.

orthotics Ranging from a homemade arm sling to corsets and finger splints, orthotic devices mechanically stabilize, support, or protect weakened structures of the body. For example, an orthotic shoe insert, when properly fitted, provides postural support and relieves stresses caused by abnormalities in the skeletal system. By guiding the foot into normal patterns, these custom-made inserts assist structural and functional relationships throughout the body as the pelvis and spine become more stable and balance is restored. Otherwise, misalignment of the vertebrae can eventually develop into chronic conditions, such as ARTHRITIS, DEGENERATIVE DISK DISEASE, or assorted muscle pains and ailments.

As authors Dorothy D. Aiello, P.T., M.S., and Patrick George, C.P.O., summarized, "Any patient who presents with back pain should have their feet assessed." They explained, "The art of orthotics is to achieve a balance between stability and mobility." Once a physician or therapist has considered various factors, such as range of motion, strength, tone, dexterity, gait, and pain, appropriate bracing can then be prescribed with extra precaution taken for patients experiencing edema or impaired sensation, as may occur in cases of DIABETES. In addition to FOOTWEAR, biomechanical alignment may be needed in ankle-foot orthoses designed to provide support or alleviate the pain of arthritis. For knee orthoses, a variety of shapes (H, half-moon, U, and doughnut) come with and without hinges, so the therapeutic choice depends on the condition and amount of control needed for protection, external stability, or relief of pain. Similarly, a back brace, body jacket, or corset may be prescribed to aid recovery following back surgery or a vertebral fracture.

A National Institutes of Health Osteoporosis and Related Bone Diseases National Resource Center fact sheet cautioned about the tendency of back muscles to weaken with prolonged use of orthotic devices. Nevertheless, until therapeutic exercises can be resumed, spinal supports can help to reduce pain and provide protection with the specific type and design depending on the need. For instance, several designs address thoracolumbar support alone since vertebral fractures caused by OSTEOPOROSIS most often occur in this spinal region. If multiple fractures or severe cases of KYPHOSIS or SCOLIOSIS require bracing, a full-body jacket or a thoracolumbar corset will usually be prescribed. To maintain correct shoulder positioning, a posture support device may be needed. Although this particular orthotic comes with adjustable shoulder straps, other devices may employ zippers, snaps, buckles, or Velcro to enable a patient to get an orthotic on and off easily.

Aiello, Dorothy D. and Patrick George. "Orthotic Options." Available online. URL: http://www.rehabpub.com Downloaded on May 2, 2003.

Danchik, John. "Going the 'Extra Mile' with the Orthotics Process." *The American Chiropractor* 24, no. 6 (2002): 38.

National Institutes of Health Osteoporosis and Related Bone Diseases National Resource Center. "Supports for Spinal Osteoporosis." Available online. URL: http://www.osteo.org/newfile.asp Downloaded on February 19, 2003.

Osgood-Schlatter disease An American Academy of Family Physicians fact sheet called this disease "one of the most common causes of knee pain in young athletes," especially in boys during a growth spurt. As the fact sheet further explained, "It is believed that Osgood-Schlatter disease results from the pull of the large powerful muscles in the front of the thigh (called the quadriceps). The quadriceps join with the patellar tendons, which run through the knee and into the tibia, to connect the muscles to the knee. When the quadriceps contract, the patellar tendons can start to pull away from the shin bone, causing pain." Fortunately, most instances will resolve themselves as the patellar tendons develop and become stronger in the mature body. Until then, the RICE METHOD of Rest, Ice, Compression, and Elevation can help to alleviate pain, while therapeutic exercises, such as straight-leg raises and leg curls, may be prescribed.

American Academy of Family Physicians. "Osgood-Schlatter Disease: A Cause of Knee Pain in Children." Available online. URL: http://familydoctor.org Downloaded on March 3, 2003.

osteitis deformans See PAGET'S DISEASE.

osteo- This prefix means *bone.* For example, osteoarthropathy refers to any disease of the bones and joints, osteochondrous indicates involvement of bone and cartilage, and osteodermia concerns bony deposits in the skin.

osteoarthritis The most common form of arthritis, osteoarthritis (OA) typically begins as cartilage wears or becomes misshapen, thereby changing both the structure and the ability of bones and joints to function as the condition progresses from painful to a potential disability. The commonly found estimate of 20–21 million Americans with OA includes men and women of all ages with the over-50 age group comprising the largest numbers. However, OA does not inevitably come with aging. Other factors, such as weight, injury, the prior infection of a joint, a genetic predisposition to cartilage wear (primarily in the hands or knuckles), and prolonged stress on joints through work conditions or strenuous physical activity greatly increase the risks, not only of developing OA but also the degenerative problems it can cause. According to the Arthritis Foundation Research Web site, "OA accounts for more than half of the total hip replacements and 85 percent of the total knee replacements done in the United States," with medical costs "estimated from $15.5 billion to $28.6 billion annually."

Calling OA a "degenerative joint disease," the American College of Rheumatology (ACR) fact sheet "Osteoarthritis" said, "It most often affects middle-aged and older people, involving the neck, lower back, knees, hips and fingers. Nearly 70 percent of people over the age of 70 have x-ray evidence of the disease, but only half of these people ever develop symptoms." For those who do, the ACR health information also said, "Therapy for OA includes both medication and other treatments that help to relieve pain and improve joint function. Drug therapy should begin with simple pain relievers (acetaminophen) and progress to nonsteroidal anti-inflammatory drugs and/or intermittent corticosteroid injections. Recently, several thick liquids that resemble normal joint fluid have been approved for use by repeated injection in the knee joints. In addition, there is some evidence suggesting that some dietary constituents may have a beneficial effect."

An extensive report published in the ACR journal *Arthritis & Rheumatism* said, "The goals of the contemporary management of the patient with OA continue to include control of pain and improvement in function and health-related quality of life, with avoidance, if possible, of toxic effects of therapy." Specific suggestions in "Table 1. Nonpharmacologic Therapy for Patients with Osteoarthritis" of the report included patient education, self-management programs, weight loss (if overweight), aerobic exercise, physical therapy (particularly, range of motion and muscle-strengthening exercises), devices to assist ambulation, appropriate footwear, lateral-wedged insoles or bracing as needed, occupational therapy, joint protection, and energy conservation. Since OA often involves weight-bearing joints, the report further said, "Individuals with OA of the lower extremity may have limitations that impair their ability to perform activities of daily living such as walking, bathing, dressing, use of the toilet, and performing household chores. Physical therapy and occupational therapy play central roles in the management of patients with functional limitations. The physical therapist assesses muscle strength, joint stability, and mobility; recommends the use of modalities such as heat (especially useful just prior to exercise); instructs patients in an exercise program to maintain or improve joint range of motion and periarticular muscle strength; and provides assistive devices, such as canes, crutches, or walkers, to improve ambulation. Similarly, the occupational therapist can be instrumental in directing the patient in proper joint protection and energy conservation, use of splints, and other assistive devices, and improving joint function. In addition, the input of a vocational guidance counselor may be important to patients who are still actively employed."

Another comprehensive report, published by the Agency for Healthcare Research and Quality (AHRQ), gave particular emphasis to "Managing Osteoarthritis: Helping the Elderly Maintain Function and Mobility." Although AHRQ has funded various studies, one focus included the Chronic Disease Self-Management Program to help patients deal with their symptoms, thus reducing the need for health care. AHRQ research also investigated the high use—and high costs—of nonsteroidal anti-inflammatory drugs (NSAIDs) for osteoarthritic conditions, finding that "NSAIDs provided very little relief of pain or improvement in function, and they were associated with ulcers, bleeding, and gastrointestinal perforation." Therefore, "Patients who used NSAIDs utilized more hospital and emergency services than nonusers. . . ." With attention given to self-knowledge, AHRQ continued to "Encourage patients to change their behavior to improve symptoms or slow disease progression" with suggestions including appropriate dietary changes and exercise. As the report stated, "Regular exercise helps patients retain mobility and counteracts loss of muscle strength. Exercise such as walking or aquatics improves aerobic capacity and stamina while decreasing depression and anxiety." The report interestingly added, "If patients attribute pain to the progression of osteoarthritis, then they may avoid activities that increase pain. However, if patients attribute pain to loss of muscle tone and strength, then they may increase physical activity."

Since NSAIDs have been implicated in affecting joint cartilage metabolism, other options may be introduced for pain relief. "Topical therapy, such as capsaicin cream, has been shown to be appropriate for patients with knee osteoarthritis who did not respond to or did not want to take oral analgesics. Corticosteroid injections into the joint were helpful in diminishing symptoms in patients with knee osteoarthritis who had swelling and inflammation, but they were not recommended for hip osteoarthritis because of progressive cartilage damage from repeated injections. Patients who do not respond to medical therapy or who require more than three or four joint injections each year to control symptoms of knee osteoarthritis are candidates for surgical intervention." When an orthopedic specialist or physician has deemed surgery advisable, "AHRQ research revealed that the elderly face higher risks of complications and mortality than younger people when they have surgery, including surgical knee repair. However, AHRQ studies also showed: The elderly reported better quality of life, less pain, and better physical function after knee replacement surgery; Surgical complications and mortality rates were lower for surgeons and hospitals that performed more knee replacement surgeries."

Meanwhile, the Mayo Clinic reported on the opposite extreme of treatment and cautioned patients to talk to a primary care physician about herbals or other substances, including natural foods, to assure compatibility with prescribed medications. Furthermore, any new treatment should be carefully evaluated beforehand, particularly if scientific evidence—or good sense—seems to be lacking. For instance, some naturalists believe in the effectiveness of bee venom in relieving arthritic pain either because of its enzymatic action or its ability to bump up the body's production of natural steroids. However, if the patient happens to be allergic to bee stings, that treatment would be foolish and could be fatal. More sensible might be supplementation of vitamins A, C, and E, which "may help prevent the cell damage that leads to joint pain," but, "taking too much vitamin A may worsen OA." A safer choice might be the inclusion of foods high in those vitamins, assuming, of course, they do not interfere with the prescribed medical treatment. Similarly, a diet rich in the omega-3 fatty acids believed to help joint inflammation can be found in cold-water fish, such as salmon or cod, which, on several levels, could be preferable to gagging on the smell and taste of cod liver oil. Although many believe that turmeric, cumin, celery, cinnamon, and capsicum (cayenne pepper) contain anti-inflammatory properties, scientific studies have not adequately focused on their medicinal value. However, the Mayo report offered a sprig of herbal hope by saying, "A trial of ginger as a treatment for osteoarthritis found it may be helpful."

See also NUTRITION.

Agency for Healthcare Research and Quality. "Managing Osteoarthritis: Helping the Elderly Maintain Function and Mobility." Available online. URL: http://www.ahrq.gov Downloaded on September 4, 2003.

American College of Rheumatology. "Osteoarthritis." Available online. URL: http://www.rheumatology.org/research/guidelines/0a-mgmt/oa-mgmt.html Downloaded on February 17, 2003.

Arthritis Foundation Research. "Delivering on the Promise in Osteoarthritis." Available online. URL: http://www.arthritis.org Downloaded on September 4, 2003.

Mayo Clinic. "Complementary and Alternative Arthritis Treatments." Available online. URL: http://www.mayoclinic.com/invoke.cfm Downloaded on November 8, 2002.

osteoblasts Born during the ongoing processes of BONE DEVELOPMENT, these newly grown cells attach to calcified matrix and help living BONE continue to form. For this natural progression to work well, however, the body must perform a balancing act as each bone poises between the growth of new bone tissue and the cellular demolition required for OSTEOCLASTS to get on with their task of remodeling the skeletal system.

osteochondritis dissecans An inadequate blood supply to a bone can cause various types of problems. However, when the outcome involves a separation of bone and cartilage, osteochondritis dissecans occurs. Although this condition can affect all ages, its severity and length of duration may depend on the person's age. For instance, in growing children—especially boys from age 10 to 20—a period of rapid growth combined with high physical activity can cause a temporary loss of blood supply to a bone, which eventually results in the loosening of bone and cartilage. As explained by an American Academy of Family Physicians fact sheet, "The loose piece may stay in place or fall into the joint space, making the joint unstable. This causes pain and feelings that the joint is 'catching' or 'giving way.' These loose pieces are sometimes called 'joint mice.'" By commonly pestering knees and elbows, the joint mice generate pain and make a joint less stable. To evaluate the extent of the condition, X-rays or magnetic resonance imaging (MRI) may be ordered to see if the piece of bone has completely dislodged. If so, surgery may be required. If not, other therapies will be suggested to keep the condition from worsening, particularly in growing children who, thankfully, may grow into the cure of time-strengthened bones.

American Academy of Family Physicians. "Osteocondritis Dissecans." Available online. URL: http://familydoctor.org/handouts/488 Downloaded on September 2, 2003.

osteoclasts These large cells—formed in marrow before relocating to the surface of a bone—have a career of repairing living BONE by removing old cellular debris. Besides being activists in remodeling or other bone-healing processes intended to tend or mend an injured or fractured bone, osteoclasts also lend their name to the technological device clinically used to fracture bones, on purpose, for therapeutic goals.

See also BONE DEVELOPMENT; OSTEOBLASTS.

osteodystrophy With changes in the bones similar to those that occur in OSTEOPOROSIS, this condition results from a defect in BONE DEVELOPMENT. In renal osteodystrophy, those changes can begin many years before presenting noticeable symptoms—particularly in adults unaware of a kidney problem—thus making this a silent crippler.

In April 2003, the National Institute of Diabetes and Digestive and Kidney Diseases published health information in a four-page brochure, which stated that 90 percent of the dialysis patients encounter renal osteodystrophy as the kidneys fail to maintain the proper blood levels of calcium and phosphorus. This means, "When the kidneys stop working normally, phosphorus levels in the blood can become too high, leading to lower levels of calcium in the blood and resulting in the loss of calcium from the bones." In growing children, renal osteodystrophy can cause even greater concern because, as the publication further explained, "The condition slows growth and causes deformities. One such deformity occurs when the legs bend inward or outward (toward or away from the body); this deformity is referred to as 'renal rickets.' Another important consequence is short stature. Symptoms can be seen in growing children with renal disease even before they start dialysis."

Once a diagnosis has been made, a blood sample can help the physician assess mineral levels and decide if medication, dialysis, or simply a change in diet is needed. For the latter, emphasis will be on reducing dietary intake of phosphorus, especially dark soft drinks, beer, dairy, nuts, and dried beans. Calcium supplements may also be recommended, excluding those that aim to reduce stomach acids since, like other over-the-counter medications, they usually contain high levels of phosphorus.

National Kidney and Urologic Diseases Information Clearinghouse. "Renal Osteodystrophy." Available online. URL: http://www.niddk.nih.gov Downloaded on July 21, 2004.

osteogenesis imperfecta Commonly known as brittle bone disease, this form of osteoporosis most often affects children rather than adults. Although the types and severity of symptoms vary, osteogenesis imperfecta (OI) generally has a genetic cause, whether by a spontaneous genetic mutation or an inherited genetic flaw. In either case, a defect in the body's ability to produce and utilize collagen causes bones to break easily, sometimes even during simple everyday activities. In severe cases, OI may also cause the whites of the eyes to turn blue and become more prone to damage in drying conditions, such as harsh lighting, sun, and wind.

Information from the Center for Metabolic Bone Disease and Molecular Research, of the St. Louis Shriners Hospital, explained, "Patients may suffer fractures and the skeleton may be deformed. Because collagen is found throughout the body, other areas of the body are affected, such as ligaments, teeth and sclera (whites of eyes). Affected small bones in the ear may cause hearing difficulties. This disorder ranges from very mild with the child appearing normal height and with a normal skeleton, to severe in which hundreds of fractures can occur over the child's lifetime and result in severe skeletal deformity." Unfortunately, the latter instances may further exacerbate a parent's frustration and anguish if frequent fractures lead to accusations of child abuse. However, a February 27, 2003 news release offered a new measure of hope. That article, entitled "Shriners Hospitals Lead in the Research for Children with Osteogenesis Imperfecta," announced a two-year study of the effects of a drug used for treatment of osteoporosis "to see if alendronate can increase bone density, decrease fractures, and lessen pain."

The Osteogenesis Imperfecta Foundation groups the clinical features of OI into four identifiable categories. Type I is the most common and mildest form. Bone fractures usually occur before puberty. Loose joints, low muscle tone, and a blue or purplish tint to the whites of the eyes also characterize Type I, yet these children will usually reach normal stature as adults. Type II presents the most severe instances of OI, often with respiratory problems and bone deformities resulting in infant mortality. Types III and IV range in severity between the first two categories, with shorter stature often present in both. With no present cure, treatment typically aims to prevent or control symptoms, "maximizing independent mobility and developing optimal bone mass and muscle strength." Surgical and dental procedures and the use of mobility aids may be more common among severe instances of OI. However, "people with OI are encouraged to exercise as much as possible to promote muscle and bone strength, which can help prevent fractures. Swimming and water therapy are common exercise choices for people with OI, as water allows independent movement with little risk of fracture. For those who are able, walking (with or without mobility aids) is excellent exercise. Individuals with OI should consult their physician and/or physical therapist to discuss appropriate and safe exercise."

In addition to encouraging doctor-approved EXERCISE, the Osteogenesis Imperfecta Foundation focused on foods in another fact sheet, "OI Issues: Nutrition." Although foods and supplements offer no cure or prevention of symptoms, "Nevertheless, it is clear that to maintain optimal health, children and adults with OI should eat a balanced diet, which includes a variety of vitamins and minerals, and is low in fat and added sugar. Excessive weight gain should be avoided. Portion size, meal frequency, and total caloric intake may need to be adjusted depending on the severity of OI, body size, and activity level. Dental health may also affect what kind of foods a person with OI can eat, and how they are prepared." With proper exercise, NUTRITION, and medical assistance, OI patients can usually lead productive—and, perhaps, extraordinarily ordinary—lives.

Center for Metabolic Bone Disease and Molecular Research, of the St. Louis Shriners Hospital. "News From the Shriner's Hospital." Available online. URL: http://www.shrinershq.org Downloaded on February 18, 2003.

Center for Metabolic Bone Disease and Molecular Research, of the St. Louis Shriners Hospital. "Shriners Hospital Lead in the Research for Children with Osteogenesis Imperfecta." Available online. URL: http://www.shrinershq.org Downloaded on February 27, 2003.

Osteogenesis Imperfecta Foundation. "Fast Facts On Osteogenesis Imperfecta." Available online. URL: http://www.oif.org/site Downloaded on February 26, 2003.

Osteogenesis Imperfecta Foundation. "OI Issues: Nutrition." Available online. URL: http://www.oif.org/site Downloaded on September 6, 2003.

osteomalacia This adult form of RICKETS presents softened bones resulting from either digestive malabsorption or a lack of vitamin D. In osteomalacia, however, another common causative involves the kidneys as high acidity or acidosis softens and thins the bones. Treatment, therefore, depends on adequately addressing the underlying condition as determined by blood tests and the diagnosis of a rheumatologist or other physician.

osteomyelitis A generic term for bone infection, osteomyelitis can be acute or chronic. In either case, microorganisms, such as bacteria or fungi, invade a bone from one of three directions: through the blood, from a nearby infection, or via direct contact. For instance, the piercing or skin-muscle penetration caused by a needle, nail puncture, thorn, wound, cut, or insect bite could introduce the microorganism. The most serious infections will often be introduced into the bone by a fungal infection, syphilis, or tuberculosis. In most cases, treatment relies heavily on a full course of antibiotics with the choice depending on the primary causative.

Robert C. Mellors, M.D., Ph.D., of Weill Medical College of Cornell University, said, "Osteomyelitis of children usually begins in the metaphysis of long bones. The blood-borne bacteria are carried to the marrow space by way of the nutrient artery." In adults, a more likely route goes through highly vascular vertebrae. There, blood vessels allow the infection to spread "by way of the nutrient branches of the spinal artery or by flow from the pelvic veins to the lumbar veins." However, this vertebral infection may be "secondary to a primary bacteremia caused by genitourinary tract infection, soft tissue and respiratory infections, and those contrived by i.v. drug abusers." Although the symptoms may be subtle—even unnoticed—in adults, children usually experience sudden onset. As Dr. Mellors described it, "The early symptoms of childhood osteomyelitis are those of infection and inflammation: fever, bone pain often throbbing and severe and referred to the metaphysis, tenderness to pressure, limitation of movement which in the extreme may render the limb immobile ('pseudoparalysis'), local erythema, swelling, and heat. Blood cultures are positive in about 50% of pediatric cases," with a clinical diagnosis "supported by a bone scan."

Prior to antibiotics, the mortality rate for patients with osteomyelitis reached 20–40 percent. Today, however, the lack of diagnosis or prompt treatment continues the threat and can transform the infection into a chronic condition. As Dr. Mellors explained, "In chronic osteomyelitis, the avascular dead tissue, pus and bacteria may remain isolated within an area of bone fibrosis and sclerosis and give rise to recurrent episodes of acute osteomyelitis. The treatment of chronic bone infections usually requires, in addition to antimicrobial therapy, surgical intervention to drain abscesses and remove necrotic tissue."

According to the National Institutes of Health (NIH), "When the bone is infected, pus is produced within the bone, which may result in an abscess. The abscess then deprives the bone of its blood supply. Chronic osteomyelitis results when bone tissue dies as a result of the lost blood supply. Chronic infection can persist intermittently for years." When tests, such as a bone scan, blood culture, biopsy, or X-ray indicate osteomyelitis, NIH health information further stated, "In chronic infection, surgical removal of dead bone tissue is usually necessary. The open space left by the removed bone tissue may be filled with bone graft or by packing material to promote the growth of new bone tissue. Antibiotic therapy is continued for at least 3 weeks after surgery." If the surgical patient has poor circulation, the prognosis may remain poor due to the increased possibility of the eventual loss of the affected limb. With adequate treatment, however, acute cases of osteomyelitis usually have a more promising outcome as the bone resumes its normal processes of remodeling and repair.

See also BONE; BONE DEVELOPMENT.

Mellors, Robert C. "Bone." Available online. URL: http://edcenter.med.cornell.edu Downloaded on July 30, 1999.

National Library of Medicine. "Osteomyelitis." Available online. URL: http://nlm.nih.gov/medlineplus/print/ency/article/000437.htm Downloaded on September 5, 2003.

osteonecrosis A type of NECROSIS, this condition results from a temporary—or permanent—disruption of blood flow to a bone, ultimately leading to its death. If this involves bones articulating in a joint, the joint itself may collapse. The National Institute of Arthritis and Musculoskeletal and Skin Diseases stated, "The amount of disability that results from avascular necrosis depends on what part of the bone is affected, how large an area is involved, and how effectively the bone rebuilds itself."

With orthopedic physicians most likely to diagnose the disease, about 10,000 to 20,000 people develop osteonecrosis each year. Common sites are in the long bones, such as the femur, or in the knees and other primary joints. Although any age can be affected, most incidents occur in a person's 30s or 40s with causatives including injury, steroids, blood disorders, excessive use of alcohol, and radiation. If X-ray or magnetic resonance imaging (MRI) confirm a diagnosis, treatments will consider the patient's age, the stage of the disease, and its location with a therapeutic focus on stopping further damage, reducing pain, and improving the patient's use of the affected bone or joint.

National Institute of Arthritis and Musculoskeletal and Skin Diseases. "Health Topics: Questions and Answers About Avascular Necrosis." Available online. URL: http://www.niams.nih.gov/hi/topics Downloaded on July 23, 2003.

osteopathy Although this word can refer to bone diseases in general, osteopathy most commonly denotes a medical system of conservative health maintenance and disease prevention. To signify this specialty, the primary care physician receives a medical degree indicated by a D.O. rather than an

M.D. Often, the main distinction between these two practices has to do with an osteopath's emphasis on maintaining equilibrium in the musculoskeletal system with treatments sometimes involving spinal manipulation similar to a chiropractic adjustment but also including pharmaceutical prescriptions.

As further clarification, Donald Siehl, D.O., stated, "Illness is a disparity between the neuromuscular system and the visceral system in many instances, and this forms a cycle which must be broken into in order to adequately treat the problem. Therefore, we treat by all means possible, but recognize as osteopathic physicians that the most effective treatment is directed to the area of pathology, the lesioned area, or the area of somatic dysfunction in the spinal region. The aim of treatment is to normalize structure in these areas and thus normalize function. Then the body tends to return other tissues to normal. We cannot always normalize all tissues and have to be content with partial normalization. This is why in many instances regular osteopathic manipulative treatment is needed, and why in many instances we have to assist the manipulative aspect of treatment with other measures such as medication, diet and nutrition, rest and physiotherapy modalities."

Siehl, Donald. "The Andrew Taylor Still Memorial Lecture: The Osteopathic Difference—Is It Only Manipulation?" *JAOA: The Journal of the American Osteopathic Association* 101, no. 10 (October 2001): 630–634.

osteoporosis In most people, BONE MASS peaks in the young-adult years and then naturally declines. However, if that peak never gets very high and other demands on the musculoskeletal system occur, osteoporosis—or porous bones—can result in sudden fractures. In Asian and Caucasian women especially, bone mass may diminish by 30 percent within the first five years following menopause, mainly because of a decrease in the body's production of bone-strengthening estrogen. Yet men, children, and women of all ages and races can develop osteoporosis too, particularly if they have certain diseases or take medications that impact bones adversely. For instance, RHEUMATOID ARTHRITIS interferes with calcium absorption as do the corticosteroids commonly prescribed for that and other diseases, thus tipping the scales toward the likelihood of bone imbalances. Fortunately, a rheumatologist can take into account both the individual and the medical variables before developing an effective course of treatment for a patient's needs.

As with many musculoskeletal disorders, however, osteoporosis often can be avoided. The American College of Rheumatology explained, "The best treatment for osteoporosis is prevention. Adequate calcium consumption (more than 1,200 mg per day) and weight-bearing exercise by adolescent and young adult women can increase peak bone mass, which can lower the risk of fractures in later years. Weight-bearing exercise improves bone strength throughout life. Adequate consumption of calcium and vitamin D is essential throughout adulthood for healthy bones. The elimination of risk factors such as smoking, heavy alcohol and caffeine intake, along with the appropriate use and close monitoring of medications known to produce bone loss are considered important adjuncts in the prevention of osteoporosis."

According to "Fast Facts on Osteoporosis," by the National Institutes of Health (NIH) Osteoporosis and Related Bone Diseases National Resource Center, "Osteoporosis is a major public health threat for more than 44 million Americans, 68 percent of whom are women. In the U.S. today, 10 million individuals already have the disease and almost 34 million more are estimated to have low bone mass, placing them at increase risk for osteoporosis." Often called a silent disease, a bone density test, such as the often-recommended DUAL X-RAY ABSORPTIOMETRY (DEXA or DXA), can make osteoporosis more detectable by predicting the chances of bone fracture. However, as the NIH information stated, "People may not know that they have osteoporosis until their bones become so weak that a sudden strain, bump, or fall causes a fracture or a vertebra to collapse. Collapsed vertebrae may initially be felt or seen in the form of severe back pain, loss of height, or spinal deformities such as kyphosis (stooped posture)." Once a diagnosis has been made, the patient may take FDA-approved medications including bisphosphonates (such as alendronate or risedronate), calcitonin, or HORMONE REPLACEMENT THERAPY. Other treatments are continuously being investigated.

Another NIH fact sheet, "Osteoporosis and Arthritis: Two Common but Different Conditions," contrasted treatments by saying, "Everyone with arthritis will use pain management strategies at some time. This is not always true for people with osteoporosis." Although the latter group may need pain control when recovering from a fracture, the quieter condition does not typically voice its painful possibilities. Nevertheless, "osteoporosis and arthritis do share many coping strategies. With either or both conditions, people benefit from exercise programs that may include physical therapy and rehabilitation. In general, exercises that emphasize stretching, strengthening, posture, and range of motion are appropriate," for instance, low-impact aerobics and swimming. As another interesting, and, perhaps, encouraging note, the NIH comparison also said—with italicized emphasis theirs, "While it is possible to have both osteoporosis and arthritis, studies show that people with osteoarthritis are *less likely* to develop osteoporosis. On the other hand, people with rheumatoid arthritis may be *more likely* to develop osteoporosis, especially as a secondary condition from medications used to treat RA."

The ability of medications to disturb the body's balance in processes such as BONE DEVELOPMENT (remodeling) may often be the case in men who acquire osteoporosis. According to still another fact sheet from NIH, "Osteoporosis in Men," "At least half of men with osteoporosis have at least one (sometimes more than one) secondary cause. In cases of secondary osteoporosis, the loss of bone mass is caused by certain lifestyle behaviors, diseases or medications. The most common causes of secondary osteoporosis in men include exposure to glucocorticoid medication, hypogonadism (low levels of testosterone), alcohol abuse, smoking, gastrointestinal disease, hypercalciuria and immobilization."

Although men typically accumulate a greater bone mass density than women, diet or disease-produced malabsorption of nutrients can result in bone loss as can inactivity. University of Arkansas researchers "looked at the physical activities of more than 3,300 women aged 50+," and found "that gardening was one activity strongly related to maintaining healthy bones." As lead researcher Lori Turner, Ph.D., reportedly said, "There's a lot of weight-bearing motion going on in the garden: digging holes, pulling weeds, pushing a mower." Meanwhile, a study from the Penn State University College of Medicine traveled in the opposite direction by "Studying Bears to Fight Human Osteoporosis." "Understanding a bear's long winter nap might yield the key to fighting osteoporosis in humans," particularly as researchers "determine why bears continue to regenerate bone" during that ultimate inactivity—hibernation. Until the mysteries of immobility can be unlocked, however, a sensible exercise program may be preferable to tampering with the key.

See also EXERCISE; NUTRITION.

American College of Rheumatology. "Osteoporosis and Coricosteroid-Induced Osteoporosis." Available online. URL: http://www.rheumatology.org Downloaded on February 17, 2003.

Andrews, Linda Wasmer. "Digging for Bones." *Mature Outlook* (April 2001): 28.

Lewerenz, Dan. "Studying Bears to Fight Human Osteoporosis." *The Union Leader* (March 6, 2003): D 12.

Osteoporosis and Related Bone Diseases National Resource Center. "Osteoporosis and Arthritis: Two Common but Different Conditions." Available online. URL: http://www.osteo.org Downloaded on February 19, 2003.

Osteoporosis and Related Bone Diseases National Resource Center. "Osteoporosis in Men." Available online. URL: http://www.osteo.org Downloaded on February 19, 2003.

osteosarcoma Also referred to as osteogenic sarcoma, this cancerous tumor of the bone has been called the most common primary BONE CANCER, particularly in youths. According to the National Library of Medicine and the National Institutes of Health, a list of symptoms included bone pain, tenderness, swelling, and possibly bone fracture as the first sign. Although its causes remain unknown, the MEDLINEplus information further indicated, "In some cases, osteosarcoma runs in families and at least one gene has been linked to increased risk." For a medical diagnosis, testing generally relies on X-ray or computed tomography (CT) scan of the affected area with appropriate blood tests. Once the need for surgical removal of a tumor has been confirmed, chemotherapy usually begins beforehand with injections into the vein in hopes of tumor shrinkage.

To address the potential outcome of standard treatment, the National Cancer Institute said, "The chance of recovery (prognosis) and choice of treatment depend on the size, location, type, and stage of the cancer (how far the cancer has spread), how long the patient had symptoms, how much of the cancer is taken out by surgery and/or killed by chemotherapy, and the patient's age, blood and other test results, and general health." For patients who have not been helped by standard medical efforts, the www.cancer.gov Web site recommends calling (800) 4-CANCER for information about participation in ongoing clinical trials around the country.

National Cancer Institute. "Osteosarcoma/Malignant Fibrous Histiocytoma of Bone." Available online. URL: http://www.cancer.gov Downloaded on September 10, 2002.

National Library of Medicine. "Medical Encyclopedia: Osteosarcoma." Available online. URL: http://www.nlm.nih.gov/medlineplus Downloaded on July 11, 2002.

osteotomy This operation or incision involving bone may be used for various types of surgical corrections.

See also SURGERY.

oxygen, effects of The amount of oxygen a person takes in will directly affect the level of energy expended by the musculoskeletal system and, therefore, the whole body. For instance, fast-twitch muscle fibers depend on energy acquired during anaerobic use of glycogen, the main type of carbohydrate stored in the body. Conversely, slow-twitch muscle fibers rely on aerobic processes that require oxygen to tap into the energy the body stores in the form of carbohydrates, proteins, and fats. So, if oxygen levels decrease, slow-twitch muscles may be less likely to function well.

See also GRAVITY, EFFECTS OF.

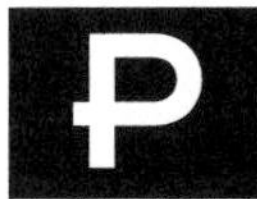

Paget's disease As the second most common bone disease in the world, this chronic, and perhaps hereditary, condition affects the BONE DEVELOPMENT (remodeling) process as abnormally large OSTEOCLASTS cause OSTEOBLASTS to work frantically in an effort to rebuild bone tissue. In the resulting disorderly process, bones thicken but weaken. Pain usually occurs in any affected bone. It most likely occurs in the spine, skull, pelvis, or long bones of the leg as the progressive disorder gradually produces deformities, fractures, or other complications, sometimes in more than one family member. Since early treatment affects the prognosis and quality of life, anyone over age 40 with a blood relative who has been diagnosed with Paget's disease might consult a rheumatologist, endocrinologist, or other specialist to arrange for an alkaline phosphatase blood test every two or three years. If results exceed the normal range, an X-ray or bone scan can be performed to confirm a diagnosis.

The National Institutes of Health (NIH) Osteoporosis and Related Bone Diseases National Resource Center, described the disease's progress by saying, "Paget's disease displays three distinctive stages. In the earliest stage of the disease, an osteolytic lesion may be observed in the skull or a long bone. In the second stage of the disease, x-rays reveal both osteolytic and sclerotic changes in the same bone. In the last stage of the disease, the sclerotic lesion dominates the bone and there may be an increase in the dimensions of the bone itself." When skeletal deformities occur, the location usually influences the type and severity. For instance, long bones may bow while an enlarged skull may lead to headaches or hearing loss. In the spine, compression can impinge on nerve endings, resulting in intense pain and impaired neurological function. In about 1 percent of the cases, the bone develops malignant OSTEOSARCOMA. This means, however, that 99 percent of patients with Paget's disease do not develop BONE CANCER. For that highly predominate group, the NIH report stated, "Four main methods of treatment exist for a patient with Paget's disease: non-pharmacological therapy (focusing mainly on physical therapy as a means of improving muscle strength to help control some types of pain); pharmacological therapy using either bisphosphonates or calcitonins; pain management using analgesics; or surgery."

Often, a mild form of Paget's disease can be suppressed by bisphosphonates that work toward reducing bone resorption by osteoclasts. For those who cannot tolerate that medication, calcitonins may be used for similar purposes. However, another NIH patient information sheet, "Paget's Disease of Bone," recommended "1000–1500 mg of calcium, adequate sunshine, and at least 400 units of vitamin D daily. This is especially important in patients being treated with bisphosphonates. Patients with a history of kidney stones should discuss calcium and vitamin D intake with their physician. Exercise is very important in maintaining skeletal health, avoiding weight gain, and maintaining joint mobility. Since undue stress on affected bones should be avoided, patients should discuss any exercise program with their physician before beginning." Assuming treatments precede any major changes in the bones, NIH also reported, "The outlook is generally good."

Osteoporosis and Related Bone Diseases National Resource Center. "The Management of Paget's Disease of Bone," National Institutes of Health. Available online. URL: http://www.osteo.org/newfile Downloaded on February 19, 2003.

Osteoporosis and Related Bone Diseases National Resource Center. "Paget's Disease of Bone," National Institutes of Health. Available online. URL: http://www.osteo.org/newfile.asp?doc=p110i Downloaded on February 19, 2003.

pain See ACUTE PAIN; CHRONIC PAIN.

pain management Apparently, the diverse peoples of the U.S. have found a unifier: pain. According to the survey "Pain in America," developed for Merck by Ogilvy Public Relations and conducted May/June 1999 by the Gallup Organization, nine in 10 Americans regularly experience pain with almost 26 million classifying theirs as severe. Four in five assumed this has to do with getting older, and 55 percent felt uncomfortable with the prospect of regularly using medication. About half the sufferers said pain puts them in a bad mood, which may account for the 54 percent who said they prefer to be left alone when they are not feeling well.

Another 1999 survey entitled "Chronic Pain in America: Roadblocks to Relief," conducted by Janssen Pharmaceutica for the American Pain Society and the American Academy of Pain Medicine, offered outcomes in "Pain Issues: Pain Is An Epidemic." It said, "The most common types of pain include arthritis, lower back, bone/joint pain, muscle pain, and fibromyalgia." With these and other discomforts disturbing concentration, sleep, and the performance of daily tasks, such as chores and exercise, "an unrelenting downward spiral of depression, isolation and loss of self esteem," also occurs. As mental stress and anxiety complicate issues with which researchers and clinicians have become painfully aware, "no single health care profession holds the puzzle piece that solves this puzzle; rather, each health care profession holds a critical piece that contributes." Indeed, numerous therapeutic options can address individual preferences as patients choose from traditional allopathic medicine or MEDICAL ALTERNATIVES, such as BIOFEEDBACK, COLD THERAPY, HEAT THERAPY, CHIROPRACTIC adjustments, OSTEOPATHY, or NUTRITION.

For instance, the Department of Health and Human Services claimed, "A Mediterranean diet high in olive oil, cooked vegetables, and fish appears to ease symptoms of rheumatoid arthritis." Although results might not be discernible at six weeks, "By the end of the 12-week period, physical function, vitality, and various other measures had improved in the Mediterranean-diet group but not in the control group." An average weight loss of 6.6 pounds may have contributed to this outcome as may have the anti-inflammatory properties of fish oil. Reduction of red meat, dairy, and other high-fat products found in most American diets probably helped, too. However, patients with rheumatoid arthritis—and any other musculoskeletal disorder requiring medication—need to continue with those treatments for good health's sake.

As with other alternatives, sensible nutrition offers complementary—but not replacement—sources of doctor-advised therapies and medication. For pain sufferers who have been told to take over-the-counter analgesics, some HERBS FOR MUSCLES AND BONES can also prove useful. For others, a physician or pharmacist must assess each patient and affirm the safe use of an herb in conjunction with other medicinal products. In addition, clinical studies have not yet offered adequate proof of pain relief nor, in many instances, have they determined a standard dosage for a recommended herb.

With those disclaimers taken into consideration, most holistic practitioners would agree with Herb Research Foundation findings, which said, "To clarify dosage issues, a team of German researchers conducted a four-week clinical trial designed to compare the effectiveness and safety of two different dosages of willow bark extract for alleviating flare-ups of low back pain. . . . Results showed that both the high and low doses of willow bark extract afforded significantly more pain relief than placebo, but the higher dose of willow bark (240 mg/day) was significantly more effective than either the low-dose treatment or the placebo." Of the 210 participants in that study, one patient reacted with swollen eyes and itching assumed to be an allergic response to the herbal treatment.

The Herb Research Foundation also proclaimed "Devil's Claw as Effective as Drug in Relieving Osteoarthritis." With the drug in this particular study referring to diacerhein, "Results showed that the two treatments were equally effective in relieving spontaneous pain. However, by the end of the study, significantly fewer people in the devil's claw group needed to take additional analgesics for 'rescue' pain relief. The frequency of side effects was also significantly lower among people in the devil's claw group."

Often, the side effects of pharmaceuticals—including over-the-counter products—initially persuade medicine-sensitive patients to try herbs and other nutritional aids. Ironically though, some believe that rheumatoid arthritis and other musculoskeletal conditions stem from food allergies affecting the muscles and bones instead of the more commonly noted stomach upset or skin eruption. If any possibility of this exists at all, it is easy enough to check out with an elimination diet that immediately removes the most likely culprits, such as shellfish, chocolate, wheat, eggs, nuts, and dairy. After remaining on this diet for a few weeks to see if any improvement can be detected, each food can then be added back, one at a time, with a week given to note any differences. If all goes well, the next food item can be returned to the diet and so on.

Natural foods often work for or against the production of pain and can also interfere with medication. For example, herbalists and nutritionists laud alfalfa in tablet form or, better yet, heaped fresh into a salad to reduce inflammation and help those with osteoarthritis assimilate nutrients, such as calcium. This natural food source rates high in many vitamins, including vitamin K, which then makes alfalfa a problem for anyone taking a blood thinner. Similarly, ginger and cayenne help to alleviate pain—internally and externally—by increasing circulation, but this can be problematic for those patients with a stomach or skin disorder. Also, turmeric has cortisone-like properties to assuage pain, but again, some people react to this culinary herb or just do not like it.

Because each person has such individual tastes, needs, and reactions, the best pain management will be what is most effective with the least side effects, including those caused by water. Most people, for example, need much more fresh, filtered water than they drink each day, so their systems often remain in an uncomfortable state of near dehydration. Then, if they take an herb, pharmaceutical, or nutritional supplement without a full cup of water for each tablet or capsule, further dehydration creates drought conditions in bones and joints, escalating friction and pain. Conversely, a patient with a kidney dysfunction or condition requiring several medicinal supplements can experience too much hydration by drinking one cup of water per pill or herb, so even the general recommendation of ingesting lots and lots of fresh water has its limitations.

For most of the people most of the time, water and nutritional foods will normally be safer than laboratory products. However, these natural sources do not always provide enough pain relief. According to the National Institutes of Health Osteoporosis and Related Bone Diseases National Resource Center, other means of pain management include the use of heat and ice, braces or other supportive devices, EXERCISE, PHYSICAL THERAPY, ACUPUNCTURE, ACUPRESSURE, MASSAGE THERAPY, and the use of a TRANSCUTANEOUS ELECTRONIC NERVE STIMULATOR. Techniques, such as visual distraction or imagery and relaxation training, can also provide relief, particularly if anxiety has increased a patient's discomfort.

Because people have different levels of pain tolerance and the pain has different causes, treatments require personalization too. For instance, the Massachusetts Medical Society reported, "In March, the FDA approved a device to treat tennis elbow, a painful condition caused by repetitive arm movements such as thwacking tennis balls, golfing, painting, or using tools. Called the Ossa Tron, the device delivers high-energy shock waves to break up scar tissue in the elbow. The noninvasive procedure requires a single, 20-minute treatment. In a study of 225 people treated with the device, 90 percent improved, and 64 percent rated their outcome good or excellent."

Identifying the particular type of pain offers a master key for its removal. Only a physician aware of an individual's symptoms and situation can address this one to one. However, a checklist of pain syndromes would typically include ARTHRITIS, BACKACHE, BONE CANCER, burn pain, HEADACHE, facial pain (such as caused by dental problems), muscle pain, MYOFASCIAL PAIN (such as FIBROMYALGIA), REPETITIVE MOTION DISORDERS, SCIATICA, sports INJURY, SPINAL STENOSIS, TEMPOROMANDIBULAR JOINT problems, neuropathic pain (such as may follow a spinal trauma), and circulatory problems.

Although pain relief with NONSTEROIDAL ANTI-INFLAMMATORY DRUGS and other analgesics may be helpful on an irregular basis, recent research has called their prolonged use into question along with any idea that one pill fills all. The options of elective SURGERY and inadequately tested devices, such as MAGNET THERAPY, to alleviate pain also stir controversy. In general, most reputable forms of therapy continue to incorporate a RICE METHOD of Rest, Ice, Compression, and Elevation. Even this generates questions as to the body's need to set its own thermostat during a healing or pain-coping process. To add frustration to injury, the body's coping devices can also have flaws—for instance, in perpetuating a neural or muscular response long after an injury has healed. In this and other chronic cases, a biofeedback specialist or an occupational therapist can usually identify activities and behaviors that arouse discomfort and then demonstrate techniques to lessen the occasions and intensity of pain.

With the Decade of Pain Control and Research beginning at the start of the 21st century, new health care standards have been set, such as declaring pain a vital sign to be assessed regularly by physicians along with routine gauging of body temperature, blood pressure, pulse, and respiration. Ronald C. Hamdy, M.D., F.R.C.P., F.A.C.P., said, "Health care professionals have a great deal to learn about pain and pain control. Foremost, however, is the need to change our attitude toward pain. In most instances there is no longer any need to let patients suffer. One should not wait for the patient to complain about pain; instead, one should enquire about this symptom and to what extent it is interfering with the patient's daily activities and mental state. In this respect, it is worthwhile to remember the World Health Organization's definition of 'health.' It is a state of complete social, mental, and physical well-being, and not merely the absence of disease. Pain interferes with the patient's well-being and should be adequately addressed."

American Pain Society and the American Academy of Pain Medicine. "Chronic Pain in America: Roadblocks to Relief." Available online. URL: http://aapainmanage.org Downloaded on September 10, 2003.

Hamdy, Ronald C. "The Decade of Pain Control and Research." *Southern Medical Journal* 94, no. 8 (August 2001): 753.

Herb Research Foundation. "Devil's Claw as Effective as Drug in Relieving Osteoarthritis." Available online. URL: http://www.herbs.org/current Downloaded on September 10, 2003.

Herb Research Foundation. "Willow Bark Extract Reduces Low Back Pain." Available online. URL: http://www.herbs.org/current Downloaded on September 10, 2003.

Massachusetts Medical Society. "Shock Waves Tame Tennis Elbow." *Health News* (2003).

Osteoporosis and Related Bone Diseases National Resource Center. "Strategies for Osteoporosis: Coping with Chronic Pain." Available online. URL: http://www.osteo.org/newfile Downloaded on February 19, 2003.

Pain Foundation. "1999–2000: Pain in America: A Research Report." Available online. URL: http://www.painfoundation.org/gain.asp?menu=1&item=3&file=documents/doc055.htm Downloaded on February 10, 2004.

paralysis The opposite of pain, paralysis shuts down the sensation of feeling and causes complete or partial dysfunction of the musculoskeletal system as affected areas of the body fail to respond or move. Some causatives include spinal injury, brain trauma, MULTIPLE SCLEROSIS, stroke, POST-POLIO SYNDROME, and certain types of MUSCULAR DYSTROPHY. Patients having Bell's palsy or a stroke—as well as newborns experiencing a BIRTH INJURY—frequently experience paralysis on one side of the face as evidenced by a drooping mouth or excessive tearing from one eye.

A neurotoxin produced by an embedded tick can also cause paralysis, particularly in children. In those cases, the National Library of Medicine and the National Institutes of Health stated, "The resulting paralysis is ascending (starting in the lower body and moving up) and is similar to that seen in Guillain-Barré syndrome and opposite that seen in botulism and paralytic shellfish poisoning (descending). Affected children develop an unsteady gait (ataxia) followed several days later by lower extremity weakness that gradually moves up to involve the upper limbs. Paralysis may cause loss of respiratory ability and ventilatory assistance may become necessary." Most of the time, however, "Removing the tick removes the source of the neurotoxin. . . ." with rapid and full recovery then expected.

In the case of periodic paralysis, a genetic disorder may be the primary causative as temporary episodes of weakness affect the limbs or the entire body for a few hours up to several days. However, long-term instances of paralysis often involve a spinal injury with a trauma above the fourth vertebra resulting in the most devastating form of paralysis, as experienced by the actor Christopher Reeve. Subsequently, the superman and superwoman efforts of Reeve and his wife Dana resulted in the founding of the Paralysis Resource Center, devoted to treatments for spinal cord disease, trauma, and degenerative musculoskeletal conditions such as AMYOTROPHIC LATERAL SCLEROSIS (ALS.) The article "About Paralysis" on www.paralysis.org/news raised the question, "Is there hope for a cure?" The response offered a realistic yet hopeful view, "In the short term the cure is more likely to mean better bowel and bladder and perhaps sexual function for people with paralysis, reduced pain, improved breathing and/or hand function for quadriplegics. People with ALS may gain years of life; people with MS [multiple sclerosis] might have greater stamina and less frequent exacerbations. Some people may gain functional ambulation; some might even be able to toss out their wheelchairs."

Paralysis Organization. "About Paralysis." Available online. URL: http://www.paralysis.org/m/news Downloaded on April 19, 2002.

National Library of Medicine and National Institutes of Health. "Tick Paralysis." Available online. URL: http://www.nlm.nih.gov/medlineplus/print/ency/article Downloaded on November 9, 2001.

Parkinson's disease Not a musculoskeletal but a neurological disorder, Parkinson's disease nevertheless affects muscles, gait, and balance as cells in the midbrain progressively degenerate. Tremors of the limbs and unmanageable movements also occur. Although prolonged use of some drugs can result in Parkinson-like symptoms, primary forms of the disease have unknown causes. According to the National Parkinson Foundation, "Parkinson's disease affects one of every 100 persons over the age of 60." These 1.5 million Americans comprise a larger group than those with MULTIPLE SCLEROSIS and MUSCULAR DYSTROPHY combined. At present, treatments often focus on physical, speech, and occupational therapies in conjunction with a greater availability of effective medication. As the foundation Web site emphasized, "Good medical management helps restore lost functions in an untreated patient and protects against secondary symptoms that could otherwise develop." Assuming that treatment effectively prevents those secondary conditions, Parkinson's disease is not a fatal illness.

National Parkinson Foundation, Inc. "What the Patient Should Know." Available online. URL: http:/www.parkinson.org Downloaded on February 26, 2003.

patella See KNEE.

patellofemoral syndrome A KNEE is no simple matter. The kneecap (patella) needs to slide smoothly in grooves provided by the thighbone, thereby transmitting power from the upper quadriceps muscle into the lower leg. The knee also needs to keep cartilage together with the knee joint clearly articulating so the leg can bend with no excessive stress on either side. If something—such as a training error, biomechanical flaw, overuse, or muscle tension—prevents the performance of this concerted effort, patellofemoral syndrome (PFS) can occur with plenty of patellofemoral pain. Treatment may then include the RICE METHOD of PAIN MANAGEMENT with occasional taping to align, correct, and protect the patella.

According to a joint endeavor of the American Orthopaedic Society for Sports Medicine and the National Athletic Trainers' Association and Sports Physical Therapy Section, "If the soft tissues (retinaculum, tendon or muscle) are the source of the pain, stretching particularly in the prone (face down) position, can be very helpful to make the support structures more resilient and flexible. One simple stretch is to lie prone, grab the ankle of the affected leg with one hand and gently stretch the front of the knee." With modification of physical activity recommended until the pain subsides, gentle warm-ups can be followed by therapeutic exercises aimed to build up the QUADRICEPS muscle. Sometimes, though, surgery may be needed. "If the cartilage under the kneecap is fragmented and causing mechanical symptoms and swelling, arthroscopic removal of the fragments may be helpful. If the patella is badly aligned, however, a surgical procedure may be needed to place the kneecap back into proper alignment, thereby reducing abnormal pressures on the cartilage and supporting structures around the front of the knee."

Fulkerson, John P., M.D. "Patellofemoral Pain." Available online. URL: http://www.sportsmed.org Downloaded on July 5, 2003.

pectoral region The pectoral muscles of the chest and the pectoral or SHOULDER girdle consist of the scapula and CLAVICLE or collarbone. These muscles and bones assist breathing, chest expansion, arm movement, and the exertion of strength, which often makes the pectoral region take the fall as ROTATOR CUFF muscles strain and collarbones break. As pertains to the chest, the interwoven layers of pectoral muscles provide a protective and, often, decorative device over the thoracic ribs, covering the heart like a breastplate.

pediatric studies The September 2002 death of 10-year-old Taylor Davison in Illinois revealed a belated need for pediatric policies to protect children from sports injuries. An article reporting on this in *Newsweek* quoted Dr. Reginald Washington, a pediatric cardiologist and chairman of the American Academy of Pediatrics Committee on Sports Medicine and Fitness, as saying, "There is a serious lack of data about what types of injuries are occurring." Such investigations could take years. Yet researchers from the University of Pittsburgh contend that reduction of risk and injury would be immediately possible if leagues required first aid training to equip coaches to recognize and correctly respond to traumas, especially those involving the head, neck, or spine. Again according to the *Newsweek* article, enforceable rules need to address a child's return to play if the potential of serious injury, such as a concussion, even mildly exists.

In addition to the seriousness of sports injuries among both boys and girls, the American Academy of Pediatrics expressed concern over backpack injuries, stressing that no child should carry more than 10–20 percent of his or her body weight. As 1999 statistics by the Consumer Product Safety Commission suggest, this general guideline may be unknown or unheeded since, in that year alone, over 6,000 children suffered backpack-related injuries, with 56 percent in the five to 14 age group. For security reasons, some schools no longer offer lockers for textbook storage at a time when notepads, calculators, or other electronic devices add to a backpack's weight, putting more stress on a child's growing musculoskeletal system. As an easy reference for knowing how much is too much, an article in *USA Today* quoted Scott Bautch, former president of the American Chiropractic Association's Council on Occupational Health, as saying, "If they're leaning forward, that backpack is too heavy."

Still another primary cause of musculoskeletal injuries and death in children involves vehicular accidents. Although the number of such instances decreased as public awareness of the importance of child restraints increased, the National Highway Traffic Safety Administration (NHTSA) recommends that children who have outgrown a safety seat be provided a booster seat at least until they are 4'9" or eight years old. The NHTSA reports, "Today, 95 percent of infants and 91 percent of toddlers, age one to age four, are restrained in safety seats," but only 10 percent of the children between four and eight continue to have proper safety equipment while riding in a car.

Many children, of course, might do well to walk. Despite recommendations that young people exercise or otherwise participate in moderate physical activities for a minimum of 30–60 minutes each day, those numbers come closer to a typical weekly total. In 2003 the National Institute of Child Health and Human Development (NICHD) issued a news release entitled "Study Suggests Schools Lacking in Exercise Programs for Children." The ongoing NICHD study involves observations and evaluations of over 1,300 children around the United States. However, this particular investigation assessed the physical activities of 814 third graders from 648 schools across the country, finding that, "on average, children had 2.1 PE classes per week, totaling 68.7 minutes." These low numbers seem especially troubling in light of an earlier report from the Department of Health and Human Services "which estimated that 300,000 Americans die each year as a result of sedentary lifestyle and poor eating habits." Although that report focused on adults, the ability to build BONE MASS begins in the formative years and either assists or hinders a person's bone health throughout life.

In addition to that long-term concern, poor habits can have a more immediate impact. For example, the NICHD, announced, "The proportion of children ages 6 to 18 that were overweight increased from 6 percent in 1976–1980 to 11 percent in 1988–1994 to 15 percent in 1999–2000." Although the reasons remained unclear, the report suggested, "Eating out, diets low in fruits and vegetables, and lack of exercise probably play a role." Indeed, a 2001 National Institutes of Health news release reported, "Only 13.5 percent of girls and 36.3 percent of boys age 12 to 19 in the United States get the recommended daily allowance (RDA) of calcium, placing them at serious risk for osteoporosis and other bone diseases, according to statistics from the Department of Agriculture. Because nearly 90 percent of adult bone mass is established by the end of this age range, the nation's youth stand in the midst of a calcium crisis."

With good NUTRITION and EXERCISE being crucial to healthy BONE DEVELOPMENT in children, another factor involving young musculoskeletal systems concerns not only malnutrition but maltreatment. The NICHD said, "Researchers at the University of Wisconsin have found that low-income children who receive pre-school and early-grades learning assistance, coupled with services for parents, are less likely than those who do not receive these services to be victims of child maltreatment." According to this study, "Children who attended the preschool intervention program had a 52 percent lower rate of maltreatment, compared with a control group of children who did not attend."

Too often, child abuse results in wrenched arms and broken bones, but NICHD released more sad news in 2003. After evaluating the data from 15,686 students in grades six through 10 in public and private schools around the country, the results showed, "Both children who bullied and their victims were more likely than youth who had never been involved in bullying to engage in violent behaviors themselves. However, the association between bullying and other forms of violence was greatest for those who bullied others." While this may be the very first study to examine how bullying relates to other forms of violence, one conclusion seems obvious: what is given out and received will more readily be passed on, whether a bad habit or a good one.

National Institute of Child Health and Human Development. "Bullies, Victims at Risk for Violence and other Problem Behaviors." Available online. URL: http://www.nichd.nih.gov Downloaded on April 14, 2003.

National Institute of Child Health and Human Development. "Federal Interagency Forum on Child and Family Statistics: Teen Birth Rate Down, Exposure to Secondhand Smoke Drops, Kids More Likely to Be Overweight." Available online. URL: http://www.nichd.nih.gov Downloaded on July 18, 2003.

National Institute of Child Health and Human Development. "Study Suggests Schools Lacking in Exercise Programs for Children." Available online. URL: http://www.nichd.nih.gov Downloaded on February 10, 2003.

Noonan, David. "How Safe Are Our Youngest Athletes?" *Newsweek* (September 16, 2002): 50.

Spector, Mike. "Kids' Backpacks Pack a Load of Problems." *USA Today* (September 11, 2002): 6D.

pelvic region In the human body, this bottom part of the trunk comes muscle packed around the bony frame of the pelvic girdle. Those bones, which comprise the lower portion of the APPENDICULAR SKELETON, include the right and left HIP, the SACRUM, and the COCCYX (tailbone). Naturally, women have wider, shallower pelvic bones suitable for childbearing. Otherwise, the pelvic structure for both sexes protects the reproductive, urinary, and digestive systems; provides a foundation for the upper body; and offers the pelvic floor muscles a good place to sit. If those muscles need strengthening, a simple exercise—Kegels—is to squeeze or hold as though trying to avoid voiding. Hold for about 10 seconds, and then rest for another 10 seconds. The exercise can be performed while sitting, standing, or lying around. If done three or four times a day, a set of 10 contractions will build up weakened muscles in the pelvic floor and assist bladder control, too. This same exercise can also help to prevent muscle injuries if a person squeezes together the pelvic muscles while lifting weighty objects.

Despite the strength of the pelvic floor, hip bones receive a high share of fractures. According to the American Academy of Orthopaedic Surgeons, "A pelvic fracture is often associated with substantial bleeding, sensory and motor dysfunction, and other injuries." Growing teens, participants in sports, the elderly, or people with osteoporosis remain at high risk for muscle tears and fractures of individual bones. "However, most pelvic fractures involve high-energy forces, such as those generated in a motor vehicle accident, crush accident or fall. Depending on the direction and degree of the force, these injuries can be life-threatening." Following emergency assistance and stabilization of the injury, "All pelvic fractures require X-rays, usually from different angles, to show the degree of displacement to the bones. A computed tomography (CT) scan may be ordered to define the extent of other injuries. The physician will also examine the blood vessels and nerves to the legs to see if they have been injured." If so, impaired mobility and sexual function may result even after surgery. However, stable pelvic fractures usually mend well.

American Academy of Orthopaedic Surgeons. "Fracture of the Pelvis." Available online. URL: http://orthoinfo.aaos.org/fact Downloaded on September 13, 2003.

periosteum Except for the actual joint where the extremities of bones articulate with one another, this fibrous membrane encases each bone, providing a thin but nicely layered surface. Within the periosteum sheath, nerves provide sensation and enervation to the particular bone they assist while blood vessels bring nutrients and life. Also housed within the periosteum is an inner layer of connective tissue that actively functions in forming new bone tissue and repairing injuries. However, the sheath itself can experience various types of wounding. For instance, periosteophyte refers to a bony growth on the otherwise typically smooth surface, and periosteomyelitis presents with inflammation. When a trauma or infectious disease affects the sheath, periostitis can cover the affected bone with pain, inflammation, and fever. If all works according to plan, however, fibers of protein will link the appropriate tendons to skeletal bones by passing through the surface membrane of the periosteum and making a strong connection for muscles to become attached, moving their favored bones effectively.

PET scan See POSITRON EMISSION TOMOGRAPHY.

phalanges See FINGER OR FINGERS.

phosphorus See NUTRITION.

physical activity See ACTIVITY; EXERCISE.

physical therapy As one of the medical professions devoted to the musculoskeletal system, physical therapy—or physiotherapy—is most known as a course of rehabilitative action intended to increase a patient's range of motion, coordination, strength, balance, gait, and/or mobility. Generally, a physical therapist (PT) will be called in by a physician or an orthopedic specialist to assist in a patient's recovery after a stroke, injury, or surgery. However, a PT can help to prevent disabilities too, as pointed out by Dagny Scott Barrios in *Runner's World.* Although most insurance companies will not cover therapy except by a doctor's referral, Barrios contends, "Physical therapists are a runner's first line of defense against injury, yet they don't just heal. They can keep you from getting injured in the first place." For example, a PT might check the shoes of a runner or other athlete to evaluate a need for orthotics and other supportive equipment. A PT might customize a program of stretches and exercises to target a specific muscle group. If an injury has occurred, a PT might use ultrasound to treat tendinitis or a sprain and, perhaps, apply deep-tissue massage to a runner's knee. Although some overlapping exists in treatments provided by an OCCUPATIONAL THERAPIST (OT) and a PT, an OT often focuses on helping a patient to develop or regain fine-motor skills, such as those needed for writing, dressing, and performing daily tasks. In contrast, a PT works to strengthen or rehabilitate the large muscles required for ambulation and athletic performances. In either profession, specialized studies and state examinations assure proficient training for certification or licensing.

Barrios, Dagny Scott. "Healing Hands." *Runner's World* (March 2003): 86–91.

pigeon toes See FEET OR FOOT; INTOEING.

pivot joint This type of synovial JOINT allows bones to rotate. For example, the top two cervical vertebrae form a pivot as the projection of one bone fits into the ringed socket of another, enabling a person's head to turn, normally, from side to side with interest or with a clear show of "NO!"

plantar fasciitis Running along the bottom of the foot is the tough, fibrous tissue of fascia that travels from heel to toe. If it steps into a whole lot of pain, that condition may be plantar fasciitis. According to an American Academy of Orthopaedic Surgeons (AAOS) fact sheet, this overuse injury brings inflammation to the fascia on the sole or plantar surface of the foot. "The condition starts gradually with mild pain at the heel bone often referred to as a stone bruise." Although common among overweight persons, runners, and those who spend much time on their feet, plantar fasciitis can become a chronic problem if left untreated. With the RICE METHOD of Rest, Ice, Compression, and Elevation as the first course of action, AAOS also advised, "A program of home exercises to stretch your Achilles tendon and plantar fascia are the mainstay of treating the condition and lessening the chance of recurrence." Shock-absorbing shoes, taping, and an orthotic heel pad may also be needed, but "about 90 percent of people with plantar fasciitis improve significantly after two months of initial treatment." If not, corticosteroid injections or a walking cast for a couple of weeks may help a person to avoid surgery on the involved ligament.

The American College of Foot and Ankle Surgeons concurred with the typical treatments and also emphasized predisposing factors to consider, such as ARTHRITIS, bone abnormalities, GOUT, and collagen disorders—each of which needs to be checked out by a physician or rheumatologist. About 14 percent of the adults in the U.S. experience plantar fasciitis or a similar condition, such as a heel spur. However, the common causes of high arches, PRONATION, FLATFEET, or inappropriate FOOTWEAR can often be detected and corrected, enabling the patient to step away from a more serious foot problem.

American Academy of Orthopaedic Surgeons. "Plantar Fasciitis." Available online. URL: http://orthoinfo.aaos.org Downloaded on September 15, 2003.

American College of Foot and Ankle Surgeons. "Heel Pain," URL: http://www.acfas.org Downloaded on September 15, 2003.

plantar flexion This joint movement occurs as the foot points down, placing a flexible person into a tiptoe position.

plasmacytoma See MULTIPLE MYELOMA.

podiatry This medical specialty focuses on solutions to almost every problem of the foot, ankle, and heel, from bunions and ingrown toenails to biomechanical deformities, fractures, and infections. After receiving a doctorate in podiatric care, a podiatrist must pass state and national examinations to be fully licensed. To treat foot-related problems, including those encountered by advanced cases of diabetes, a podiatrist may fit orthotics, design casts, set broken bones, prescribe medications, perform surgery, and enlist the aid of therapists. According to the Bureau of Labor statistics, about 18,000 podiatrists worked in hospitals or set up practices in 2000 as all age groups in the U.S. got more actively on their feet.

Bureau of Labor Statistics. "Podiatrists." Available online. URL: http://statsbls.gov/oco Downloaded on September 16, 2003.

pod- or podo- Not a pod but a podium for FEET, these suffixes relate to the foot in some way. For instance, podobromidrosis refers to smelly feet, and podalgia means foot pain—perhaps from cramming the toes into tightly fitted shoes like too many peas in a pod.

poliomyelitis See POST-POLIO SYNDROME.

polymyalgia rheumatica This syndrome seems to affect people over age 50, causing aches and stiffness in the neck, shoulders, and hips. Often found in conjunction with some type of underlying inflammatory disorder, polymyalgia rheumatica (PMR) can be difficult to diagnose since no specific tests presently pinpoint the problem. An American College of Rheumatology fact sheet said typical treatments aim to relieve symptoms, usually with prednisone, but with nonsteroidal anti-inflammatory medication used in milder cases. Additional symptoms, such as fatigue, low-grade fever, weight loss, or depression, may also be in need of treatment to lift a patient's spirits and quality of life.

American College of Rheumatology. "Polymyalgia Rheumatica and Giant Cell Arteritis." Available online. URL: http://www.rheumatology.org Downloaded on February 17, 2003.

polymyositis An inflammatory muscle disease, polymyositis sometimes accompanies disorders of the autoimmune system or of the connective tissue, such as RHEUMATOID ARTHRITIS. Muscle weakness occurs closest to the trunk of the body. In describing the condition, the National Institute of Neurological Disorders and Stroke (NINDS) said, "Eventually, patients have difficulty rising from a sitting position, climbing stairs, lifting objects, or reaching overhead." Fatalities rarely result except "in patients with severe and progressive muscle weakness, dysphagia, malnutrition, pneumonia, or respiratory failure." Immunosuppressants and steroid drugs accompany physical therapy, which is "usually recommended to avoid muscle atrophy." Also according to NINDS, responses to treatment vary from satisfactory to very good.

The National Institute of Neurological Disorders and Stroke. "What Is Polymyositis?" Available online. URL: http://www.ninds.nih.gov/health Downloaded on November 19, 2001.

popliteal tendinitis If the popliteus (or popliteal) tendon pops, tears, or uncomfortably stretches over time, the knee will likely feel it as popliteal tendinitis (or tenosynovitis.) Normally, the popliteus tendon extends from behind the thighbone across the back of the knee and then wraps around to the top of the shinbone to keep the lower leg from twisting when running. If a foot rolls inward on a hard step or during a downhill race, inflammation, pain, and swelling may occur on the outside of a knee that becomes tender to the touch. Ignoring the condition will not make it go away. Instead, the condition will only worsen as scar tissue forms a long-term bond with pain.

Initial treatment usually begins with the RICE METHOD—Rest, Ice, Compression, and Elevation of the leg above the heart level. Additional therapy then depends on a proper diagnosis to distinguish the problem from similar conditions, such as a tear in the kneecap, that can also cause pain near the joint line. Timothy S. Petsche, M.D., and F. Harlan Selesnick, M.D., said, "Popliteus tendinitis is important to recognize because it often is severe enough to prevent athletic participation, but it also usually responds quickly to appropriate management. Diagnosis is based on a careful history and examination. Inflammation can be treated with NSAIDs [nonsteroidal anti-inflammatory drugs], but injection is reserved for refractory cases. The key to successful and lasting improvement is inclusion of a therapy program for the quadriceps that strengthens and improves muscle endurance."

See also KNEE; TENDINITIS OR TENDONITIS.

Petsche, Timothy S., M.D., and F. Harlan Selesnick, M.D. "Popliteus Tendinitis: Tips for Diagnosis and Management." Available online. URL: http://www.physsportsmed.com Downloaded on September 17, 2003.

positron emission tomography Fondly called a PET scan, this radiographic technique offers three-dimensional colorized computer images to examine chemical substances in various body tissue and precisely locate dysfunctions or disorders, such as in the brain.

post-polio syndrome In the first half of the 20th century, the viral disease known as polio or infantile paralysis shortened young lives by the thousands as poliomyelitis struck spinal cords and shut down respiration. Those who survived the fever and searing inflammation of the nervous system often experienced muscle contractions, muscular atrophy, and permanent deformities. As the virus affected countless numbers around the world, the March of Dimes funded research that soon led to the development of the Salk vaccine and, shortly thereafter, the Sabin oral vaccine—both of which effectively eradicated polio in America. Today, however, up to a quarter-million polio survivors in the U.S. alone may have post-polio syndrome (PPS).

According to the March of Dimes, "The main symptom of PPS is new muscle weakness that gradually worsens." Breathing problems or difficulty with swallowing occur infrequently but, according to the March of Dimes report, "Even muscles that were believed to be unaffected by the previous bout with polio may be affected." The causes for this recurrent problem remain a mystery. "However, many researchers believe that PPS symptoms result, at least in part, from the unusual stress placed on surviving nerve cells. During the initial attack of polio, some of the nerve cells in the spinal cord that control muscles (called motor neurons) are damaged or destroyed. Without impulses from these nerve cells, a muscle cannot function. Fortunately, some motor neurons usually survive the polio attack and send out new nerve connections to the orphaned muscle cells in an attempt to take over the function of the nerve cells that were destroyed. This process enables an individual to regain at least some use of affected muscles. However, after many years, the overburdened nerve cells may begin to fail, resulting in new muscle weakness."

Although no definitive tests exist for PPS, a computed tomography (CT) scan or magnetic resonance imaging (MRI) can often eliminate the possibility of other disorders. Then treatment may include physical therapy, moist heat, ice packs, or massage with medications prescribed to lessen the pain. Devices that assist mobility and conservation of energy may also be advised with exercises, such as gentle stretches, uniquely designed for the individual.

A National Center on Physical Activity and Disability (NCPAD) fact sheet reported that 16–40 percent of polio survivors may encounter PPS symptoms three to four decades after the original illness. Although NCPAD soundly advised a medical evaluation before starting any exercise program, it listed the potential benefits as including "improvement in cardiovascular capacity and in performing activities of daily living; Maintenance of muscle strength, endurance and power; Greater range of motion." In general, NCPAD encouraged "short-term" exercise for formerly affected muscles that show no present indication of weakness with a full exercise program for muscles that were never affected. Another recommendation emphasized the use of a log or diary to monitor energy levels with strong warnings to "immediately STOP exercising upon experiencing weakness or discomfort after exercise" since this signals excessive activity that can further weaken muscles rather than having the strengthening effect intended.

In a comprehensive two-part article on PPS for *Geriatric Times*, Dr. Susan L. Perlman—a neurologist and the former director of the UCLA Post-Polio Clinic—said, "Although loss of independence for personal activities of daily living (ADL) is fairly rare, many people with PPS experience changes in lifestyle or activity, usually first noted with difficulty walking and climbing stairs or with instrumental ADL (e.g., cooking, cleaning, shopping and driving)." Cold intolerance and muscle cramping may also be commonly experienced. "Neurological consultation should be sought when the neurologic symptoms present are unusually severe or just unusual for PPS (e.g., seizures, changes in memory or mood, vision or hearing abnormalities, dizziness, tremor or imbalance, numbness, rapidly progressive muscle weakness and atrophy, severe headache or other non-orthopedic pain). A neurologist or physical medicine specialist can perform an electromyogram and nerve conduction studies to help confirm the presence of underlying motor unit changes from the original polio infection and to look for changes consistent with other diseases."

As mentioned in the same article, an international conference on PPS suggested an interdisciplinary team of medical specialists, including an orthopedist, rheumatologist, physical therapist (PT), OCCUPATIONAL THERAPIST (OT), and others as needed with a primary care physician coordinating both the evaluation and the treatment processes. For instance, a PT or OT might assist the patient in assessing his or her lifestyle and arranging a more ergonomically correct environment. An orthopedic specialist might prescribe a brace or walking device to aid mobility and prevent FALLING. Other treatments may involve aquatic exercises, BIOFEEDBACK, and various types of medication, from a topical ointment to a MUSCLE RELAXANT, but with careful monitoring to avoid medicating the pain caused by overuse. In those instances, the activity itself should cease. Dr. Perlman also pointed out, "The strongest medicine that a practitioner can provide to a patient with PPS is education and encouragement. Sixty percent of polio survivors with new symptoms have a medical or neurological problem that is unrelated to polio, and that problem may be treatable."

March of Dimes. "Post-Polio Syndrome (PPS)." Available online. URL: http://www.marchofdimes.com Downloaded on April 22, 2003.

National Center on Physical Activities and Disabilities (NCPAD). "Post-Polomyelitis." Available online. URL: http://www.ncpad.org/factshthtml Dowloaded on September 5, 2002.

Perlman, Susan L., M.D. "Post-Polio Syndrome, Part I: Definition and Diagnosis." Available online. URL: http://www.geriatrictimes.com/archive.html Downloaded on September 17, 2003.

Perlman, Susan L., M.D. "Post-Polio Syndrome, Part II: Treatment Strategies." Available online. URL: http://www.geriatrictimes.com/archive.html Downloaded on September 17, 2003.

posture With BONE DEVELOPMENT being such an active issue in growing children, parents often take a postural position with commands to "Stand up straight!" and "Stop slumping those shoulders!" Indeed, a person's carriage comes weighted with connotation, characterization, and body language signs, from being an upright citizen to a slouch.

In discussing the importance of posture in helping athletic performances, the January/February 2001 issue of *Sports Illustrated For Women* offered some ideas for exercises to strengthen and maintain healthy posture. For example, chin tucks, which reportedly assist the neck and shoulders, came with terse instructions to "stand tall with shoulders down and chest lifted. Tuck chin in (not down), drawing head and ears over shoulders while continuing to lift chest; look straight ahead. Hold 5 to 10 seconds, then relax; repeat 10 times." Since any exercise can easily strain an existing problem with the neck, back, or knees, a determining factor will be whether the person can maintain a neutral position in the affected joint. For instance, those with hip or knee pain would be wise to avoid the posture-strengthening exercise of isometric presses. If, however, the beginning position poses no concerns, the article instructed, "Lie face up, knees bent and feet on floor, a few inches in front of knees. Place hands under lower back so fingertips meet in the area under navel. Draw navel to spine to engage abdominal muscles. Feel the pressure of the lower back pressing against hands, but don't flatten the back—try to keep the natural curvature of the spine." After holding that pose for five to 10 breaths, the instructions continued, "Slide feet about six inches farther from butt, straightening legs slightly. Hold another 5 to 10 breaths. Continue to move feet farther away, going as far as you can without arching lower back off the floor."

Although people of all ages might enjoy exercising to enhance their athletic performances and improve posture too, a more likely occurrence has children and adults sedately seated in front of a computer screen. This has rightly aroused public health concerns about the increasingly inactive lifestyle of most Americans. Postural problems can also develop from using ill-fitting equipment. However, the ERGONOMIC chairs and work stations intended for adults may not offer the support a smaller body needs. To address this, the American Occupation Therapy Association reminded readers, "A few adjustments can be made to a child's work area to promote a healthy lifestyle free of pain." For instance, "The head should be level with the monitor and the top of the screen at eye level. The forearms should be parallel to the keyboard and held only slightly above it. The lower back should be supported while sitting in front of a computer. Place a small pillow or rolled up towel between the back of the chair and the child's lower back to provide back support. Feet should rest flat on the floor or on a footstep. If a child cannot reach a footstep, stack boxes under it to raise it until the child can rest his or her feet comfortably."

With activity needed to maintain bone health for any age group, the National Institutes of Health Osteoporosis and Related Bone Diseases National Resource Center stated, "By practicing proper posture and learning the correct way to move (called *body mechanics*), you can protect your bones while remaining physically active. One of the most important concepts in body mechanics and posture is *alignment,* which refers to the relationship of the head, shoulders, spine and hips to each other. Proper alignment puts less stress on the spine and ensures good posture. A slumped, head-forward posture puts harmful stress on the spine, as does bending forward or twisting your spine."

Since muscle strength, flexibility, and posture greatly affect quality of life, particularly for those with osteoporosis, the Osteoporosis and Related Bone Diseases National Resource Center offered the following practical suggestions for aligning the spine. "Stand with your back against a wall with your heels 2 inches from the wall. Tighten your abdominal muscles. . . . Lift your breastbone, keep your head up, and look straight ahead. Bring your shoulders back toward the wall. There should be a small hollow at the small of your back. Maintaining this position, move away from the wall and check your posture in a full length mirror from the front and side." By following those instructions, a person becomes more aware of the feel and look of proper spinal alignment. To maintain that good posture while standing, the fact sheet further recommended, "Keep your head high, chin in, shoulder blades slightly 'pinched.' Maintain the natural arch of your lower back as you flatten your stomach. Your feet should point straight ahead with your knees lined up over your second toe. If you are standing in one place for any length of time, put one foot up on a stool or in an open cupboard. Switch feet periodically." Once seated, the natural arch in the back continues to be maintained with the head, back, and hips in alignment and feet flat on the floor but with a footstool recommended for prolonged sitting. These suggestions address patients with osteoporosis but work for almost anyone interested in upholding healthy posture.

American Occupation Therapy Association. "Healthy Computing for Today's Kids." Available online. URL: http://www.aota.org/featured/area6 Downloaded on December 1, 2001.

Osteoporosis and Related Bone Diseases National Resource Center. "Strategies for Osteoporosis: Guidelines for Safe Movement." Available online. URL: http://www.osteo.org/newfile Downloaded on February 19, 2003.

Staff. "A Tall Order." *Sports Illustrated for Women.* Available online. URL: http://sportsillustrated.cnn.com/sifor women/2001/january_february/contents/ Downloaded on February 19, 2003.

potassium See NUTRITION.

poultice A hot mustard sandwich between two squares of muslin makes an age-old recipe. When universally applied to sore and achy muscles, a poultice can relieve pain and improve circulation. Other sandwiched ingredients—from warm linseed oil to stir-fried onions—are used depending on the complaint or culture from which a patient comes. The treatment differs from other home remedies, such as a mustard plaster, in that the latter can be applied to dry skin whereas a poultice is damp or downright wet with a thin cloth to protect the most sensitive skin.

pregnancy, effects of Women awaiting childbirth have unique concerns regarding their muscles and bones. One of the most worrisome is the "Effect of Pregnancy on Bone Mineral Density and Biochemical Markers of Bone Turnover in a Patient with Juvenile Idiopathic Osteoporosis." In the case report by that title published in the *Journal of Bone and Mineral Research,* a team of doctors from Scotland and the U.K. presented their findings on a 19-year-old patient whom they had diagnosed about seven years prior as having JUVENILE OSTEOPOROSIS. At that time, her pediatrician had referred the girl (LG) to them to find out what caused the persistence of a lower backache. When a series of spinal X-rays and a BONE MINERAL DENSITY test revealed multiple vertebral fractures, the doctors promptly began treatments for juvenile osteoporosis, bringing the disorder in check until her pregnancy. Despite immediate supplements of calcium and vitamin D followed up with careful monitoring, "At 32 weeks gestation, LG suffered acute onset of back pain, which was very disabling and required the use of crutches to walk. When reexamined, her height had decreased by 3 in. and her posture had changed dramatically with a marked kyphosis." X-rays taken after the cesarean delivery of an early but healthy baby "showed acute fracturing of three previously fractured vertebrae." However, no new bone breaks had occurred.

This case history demonstrated the rarity of a fracture even when one might be expected. Rarer yet would be an osteoporosis-type fracture in any woman during a normal pregnancy. According to a National Institutes of Health Osteoporosis and Related Bone Diseases National Resource Center fact sheet, "It appears that if pregnancy-associated osteoporosis does exist, it is probably quite rare. (By 1996, eighty cases had been reported in the literature.)" Of these highly unusual instances, "pregnancy-associated osteoporosis tends to be identified with the postpartum period (56%) or the third trimester (41%). Affected women usually present with back pain, loss of height, and vertebral fractures. Hip pain and fracture of the femur are less common but have been reported. The condition usually appears during the first pregnancy, tends to be temporary and usually does not recur." In the overwhelming majority of women, however, "physiologic changes during pregnancy that may actually be protective of bone include the third trimester estrogen surge and increased bone loading due to weight gain."

Regarding women who choose to nurse their infants, the report continued, "Two physiologic occurrences may be responsible for bone loss during lactation. First, there is an increased calcium demand from maternal bone. This demand varies from woman to woman based on the amount of breast milk produced and upon the duration of lactation. Secondly, because of elevated prolactin levels, women who breastfeed tend to be in a hypoestrogenic state. Though significant amounts of bone mineral can be lost during breastfeeding, the loss of bone tends to be transient. Studies have consistently shown significant trends in bone loss during lactation, with full recovery of bone density by six months after weaning."

Black, A. J., R. Reid, et al. "Effect of Pregnancy on Bone Mineral Density and Biochemical Markers of Bone Turnover in a Patient with Juvenile Idiopathic Osteoporosis." *Journal of Bone and Mineral Research* 18, no. 1 (2003): 167–171.

Osteoporosis and Related Bone Diseases National Resource Center. "Pregnancy, Lactation and Bone Health." Available online. URL: http://www.osteo.org/newfile Downloaded July 1999.

pressure points In traditional or allopathic medicine, a pressure point refers to the area where an artery nearing the skin surface can be felt in the throb of a pulse. If an INJURY OR ACCIDENT causes bleeding, direct pressure on the point can stop the flow of blood or lessen a hemorrhage as a measure of FIRST AID until professional medical help arrives. For musculoskeletal concerns addressed by the MEDICAL ALTERNATIVE of ACUPRESSURE, pressure points may be a common but incorrect way of referring to the potent points to which a trained technician applies pressure, releases tension, and relaxes bundled nerves and knotted muscles sorely in need of kneading.

pressure sores Sometimes referred to as bedsores, these sensitive patches can redden the skin if a person lounges for hours without moving or remains seated on a long flight with no bed in sight. The Mayo Foundation for Medical Education and Research, pinpointed the condition "over weight-bearing parts of the body, especially where a bone is near the skin, such as the hips, shoulder blades, tailbone and heels. Some people may develop bedsores after just a few hours of constant pressure on such an area." The article continued, "If a person is unable to move without help, it's important to shift his or her position at least every 2 hours to keep pressure from remaining on just one area. Cushions or foam wedges can be used to shift the person's weight—in a bed or a chair."

A September 2000 article from the American Academy of Family Physicians said, "Deep sores can go down into the muscle or even to the bone. If pressure sores are not treated properly, they can become infected." Although circulatory problems, such as DIABETES and hardening of the arteries, can complicate the condition, most pressure sores heal by "relieving the pressure that caused the sore. Treating the sore itself. Improving nutrition and other conditions to help the sore heal." To treat the ulcerated area, rinse it in salt water to remove dead tissue and use a sterile dressing covered with a bandage or gauze. "Newer kinds of dressings include a see-through film and a hydrocolloid dressing . . . a bandage made of a gel that molds to the pressure sore." The latter can be kept on for a few days, whereas other types of bandages usually need replacing daily. Unless a fever, swelling, or some other evidence of an infection exists, most pressure sores will heal in two to four weeks.

American Academy of Family Physicians. "Pressure Sores." Available online. URL: http://www.familydoctor.org Downloaded on March 3, 2003.

Mayo Foundation for Medical Education and Research. "Preventing Bedsores." Available online. URL: http://www.mayoclinic.com Downloaded on June 5, 2001.

prolapsed disk See HERNIATED DISK.

pronation As it relates to the entire body, pronation humbly places a person in a prone or face-down position. As a joint movement opposite that of supination, pronation positions a hand palm down or lowers the sole of a foot downward and back. If a person has overpronation in walking, the foot rolls inward too much, stressing the legs, ligaments, and hip bones. Unless the problem involves a neurological factor, well-designed FOOTWEAR or an ORTHOTIC shoe insert can often correct the gait. If not, an orthopedic specialist may recommend PHYSICAL THERAPY, SURGERY, or another corrective device.

prosthesis As a means of replacing a natural device with a synthetic one, a prosthesis can refer to anything from a set of dentures to a hearing aid to an artificial organ. As regards the musculoskeletal system, a prosthesis usually means the introduction of an artificial limb following an AMPUTATION.

In discussing this mixed bag of supportive devices, C. A. Wolski said, "Orthotics and prosthetics today incorporate technology and engineering for better functioning, but there are no quick fixes." For example, the advent of such offerings as a myoelectric arm prosthesis can increase the patient's control while using that very sensitive electrode-operated device. However, the flexibility or maneuverability of moving fingers into a pinching grip still belongs to the bionic arm of science fiction. Therefore, an artificial arm or hand may be used primarily for cosmetic purposes, an exception being the assistance a prosthesis brings for balance and sitting, especially when used by a young child.

Greater technological strides have been made in walking. As Wolski reported, "Where prosthetic science has made advances in returning normal function is in the lower extremities, with the introduction of microprocessor knee units." Presently costing about $15,000, these units can keep step with more active patients in changing speed of movement. Stronger but lighter-weight materials also assist mobility as do silicone liners and ease of use. "Lifestyle as much as a patient's injury informs what type of prosthetic they will be issued." While such options and materials certainly help with ambulation, an ill-fitting prosthesis reportedly remains a common occurrence since the measurements usually change from those taken before the swelling subsides after surgical amputation.

As methods of assisting patients continue to improve, more options fit the very specific needs of individuals who have experienced a life-altering event. For example, according to the Department of Veterans Affairs, "The losses of an eye, ear, nose, cheek, hand, foot, are examples of items replaced with removable custom fabricated prostheses at the Restoration Clinics. Composed of plastic and/or silicone, maintained by the beneficiary or guardian, the prostheses are made to last from one to three years. The plastic eye prostheses are made to last 3 to 5 years; however, some persons are able to wear them for a period of 10 years. Patients should have their ocular prosthesis replaced at least every 5 years. Longer wear increases the risk of giant papillary conjunctivitis which is very difficult to treat." To construct an implant, the process involves "a custom fitted prosthesis made of medical grade silicone, acrylic, or metal used as volume replacement and insert for areas of the body." To do this, impressions are first made for "duplication of defected areas of the body by use of alginate (seaweed) or silicone base materials. It gives the provider a negative mold which is used to create a positive cast. The positive cast is modified to form the final prosthesis." If this happens to be a maxillofacial prosthesis fabricated with silicone, that custom-fitted process involves "replacement of anatomical structures of the face and oral cavity which integrates function and replaces the natural appearance."

Department of Veteran Affairs. "Ocular Prostheses and Facial Restoration," *VHA Handbook 1173.11, Transmittal Sheet.* Washington, D.C.: Veterans Health Administration, (November 2, 2000).

Wolski, C. A. "A Mixed Bag," Available online. URL: http://www.rehabpub.com/features Downloaded on April 16, 2003.

protein These large molecules, composed of amino acids, are essential to all human and animal life processes. Long considered to be building blocks by nutritionists, the many shapes of protein molecules intrigue structural biologists who want to discover how each design can affect and assist the work of protein in upbuilding the human body. According to the National Institutes of Health publication "The Structures of Life," scientists also hope to understand the purpose behind the structural designs of protein molecules and then use that information to develop new medical helps and diagnostic tools.

A follow-up news release in 2003 from the Department of Health and Human Services said, "In a step toward charting the protein structure universe, scientists funded through the National Institute of General Medical Sciences' Protein Structure Initiative have just created a map of the protein shapes that nature repeats over and over again to construct the billions of complex proteins that make up life. The three-dimensional map shows similarities and differences among the protein shapes, letting scientists visualize the organization of all protein structures—the many possible twists, turns and shapes—and see evolutionary changes that may have occurred with time. This new depiction of the protein universe provides a global view of the relationships between protein shapes. It has definite potential to help us predict the structure of protein." Apparently, scientists hope this inventory will "expand our knowledge of basic biology and . . . be a valuable medical and pharmaceutical research tool in the future." With this telescopic exploration of inner space continuing, protein research may be the key in locating and repairing flaws in a cosmos of GENETIC FACTORS.

Meanwhile, microscopically, the protein tests done in a medical laboratory can view a blood sample from an individual to ascertain his or her present nutritional status and the indication of a condition, such as a liver disorder, digestive problem, or kidney disease, as shown by abnormal protein levels. This can have particular significance to the musculoskeletal system since proteins affect the health of every part of the body—from muscles and bones to skin, fingernails, and hair. A lack of protein, however, can cause muscle mass to diminish, bone repairs to cease, and immune systems to fail.

While studying the topic, the Harvard School of Public Health released findings in 2003 that said, "Adults need a minimum of 1 gram of protein for every kilogram of body weight per day to keep from slowly breaking down their own tissues. That's about 9 grams of protein for every 20 pounds." As a sample of a simple diet offering about 70g of protein, a suggested menu began with cereal and milk followed by a peanut butter and jelly sandwich at lunch and a piece of fish with a side dish of beans for dinner. Other foods, such as fresh fruit and greens, would be needed, of course, for balanced NUTRITION. However, this report focused on the daily need for protein and then considered how much might be too much. As the article explained, "The digestion of protein releases acids that the body usually neutralizes with calcium and other buffering agents in the blood. Eating lots of protein, such as the amounts recommended in the so-called no-carb diets, requires lots of calcium. Some of this may be pulled from bone. Following a high-protein diet for a few weeks probably won't have much effect on bone strength. Doing it for a long time, though, could weaken bone. In the Nurses' Health Study, for example, women who ate more than 95 grams of protein a day were 20 percent more likely to have broken a wrist over a 12-year period when compared to those who ate an average amount of protein (less than 68 grams a day). . . . While more research is clearly needed to define the optimal amount of daily protein, these results suggest that high-protein diets should be used with caution, if at all."

Harvard School of Public Health. "Protein Moving Closer to Center Stage." Available online. URL: http://www.hsph.harvard.edu/nutritionsource/protein Downloaded on June 16, 2003.

National Institutes of Health. "The Structures of Life." Available online. URL: http://www.nih.gov/news Downloaded on March 3, 2003.

protraction The opposite of retraction, this type of joint movement moves a part away from the body as when the chin juts forward in a determined gesture or stubborn stance.

pseudogout This condition imitates GOUT by presenting localized swelling and discomfort. In pseudogout, calcium crystals (not uric acid crystals as found in gout) become painfully deposited in the joints and, sometimes, in cartilage too. A rheumatologist or other specialist may want to rule out an infection, a systemic disease, or another disorder, such as of the thyroid. Generally, though, the diagnostic tests will include X-rays and JOINT ASPIRATION to confirm the presence of calcium crystals and assess the involved joint. According to an American College of Rheumatology (ACR) fact sheet, "Pseudogout affects about 3% of people in their 60s and increases with age to as high as 50% in people over 90." The treatment may consist of oral anti-inflammatory drugs and corticosteroid joint injections with other medication useful in preventing future attack. As ACR added, "Unfortunately, no treatment is available to dissolve the crystal deposits. Controlling inflammation helps to halt the progression of joint degeneration that often accompanies pseudogout."

Information from the Arthritis Society explained the typical progression. "The calcium deposits and chronic inflammation can cause parts of the joint structure to weaken and break down. Cartilage, the tough elastic material that cushions the ends of the bones, can begin to crack and get holes in it. Bits of cartilage may break off into the joint space and irritate soft tissues, such as muscles, and cause problems with movement. Much of the pain of pseudogout is a result of muscles and the other tissues that help joints move (such as tendons and ligaments) being forced to work in ways for which they were not designed, as a result of damage to the cartilage. Cartilage itself does not have nerve cells, and therefore cannot sense pain, but the muscles, tendons, ligaments and bones do."

Although pseudogout comes on without warning, the symptoms may just as suddenly disappear—in a few days or a few weeks—only to appear again elsewhere. Fortunately, however, "The attacks will usually affect only one joint at a time." With the instigation of low-impact exercises, such as swimming, walking, and using a stationary bicycle, patients will be more apt to maintain bone strength and joint flexibility. Also, COLD THERAPY can help to reduce swelling and pain, while HEAT THERAPY encourages achy muscles to relax. In addition, assistive devices, such as grab bars or walkers, can aid in the performance of daily routines. To prevent wearing down the musculoskeletal system, however, conservative habits can be designed to pace activities, avoid awkward positions, and maintain optimal body weight, thus taking a load off the weight-bearing joints.

American College of Rheumatology. "Pseudogout." Available online. URL: http://www.rheumatology.org/patients/factsheet/pseudo-g.html Downloaded on February 17, 2003.

Arthritis Society. "Pseudogout." Available online. URL: http://www.arthritis.ca/types Downloaded on February 18, 2003.

pubis bone See PELVIC REGION.

quadriceps As the familiarly abbreviated version of this muscle group may hint at, quads come in four parts. The quadricep femoris are major leg EXTENSOR MUSCLES located on the front of each thigh. This extensive muscular action can sometimes mean a tug-of-war with the FLEXOR MUSCLES pulling from the lower back of the leg as both muscle groups compete somewhere along the lines of the kneecap.

When the quadriceps overpower the lower leg, according to *The Johns Hopkins Medical Letter, Health After 50,* "Strong thigh muscles (quadriceps) have long been viewed as an important factor in maintaining knee function. Consequently, exercises to strengthen the quadriceps are often recommended to help stabilize the knee joint, reduce pain, and improve function in patients with knee OA [osteoarthritis]. In a study reported in the April issue of the *Annuals of Internal Medicine,* however, researchers assessed the possible impact of strong quadriceps on the course of knee OA in 171 people whose average age was 64." The Johns Hopkins article summarized, "The researchers found that patients who at the start of the study had the strongest quadriceps along with misaligned or loose knees were at greater risk for progression of knee OA. (For patients whose knees were not misaligned, the strength of the quadriceps muscle at baseline had no effect on disease progression.) The findings are still considered preliminary. However, they suggest that quadriceps-strengthening exercises may not benefit all patients with knee OA and that special exercise programs may need to be developed for people with misaligned or lax knees."

While that report considered the effects of misalignment on osteoarthritic knees and also the importance of a personally tailored EXERCISE program, Dr. Mrugeshkumar K. Shah, of the Department of Physical Medicine and Rehabilitation at Harvard Medical School, said, "Unilateral rupture of the quadriceps tendon is a common injury and has been well reported. However, simultaneous bilateral rupture of the quadriceps tendons is uncommon. It generally occurs from a fall down stairs or is spontaneous." Although such a damaging fall would be quite obvious, this type of injury might otherwise indicate the possibilities of other medical concerns, which often depend on a person's age. "Also, patients presenting with quadriceps tendon rupture should be evaluated for an underlying chronic medical condition, such as renal disease, diabetes, or rheumatologic disease, since the rupture may be the first sign of underlying illness."

Johns Hopkins University. "Knee Arthritis: Flawed Therapies." *The Johns Hopkins Medical Letter, Health After 50* 15, no. 6 (August 2003): 1–2.

Shah, Mrugeshkumar K. "Simultaneous Bilateral Rupture of Quadripceps Tendons." *Southern Medical Journal* 95, no. 8 (August 2002): 860–866.

quadriplegia Usually caused by a spinal cord injury, quadriplegia results in PARALYSIS of all four limbs. The higher on the cervical vertebrae the injury occurs, the greater the likelihood of paralysis affecting respiration, in which case, breathing must be artificially maintained immediately.

quantitative computed tomography Multiple X-rays collect computerized images that go into a computed tomography (CT or CAT) scan.

Numerous CT scans provide the images comprising quantitative computed tomography, or QCT. More pictures do not necessarily mean better or sharper images, but they do offer an average view of photogenic subjects, such as BONES and BONE MINERAL DENSITY, to assist a physician or specialist of the musculoskeletal system in reaching an accurate diagnosis.

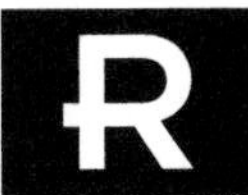

rachiocentesis See LUMBAR PUNCTURE.

radiation As the source of electromagnetic energy supplied by the sun, radiation radiates in or around almost everything in life. Radiation arrives at the Earth as particles or rays, as visible ultraviolet, or infrared light; X-rays; gamma rays; or alpha and beta particles. Frequently, these radioactive elements have been effectively harnessed. For example, radiation offers an aggressive, and sometimes radical, course of treatment in BONE CANCER therapy as radium works to eradicate a tumult of malignant cells. Low levels of radiation also bring medical means for X-RAYS or other RADIOGRAPHS. These diagnostic tools produce light and shadow to clarify or reveal conditions of the musculoskeletal system, including the mouth and jaw. With its persuasive power, energy, and often incredible longevity, radiation can discharge health or harm, depending on its use and other variables, known or unknown.

According to the Environmental Protection Agency (EPA), "Radioactive materials that decay spontaneously produce ionizing radiation, which has sufficient energy to strip away electrons from atoms (creating two charged ions) or to break some chemical bonds. Any living tissue in the human body can be damaged by ionizing radiation. The body attempts to repair the damage, but sometimes the damage is too severe or widespread, or mistakes are made in the natural repair process. The most common forms of ionizing radiation are alpha and beta particles, or gamma and X-rays."

Generally, the amount and duration of radiation exposure determine the type and severity of its effects on each individual. For example, "Stochastic effects are associated with long-term, low-level (chronic) exposure to radiation," such as may arise with radon gas and other forms of pollution. In the ongoing presence of these stochastic effects, radium can collect in calcium-rich areas of the body, such as the bones and teeth. In addition, "Radiation can cause changes in DNA, the 'blueprints' that ensure cell repair and replacement produces a perfect copy of the original cell." As these genetic mutations occur, cellular changes can be passed to offspring. Conversely, "Non-stochastic effects appear in cases of exposure to high levels of radiation, and become more severe as the exposure increases. Short-term, high-level exposure is referred to as 'acute' exposure."

Unlike bone cancer or other malignancies that can be slowly produced by stochastic effects, "effects from 'acute' exposure to radiation usually appear quickly. Acute health effects include burns and radiation sickness," which can cause "premature aging and even death. If the dose is fatal, death usually occurs within two months. The symptoms of radiation sickness include: nausea, weakness, hair loss, skin burns or diminished organ function. Medical patients receiving radiation treatments often experience acute effects, because they are receiving relatively high 'bursts' of radiation during treatment." Those high doses, however, are measured in rems rather than millirems (mrem). In contrast, the X-rays used for dental and orthopedic purposes deliver less than 10 mrem each time—well below the annual maximum of 100 mrem that the EPA and other regulatory agencies deem a safe level of exposure for most adults.

One of the regulatory agencies that sets standards for public safety is the Center for Devices and Radiological Health of the U.S. Food and Drug Administration (FDA). A 2002 fact sheet explained,

"This advisory committee was established in accordance with the Radiation Control for Health and Safety Act of 1968. This committee advises FDA regarding proposed performance standards for electronic products which emit radiation. Mandatory performance standards currently exist for television receivers, cold-cathode gas discharge tubes, diagnostic x-ray systems and their major components, radiographic equipment, fluoroscopic equipment, computed tomography equipment, cabinet x-ray systems, microwave ovens, laser products, sunlamp products and ultraviolet lamps intended for use in sunlamp products, high-intensity mercury vapor discharge lamps, and ultrasonic therapy products."

In 2001, the same FDA Web site updated the article "Does the Product Emit Radiation?" listing additional sources often seen in clinical and other surroundings devoted to the therapeutic treatment of muscles and bones. For example, the sanitizing and sterilizing devices used in most medical facilities emit ultraviolet light, while the radiation in a diathermy unit falls into the infrared zone. Other commonly used radiation-emitting items include laser equipment and products relying on microwaves, radio waves, and infrasonic, sonic, or ultrasonic waves. With these waves and waves of radiation discharging daily in therapy centers, offices, schools, hospitals, and homes, patients might count on their own abacus or fingers to add up the levels of mrem to which they are typically exposed each year.

Center for Devices and Radiological Health. "Does the Product Emit Radiation?" Available online. URL: http://www.fda.gov.cdrh Downloaded on September 26, 2003.

Center for Devices and Radiological Health. "Technical Electronic Product Radiation Safety Standards Committee." Available online. URL: http://www.fda.gov/crdh/teprsc.html Downloaded on September 26, 2003.

Environmental Protection Agency. "Understanding Radiation." Available online. URL: http://www.epa.gov/cgi-bin Downloaded on September 25, 2003.

radiograph Radiographic equipment can record and measure radiation from the Sun and document environmental wonders, such as seeing how many seeds occupy a single pine cone—information that could come in handy for a reforestation project. In the medical community, a radiograph produces images on a sensitive photographic plate or a fluorescent screen. Unlike the typical photo emerging from a darkroom though, any old light source will not do. Instead, a radiograph makes use of small amounts of radiation emitted through the human body, producing lights and shadows that are read by a well-trained physician specializing in radiology.

Although radiologists have developed alternative diagnostic tools, such as MAGNETIC RESONANCE IMAGING (MRI) and ULTRASONOGRAPHY that do not use the standard forms of RADIATION, various types of X-RAYS still provide the most commonly favored instruments for evaluating joints and bones. As explained by the Radiological Society of North America, "X-ray images can be used to diagnose and monitor the progression of degenerative diseases such as arthritis. They also play an important role in the detection and diagnosis of cancer, although usually computer tomography (CT) or MRI is better at defining the extent and the nature of a suspected cancer. On regular x-rays severe osteoporosis is visible." Yet radiographs also have their limitations. "While x-ray images are among the clearest, most detailed views of bone, they may not provide equally revealing information about involved soft tissues. In the case of a knee or shoulder injury, for example, an MRI may be more useful in identifying ligament tears, joint effusions or other problems."

The article "Radiology's Role in Confirming Anthrax Infection Quickly" said, "As the medical community continues its pursuit of the most efficient method to confirm cases of inhalational anthrax, computed tomography (CT) has been shown to be quick and accurate in enabling detection of the condition. X-ray is the standard recommendation as the first radiologic test, followed—when appropriate—by a CT exam." According to James P. Earls, M.D., a radiologist with Fairfax Radiological Consultants, "When a patient presents with symptoms and possible exposure to anthrax, a CT scan can confirm the presence of the disease in a matter of minutes—many hours or even days before blood or sputum cultures turn positive."

Although this does not directly impact the musculoskeletal system, such techniques may have future application in utilizing technology as a comparative and instructive diagnostic tool. "To that end, radiologists now have a valuable resource on the Internet to compare patient x-rays and CT scans to identify inhalational anthrax." In other areas, the production of photographs, trial results, and case studies on countless Web sites make the Internet well on the way to weaving new resources of medical design.

Radiological Society of North America. "Bone Radiography." Available online. URL: http://www.radiologyinfo.org Downloaded on May 21, 2003.

Radiological Society of North America. "Radiology's Role in Confirming Anthrax Infection Quickly." Available online. URL: http://www.radiologyinfo.org Downloaded on September 25, 2003.

range of motion How many ways can a good joint move? Range of motion normally includes abduction, adduction, DEPRESSION, ELEVATION, DORSIFLEXION, EVERSION, EXTENSION, FLEXION, ROTATION, SUPINATION, INVERSION, PRONATION, PROTRACTION, or RETRACTION—all of which come down to four basic movements:

- Some joints glide.
- Some are capable of angular motion.
- Some move conically by CIRCUMDUCTION.
- Some rotate.

If, however, something hinders a joint's range of motion, the limitation of an expected movement usually indicates a problem. This may be due to a DEGENERATIVE JOINT DISEASE, an injury to the SPINE or nervous system, damage to the musculoskeletal system, or another underlying medical condition. Regardless, a physical examination that assesses a patient's range of motion can assist a doctor or a therapist in arriving at a diagnosis and selecting an appropriate course of treatment.

Raynaud's disease or Raynaud's phenomenon Most often affecting young women age 18–30, this vascular disorder causes arteries in the extremities to constrict, especially during cold weather, thus limiting blood flow and causing spasm. According to the National Heart, Lung, and Blood Institute of the National Institutes of Health, "Extremities—hands and feet—are most commonly affected, but Raynaud's can attack other areas such as the nose and ears. Symptoms include changes in skin color (white to blue to red) and skin temperature (the affected area feels cooler). Usually there is no pain, but it is common for the affected area to feel numb or prickly, as if it has fallen asleep." Although its causes remain unclear, a primary form of the disease can be evoked by smoking or using certain types of drugs, including prescription medications. Secondary Raynaud's, however, involves an underlying medical condition, such as SYSTEMIC LUPUS, pulmonary hypertension, a nerve problem, or RHEUMATOID ARTHRITIS. In addition to diagnosing and treating the primary condition, a doctor may prescribe a vasodilator to relax the arteries and improve blood flow. Injuries and frostbite can also cause Raynaud's. Conversely, the disease can produce frostbitelike symptoms, sometimes even resulting in GANGRENE. Therefore, a patient will be advised to avoid exposure to the cold, including grabbing frozen food from the freezer with a bare hand.

Besides the importance of wearing mittens, gloves, warm socks, and other devices designed to protect a Raynaud's patient from frigid conditions, the Centers for Disease Control and Prevention (CDC) warned of the need to avoid the use of vibrating tools. *Morbidity and Mortality Weekly Report* stated, "The major health problems associated with the use of vibrating tools are peripheral vascular and peripheral neural disorders of the fingers and hands. The signs and symptoms of these disorders include numbness, pain, and blanching of the fingers. The constellation of vibration-induced signs and symptoms is referred to as hand-arm vibration syndrome (HAVS) (sometimes called Raynaud's phenomenon of occupational origin or vibration white finger disease)." In the U.S. alone, approximately 1.5 million workers use power tools, such as chain saws, sanders, riveters, and drills. As a result, "The prevalence of HAVS in worker populations that have used vibrating tools has ranged from 6% to 100%." As the CDC report also pointed out, "The early stages of HAVS are usually reversible if further exposure to vibration is reduced or eliminated. However, for advanced stages, treatment is usually ineffective, and the disorder can progress to loss of effective hand function and necrosis of the fingers. Therefore, prevention is critical."

Centers for Disease Control and Prevention. "Notice to Readers Availability of NIOSH Criteria Document on Hand-Arm Vibration Syndrome." *MMWR, Morbidity and Mortality Weekly Report* 39, no. 19 (May 18, 1990): 27.

National Institutes of Health. "Facts About Raynaud's Phenomenon." Available online. URL: http://www.nhlbi.nih.gov Downloaded on September 22, 2003.

reactive arthritis Besides presenting arthritic symptoms, such as swollen joints and pain, this disorder can produce rash, fever, visual problems, and weight loss as the immune system reacts—and keeps on reacting—to an infection that has already been destroyed. According to an American Academy of Family Physicians information sheet, this uncommon disease most commonly affects men 20–40 years old. The initial infection may have occurred from bacterial sources as diverse as food poisoning or a sexually transmitted disease, with an antibiotic needed to treat the latter. For direct treatment of reactive arthritis or protection of the affected joints, a doctor may prescribe additional medication. Usually, the disorder will then disappear in three or four months.

See also REITER'S SYNDROME.

American Academy of Family Physicians. "Reactive Arthritis: What You Should Know." Available online. URL: http://familydoctor.org Downloaded on September 22, 2003.

reflex As involuntary and often protective responses, the body's reflexes seem fairly predictable to a trained technician and an observant eye. For example, flashing a bright light in the eyes causes the pupils to contract in an accommodation reflex that enables the person's vision to adapt while protecting the eyes from glare. A sneeze reflex clears the sinuses, and a cough reflex clears and protects the lungs from congestion. More directly involved with the musculoskeletal system is a chain reflex that involves the activation of one reflex by another. In contrast, a flexor withdrawal reflex causes the body to pull away smartly from a source of pain. Less obvious, perhaps, is a delayed reflex, which occurs a few moments after a stimulus has occurred. In small children of about four to 24 months, a neck-righting reflex causes a baby's torso to turn in the direction of the head. If someone lightly touches the underside of a tiny foot, infants of 10 months or less will curl their toes in a plantar grasp reflex. Young infants will also normally flail their extended arms in a startle reflex. If a spot on the patella gets tapped, persons of all ages will, hopefully, experience a physical knee-jerk reflex. Metaphorically speaking though, the phrase also applies to almost any reaction bypassing mental processes involving a thoughtful response. In any case, a person's automatic reflexes—or lack thereof—will be very instructive to the highly observant eye of a trained diagnostician.

regeneration From healing a FRACTURE and remodeling BONE to reproducing human life, the body has diverse ways to restore and renew itself. The opposite of a degenerative condition, a regenerative one assists in repairs and development of robust cells and tissues. Sometimes, the body does this on its own with little or no outside help, as when a clean cut or scratch mends without a trace of scarring. At other times, regeneration of cells may get a boost from the surgical ward or laboratory. For instance, a BONE MARROW transplant from a carefully matched donor may help to stimulate healthy new blood cells and bone growth in LEUKEMIA and BONE CANCER patients.

The National Institute of General Medical Sciences discussed a standard practice of removing badly burned skin and immediately replacing it with skin grafts. "Now," however, "Dr. Steven T. Boyce, of the University of Cincinnati and the Cincinnati Shriner's Burn Hospital, has succeeded in growing skin cells from a burned patient and adding them to a polymer sheet to create living skin grafts in the laboratory. In an effort to permanently close burn wounds, Boyce and his coworkers placed the laboratory-grown skin grafts on top of Integra® and bathed everything with a nutritious mix of growth factors and antibiotics to help prod the growth of new blood vessels and control infection." With the use of this artificial skin system known as Integra Dermal Regeneration Template, the natural skin of each patient "returned to its original softness, smoothness, and strength—with minimal scarring." By restoring the skin's elasticity, this innovative treatment will undoubtedly affect muscular areas of the body and limb movement, too.

Although many complicating factors will need to be resolved through RESEARCH before human application can occur, this study centered on a potentially useful premise. According to the National Institutes of Health, "Sensory nerve cells are located near the spinal cord and their axons have two branches. One branch carries signals from the skin or other parts of the body to the cell. This fiber is a part of the peripheral nervous system. The other branch is a spinal cord fiber that carries sensory signals to the brain. If the nerve fiber leading to the brain through the spinal cord is injured, inhibitory proteins normally prevent it from regenerating." By altering that response, however, "Scientists have made a key discovery that could lead to a new treatment for spinal cord injuries."

Davis, Alison. "Living Skin Grafts Enhance Burn Treatment." Available online. URL: http://www.nigms.nih.gov Downloaded on February 21, 2002.

National Institute of Neurological Disorders and Stroke. "Signaling Molecule Improves Nerve Cell Regeneration in Rats." Available online. URL: http://accessible.ninds.nih.gov/news Downloaded on August 29, 2002.

rehabilitation If an ACCIDENT, illness, or INJURY causes an impairment—whether physical, mental, or spiritual—a rehabilitative effort aims to recover what has been lost. Although this process typically includes various types of therapy, rehabilitation also involves the education of patients and their families—for example, in raising their awareness of what caused a particular problem and what corrective measures can be taken to prevent it from happening again. However, other instances too numerous to mention might include the adjustments needed when a family member experiences an ongoing medical disorder, such as one caused by BIRTH DEFECTS or MUSCULAR DYSTROPHY. In such cases, pediatric rehabilitation may include medication, medical equipment such as a brace or wheelchair, and PHYSICAL THERAPY to show young patients and their caregivers how to relax the affected muscles or increase overall musculoskeletal strength.

If a person suffers a STROKE, rehabilitation may come under the auspices of a physician specializing in rehabilitative care. According to the American Heart Association, those rehabilitative services may include rehabilitation nursing, physical therapy, OCCUPATIONAL THERAPY, speech-language therapy, NUTRITION, and counseling or support groups to help a person improve his or her independence, lessen the likelihood of FALLING, and regain skills in self-care, mobility, communication, cognition, and socialization.

Unfortunately, health care insurance may limit coverage, influencing patient services and family finances as well. To address these effects, the University of Utah Health Sciences Center said, "Financial problems due to medical bills or unemployment can occur, adding more stress on the family. Changes in living arrangements, childcare issues, and community re-entry can all pose new problems for the patient and family. By working together with the rehabilitation team, the patient and family can help reduce some of the adverse effects of disability. This can be accomplished by identifying the adverse effects of disability within the family; working together on realistic solutions; participating in family education and counseling; planning for discharge and community re-entry."

For disabled and older patients, some government assistance may be available to alleviate costs. A Centers for Medicare & Medicaid Services (CMS) fact sheet said, "Medicaid Rehabilitation services, defined in the Code of Federal Regulations at 42 CFR 440.130(d), are an optional Medicaid state plan benefit that must be recommended by a physician or other licensed practitioner of the healing arts, within the scope of practice under state law for the maximum reduction of a physical or mental disability and to restore the individual to the best possible functional level. The services may be provided in any setting (at the state's option) and can include occupational and physical therapy services, as well as mental health services, such as individual and group psychological therapies, psychosocial services, and addiction treatment services. Because rehabilitation services are an optional Medicaid benefit, not all states provide this Medicaid service." In addressing "New Medicare Limits on Therapy Services," CMS also announced, "Starting on September 1, 2003, Medicare limits how much it covers for outpatient Physical Therapy (PT), Speech-Language Pathology (SLP), and Occupational Therapy (OT.) The limits are: $1,590 per year for PT and SLP combined, and $1,590 per year for OT." Although a patient typically pays an annual deductible as well as 20 percent of the cost of rehabilitation, "The limits generally don't apply to the therapy services you get at hospital outpatient departments. Medicare should continue to pay for therapy services if you get them in a hospital outpatient department unless you reside in a Medicare-certified bed in a skilled nursing facility."

The National Institutes of Health (NIH) offered information about screening methods for rehabilitation medicine that said, "The primary function of the Department of Rehabilitation Medicine (RMD) is to diagnose and treat patients at the NIH who have problems in locomotion, activities of daily living, occupational roles, communication, swallowing, or problems with chronic pain. The major goal of this department is to help patients achieve maximal function so that they can resume their daily living activities as normal as possible." To accomplish this goal, the department uses various devices. The NIH explained, "Before a new test, evaluation technique, or piece of physical equipment can be considered for use in the treatment of patients it must be carefully studied. Researchers must make sure the test, technique, or instrument is safe, sensitive, accurate, specific, and reproducible. Therefore, all of these . . . must first undergo a trial period. Normal volunteers and patients from the RMD and outside of the RMD may be selected to participate."

In addition to the government's efforts to increase available options, medical research centers and universities around the country engage in rehabilitation clinical trials. A fact sheet issued by RehabTrials listed numerous trials in progress or recently completed. For example, a State University of New York Upstate Medical University study on "Rehabilitation After Spinal Cord Injury" actively compared "the 'body weight support (BWS)' method of training on a treadmill, versus BWS training on a track, versus comprehensive physical therapy." A two-year clinical trial with "A Comparison of Weighted Vest Training and Strength Training in Mobility Limited Elders" by Spaulding Rehabilitation Hospital said, "This proposal seeks to expand upon preliminary work evaluating potential means of improving muscle power and function in mobility limited elders." Meanwhile, Kessler Medical Rehabilitation Research & Education Corporation in New Jersey completed its study of "Music Therapy in the Treatment of Brain Injury." It concluded, "Results lend preliminary support to the efficacy of music therapy as a complementary therapy for social functioning and participation in rehabilitation and a trend towards improvement in mood during acute rehabilitation." When compared with the control group, "There was a significant improvement in family members' assessment of participants' social interaction in the music therapy group" Although a tremendous variety of clinical trials and medical RESEARCH continue around the U.S., one conclusion might be drawn: rehabilitation begins well with a cooperative team of highly trained professionals and ends well when supportive help for the entire family goes on at home.

American Heart Association. "What Is Stroke Rehabilitation?" Available online. URL: http://www.americanheart.org Downloaded on September 24, 2003.

Centers for Medicare & Medicaid Services (CMS). "Rehabilitation Services." Available online. URL: http://cms.hhs.gov/medicaid/services Downloaded on May 15, 2002.

National Institutes of Health. "Protocol Number: 94-CC-0130." Available online. URL: http://clinicalstudies.info.nih.gov Downloaded on September 24, 2003.

Rehab Trials. "Rehabilitation After Spinal Cord Injury." Available online. URL: http://www.rehabtrials.org Downloaded on December 10, 2002.

Rehab Trials. "Rehabilitation Clinical Trials." Available online. URL: http://www.rehabtrials.org Downloaded on September 24, 2003.

University of Utah Health Sciences Center. "Physical Medicine and Rehabilitation." Available online. URL: http://www.med.utah.edu/healthinfo/adult/rehab/effects.htm Downloaded on September 24, 2003.

rehydration See HYDRATION.

Reiter's syndrome A subtype of REACTIVE ARTHRITIS, Reiter's syndrome can occur when a bacterial infection belatedly causes joints to swell after a systemically irritating illness has passed. While this may keep rheumatologists on their toes in connecting the two events, Reiter's sufferers will find their own toes—or knees or ankles—painfully swollen. If a blood test shows that the patient inherited a particular type of tissue, the presence of the disease will be even more likely and may not resolve as readily. For most patients, though, Reiter's will disappear within a few weeks.

According to an Arthritis Society fact sheet, "The treatment for managing Reiter's syndrome includes medications, rest, joint protection and special exercises. Your treatment program, which should be developed by a rheumatologist, will be designed to reduce pain and inflammation, prevent or decrease the amount of joint damage, and restore the function of damaged joints." If the symptoms of Reiter's syndrome persist, "Disease modifying antirheumatic drugs (DMARDS) may be prescribed when inflammation continues for more than six weeks or when many joints are inflamed." For severe pain and swelling, cortisone injections may be needed, and, if the eyes have been affected, cortisone eyedrops may also be prescribed.

Arthritis Society. "Reiter's Syndrome." Available online. URL: http://www.arthritis.ca/types Downloaded on January 23, 2003.

relaxation training When pain erupts from inflammation of fibrous tissue, as occurs in FIBROMYALGIA, or from joint inflammation, as with ARTHRITIS, this technique of progressively relaxing muscles will probably provide little relief. If, however, a person holds and hoards muscular tension in a well-kept collection of anxiety and pain, then relaxation training may be just what the doctor orders. To relax sorely uptight muscles, the person begins at the head and works down or at the feet and works up, progressively involving one group of muscles at a time. After tensing a particular group on purpose for five seconds, the muscles are then intentionally relaxed for 10–15 seconds before the person again alternates tension with relaxation of the next muscle group.

According to Gay L. Lipchik, Ph.D., of St. Vincent Rehabilitation Associates in Erie, Pennsylvania, "Relaxation training slows down the sympathetic nervous system, which is responsible for the stress response. . . . During stress, heart rate and blood pressure increase, sweat production increases, breathing becomes shallow, and adrenaline and other hormones are released, causing blood vessels to constrict and muscles to contract." At such times, the patient may notice hunched shoulders and a tightened jaw. However, by using the systematic procedure of tensing and then relaxing muscles, "Deep relaxation reverses many of the physical responses to stress that can trigger headaches. Additionally, during deep relaxation, the relaxed person takes fewer breaths per minute, yet breathes more deeply, 'bathing' the blood cells in oxygen, which means more oxygen gets to the muscles and to the brain." Not only can this technique relieve muscular aches from head to toe, "With practice, deep relaxation changes your body's response to adrenaline and other stress hormones so that it takes a greater disruption from life stresses (and the stress response) to trigger a headache."

Likewise, the Arthritis Foundation said, "People who are in pain experience both physical and emotional stress. Pain and stress have similar effects on the body: muscles tighten, breathing becomes fast and shallow, and heart rate and blood pressure go up. Relaxation can help you reverse these effects and give you a sense of control and well-being that makes it easier to manage pain." This can be especially helpful when patients feel they have little control over their lives or bodies. For instance, the American Cancer Society reported on the reduced occurrences of nausea, pain, anxiety, and depression when patients applied some form of relaxation technique. "Not only does it help, it works even when different methods are used." In addition to progressive muscle relaxation training, other calming techniques include visualization of a pleasant image or scene, music therapy, and prayer.

American Cancer Society. "Relaxation Training Helps Patients Put Mind Over Matter." Available online. URL: http://www.cancer.org Downloaded on February 15, 2002.

Arthritis Foundation. "Practice Relaxation." Available online. URL: http://www.arthritis.org Downloaded on September 24, 2003.

Lipchik, Gay L. "Relaxation Training." Available online. URL: http://www.achenet.org/articles Downloaded on December 10, 2002.

remodeling See BONE; BONE DEVELOPMENT.

repetitive motion disorder(s) Also known as a repetitive stress or repetitive strain injury (RSI), an array of cumulative trauma disorders go by a variety of names according to the location. For instance, tarsal tunnel syndrome transmits soreness from repeatedly strained movements of the toes—similar to the way the more commonly known CARPAL TUNNEL SYNDROME starts in an overworked hand or wrist, radiating pain from the thumb and fingertips up the arm and into the neck or shoulder. In any case or body part, a repetitive strain injury stands for pain or, perhaps worse, tingling and NUMBNESS. As Dr. Lori B. Siegel said, "The hands sleep better than the patient." Whether numb or not, RSI relief chiefly comes by avoiding or preventing the ill-fitting motion of a joint. Therefore, the ongoing sources of an irritation need to be evaluated from a problem-solving mode. If this proves too puzzling, the sufferer may welcome expert evaluation by an OCCUPATIONAL THERAPIST in identifying causatives and finding workable solutions. Generally, the types, methods, and equipment involved in regularly repeated tasks or movements bear careful scrutiny by the affected individuals, their employers, and, occasionally, the U.S. government.

In July 1997, the Department of Health and Human Services of the National Institute for Occupational Safety and Health issued an extensive report entitled *Musculoskeletal Disorders and Workplace Factors*, edited by Bruce P. Bernard, M.D., M.P.H. According to the most current data involving lost workdays at that time, "705,800 cases (32%) resulted from overexertion or repetitive motion. Specifically: 367,424 injuries were due to overexertion in lifting; 65% affected the back. Another 93,325 injuries were due to overexertion in pushing or pulling objects; 52% affected the back. In addition, 68,992 injuries were due to overexertion in holding, carrying, or turning objects; 58% affected the back. Totaled across these three categories, 47,861 disorders affected the shoulder. The median time away from work from overexertion injuries was 6 days for lifting, 7 days for pushing/pulling, and 6 days for holding/carrying/turning." In addition to those statistics, "92,576 injuries or illnesses occurred as a result of repetitive motion, including typing or key entry, repetitive use of tools, and repetitive placing, grasping, or moving of objects other than tools. Of these repetitive motion injuries, 55% affected the wrist, 7% affected the shoulder, and 6% affected the back. The median time away from work was 18 days as a result of injury or illness from repetitive motion." Following reports of work-related MUSCULOSKELETAL DISORDERS (MSDs) involving the neck, shoulder, elbow, hand/wrist, hand/arm, and lower back, appendix B included this statement, "A worker's ability to respond to external work factors may be modified by his/her own capacity, such as tissue resistance to deformation when exposed to high force demands. The level, duration, and frequency of the loads imposed on tissues, as well as adequacy of recovery time, are critical components in whether increased tolerance (a training or conditioning effect) occurs, or whether reduced capacity occurs which can lead to MSDs. The capacity to perform work varies with gender and age, among workers, and for any worker over time. The relationship of these factors and the resulting risk of injury to the worker is complex and not fully understood."

Sometimes, an objective evaluation provides innovative efforts toward improving those specific work conditions, such as the ERGONOMIC designs of hand tools, lighting, chairs, keyboards, workstations, and, yes, baby carriers. In April 2002, occupational therapists Sharon Maynard and Lisa G. Blain wrote about "ErgoMOMics," including the importance of using a front carrier in "an ergonomically correct method of holding a baby. The mother should maintain neutral joint positions by keeping the arms close to her body in order to spread out the weight." To prevent repetitive strain injuries, "It is imperative that caregivers implement proper posture, body mechanics, and joint protection techniques during child care activities in order to prevent debilitating injuries." This may mean something as simple as neck and back extensions done while stretching out, prone on the floor, as the infant rests nearby on a blanket. Also, parents can often avoid shoulder or arm fatigue by distributing weight more effectively. For instance, instead of using both arms to carry a child in a car seat, the parent might use one arm to hold the baby and the other arm to carry the seat. Better yet, the car seat might be kept in the car and an infant seat used in a safe, centrally located place at home. With both arms freed for carrying the child, the baby's weight can then be shifted back and forth to avoid stressing the same side continuously.

Eventually, almost any routine or chore that regularly stresses one part of the body will present long-term damage in the form of TENDINITIS or a MUSCULOSKELETAL DISORDER. The National Institute of Neurological Disorders and Stroke explained, "Repetitive motion disorders (RMDs) are a variety of muscular conditions that result from repeated motions performed in the course of normal work or other daily activities. RMDs may be caused by overexertion, incorrect posture, muscle fatigue, compression of nerves or tissue, too many uninterrupted repetitions of an activity or motion, or friction caused by an unnatural or awkward motion such as twisting the arm or wrist. Over time, these conditions can cause temporary or permanent damage to the soft tissues in the body, such as the muscles, nerves, tendons, and ligaments." Treatment for RMD usually involves "reducing or stopping the motions that cause symptoms. Splints may relieve pressure on the muscles and nerves. Medication such as pain relievers, cortisone, and anti-inflammatory drugs may reduce pain and swelling. Physical therapy may relieve the soreness and pain in the muscles and joints. In rare cases, surgery may be required to relieve symptoms and prevent permanent damage. Other treatment options may include taking breaks to give the affected area time to rest, stretching and relaxation exercises, and applying ice to the affected area to help reduce pain and swelling. Many companies have developed ergonomic programs to help workers adjust their pace of work and office equipment to minimize problems."

Repetitive motion disorders, however, are not confined to working conditions that no longer work. Cervical vertebrae can lose their natural S curve as a person bends too long over books or crochet hooks. Repetitive stresses on the ACHILLES TENDON OR HEEL can elevate with each poor choice of FOOTWEAR, such as high-heeled shoes. Carpal tunnel syndrome can put a brush with pain into a painterly artist's hand. Musicians also are not exempt from the jarring effect of potentially discordant muscles.

Dr. Steven Liu and Dr. Gregory F. Hayden, of Charlottesville, Virginia, said, "Maladies in musicians may range in severity from an incidental asymptomatic finding in a casual and occasional player to a serious injury that significantly disables a professional musician from practicing or performing. The most prevalent medical problems among musicians relate to overuse of muscles involved in the repetitive movements of playing, often in combination with prolonged weight bearing in an awkward position. . . . Overuse syndromes are caused by excessive or unaccustomed use, are characterized by pain and loss of function in muscle units, and are manifested by weakness, loss of control (accuracy), and loss of agility (speed). This problem has been associated with increased time and intensity of practicing, a predisposing musculoskeletal condition at baseline, and overly tense technique." With each musical instrument being instrumental in the type of repetitive motion disorder that occurs, variety may be key. For instance, a violinist suffering with TEMPOROMANDIBULAR JOINT (TMJ) disorder might switch to fiddling with a piano for a while to give the jaw a rest. A clarinet player with an overloaded thumb injury might learn to love playing a triangle—temporarily, of course. As trumpet players may know, Satchmo's syndrome received its name from "Louis Armstrong because it matched the symptoms he experienced in his lips in 1935 that forced him to stop playing the trumpet for 1 year." As musical history records it, that one year did not last forever. A heavy refrain of repeated motion disorders does not have to linger over the musical world. Just as research has led to improved conditions and ergonomic equipment in other fields, so too can music score. To relieve the malady in music, doctors Liu and Hayden concluded their problem-solving composition on this note of levity, "Research in medical engineering could also be applied to instrument construction in hopes of lowering the incidence of certain instrument related injuries. Lighter weight instruments with new designs promoting more comfortable playing positions could decrease the incidence of overuse syndrome or entrapment neuropathies and could provide alternatives for affected musicians. We hope that medical progress will be able to take the sour notes out of making sweet music."

Bernard, Bruce P., ed. *Musculoskeletal Disorders and Workplace Factors.* National Institute for Occupational Safety and Health (July 1997): 1–3.

Liu, Steven and Gregory F. Hayden. "Maladies in Musicians." *Southern Medical Journal* 95, no. 7 (July 2002): 727–734.

Maynard, Sharon and Lisa G. Blain. "ErgoMOMics." Available online. URL: http://www.rehabpub.com/features Downloaded on April 16, 2003.

National Institute of Neurological Disorders and Stroke (NINDS). "NINDS Repetitive Motion Disorders Information Page." Available online. URL: http://www.ninds.nih.gov/health Downloaded on September 25, 2003.

repetitive stress injury See REPETITIVE MOTION DISORDERS.

research Somewhere around the time people discovered they have muscles and bones, research undoubtedly began. Initially, this may have meant identifying, classifying, and naming bones and muscles. Eventually, someone had to try that first herb for medical purposes, set that first fractured bone, or lay sore muscles onto the flat bed of a sun-heated rock. Times have changed, of course, with infinite but infinitesimal possibilities. Nevertheless, when ill or hurting people search for relief and find none, they are often willing to research into unknown areas. Instead of going around and around reinventing an investigative process, however, many choose to participate in ongoing clinical trials. Usually, this research will be sponsored and/or conducted by a pharmaceutical company, hospital, university center, government agency, or other research group, such as a manufacturing company, with a vested interest in new inventions, products, and designs. Therefore, finding out who is doing the research and why can help a patient know whether to become involved.

To help patients better understand what their participation in medical research may require, the National Institutes of Health (NIH) Department of Health and Human Services stated, "Choosing to participate in a clinical trial is an important personal decision," with patients encouraged "to talk to a physician, family members, or friends about deciding to join a trial. After identifying some trial options, the next step is to contact the study research staff and ask questions." For example, an interested person might want to clarify the specific type of study, its purpose or goal, the sponsorship, and the expected risks or side effects. Other questions might address what follow-up tests and treatments will be needed, whether hospitalization will be required, how much time will be involved from start to finish, and who is picking up the tab. Some studies, for example, offer to pay the participants for their involvement with additional reimbursements given for the related expenses (like travel costs) they incur.

To differentiate between clinical, interventional, or observational trials, the NIH explained, "A clinical trial (also known as clinical research) is a research study in human volunteers to answer specific health questions. Carefully conducted clinical trials are the fastest and safest way to find treatments that work in people and ways to improve health. Interventional trials determine whether experimental treatments or new ways of using known therapies are safe and effective under controlled environments. Observational trials address health issues in large groups of people or populations in natural settings." Although most patients, understandably, would not want to become a guinea pig in an ill-advised project, the NIH explained the advantages of highly regarded research by saying, "Participants in clinical trials can play a more active role in their own health care, gain access to new research treatments before they are widely available, and help others by contributing to medical research."

Although each study will come with its own set of requirements, the criteria for patient participation might include the type and severity of a disease or disorder, the length of endurance, and even the person's proximity to the research facility where tests will be conducted or information gathered at scheduled intervals. Unless the research focuses on a genetic characteristic or a pregnancy-related issue, pregnant women will usually be excluded. Other limiting factors may involve economic impacts or culturally related influences on patient health and care. In general though, once a participant has qualified for the study, a medical history will be taken, a physical exam performed, and a baseline established for measuring the effectiveness of the treatment.

When describing the typical process, authors Cary P. Gross, Raburn Mallory, Asefeh Heiat, and Harlan M. Krumholz said, "When researchers perform clinical studies comparing one treatment with another, they often use an experimental design known as a randomized, controlled trial (RCT). This design ensures that patients are randomly assigned to treatment groups in a way that will not bias the results by putting many people who are likely to respond favorably into one group and many who are not likely to respond into another. Although RCTs are generally accepted as the strongest way to design a clinical study, the usefulness of the findings depends not only on the strength of random assignment but also on how well the experimental patients represent all patients with the particular disease being studied."

Occasionally, these studies focus on pharmaceutical treatments that may alleviate symptoms or offer a potential cure. The CenterWatch Web site clarified this aspect of research: by saying, "Before a pharmaceutical company can initiate testing in humans, it must conduct extensive preclinical or laboratory research. This research typically involves years of experiments in animal and human cells." If this stage proves successful, the company gives the collected data to the U.S. Food and Drug Administration (FDA) with a request to test the new drug on people. When that approval comes, Phase I investigates the drug's safe use on healthy individuals by assessing the body's responses, from absorption to side effects. Also according to CenterWatch, "This initial phase of testing typically takes several months. About 70 percent of experimental drugs pass this initial phase of testing." Phase II then involves randomized trials, whereas Phase III tests a new drug on hundreds—sometimes thousands—of patients. With about 70–90 percent of those drugs passing this Phase III, the final one analyzes similar medicines on the market with comparatives ranging from the new drug's long-term impact on patients to its cost effectiveness.

Since tests performed on a product by its own manufacturer could, conceivably, be compromised, the U.S. government established numerous guidelines and protocols. According to the National Center for Research Resources (NCRR), "The General Clinical Research Centers (GCRSs) are a national network of 78 centers that provide optimal settings for medical investigators to conduct safe, controlled, state-of-the-art, in-patient and out-patient studies of both children and adults. . . . Investigators who have research project funding from NIH and other peer-reviewed sources may use GCRCs. . . . To ensure research diversity at the GCRCs, no single group of investigators at a center may utilize more than 33 percent of the resources." The NCRR information also assured, "Federal regulations and policies protect subjects in clinical research protocols, ensuring that their safety is given the highest priority. These regulations complement the policies of academic institutions that host the GCRCs."

Those regulations may be even more stringent when children become involved. The Mayo Foundation for Medical Education and Research (MFMER), said, "The involvement of children in studies—also known as clinical trials—is becoming much more common than in the past. In 1997, Congress passed the FDA Modernization Act. This law gave the FDA the right to request that drug manufacturers perform studies in children if such studies hadn't been done previously." Again, with the NIH establishing guidelines, the decision to include children in research came about "because very little research has been published about the effects of drugs on children." Such investigations could be valuable if for no other reason than to show the different ways a child's system reacts to drugs than an adult's—for example, caffeine. Nevertheless, researchers cannot force the issue. As the MFMER article pointed out, "Even when there is a possibility of death and only the experimental therapy offers a chance of survival, a child's parents still must give permission for the child to receive the experimental treatment." This, however, will not be the only consent sought, "If the parents agree to let their child enroll in a study, the researchers then seek the child's assent." In addressing those times, the MFMER article included this essential passage, "The American Academy of Pediatrics Committee of Bioethics notes that assent should include at least these elements: Helping the child to achieve an understanding appropriate for his or her age of the illness; Telling the child what to expect from tests and treatments; Assessing the child's understanding of the condition and the things that influence how he or she responds to the request for assent—influences such as pain that is not controlled adequately or pressure from parents; Asking the child whether he or she is willing to accept the proposed treatment." These guidelines assist adults in an honest discussion with a child. "Like adults, children can refuse to participate, and their refusal must be accepted. They can also drop out of a study at any time without negative consequences."

An exception, of course, would be a prelinguistic child—the youngest of whom may be involved, not in a clinical trial, but in research of another kind. Instead of discarding the umbilical cord and placenta after a child's birth, "during the 1970s, researchers discovered that umbilical cord blood is a rich source of blood-forming (hematopoietic) stem cells," reported KidsHealth. Basically, "these primitive (early) cells found primarily in the bone marrow . . . are capable of developing into the three types of mature blood cells present in our blood—red blood cells, white blood cells, and platelets. Cord-blood stem cells may also have the potential to give rise to other cell types in the body." This could prove crucial, for instance, to a child or sibling who later develops a major illness, such as BONE CANCER or LEUKEMIA. Then, instead of relying on a bone marrow transplant, STEM CELLS from the cryogenically stored umbilical cord blood could be used. Although that process of freezer storage began only recently, "Blood-forming stem cells that have been stored up to 14 years have been used successfully in transplants." Since most hospitals do not have cryogenic facilities, however, prior arrangements would be needed. Also, parents can expect to pay both up-front and annual storage fees. If such costs prove unaffordable or if family genetics offer no concern, another KidsHealth idea suggested donating umbilical cord blood to a research center, the American Red Cross, or the National Marrow Donor Program.

Besides finding productive and, perhaps, curative uses for previously discarded placentas, other areas of research offer challenging frontiers. Not only do clinical studies let patients actively participate in their own care, but research provides medical minds with pioneering possibilities. The University of Miami School of Medicine announced, "The Miami Project to Cure Paralysis has been designated by the National Institutes of Health as a Facility of Research Excellence in Spinal Cord Injury (FORE-SCI)." From a researcher's point of view, FORE-SCI proposed to "promote the recruitment of outstanding investigators into the field of SCI research; Enhance research collaborations between different laboratories; Increase the number of scientists working on this field; Compare the efficacy of different treatments with a minimum of variability; Assess and replicate promising, published studies that could lead to treatments for SCI; Obtain the necessary data and knowledge to initiate clinical trials targeting paralysis."

Elsewhere, the Department of Neurology at Baylor College of Medicine has been focusing "on the structure and assembly of myosin-containing filaments and on the control of gene expression for myosin and other genes related to muscle development." According to Baylor research, "The mechanisms controlling expression of active myotonic dystrophy protein kinase at molecular and cellular levels are being pursued in order to understand its roles in development, regulation, and the pathogenesis of the multi-system disease affecting heart, brain, and eye as well as muscle." At the Muscle Mechanics Laboratory of the University of Michigan Institute of Gerontology, a September 2003 list of research topics announced such diverse areas as sarcomere dynamics, tissue engineering, nerve regeneration, age-related changes, denervated muscle, muscle development, single muscle fiber mechanics, muscle conditioning, contractility of dystrophic muscle, and pathogenesis of muscular dystrophy.

Meanwhile, government studies continue under the auspices of various departments of the National Institutes of Health. For example, the National Institute of Arthritis and Musculoskeletal and Skin Diseases (NIAMS) sponsors clinical research to "explore how genes—units of heredity—may influence the severity of Ankylosing Spondylitis." In August 2003, www.clinicaltrials.gov last reviewed information for another NIAMS study, "Electromagnetic Treatment for Bone Loss After Fractures." Also in August 2003, www.ClinicalTrials.gov announced a study sponsored by Wake Forest University Research Base in conjunction with the National Cancer Institute. Entitled "Survival TRaining for ENhancing Total Health (STRENGTH)," the rationale for that 16-month study proposed, "A home-based exercise and/or diet program may improve the quality of life of breast cancer patients by preventing an increase in body fat and weight, and a loss of lean body tissue."

Not weight loss but bone loss has received ongoing attention at the National Space Biomedical Research Institute (NSBRI) as has the alteration of muscle fibers in weightless environments. With information regarding both areas of study, NSBRI explained, "Weightless environments place a reduced load on leg muscles and on the back's muscles used for maintaining posture on Earth. These muscles begin to weaken or reduce in size. The loss of muscle strength during an extended mission could pose dramatic problems in the event of an emergency situation upon landing. While astronauts exercise in space, exercise alone will not counteract the muscle loss experienced on long-duration missions. It is possible astronauts on long missions may lose up to 25 percent of their muscle mass unless more effective solutions are devised." As NSBRI research focuses on the effects of GRAVITY and the "genetic, cellular and physiological processes involved in muscle function." Researchers hope the methods developed "to prevent or reduce muscle loss" will present good solutions for patients confined to a bed or wheelchair here on Earth.

CenterWatch. "Background Information on Clinical Research." Available online. URL: http://www.centerwatch.com/patient/backgrnd.html Downloaded on September 26, 2003.

Department of Health and Human Services. "Introduction to Clinical Trials." Available online. URL: http://clinicaltrials.gov Downloaded on June 30, 2003.

Department of Neurology. "Muscle Development and Disease." Available online. URL: http://www.bcm.tmc.edu/neurol/research/basic Downloaded on September 26, 2003.

Gross, Cary P., Raburn Mallory, et al. "Reporting the Recruitment Process in Clinical Trials: Who Are These Patients and How Did They get There?" *Annals of Internal Medicine* 137, no. 1. (July 2, 2002): 1–38.

Mayo Clinic. "Kids in Research: Making the Decision." Available online. URL: http://www.mayoclinic.com Downloaded on July 17, 2001.

Muscle Mechanics Laboratory. "Research Topics." Available online. URL: http://www.iog.umich.edu/research Downloaded on September 23, 2003.

National Center for Research Resources. "General Clinical Research Centers." Available online. URL: http://www.ncrr.nih.gov/clinical Downloaded on September 26, 2003.

National Institute of Arthritis and Musculoskeletal and Skin Diseases. "Electromagnetic Treatment for Bone Loss After Fractures." Available online. URL: http://clinicalstudies.info.nih.gov Downloaded on September 26, 2003.

National Institute of Arthritis and Musculoskeletal and Skin Diseases. "General Clinical Research Centers."

Available online. URL: http://clinicalstudies.info.nih.gov Downloaded on September 26, 2003.

National Space Biomedical Research Institute (NSBRI). "Muscle Alterations and Apathy." Available online. URL: http://www.nsbri.org/Research Downloaded on September 26, 2003.

Trigg, Michael. "Banking Your Newborn's Cord Blood." Available online. URL: http://kidshealth.org Downloaded on September 23, 2003.

University of Miami School of Medicine. "Training Opportunities for Researchers." Available online. URL: http://www.miamiproject.miami.edu/fore-sci.htm Downloaded on June 10, 2003.

resistance training Also known as strength training or weight training, the success of a program depends on the goal. For instance, an athlete may want to improve performance by increasing strength, while a desk-bound worker might want to enhance muscle tone. People of all types and ages may need resistance training to assist REHABILITATION after an ACCIDENT or SURGERY. To avoid contributing to another injury, however, proper lifting techniques can help to prevent TENDINITIS or REPETITIVE MOTION DISORDERS.

Dr. Michael Bird said, "Proper lifting technique is based on knowledge of what joints and muscles a lift is specifically designed to emphasize. Correct lifting techniques will only use those joints and muscles and not others." Similarly, "Proper range of motion for the joints involved is also important in safely performing lifts." Obviously, overextending the range of a joint can cause musculoskeletal problems but, reportedly, fewer ones. Conversely, "Using less range of motion allows lifters to achieve greater weights sooner, but sacrifices the overall development of the muscle and increases the likelihood of injury when the muscle is stressed." With other factors to consider, such as maintaining body balance and handling manageable weights, "most lifts should occur in slow, controlled manners." Other considerations included "warm up exercises emphasizing the same muscles involved in the lifting," and the use of safety items, such as protective collars, to decrease the risk of injuries. Also, "Using a spotter allows technique, range of motion, and balance to be maintained with a small amount of guidance rather than the lifters stressing muscles, ligaments, or tendons beyond their capability."

The Mayo Foundation for Medical Education and Research recommended water workouts as a good way to avoid stressing joints, bones or muscles. By using weighted boots, barbells, and the natural resistance of water, strength-training exercises might include "upper and lower body moves—such as squats and biceps curls . . . performed in the water." Such exercises may be especially helpful for persons with arthritis or some type of disability where the water's buoyancy would provide uplifting assistance. As the Mayo article added, "Another benefit of water workouts is the fact that they incorporate resistance training—which keeps you from losing muscle and strength as you age. Water offers resistance, which strengthens your muscles as you push against it. Simply walking in water with correct posture will work your abdominal muscles. That not only beats doing sit-ups, but may offer you greater benefits because you're strengthening your abdominal muscles in the same way you use them—by holding yourself upright."

Another Mayo article said, "Weight training most benefits preteens who have a focused interest in a particular sport." However, "research shows weightlifting increases a young child's muscle strength and endurance. The American Academy of Pediatrics, the American College of Sports Medicine, and the National Strength and Conditioning Association all support weightlifting for kids—if it's done properly. Today's children are increasingly overweight and out of shape. Weight training can help put them on the lifetime path of better fitness and health." As with adults who need to be especially careful of weakened muscles or joints, "Lighter weights with more repetitions make children stronger. It's also safer." To accommodate these special needs, equipment can appropriately be improvised. For example, "Try milk jugs filled with water or large resistance rubber bands." While hefty weights with fewer repetitions can build up muscles in heartier folks, lighter weights lifted more frequently can increase just about anyone's endurance and strength, making resistance training almost irresistible.

Bird, Michael. "Building Strength Safely: Focus on Proper Technique in Resistance Training." *ACSM Fit Society* Available online. URL: http://www.acsm.org/health+fitness/pdf/fitsociety/fitsc402.pdf Downloaded on June 30, 2004.

Mayo Foundation for Medical Education and Research. "Water Workouts: A Cool Way to Exercise Without Stressing Your Joints, Bones or Muscles." Available online. URL: http://www.mayoclinic.com Downloaded on July 8, 2002.

Mayo Foundation for Medical Education and Research. "Weight Training for Kids: Technique is Key." Available online. URL: http://www.mayoclinic.com Downloaded on September 19, 2001.

resorption Before a new building can begin on a previously occupied site, some clearing must first be done to rid the area of old debris. Similarly, the resorption process clears away old cellular matter to allow room for the growth of healthy new tissue in the ongoing renovation project of BONE DEVELOPMENT. If too many new cells arrive too soon, overgrowth can cause a problem, such as BONE SPURS. If too many cells undergo resorption before the new cells catch up, BONE MASS will lessen and a disorder, such as OSTEOPOROSIS, will be more likely to occur.

respiratory muscles As Adam and Eve may have hinted with this ribbing, inspiration comes with some thanks due the respiratory muscles between the intercostal RIBS. The inhalation half of breathing also involves the diaphragm and muscles of the PECTORAL REGION with backup as needed by the ACCESSORY MUSCLES. To aid the other half of the respiration process in the expulsion of air from the lungs, rectal and ABDOMINAL MUSCLES exert an expiring influence. With these opposite sets of respiratory muscles attracting a balance between inhalation and exhalation, air flows in and out of the body, effectively alternating inspiration with expiration—for most people, that is.

For some, breathing may be difficult and conditional with shortness of breath medically referred to as dyspnea. To address this frightening circumstance of gasping for air, the Warren Grant Magnuson Clinical Center at the National Institutes of Health published a two-page patient information brochure, *Living With Dyspnea—4 Ways to Breathe Easier.* For example, to relieve labored breathing, the brochure suggested pursed-lip breathing with the mouth in a whistling position to expel air. "One way to do this is to take twice as long to breathe out as you breathe in. For example, count 'one . . . two,' as you breathe in. Purse your lips, then count 'one . . . two . . . three . . . four,' as you breathe out." If exertion causes muscles to tighten, thereby hindering respiration, the NIH brochure then recommended positioning. To do this, "1. Rest against the wall and lean forward with your hands on your thighs. This position relaxes your chest and shoulders, freeing them to help you breathe. Use pursed-lip breathing. 2. If you can, sit down with your arms resting on your legs. Continue to do pursed-lip breathing." When walking or lifting objects, paced breathing may alleviate shortness of breath. "For walking: 1. Stand still and breathe in. 2. Walk a few steps and breathe out. 3. Rest, and begin again." Similarly, "For lifting: 1. Hold the object, but do not lift it. Breathe in. 2. Lift the object and breathe out. If possible, use your breathing muscles for one activity at a time." Easier breathing involves "desensitization," too, which means relying on the prior suggestions and remembering something can usually be done to improve the situation. This reminder also helps to lessen fears, thus enabling a person to relax.

Cause for alarm, however, often occurs among patients with chronic obstructive pulmonary disease (COPD) as lungs hyperinflate, further taxing physical energy and air reserves. Therefore, research has focused on breathing methods and equipment for this critical area. A team of doctors from Switzerland reporting in the *American Journal of Respiratory and Critical Care Medicine* stated, "A recently developed training device allows respiratory muscle training (RMT) with normocapnic hyperpnea at home. Studies with healthy subjects using this device resulted in increased cycling endurance and decreased perceived respiratory exertion during exercise. On the basis of these results, we wanted to test the feasibility and effectiveness of home training with this device in a randomized, controlled study of subjects with COPD.

The aim was not only to assess the effects on respiratory muscle and exercise performance, but also to include the important variables of dyspnea and health-related quality of life." With the study protocol approved by the ethics committee of the Triemli Hospital in Zurich, the team concluded, "In summary, the results of the present study show that respiratory muscle endurance training with normocapnic hyperpnea improves respiratory muscle and exercise performance, health-related quality of life, and dyspnea. The new portable training device used in the study makes home-based endurance training with normocapnic hyperpnea feasible, and allows its widespread application."

Although this study of respiratory training focused on COPD, other conditions can hinder air flow—overexertion, alcohol consumption, nasal obstructions, chest damage, and neurological dysfunctions. Regardless, "If the respiratory muscles are inefficient for mechanical reasons . . . the magnitude of tension in the muscle produced by a given amount of muscle contraction is proportionately lower than in the normal state." Brendan Caruana-Montaldo, Kevin Gleeson, and Clifford W. Zwillich explained, "The respiratory muscles consist of the diaphragm and the intercostals, abdominal, and accessory muscles of respiration. The diaphragm is responsible for the majority (75%) of air movement during quiet inspiration, while the intercostals, abdominal, and accessory muscles (sternocleidomastoid and other neck muscles) account for the remainder. Inspiration at rest is active and expiration is a passive event in patients with normal lungs. During exercise or in patients with airway obstruction, both inspiration and expiration become active, with expiratory contraction of the abdominal wall and internal intercostals muscles." While using the premise that "the measurement of the ventilatory response to exercise is a useful clinical tool that is often used to evaluate the cause of dyspnea or exercise limitation," the researchers concluded with the following. "Our knowledge of the control of ventilation is constantly evolving through continued clinical and basic research. Abnormalities of respiratory drive are often overlooked in clinical practice. They should be considered whenever the level of respiratory muscle weakness, intrapulmonary gas exchange abnormalities, or lung mechanical dysfunction cannot explain deranged blood gases. Breathing abnormalities tend to be more severe during sleep than during wakefulness, and they have serious consequences. The effective management of ventilatory control abnormalities has important prognostic implications in the setting of both acute and chronic disease."

At another end of the health spectrum, William E. Amonette and Terry L. Dupler of the Fitness and Human Performance Laboratory, University of Houston-Clear Lake, studied maximal oxygen consumption (VO_2 max) in healthy athletes. Subsequently, the American Society of Exercise Physiologists published their findings, which said, "The effects of resistance training on skeletal muscle are well documented. When performed with the correct repetition scheme and load assignment, resistance training can produce skeletal muscle hypertrophy, strength, or local muscle endurance. Traditionally, strength and power athletes have used resistance training to augment sport performance while endurance athletes have avoided resistance exercise believing that increased muscle would decrease aerobic performance. However, skeletal muscle also controls many crucial elements of aerobic conditioning including lung ventilation. The diaphragm, external and internal intercostals, scalene, and abdominal muscles (i.e., respiratory muscles) help to facilitate the increased ventilation needed to sustain blood oxygenation during exercise. If these muscles play such a crucial role in exercise, logically one would think we should train them just as we would any other skeletal muscle." With that interesting premise in mind, the researchers concluded, "When doing further research with highly trained athletes, one might also consider trying different training protocols. In all forms of resistance training, not only is the intensity increased, but the overall volume and duration is also varied. Perhaps training at a higher volume (i.e. more reps) might produce more favorable metabolic changes in the respiratory muscles. As long as athletes and scientists strive to push the limits of human performance, every avenue of training will be explored. Pulmonary resistance training with athletes is still relatively new and has seen only minimal research. As records continue to fall in the athletic world, research should continue on pulmonary resistance training along with all other aspects of exercise performance." Since other areas of research focusing on sports have aided understanding of the musculoskeletal system, these new athletic challenges may bring forth findings that assist at least some heavily labored persons to catch their breath.

Amonette, William E. and Terry L. Dupler. "The Effects of Respiratory Muscle Training on VO2 Max, the Ventilatory Threshold and Pulmonary Function." Available online. URL: http://www.css.edu/users/tboone2/asep/May2002JEPonline.html Downloaded on February 10, 2004.

Boutellier, Vrs, Thomas A. Scherer, et al. "Respiratory Muscle Endurance Training in Chronic Obstructive Pulmonary Disease." *American Journal of Respiratory and Critical Care Medicine* 162 (2000): 1,709–1,714.

Caruana-Montaldo, Brendan, Kevin Gleeson, et al. "The Control of Breathing in Clinical Practice," *CHEST* 117, no. 1 (2000): 205–225.

Warren Grant Magnuson Clinical Center. "Living with Dyspnea—4 Ways to Breathe Easier," National Institutes of Health (January 2001): 1–2.

rest During relaxing times, which may or may not include SLEEP, the body repairs itself. During a state of rest, the mind clears and so does the musculoskeletal system. By sloughing off worn cells and eliminating wastes, the body avoids toxic buildups. Conversely, a lack of rest interferes with those natural cleansing processes, thus adding to the day's fatigue. If weariness goes on too long, pain and disease will often result. This can be particularly unsettling and even dangerous for patients who already experience health problems. The American Heart Association explained, "Rest times are essential because they give the heart a chance to pump more easily." To assist patients in relaxing more frequently, the site suggested, "You might try napping after lunch, putting your feet up for a few minutes every couple of hours, or sitting down while doing certain household tasks, such as preparing food or ironing." Of course, a person might skip gleefully pass the latter and pass directly into nap time if dressed in denim or permapress.

American Heart Association. "The Importance of Rest." Available online. URL: http://www.americanheart.org Downloaded on October 2, 2003.

restless leg syndrome Involuntary movements sometimes occur in legs tired out by too much standing or walking. If, however, legs jerk, twitch, or have crawly sensations at times of inactivity, including sleep, restless leg syndrome (RLS) could be the cause. According to a Restless Legs Syndrome Foundation fact sheet, "Up to 8% of the U.S. population may have this neurological disorder." As a primary condition, the strong urge to move the legs "may become irresistible," and the discomfort "deep in the legs" can become quite painful. Since these symptoms often worsen during nighttimes of rest, RLS patients may have difficulty sleeping followed by "trouble concentrating during waking hours." About 15 percent of pregnant women develop secondary RLS, which often disappears after delivery. Anemia or low iron may be associated with RLS symptoms, too, as "are chronic conditions such as peripheral neuropathy (damage to the nerves in the legs and feet) and kidney failure. Recent literature also points toward an association between RLS and symptoms of attention-deficit hyperactivity disorder." Although the syndrome typically becomes apparent in the "middle years, many individuals with RLS, particularly those with primary RLS, can trace their symptoms back to childhood. These symptoms may have been called growing pains or the children may have been thought to be hyperactive because they had difficulty sitting still." RLS frequently runs in families as do sensitivities to certain medications, including those for colds or allergies, which may worsen the condition. In general, the Restless Legs Syndrome Foundation recommended, "Low-risk therapies involve treating symptoms that are caused by underlying disorders and making lifestyle changes." Good NUTRITION may help as will walking, stretching, taking a warm bath, or massaging the legs. Other suggestions included COLD THERAPY, HEAT THERAPY, EXERCISE, ACUPRESSURE, BIOFEEDBACK, and RELAXATION

TRAINING. Additionally, an article in *Arthritis Today* said, "What causes RLS is still unknown, but dopamine drugs, such as those prescribed for Parkinson's disease, and some seizure and sedative drugs reportedly offer relief. RLS symptoms also appear lessened in people who stay on a regular sleep schedule that includes getting enough rest each night."

DiMartino, Christina. "Getting Rid of the Creepy Crawlies," *Arthritis Today* (May/June 2002): 33.

Restless Legs Syndrome Foundation, Inc. "Living with Restless Leg Syndrome," Available online. URL: http://www.rls.org Downloaded on September 12, 2003.

retraction This type of joint movement pulls a part toward the body, such as when the fingers fold or the chin tucks toward the neck rather than away as in PROTRACTION.

rhabdomyolysis Heat stress, chills, alcoholism, crush injuries, and marathon running seem to have little in common. Yet each can release so many damaged muscle cells into the bloodstream that the overworked kidneys succumb to the toxins. The results may then be rhabdomyolysis—a disorder that can lead to kidney failure.

While discussing yet another potential causative, the Muscular Dystrophy Association warned, "Rhabdomyolysis, which not only destroys muscles but can lead to death as a result of the effects on kidneys and circulation of muscle breakdown, has been associated with cholesterol-lowering drugs that belong to a class known as statins." Because "High doses of Baycol and its use in elderly people have also been noted as risk factors for muscle damage," its manufacturer, the Bayer Corporation of Pittsburgh, voluntarily pulled that particular statin from the market in August 2001. Patients taking other types of statins, however, would be well-advised to report any new concerns to their physician. For instance, "Signs and symptoms of rhabdomyolysis include muscle pain and cramps, weakness, malaise, fever, nausea, vomiting, cola-colored urine and elevated levels of the enzyme creatine kinase (CK) in the blood." Often, these signs repeat those of other muscle disorders and inflammatory or metabolic diseases, so a more identifying sign may be dark urine—a color that "can signal the presence of the protein myoglobin, a product of muscle breakdown, which can quickly damage the kidneys." Since myoglobin shows on a urine dipstick test as blue, this simple screening process can help to confirm a doctor's diagnosis.

Doctors John M. Sauret and George Marinides, of New York, and Gordon K. Wang, of Florida, explained, "Rhabdomyolysis, which literally means striated muscle dissolution or disintegration, is a potentially lethal clinical and biochemical syndrome. Approximately 26,000 cases of rhabdomyolysis are reported annually in the United States. Prompt recognition and early intervention are vital. Full recovery can be expected with early diagnosis and treatment of the many complications that can develop in patients with this syndrome." Although diverse factors may be involved, "The most common causes are alcohol abuse, muscle overexertion, muscle compression and the use of certain medications or illicit drugs. . . . Other significant causes of rhabdomyolysis include electrical shock injury and crush injury. In crush injury, rhabdomyolysis occurs because of the release of necrotic muscle material into the circulation after compression is relieved in, for example, persons trapped in crashed cars or collapsed buildings. Heatstroke and sporting activities especially in previously untrained persons, are also common causes of the syndrome. Heat dissipation impairment from wearing heavy sports equipment or exercising in humid, warm weather increases the risk of rhabdomyolysis." Additionally, "Numerous infectious and inflammatory processes can lead to rhabdomyolysis. Certain metabolic and endocrinologic disorders can also increase the risk of developing the syndrome." Since treatment primarily aims to preserve renal function, "Intravenous (IV) hydration must be initiated as early as possible. In the patient with a crush injury, IV fluids should be started even before the trapped limb is freed and decompressed, and certainly no later than six hours after decompression. The longer it takes for rehydration to be initiated, the more likely it is that oliguric renal failure . . . will be established."

While discussing similar treatment, Dr. Andrew Koren, of the Department of Nephrology at the NYU–Mount Sinai Medical Center in New York, explained, "Early and aggressive hydration may prevent complications by rapidly eliminating the myoglobin out of the kidneys. The hydration needs with muscle necrosis may approximate the massive fluid volume needs of a severely burned patient. This may involve intravenous administration of several liters of fluid until the condition stabilizes. Diuretic medications such as mannitol or furosemide may aid in flushing the pigment out of the kidneys. If the urine output is sufficient, bicarbonate may be given to maintain an alkaline urine state. This helps to prevent the dissociation of myoglobin into toxic compounds."

Andrew Koren, M.D. "Rhabdomyolysis." Available online. URL: http://www.nlm.nih.gov/medlineplus/print Downloaded on November 30, 2001.

Muscular Dystrophy Association. "Muscle-Related Effects of Anti-Cholesterol Drugs Warrant Attention." Available online. URL: http://www.mdausa.org/research Downloaded on August 31, 2001.

Sauret, John M., George Marinides, et al. "Rhabdomyolysis." *American Family Physician* 65, no. 5 (March 1, 2002): 907–912.

rheumatism Generalized symptoms of achy joints and muscles seem as vague as this condition. With similarities to FIBROMYALGIA, ARTHRITIS, BURSITIS, GOUT, and other MUSCULOSKELETAL DISORDERS, rheumatism may involve none of the above or various combinations of them all. For example, the *Johns Hopkins Family Health Book* shows "Rheumatism of the Soft Tissue" as "bursitis, tendinitis, tendosynovitis, and chondritis," with appropriate information on each. However, current editions of most major medical home health guides do not even list the topic. Indeed, the Greek word *rheuma,* which refers to swelling—as in the swollen joints of rheumatism—is considerably older than the timeworn treatments most often recommended.

Alternative treatments listed on www.healthlibrary.com included a cleansing fast of orange juice and water for three or four days followed by a couple of weeks of a fresh fruit and vegetable diet. After this comes the slow addition of seed foods, such as nuts and grains, with celery used in extract form or as seeds in a condiment. Soured dairy, such as low-fat or fat-free yogurt and buttermilk, can then be added too. Although a doctor should always be consulted prior to making any major changes, a well-balanced diet can often decrease rheumatic symptoms if for no other reason than a variety of foods gets the body's optimal levels of acids and alkalines into a better balance. As the same article rather ardently explained about a typical nutritional imbalance, "The chief cause of rheumatism is the poisoning of the blood with acid wastes, which results from imperfect elimination and lowered vitality. Meat, white bread, sugar, and refined cereals . . . leave a large residue of acid toxic wastes in the system. These acid wastes are not neutralized due to the absence of sufficient quantities of alkaline mineral salts in the foods eaten. This upsets the acid-alkaline balance in the body and produces the condition described as acidosis." With an accumulation of acid wastes usually occurring around the joints, chronic muscular pain and stiffness increase even more with movements or the exposure to cold. Besides avoiding a cold or damp environment, "Other helpful methods in the treatment of rheumatism are application of radiant heat and hot packs to the affected parts, a hot tub bath, cabinet steam bath, dry friction and a sponge bath."

In addition to HEAT THERAPY and the recommendations of a rheumatologist, an old-fashioned soaking in a warm bath of Epsom salt can often wring out rheumatic pain. The most natural preventative, however, involves neither slowly soaking oneself in salts nor initiating a fast cleansing but regularly maintaining a well-balanced diet based on solid principles of good NUTRITION.

Nature Cure. "Rheumatism." Available online. URL: http://www.healthlibrary.com Downloaded on October 3, 2003.

rheumatoid arthritis This chronic disease causes joint swelling, pain, and stiffness. Inflammation sometimes involves body organs and nodules affecting the eyes and heart. In children especially, eye involvement can lead to blindness.

According to the American College of Rheumatology (ACR), rheumatoid arthritis (RA) affects over 2 million Americans of all ages—75 percent of which are women. With symptoms often beginning in the 20–45 age group, RA patients may later experience osteoporosis—particularly if the disease has not been promptly detected and treated. Timeliness will not stop the disease but can affect its outcome. For example, the ACR said, "Initial aggressive drug treatment may prevent work disability in patients with early stage rheumatoid arthritis, according to research presented this week at the American College of Rheumatology Annual Scientific Meeting in New Orleans, Louisiana." Referring to a five-year study in Finland where "researchers obtained data of the patients' sick leave and arthritis-related retirement by utilizing the national social insurance registers and case records," results showed that "work disability lasted far longer in the single-drug group than in the combination-drug group."

Aggressive treatment, of course, requires an accurate diagnosis. Therefore, to address the features that differentiate RA from other arthritic disorders, the National Institute of Arthritis and Musculoskeletal and Skin Diseases (NIAMS) of the National Institutes of Health described RA symptoms by saying, "It has several special features that make it different from other kinds of arthritis. . . . For example, rheumatoid arthritis generally occurs in a symmetrical pattern. This means that if one knee or hand is involved, the other one is also. The disease often affects the wrist joints and the finger joints closest to the hand. It can also affect other parts of the body besides the joints. . . . In addition, people with the disease may have fatigue, occasional fever, and a general sense of not feeling well (malaise). Another feature of rheumatoid arthritis is that it varies a lot from person to person." For some, symptoms may occur for a few months—or even a couple of years—before vanishing without any noticeable damage. "Other people have mild or moderate disease, with periods of worsening symptoms, called flares, and periods in which they feel better, called remissions. Still others have severe disease that is active most of the time, lasts for many years, and leads to serious joint damage and disability."

Because a person's own immune system attacks the joint capsule, this systemic condition can quickly erode, not only the joint, but the bone. As the NIAMS brochure described that process, "A joint (the place where two bones meet) is surrounded by a capsule that protects and supports it. The joint capsule is lined with a type of tissue called synovium, which produces synovial fluid that lubricates and nourishes joint tissues. In rheumatoid arthritis, the synovium becomes inflamed, causing warmth, redness, swelling, and pain. As the disease progresses, abnormal synovial cells invade and erode, or destroy, cartilage and bone within the joint. Surrounding muscles, ligaments, and tendons become weakened. Rheumatoid arthritis can also cause more generalized bone loss that may lead to osteoporosis (fragile bones that are prone to fracture)." In addition, "Some people also experience the effects of rheumatoid arthritis in places other than the joints. About one-quarter develop rheumatoid nodules . . . bumps under the skin that often form close to the joints." Other serious complications may include anemia, neck pain, dry eyes or mouth, and inflammation of the blood vessels, lining of the lungs, or the sac enclosing the heart.

Besides a physical examination and case history taken by a rheumatologist or other medical specialist, "One common test is for RHEUMATOID FACTOR, an antibody that is eventually present in the blood of most rheumatoid arthritis patients." X-rays may be used to assess the condition of the affected joints with treatments depending on the optimal combination of medications for a particular patient. As the NIAMS brochure pointed out, "No matter what treatment the doctor and patient choose, however, the goals are the same: relieve pain, reduce inflammation, slow down or stop joint damage, and improve the person's sense of well-being and ability to function." Generally, this involves alternating periods of rest with EXERCISE. Adequate care of the FEET with proper FOOTWEAR will provide protection for the lower extremities, while healthful NUTRITION and techniques to reduce STRESS will assist the whole body.

American College of Rheumatology. "Arthritis News." Available online. URL: http://www.rheumatology.org Downloaded on October 25, 2002.

American College of Rheumatology. "What Is Rheumatoid Arthritis?" Available online. URL: http://www.rheumatology.org Downloaded on February 17, 2003.

National Institute of Arthritis and Musculoskeletal and Skin Diseases. "Handout on Health: Rheumatoid Arthritis." Available online. URL: http://www.niams.nih.gov Downloaded on February 10, 2004.

rheumatoid factor Everybody has antibodies—those normal proteins in the blood with a particular role in the immune system. If, however, a blood test reveals rheumatoid factor (RF) present among those antibodies, further investigation will be needed. Although some healthy individuals have occasionally been shown to have RF, its presence usually indicates RHEUMATOID ARTHRITIS but can also point to other conditions, such as infectious diseases or connective tissue disorders. In any case, RF is not an actual antibody but an autoantibody.

According to Lab Tests Online, "An antibody is a protective protein that forms in the blood, typically in response to a foreign material, usually another protein known as an antigen. Autoantibodies, however, are antibodies . . . capable of targeting one's own proteins rather than those of an outside agent, such as bacterial protein." In addition to rheumatoid arthritis and a related condition, SJÖGREN'S SYNDROME, a positive RF test may reveal endocarditis, SYSTEMIC LUPUS ERYTHEMATOSUS, a viral infection, cancer, or tuberculosis. Whatever the reason, RF in the blood bears thorough checking by a rheumatologist or other specialist.

Lab Tests Online. "Rheumatoid Factor." Available online. URL: http://www.labtestsonline.org Downloaded on February 21, 2002.

rheumatology This nonsurgical specialty of medicine focuses on treatments of systemic disorders and rheumatic diseases, such as RHEUMATOID ARTHRITIS, OSTEOARTHRITIS, GOUT, and FIBROMYALGIA as well as the 100 or more types of ARTHRITIS. Pediatric rheumatologists have particular interest in children's forms of these conditions, such as JUVENILE ARTHRITIS, JUVENILE OSTEOPOROSIS, and JUVENILE RHEUMATOID ARTHRITIS. Besides the training and certification required for any physician of internal medicine, a rheumatologist must also receive board certification in rheumatology. According to the University of Miami School of Medicine, "Rheumatologists have special interests in unexplained rash, fever, arthritis, anemia, weakness, weight loss, fatigue, joint or muscle pain, autoimmune disease, and anorexia. They often serve as consultants, acting like detectives for other doctors."

University of Miami School of Medicine. "Rheumatologist." Available online. URL: http://www.med.miami.edu Downloaded on June 14, 2003.

ribs To shield the lungs, these headband-shaped bones curve down from the STERNUM (breastbone) and around the back to the vertebral column of the SPINE. With the flexible bones being part of the main AXIAL SKELETON and the muscles part of the RESPIRATORY MUSCLE system, the ribs and their attached muscles expand with inspiration and contract with exhalation. This allows the whole rib cage to go in and out as a person breathes. If the system functions less noticeably than a new accordion, all will probably play out well. If, however, a rib hums with pain, especially if the area is pressed or a deep breath taken, the cause may be a broken rib or FRACTURE. A compression wrap can limit chest expansion, but that also limits breathing, which can then lead to a lung infection. Therefore, "Doctors typically do not recommend compression wraps unless necessary for pain," according to the Mayo Foundation for Medical Education and Research. To relieve the discomfort, the site recommended pain medication with reassurance that "a broken rib usually heals completely in about two months."

Mayo Foundation for Medical Education and Research. "Broken Ribs." Available online. URL: http://www.mayoclinic.com. Downloaded on September 2, 2003.

RICE method This formula for PAIN MANAGEMENT offers no recipe for fluffy rice but, instead, issues an acrostic reminder to use Rest, Ice, Compression, and

Elevation to relieve swelling and discomfort, particularly after an INJURY. Effectively used for bruising too, the RICE method can also be helpful in treating conditions such as a sprained ANKLE, LIMPING, PLANTAR FASCIITIS, or POPLITEAL TENDINITIS. The application of ice or a cold compress usually continues for about 10 or 15 minutes with twice as much time in between to keep from freezing or otherwise damaging the surrounding soft tissue. Although not recommended at all when an injury involves bleeding, compression generally keeps swelling to a minimum as does elevating the area above heart level.

rickets An unusual occurrence in industrialized nations, this disorder softens bones and weakens muscles of children who lack vitamin D, CALCIUM, and phosphate in their diets. The National Library of Medicine and the National Institutes of Health (NIH) clarified the surrounding factors by saying, "When the body is deficient in vitamin D, it is unable to properly regulate calcium and phosphate levels. If the blood levels of these minerals become too low, other body hormones may stimulate release of calcium and phosphate from the bones to the bloodstream to elevate the blood levels." This deficiency then "causes progressive softening and weakening of the bones' structure. There is a loss of calcium and phosphate from the bones, which eventually causes destruction of the supportive matrix." Although hereditary factors and a kidney or liver disorder can produce rickets, too, improper NUTRITION characteristically causes this condition, which begins with pain and muscle cramps but, if left untreated, can impair growth and gradually produce skeletal deformity. Therefore, the NIH article advised, "The replacement of deficient calcium, phosphorus, or vitamin D will eliminate most symptoms of rickets." This treatment primarily occurs with dietary supplements and natural food sources, such as fish, liver, and milk. Regular exposure to sunlight in small increments of time also encourages the body's synthesis and utilization of vitamin D.

The Agency for Healthcare Research and Quality explained, "Vitamin D is necessary for proper bone growth, but it is not found in many foods naturally. It is synthesized in the skin with exposure to sunlight, but many babies do not get much exposure to the sun for a number of reasons, such as not spending time outdoors and wearing clothes, hats, or sunscreen." In general, protective devices against too much sunlight remain highly recommended. However, parents need to be aware that, "the darker an infant's skin, the more sun exposure is needed to synthesize vitamin D. Although breastfeeding is the ideal form of nutrition for infants, it does not supply the vitamin D needed for healthy bone growth." In such cases, a vitamin D supplement provides a good alternative to give a nursing infant. For babies fed an enriched formula, however, added doses of vitamin D would provide too much of a good thing.

Agency for Healthcare Research and Quality. "Vitamin D Supplementation to Prevent Rickets in Breast-Fed Babies." Available online. URL: http://www.ahrq.gov Downloaded on October 7, 2003.

MedlinePlus. "Medical Encyclopedia: Rickets." Available online. URL: http://www.nlm.nih.gov/medlineplus Downloaded on October 7, 2003.

rodding surgery Used to assist extreme cases of OSTEOGENESIS IMPERFECTA or to speed the healing of FRACTURES in long bones that refuse to mend, this surgical method offers a strong measure of control. The Osteogenesis Imperfecta Foundation explained, "Rodding surgery involves internal 'splinting' of the long bones by means of the insertion of a metal rod. Under general anesthesia, a long bone (e.g., a leg or arm bone) may be cut in one or several places, straightened and 'threaded' onto a metal rod." With the rods consisting of an appropriate length and thickness of either stainless steel or titanium, "The surgery generally requires an incision long enough to expose the bone where it is deformed. Alternatively, small incisions can be made at the end of the deformed bone, and the rod may be introduced through the skin and moved through the bone under x-ray guidance. When the bone is acutely fractured, rodding can often be done without opening the fracture site." Following this procedure, the recuperative time depends on a patient's age and level of activity, but "the limb is often supported by a lightweight cast or a splint for about four weeks." Well-chosen exercises approved by the primary care physician come recommended during recovery to maintain the patient's overall muscle tone. Then PHYSICAL THERAPY and water workouts involving the affected area may be used "after the cast is removed to help the individual regain strength."

Osteogenesis Imperfecta Foundation. "OI Issues: Rodding Surgery." Available online. URL: http:// www.oif.org Downloaded on February 19, 2003.

rotation This JOINT movement allows a bone to pivot on its axis, as when arm or hand moves in a circle.

rotator cuff In conjunction with the triangular deltoid muscles of the SHOULDER, the four muscles and corresponding tendons known as the rotator cuff enable the arm to lift and rotate. With many activities—from hanging heavy clothes to swimming, hitting an overhead shot with a racquet, or winding up for a baseball pitch—the rotator cuff can get quite a workout. Indeed, overuse, STRAINS, BURSITIS, TENDINITIS, and tearing can injure any or all of those four muscles tucked beneath the shoulder blade, as can a fall.

According to the Yale Sports Medicine Center, "Rotator cuff tears . . . essentially involve separation of their attachment onto their respective bony prominences." In most cases, "Symptoms include pain along the outside aspect of the shoulder more significant at night and with attempts at raising the arm." As a further indication of shouldering too many troubles, "Patients show traditional weakness in elevating and externally rotating the arm. Plain x-ray examination can sometimes show degeneration along the attachment site of the specific muscle." MAGNETIC RESONANCE IMAGING (MRI) may be used to determine the extent of tearing. Typical treatments then aim toward eliminating pain.

With the arm and shoulder's remarkable range of motion, not surprisingly the American Academy of Orthopaedic Surgeons (AAOS) reported over 4 million shoulder problems receiving medical attention each year. However in December 2000, the AAOS offered assurances that "in most cases, the initial treatment is nonsurgical and involves several modalities." These generally include REST, NONSTEROIDAL ANTI-INFLAMMATORY DRUGS, and strengthening and stretching EXERCISES in PHYSICAL THERAPY. In addition, the AAOS advised, "Corticosteroid injections can help reduce pain but cannot be repeated frequently because they can also weaken the tendon. Ultrasound can enhance the delivery of topically applied drugs and has thermal effects that may also help in the healing process." When surgery seems warranted, this option may involve ARTHROSCOPY "to remove bone spurs of inflammatory portions of muscle and to repair lesser tears." Other surgical procedures include "A mini-open repair that combines arthroscopy and a small incision . . . to treat full-thickness tears. . . . In more severe cases, open surgery is required to repair the injured tendon. Sometimes a tissue transfer or a tendon graft is used. Joint replacement is also an option." Regardless of the surgical method, "Full functioning may not return for six months or more." After an appropriate time-out for recovery, the orthopedic surgeon will usually suggest a therapeutic exercise program to strengthen the rotator cuff and restore the shoulder joint's amazing mobility.

American Academy of Orthopaedic Surgeons. "Rotator Cuff Tears." Available online. URL: http://orthoinfo. aaos.org/fact Downloaded on October 10, 2003.

Yale Sports Medicine Center, Sports Injuries. "Shoulder-Rotator Cuff Tear." Available online. URL: http:// info.med.yal.edu/ortho Downloaded on October 10, 2003.

runner's knee See TENDINITIS OR TENDONITIS.

S

sacro- This prefix connects a word to the SACRUM—that triangular bone just below the back of the waist. The sacroiliac, for example, refers to the joint where the sacrum and pelvis articulate. Also in that area, sacralgia and sacrodynia point to pain while sacroiliitis spells inflammation and the prospect of a frequent BACKACHE.

sacroiliac joint pain syndrome Although the RANGE OF MOTION of the sacroiliac joint involves only a simple ROTATION movement, this basic swivel action works in union with the more mobile musculoskeletal areas, such as the SPINE, HIPS, LEGS, and PELVIC REGION. To describe what happens when an INJURY or REPETITIVE MOTION DISORDER puts a stop to this smooth move, doctors Yung C. Chen, Michael Fredericson, and Matthew Smuck said, "Various athletic activities, including walking, running, jumping, leaping, and squatting, can produce unwanted motion or stress in the sacroiliac joint (SIJ) and surrounding tissues. Soft-tissue failure, overload injuries, and direct trauma provide mechanisms for the evolution of SIJ pain syndrome. Clinical symptoms or dysfunction may directly relate to intra-articular SIJ sources, extra-articular sources, or soft tissues around the SIJ, including muscles, tendons, ligaments, and neurovascular structures. . . . SIJ pain syndrome may also be a distant manifestation of a musculoskeletal injury in other parts of the kinetic chain that are stressed during sports activities." For that reason, "patients may report a history of ankle, foot, knee, hip, or spine injuries before the SIF pain syndrome manifests." To diagnose this possibility, the article stated that X-RAY, COMPUTED TOMOGRAPHY, and MAGNETIC RESONANCE IMAGING offer little diagnostic value. However, "The gold standard for the diagnosis of SIJ pain syndrome is diagnostic injection under fluoroscopic guidance," but the invasiveness of that procedure makes a "controlled-block technique . . . preferred." By "reproducing symptoms with provocative analgesic injection and relieving symptoms with an anesthetic block," the authors determined, "this is the most reliable method to establish the diagnosis of intra-articular SIJ pain and allows immediate interpretation of SIJ arthrography." Assuming that sacral stress fractures and conditions, such as GOUT or ANKYLOSING SPONDYLITIS, have been ruled out, treatments may focus on REHABILITATION or therapeutic EXERCISE to strengthen and stabilize the sacral area. Also, "Weakness or inhibition of the hip muscles, especially the hip abductors, should be addressed." For additional support, pelvic belts and ORTHOTICS, such as heel lifts or other special types of FOOTWEAR, may be beneficial with injections of corticosteroids used only as needed to reduce the pain.

For athletic reasons or not, low back pain and morning stiffness—especially in young men—may not be the result of a sports injury but an indicator of one of the inflammatory conditions belonging to the spondyloarthritis group. If so, a thorough medical history, a physical examination, and appropriate tests, such as an X-ray of the sacroiliac joint, by a rheumatologist or other specialist can present an early diagnosis with early treatment preventing the possibility of a future deformity.

Chen, Yung C., Michael Fredricson, et al. "Sacroiliac Joint Pain Syndrome in Active Patients: A Look Behind the Pain." Available online. URL: http://www.physsportsmed.com Downloaded on October 14, 2003.

sacrum Here is a puzzle: what is fused but rarely confused about where it fits or sits? What forms a large, heavy base yet is not used for weight bearing of an upright structure? What is itself a puzzle piece between the upper and lower regions of the axial skeleton? The answer adds another riddle since the Latin word, *sacrum*, means "holy bone." No one seems to know exactly why that name was chosen. One possibility points to the sacrum's placement as a protective back plate for the womb and other life-aiding organs. Regardless of the reason, this puzzling triangle-shaped piece usually widens in the female body while showing less curvature in the male. Located between the LUMBAR VERTEBRAE and the COCCYX (tailbone), the sacrum primarily carries its weight as the body sinks into a seated position, which, in today's sedentary world, may be frequent. However, the mode in which the sacrum labors with areas of the lower body makes it susceptible to referred pain or other tribulations, such as SACROILIAC JOINT PAIN SYNDROME.

With the sacrum as the point of origination, a condition known as sacral dimple can arise in babies or young children, sometimes indicating an abnormality in the lower spine. The Mayo Foundation for Medical Education and Research said, "In very young infants, a doctor may recommend an ultrasound of the sacrum to help determine if a problem exists. Additional imaging tests such as X-rays or magnetic resonance imaging (MRI) also may be needed. If these tests detect a problem affecting the spinal cord, the child may require surgery." The primary identifying sign for parents to look for includes a large or deep area of dimpling below the lower curve of the back that is sometimes covered with a small patch of hair or a birthmark. Although an assessment by the child's pediatrician should be sought, "Most sacral dimples are small and do not indicate a serious problem."

Mayo Foundation for Medical Education and Research. "Sacral Dimple (Pilonidal Dimple)." Available online. URL: http://www.mayoclinic.com Downloaded on January 12, 2002.

safety Encompassing shelter, protection, and security, safety begins at home as families around the world safeguard the well-being of their loved ones. Despite this idyllic scene, people of all ages can be snug and safe indoors with FALLS and ACCIDENTS still happening in one sudden move. For example, an action as simple as improperly LIFTING heavy bags of groceries or getting down a hefty overhead object can pull muscles and tear LIGAMENTS, especially if a person twists from a NEUTRAL POSITION into an awkward one that stresses the joints. Even if someone sits sedately in front of a television or quietly curled up with a book, poor POSTURE and insufficient ERGONOMIC support can cause musculoskeletal STRAINS and INJURIES. In addition, too much time in the company of a computer mouse or a video game can eventually cause a REPETITIVE MOTION DISORDER, such as CARPAL TUNNEL SYNDROME. Yet each of these problems arises as home inhabitants stay "safely" indoors!

Whether indoors or out, a sensible safety program will not be inhibitive so much as preventive. For instance, as new parents venture outside with a young infant, the U.S. government joins their concerns for safety by providing regulations that cover car seats and carriers for air travel. For the latter, the Federal Aviation Administration gets on board with rules about labeling infant and toddler seats to certify their safe use in an aircraft. Since car safety vests and booster seats with shields have not been proven effective in crash tests, they will not be allowed for air travel. However, children weighing over 40 pounds can use an aircraft lap belt adjusted to accommodate their smaller size.

As children reach school age, subjects such as BACKPACK SAFETY and potential SPORTS INJURIES add to parental concerns. For the latter, safety-oriented organizations, such as the National Federation of State High School Associations and the National Collegiate Athletic Association, work toward helping parents and teachers develop protective programs for athletic youth. Likewise, the American Academy of Pediatrics (AAP) issues policies about child safety as directed by their various committees, such as one on Sports Medicine and Fitness and another on Injury and Poison Prevention. The AAP then makes recommendations accordingly, such as advising the use of full protective gear to safeguard a growing child's musculoskeletal system. *Safe Ride News* reported, "A 1996 study showed that wrist guards could reduce injury by 87 percent . . . Elbow pads are 82 percent effective, and knee pads are 32 percent effective at reducing injury."

That study did not address protective helmets, but others did. Although some researchers maintain that using inadequate helmets can actually increase the risks of cerebral damage rather than protect people of all ages against injuries in activities such as biking, heading a soccer ball, or playing a contact sport, other researchers work toward improving helmet safety standards. After themselves testing four types of lacrosse helmets, for example, Shane V. Caswell and Richard G. Deivert stated, "We believe that future research is needed to assist in the development of new helmet testing standards with increased validity and reliability. These studies should include impact force and frequency measurements during game situations, the effects of repetitive impacts on a larger sample, and longitudinal studies involving helmet wear and reconditioning practices on concussion rates in men's lacrosse athletes." With an estimated 300,000 sport-related traumatic brain injuries in the U.S. each year, a lack of protective equipment can be a primary causative. Although many improvements have been made in construction and design, safety-related products vary considerably as can the standards to which they are held. For example, some materials may be exceptionally sturdy initially yet break down at a faster rate with frequent use, forceful impact, or regular wear and tear.

To provide a realistic assessment of these variations, the National Athletic Trainers' Association said, "The person selecting equipment today needs to understand what these standards are, how they are written to ensure specific characteristics in a piece of equipment and which standards a particular piece of equipment is purported to meet. It is also essential to note that, in many instances, only the manufacturer claims that the product meets a standard. With few exceptions, such as the Consumer Product Safety Commission (CPSC), the Snell Memorial Foundation (SNELL), the Safety Equipment Institute (SEI), and the Hockey Equipment Certification Council (HECC), no independent body is checking on the manufacturers to be sure that their claims are factual." Therefore, P. David Halstead asserted that setting and meeting safety standards will be most likely to occur if a governing body mandates it. "For example, if a piece of personal protective equipment is required for some type of play, such as an HECC-certified helmet is required by USA Hockey, then players will likely wear such equipment because they cannot participate without doing so." In baseball, football, lacrosse, and other sports arenas, "these governing bodies require that the helmets met NOCSAE (National Operating Committee on Standards for Athletic Equipment) standards, and further, that all participants playing within the control of the governing body wear equipment clearly identified as being in compliance." Even then, athletic safety equipment must be well-fitted, well-maintained, and regularly reconditioned—with all parts present and in place—in order to provide the protection sought.

Regarding safety in the workplace, the Occupational Safety & Health Administration (OSHA) invited researchers "to submit abstracts on current findings relating to moving forward in the prevention of Musculoskeletal Disorders (MSDs)," with a particular focus on "data-driven scientific research concerning the relationship between the workplace and MSDs, such as definitions and diagnoses, cause and work-relatedness, exposure-response relationships, intervention studies, and study design (including research methodology)."

In 2003, OSHA announced, "Each year, approximately 6,000 employees in this country die from workplace injuries while another 50,000 die from illnesses caused by exposure to workplace. In addition, six million workers suffer nonfatal workplace injuries at an annual cost to U.S. businesses of more than $125 billion. Effective job safety and health add value to the workplace and help reduce worker injuries and illnesses." To this end, employees in the U.S. have certain rights and employers have specific obligations in providing and maintaining a secure environment. Both perspectives of these work-related safety issues have been addressed in detailed information obtainable from the OSHA Web site, www.osha.gov, or by calling (800) 321-OSHA.

For retired workers or sedentary adults who want a more active lifestyle, other safety concerns arise. To address this, the American Academy of

Orthopaedic Surgeons and the U.S. Consumer Product Safety Commission offered these safety tips, "Always wear appropriate safety gear. . . . Wear the appropriate shoes for each sport. Warm-up before you exercise. . . . Exercise for at least 30 minutes a day. . . . Follow the 10 percent rule. Never increase your program (i.e., walking or running distance or amount of weight lifted) more than 10 percent a week. Try not to do the exact same routine two days in a row. Walk, swim, play tennis or lift weight. This works different muscles and keeps exercise more interesting. . . . Check treadmills or other exercise equipment to be sure they are in good working order. If you are new to weight training, make sure you get proper information before you begin." As yet another safety precaution, the brochure advised, "Stop exercising if you experience severe pain or swelling. Discomfort that persists should always be evaluated."

Likewise, side effects of pharmaceuticals should also be assessed. According to *Physician's Weekly,* "Data voluntarily supplied by 368 different U.S. healthcare facilities documents over 105,000 medication errors. Fortunately, less than 3% of these events reported cause any harm to the patient." However, "A study of 36 hospitals reported in the September 9, 2002 issue of *Archives of Internal Medicine* (Vol. 162, No. 16:1,897–1,903) showed 19% of medication doses to be in error; about 7% of which were deemed potentially harmful to the patient." Rather than blaming hospital staff or suing doctors, however, the article suggested, "Preventing errors and improving safety for patients requires a systems approach in order to modify the conditions that contribute to errors." Since the Institute for Safe Medication Practices "discovered that only 43% of responding hospitals can easily access patient information, and only 53% can easily access drug information," some solutions to this safety hazard have been suggested by the American Hospital Association and the Health Research Educational Trust Safety with support from the Commonwealth Fund. Referred to as Pathways for Medication Safety, three components have been "designed to help hospital leaders incorporate medication safety into an organization's strategic plan: identify specific error-prone processes and devise safer alternatives; and prepare to implement a bedside bar-coding system for administering medications." To put these medical errors behind bars, the system would implement something similar to what "has been used in the retail market since the early 1970's." With the Veterans Health Administration one of the first to use a barcode medication system, they "reported an 86% improvement rate in medication errors" as compared with the former manual or paper system. "Using a handheld device, the clinician scans his/her own ID badge, the patient's ID, and the medication. The system provides bedside verification and recording of all medications administered to the patient and also warns the clinician of any mismatches or potential medication errors." By utilizing this technology to record and communicate vital information instantaneously, medical workers may have found a workable way to protect their own safety records and to get a patient home safely.

American Academy of Orthopaedic Surgeons and the U.S. Consumer Product Safety Commission. "Keep Active: Safe at any Age." Available online. URL: http://www.cpsc.gov/cpscpub Downloaded on February 13, 2003.

Caswell, Shane V. and Richard G. Deivert. "Lacrosse Helmet Designs and the Effects of Impact Forces." *Journal of Athletic Training* 37, no. 2 (2002): 164–171.

Halstead, P. David. "Performance Testing Updates in Head, Face, and Eye Protection." *Journal of Athletic Training* 36, no. 3 (2001): 322–327.

Occupational Safety & Health Administration. "Job Safety and Health." Available online. URL: http://www.osha.gov Down-loaded on October 17, 2003.

Occupational Safety & Health Administration. "OSHA Seeks Abstracts on Ergonomic Research: Symposium on Research to be Held in Conjunction with NACE Meeting in January." Available online. URL: http://www.osha.gov/pls/oshaweb/owadisp.show_document?p_table=NEWS_RELEASE.... Downloaded on October 16, 2003.

Physician's Weekly. "Medication Safety: Putting Error Behind Bars." Available online. URL: http://www.physweekly.com Downloaded on June 16, 2003.

Safe Ride News. "AAP Issues In-Line Skating Policy." Available online. URL: http://www.saferidenews.com Downloaded on February 25, 2003.

Safe Ride News. *Safer Airplane Travel with Babies and Toddlers.* Available online. URL: http://www.saferide-news.com Downloaded on February 25, 2003.

SAPHO syndrome This chronic disorder derives its acrostic name from Synovitis, Acne, Pustulosis, Hyperostosis, and Osteitis. With various combinations of those conditions at work in SAPHO syndrome, the lining of synovial joints become irritated. Pus forms in hair follicles, particularly on the face and upper back. Blisters or pustules arise on the undersides of the hands and feet. Overgrowth of bone occurs, and bones inflame. According to information from www.MedicineNet.com, some researchers believe this disorder relates to arthritic conditions of the spine, such as ANKYLOSING SPONDYLITIS and REACTIVE ARTHRITIS.

To discuss the treatment options Dr. William C. Shiel Jr. said, "Treatment of patients with SAPHO syndrome is directed toward the individual symptoms that are present. Generally, treatment involves medications which reduce inflammation in the particular tissues affected. Examples of medications that are used for inflammation include non-steroidal anti-inflammatory drugs (NSAIDs, such as aspirin, ibuprofen, and naproxen) and cortisone medications (either in the form of topical creams, tablets, or by injection into the involved area). Topical cold applications can also help reduce inflammation of some tissues."

A group of doctors associated with the Hannover Medical School in Hannover, Germany, published the "Diagnostic Management of Patients with SAPHO Syndrome: Use of MR Imaging to Guide Bone Biopsy at CT for Microbiological and Histological Work-Up." The doctors suspected the involvement of a particular type of acne (*Propionibacterium acnes* or *P. acnes*) "since it has been isolated repeatedly through open surgical bone biopsy." This study, however, "demonstrates the role of MRI [magnetic resonance imaging] in identifying inflamed bone areas in patients with SAPHO syndrome and the role of CT [computed tomography]-guided bone biopsies in obtaining samples from these areas for microbiological and histopathological investigations." With MRI used to show "acute inflammatory changes" in bone, CT-guided biopsies then examined the areas identified. Subsequently, "Patients positive for *P. acnes* were started on long-term antibiotic therapy according to antibiotic susceptibility." Although some of the SAPHO patients who participated in this study showed no evidence of the bacteria, the use of MRI and CT-guided bone biopsies provided "a minimally invasive alternative to open surgery in the detection of *P. acnes* leading to the institution of a specific antibiotic therapy."

Kirchoffi T., S. Merkesdal, et al. "Diagnostic Management of Patients with SAPHO Syndrome: Use of MR Imaging to Guide Bone Biopsy at CT for Microbiological and Histological Work-Up." *European Radiology* 13, no. 10 (October 13, 2003): 2,304–2,308.

Staff. "SAPHO Syndrome." Available online. URL: http://www.MedicineNet.com Downloaded on March 30, 2002.

sarcoidosis This inflammatory disease can attack the musculoskeletal system and any organ anywhere, but the most frequent location is the lungs. As tiny clusters of inflamed cells known as granulomas characteristically appear inside and/or outside the body, the person's lung volume decreases, causing shortness of breath, a dry cough, or chest pain. If exterior evidence occurs, red bumps or a scaly rash erupts. A fever or other symptoms, such as swollen ankles, may be present. Potential triggers include viral infection, environmental toxins, and exposure to allergens with a diagnosis aided by a physical examination, chest X-ray, and laboratory tests, such as a pulmonary function study. To confirm sarcoidosis, a biopsy of the granuloma will probably be needed, and corticosteroids may be prescribed.

According to an information sheet produced by the American Lung Association, "In over half the cases, sarcoidosis appears briefly and heals naturally. Sometimes the patient does not even know or do anything about it. From 20 to 30 percent of pulmonary sarcoidosis patients are left with permanent lung damage. And for a small percentage of patients, their sarcoidosis can become chronic, lasting for many years."

As breathing capacity diminishes, skeletal muscles become affected, too. After studying "Respiratory

Muscle Strength, Lung Function, and Dyspnea in Patients with Sarcoidosis," a team of doctors from the University of Southern California Medical Center found, "Sarcoidosis is a systemic granulomatous disorder that is estimated to involve the skeletal muscles in up to 50% of patients." With those estimates going as high as 80 percent, this translates to pain, weakness, and muscle atrophy. Furthermore, "In the absence of systemic or metabolic factors that might contribute to generalized muscle weakness, decreased lung volume in patients with sarcoidosis may contribute to diminished inspiratory and expiratory muscle strength and dyspnea." With a correlation found between RESPIRATORY MUSCLE strength and endurance, the resulting fatigue can adversely affect a patient's quality of life. However, by measuring respiratory muscle function, a physician can assess and address the individual's level of weakness and then recommend the most appropriate therapies.

American Lung Association. "Sarcoidosis." Available online. URL: http://www.lungusa.org Downloaded on October 15, 2003.

Baydur, Ahmet, et al. "Respiratory Muscle Strength, Lung Function, and Dyspnea in Patients with Sarcoidosis." *CHEST* 120, no. 1 (July 2001): 102–108.

sarcomere Unless they are interfered with by a gene mutation or injury of some kind, these functional and structural units make up the basic contraction system for myofibrils of striped or striated muscle tissue. As muscular tension changes, so does the length of the sarcomere. Comprised of protein filaments of either myosin or actin between two dense plates of Z DISKS, the sarcomere attaches to BONE, thus enabling JOINTS to move with the appropriate RANGE OF MOTION in both the APPENDICULAR SKELETON and the AXIAL SKELETON.

sarcopenia See MUSCLE LOSS.

scams In the presence of acute and chronic musculoskeletal pain, consumers may become especially vulnerable to false promises of products that can alleviate suffering. With loss of sleep often an issue, scams concerning beds or mattresses have been on the rise with a current trend toward exorbitantly priced magnetic beds or mattress pads. In an interview with Carole Fleck, the assistant director of the Federal Trade Commission reportedly said the agency found "inadequate scientific evidence to support therapeutic claims for static magnets." Investigations also show that pricing for such products may be 10 times higher than the actual cost of production with magnetic promises sometimes wrapped in an airy cushion of words.

Although recent studies show some types of MAGNET THERAPY to be of actual help, getting pulled into a scam offers no help at all. To prevent such entanglements, a good rule of thumb advises wariness of any undocumented claims and/or companies with no history or locatable presence within a community. Furthermore, if something sounds too good to be true, it well may be. To ask questions or report complaints of fraud, a concerned citizen can contact the Federal Trade Commission's toll-free number, (877) 382-4357, or write to the office of the state attorney general.

Fleck, Carole. "Scam Alert: Magnetic Delusion." Available online. URL: http://www.aarp.org/bulletin/yourhealth/Articles/a2003-06-30-magnetic.html Downloaded on July 21, 2004.

scapula See SHOULDER.

Scheuermann's disease This type of KYPHOSIS causes the upper spine to round or hump but usually with no pain unless the condition becomes severe. For unknown reasons, the typically rectangular-shaped thoracic vertebrae develop a wedgelike appearance or the spinal bones grow at an abnormal rate during adolescence, causing a deformity in the upper back. Although Scheuermann's disease is not the same as poor POSTURE, treatments may be similar with EXERCISES intended to straighten and strengthen the spine and a back brace prescribed to realign the misshapen vertebrae.

sciatica Sometimes searing, sciatic pain can shoot from the lower back, down the leg, and into a scream of irritated nerves. At other times, the legs may tingle or feel numb. Often, the type and severity of the symptoms depend on the cause, which may be trauma, a HERNIATED DISK, nerve compression in the area of the SACRUM, INFLAMMATION, or a chronic underlying medical condition, such as DIABETES.

As Dr. Peter C. Wing reported, "Back and radiating pain may result from disease processes elsewhere, such as the liver, bowel or kidney, or from pathological processes arising in or close to the spine." For instance, "After 1 month of back pain, 4%–5% of patients will be found to have a disc hernia, 4%–5% will have symptoms of spinal stenosis and perhaps 1% will be diagnosed with a visceral disorder or a renal or gynecological problem." When the pain becomes chronic, "long periods of disability may result." A medical history and a physical examination help to determine the appropriate tests as well as the type of medical specialist to whom the patient may be referred. For example, if an indication of nerve damage exists, a neurologist may request magnetic resonance imaging (MRI). If ARTHRITIS or OSTEOARTHRITIS seem the likely cause of sciatic pain, a rheumatologist will prescribe relevant tests, including radiographs, before determining a course of treatment. Spinal misalignment manifesting no signs of degenerative disk disease or DEGENERATIVE JOINT DISEASE may require manipulation by an osteopath or chiropractor, while evidence of SPINAL STENOSIS can be accessed by an orthopedic specialist.

According to http://spine-health.com, "Most cases of sciatica are caused by a simple irritation to the nerve and will get better with time and conservative care. However, some sciatica symptoms may indicate a potentially serious injury to the nerve." For example, loss of bladder and/or bowel control needs to be checked out immediately since this may indicate some disturbance to the spinal cord. Similarly, "If weakness or numbness is present, the nerve may be damaged and it is important to seek attention from a health care professional. If the nerve is compressed and the pain and symptoms are severe, surgery may be warranted."

According to health information on sciatica reviewed by the faculty of the Harvard Medical School, radiant pain from this longest nerve in the body "usually clears on its own following a period of rest and limitation of activities. Most people with sciatica feel better within six weeks. . . . Once the pain of sciatic has passed, there are exercises, stretches and other measures that may prevent its return." Some examples include practicing good POSTURE, exercising ABDOMINAL MUSCLES, going for walks, swimming, and avoiding irritants, such as improper FOOTWEAR and prolonged periods of sitting.

Regarding the latter, the Mayo Foundation for Medical Education and Research offered these helpful tips for avoiding sciatic pain, "Use chairs with firm support. Sit back in your chair to avoid concentrating pressure on your sciatic nerve, which runs from your lower back to your feet. Avoid crossing your legs. Plant your feet on the floor or on a footrest. Take frequent breaks. Walk around about once every hour. Get regular exercise to strengthen your back muscles and improve your posture. Adjust your car seat so your legs are bent at the knees and hips. Use a lumbar support or a rolled-up towel to support your lower back."

Harvard Medical School. "Sciatica." Available online. URL: http://www.intelihealth.com Downloaded on December 18, 2002.

Mayo Foundation for Medical Education and Research. "Sitting and Sciatica." Available online. URL: http://www.mayoclinic.com Downloaded on September 19, 2001.

Spine Health. "Sciatica and the Sciatic Nerve." Available online. URL: http://spine-health.com Downloaded on September 26, 2003.

Wing, Peter C. "Minimizing Disability in Patients with Low-Back Pain," *Canadian Medical Association, CMAJ* 164, no. 10 (May 15, 2001): 1,459–1,468.

scoliosis This abnormal curvature of the spine redirects the natural S CURVE of the shoulders, lower back, and upper buttocks as seen from the side in profile. When viewed directly from the back, the vertebral column no longer appears straight as it normally does from that perspective but instead twists into an out-of-line *S* or *C*. As Dr. John

Grayhack described the condition, "Scoliosis is the curvature of the spine to the side, out of the normal plane. This curvature in spinal muscular atrophy most likely develops because of a lack of muscular support of the bones of the spinal column or muscular imbalance." With this spinal zigzag from side to side generally described as scoliosis, "A bending of the spine more backward (or hunchback) is kyphosis," while "a curve forward, or inward, is lordosis." Although evidence can begin in the first few months of life, scoliosis will more often be identified in school-aged youth. "Some very severely involved children at early ages have very marked curvature which interfere with their sitting or pulmonary functions. . . . Initially, conservative treatment such as seating changes, support, or even brace wear would be probably warranted." For example, a brace or body jacket may be prescribed to support the spine and enable the child to engage in daily activities. Seating devices or molds can provide additional stability, too. "Failing this, more conservative surgical treatments, such as limited fusion (surgery just at the apex of the curvature), subcutaneous rodding (a supporting rod without a fusion, with hooks only at the top and the bottom), or a 'growing construct' (a rod with cables around the spine but no fusion, with the idea that the spine can grow along the rod like a trolley). None of these options is perfect, and each has its own difficulties."

According to statistics from the Information and Support page of the National Scoliosis Foundation, these difficulties affect 2–3 percent of the population with an estimated 6 million people in the U.S. receiving no cure. "The vast majority of people with this condition are not expected to require treatment. The problem is we do not know who will get it, why they get it, which will progress, or how far they will progress. Each year scoliosis patients make more than 600,000 visits to private physician offices, and an estimated 30,000 children are put into a brace for scoliosis, while 38,000 patients undergo spinal fusion surgery."

According to the *Journal of the American Chiropractic Association,* "There are four major types of scoliosis: congenital, which is caused by a fairly rare malformation of the spine that manifests itself at birth or shortly afterward; juvenile, also relatively unusual and appearing in childhood; degenerative or adult, caused by the deterioration of joints in the spine later in life; and idiopathic or adolescent, which usually manifests itself and progresses primarily during the adolescent growth spurt." Curvatures in girls progress about 10 times more than in boys with the emotional effects devastating for both sexes, especially if bracing first becomes needed during the sensitive years of puberty. To keep spinal curvature from progressing to that point, some think that electrical stimulation may have therapeutic value, while others "believe scoliosis to be symptomatic of severe underlying abnormalities in the central nervous system." In instances where bone strength and stability have not been compromised, gentle spinal manipulation by a chiropractor or an osteopath can help to balance the SACRUM, offering yet another possibility of slowing the progression of scoliosis.

Grayhack, John, M.D. "The Hidden Twist . . . Scoliosis." Available online. URL: http://www.fsma.org Downloaded on May 29, 2002.

National Scoliosis Foundation. "Information and Support Page." Available online. URL: http://www.scoliosis.org Downloaded on October 18, 2003.

Staff. "Grading on the Curve: What We Know About Scoliosis." *Journal of the American Chiropractic Association.* Available online. URL: http://www.acatoday.com/pdf/focus_february2002.pdf Downloaded on June 30, 2004.

S curve When seen squarely from the back, a properly aligned spinal column looks like a lowercase *L.* When seen from the side, the lettering changes as one S curve draws a line from the top of the HEAD, down the back of the NECK, and onto the top arc of the SHOULDERS. Another naturally S-shaped curve then moves along the roundness of the shoulders to the inward dip of the lower back and onto the arc of the upper buttocks.

The American Physical Therapy Association, reported, "Good posture has only one appearance, but poor posture comes in many unattractive styles." Besides the advantageous way in which a "person with good posture projects poise, confidence, and dignity," correct alignment helps a body to "function at top speed. It promotes movement efficiency and endurance and contributes to an overall feeling of well-being." Conversely, a vertebral column that is bent out of shape will add undue stress to joints, muscles, ligaments and, eventually, bones and internal organs. Therefore, the body's picturesque S curve provides the musculoskeletal standard of an ideal profile, enabling a physical therapist osteopath, chiropractor, surgeon, or other orthopedic specialist to evaluate and treat what just does not line up.

See also POSTURE; SCOLIOSIS.

Annette Iglarsh, Florence Kendall, et al. "Secret of Good Posture." Available online. URL: http://www.apta.org Downloaded on October 14, 2003.

septic arthritis Sometimes referred to as bacterial arthritis or infectious arthritis, this one in 100 or more types of ARTHRITIS begins with the invasion of a bacteria or a virus in one or more of the joints. For example, the bacteria from a tick bite can result in infectious arthritis as can some sexually transmitted diseases, such as gonorrhea. Since the prognosis and treatment vary according to the causative, accurately classifying the organism becomes a primary and immediate task.

As explained by rheumatologist Dr. Lori B. Siegel, "The diagnosis of septic arthritis, like most diseases, resides with a detailed history and physical exam. The history must include a history of joint trauma or prior joint disease, intravenous drug abuse, localized joint infections, sexual activity, and a thorough social history. Intra-articular processes can be differentiated from extra-articular processes based on both the history and physical exam. Physical examination will often reveal tenderness, erythema, localized warmth, and edema. There is usually a decrease in both passive and active range of motion in the septic joint." Additionally, "In the neonatal patient, common accompanying signs include fever, lethargy, pseudo-paralysis of the extremity, and failure to feed, while in the adult, the symptoms tend to be more localized." In the latter case, "The presence of constitutional symptoms, including fever, chills, and rigors, is present in less than half of all adult cases of confirmed bacterial arthritis." Besides an assessment of the symptoms, a patient's history offers clues for putting a stop to this "rapidly destructive joint disease, which is characterized by microbial invasion into the joint space. The organisms most commonly enter the joint space via hematogenous spread from a distant source." With blood transport a likelihood, "Other common portals of entry include direct implantation via a puncture wound or intra-articular injection, surgical incisions and spread from contiguous infection, such as cellulites, septic bursitis, and osteomyelitis." Spread of microbes through the blood can also occur with intravenous drug use. "In addition, a frequently forgotten source of septic arthritis is puncture wound by a human tooth over the 2nd or 3rd metacarpophalangeal joint of a clenched fist, as can occur during a fight," whereas infants may be predisposed through maternal sources leading to the placenta. With the disease more common in children than adults, "The incidence of septic arthritis ranges from 2–10 per 100,000 individuals, yet among patients with rheumatoid arthritis or prosthetic joints, the incidence rises to 30–70 per 100,000." About half the cases involve the knee. "The second most commonly involved joint is the hip, followed by the shoulder . . . , ankle, wrist, and elbow. Septic arthritis of the interphalangeal joints are relatively rare except when there is direct penetration following a human or animal bite," but much more frequent among intravenous drug abusers. Other predisposing factors include a previous joint trauma, a prosthetic device, DIABETES, RHEUMATOID ARTHRITIS, alcoholism, and the use of corticosteroids in managing another medical condition. In the latter case, an X-ray can be useful in providing "the ability to monitor the joint for changes over time." However, magnetic resonance imaging or "MRI has the additional benefit of being able to demonstrate cellulites around an infected joint, as well as showing articular cartilage destruction. Computerized tomography (CT) is excellent for joints with complex configurations. In addition, for joints that are difficult to aspirate, . . . CT can be used to guide the aspiration." To treat the condition, Dr. Siegel advised, "Any acutely inflamed joint should be suspected of having septic arthritis until proven otherwise. Thus, the joint needs to be immobilized for a maximum of forty-eight hours in the position of comfort. While septic arthritis can be managed either surgically or medically, an early diagnosis and definite treatment is more important for cure than is the method of drainage. In the cases of septic arthritis involving the hip or poorly accessible joints, as well as those not responding to antimicrobial therapy, surgical management is required, especially when the infection occurs in children. Infections caused by spread from adjacent tissue infection should also be managed surgically. If the septic arthritis involves a joint with a prosthesis, treatment will frequently necessitate the surgical removal of the prosthesis." If this does not prove feasible, "The patient should be treated with six weeks of parenteral antibiotics," with the particular choice of medication "based on a definitive identification of the infecting organism."

Although the prognosis varies according to the type and, especially, the promptness of a course of treatment, Mark E. Shirtliff and Jon T. Mader discussed potential outcomes patients might expect. "A permanent reduction in joint function is seen in approximately 40% of patients with nongonococcal septic arthritis but ranges between 10 and 73%. This wide range of observed morbidity reflects the dependence of therapy success on host, bacterial, and diagnostic and treatment factors. The mortality associated with this disease is usually between 5 and 20% and is often a result of the transient or chronic bacteremia that causes most cases of septic arthritis." Therefore, "Patients who start treatment after experiencing symptoms for 7 days or more demonstrate a poor outcome." Besides the need for immediate medical attention, "Early physical therapy and aggressive mobilization are important for optimal recovery."

Shirtliff, Mark E. and Jon T. Mader. "Acute Septic Arthritis." *Clinical Microbiology Reviews: The Journal of the American Society for Microbiology* 15, no. 4 (October 2002): 527–544.

Siegel, Lori B., M.D. "A Swollen Joint: Why All the Fuss?" *American Journal of Therapeutics* 10, no. 4 (July/August 2003): 219–224.

sesamoid bone ARTICULATION usually connects one BONE to another, creating a JOINT. However, a few bones nestle into muscle or attach to TENDONS rather than other bones. The biggest example would be in the kneecap or patella, with smaller sesamoid bones—about the size or shape of sesame seeds—found in the foot. These little bones may be small, but they have a large part in enabling tendons to slide with ease, conveying muscle power and assisting movement.

sesamoiditis Since SESAMOID BONES occur in weight-bearing areas of the body, such as the KNEES and FEET, they receive frequent stresses that expose them to the possibilities of INFLAMMATION and TENDINITIS. These irritating instances of sesamoiditis can usually be treated without surgery, according to the American Academy of Orthopaedic Surgeons (AAOS). The AAOS differentiated between this condition and the breakage of a sesamoid bone by saying, "With sesamoiditis, pain may develop gradually; with a fracture, pain will be immediate." Although "Swelling and bruising may or may not be present," during a physical exam, "the physician will look for tenderness," usually by manipulating the affected area and assessing RANGE OF MOTION in the affected joint. In addition, "If the X-rays appear normal, the physician may request a bone scan." To relieve the stress on a foot or knee, treatment will typically consist of the RICE METHOD, NSAIDs, and well-fitted FOOTWEAR. If symptoms continue, a steroid injection or a brace may be warranted.

American Academy of Orthopaedic Surgeons. "Sesamoiditis." Available online. URL: http://orthoinfo.aaos.org/fact Downloaded on October 18, 2003.

Sever's disease This REPETITIVE MOTION DISORDER most commonly affects youth who become active in sports and, simultaneously, active in BONE DEVELOPMENT, thus placing the prime years for Sever's disease somewhere in puberty. During that time, feet usually grow faster than other bones and muscles, making tendons tighten uncomfortably and causing LIMPING, heel pain, or even an injury to the growth plate of the foot. Heel lifts or other ORTHOTICS often help as do ice packs or EXERCISES intended to stretch the ACHILLES TENDON. With well-timed treatment, most cases will disappear and, eventually, become outgrown.

shaken baby syndrome See HEAD INJURY.

shin See TIBIA.

shin splints No matter how it sounds, this phrase does not refer to a leg-bracing system but to pain occurring along the shinbone or TIBIA. FLATFEET and other flaws of BIOMECHANICS, such as legs of uneven length, can cause this condition. However, shin splints more likely occur after a sudden burst of EXERCISE or strenuous physical ACTIVITY. In runners, pain may develop at a snail's pace as calf muscles tighten or feet experience the ill effects of PRONATION or a lopsided trail lays a downhill path to pain. A correct choice of FOOTWEAR or the addition of ORTHOTICS can usually stop shin splints in their tracks with rest, ice, stretching exercises, and massage used to manage the existing discomfort.

shoes See FOOTWEAR.

shoulder As a BALL-AND-SOCKET JOINT, the shoulder has the greatest RANGE OF MOTION, which also offers the greatest opportunity for a DISLOCATED JOINT, REPETITIVE MOTION DISORDER, TENDINITIS, or other INJURY. According to the National Institutes of Arthritis and Musculoskeletal and Skin Diseases (NIAMS), about 4 million people in the U.S. require medical attention each year for shoulder SPRAIN or similar problems, with approximately 1.5 million annually visiting an orthopedic surgeon.

To explain the vulnerabilities of the shoulder's highly flexible design, NIAMS said, "The shoulder is the most movable joint in the body. However, it is an unstable joint because of the range of motion allowed. It is easily subject to injury because the ball of the upper arm is larger than the shoulder socket that holds it. To remain stable, the shoulder must be anchored by its muscles, tendons, and ligaments." To describe even further how the shoulder's structure affects its function, NIAMS went on to say, "The shoulder joint is composed of three bones: the clavicle (collarbone), the scapula (shoulder blade), and the humerus (upper arm bone). . . . Two joints facilitate shoulder movement. The acromioclavicular (AC) joint is located between the acromion (part of the scapula that forms the highest point of the shoulder) and the clavicle. The glenohumeral joint, commonly called the shoulder joint, is a ball-and-socket type joint that helps move the shoulder forward and backward and allows the arm to rotate in a circular fashion or hinge out and up—away from the body."

To assess the normal configurations of shoulder movement, doctors Paul A. Borsa, Mark K. Timmons, and Eric L. Sauers focused on "Scapular-Positioning Patterns During Humeral Elevation in Unimpaired Shoulders." They reported, "During dynamic arm movement, the scapula must move synchronously with the humerus to provide optimal congruence between the glenoid and the humeral head. This congruence is necessary for establishing adequate length-tension relationships for the muscles acting on the scapula and the humeral head and for maintaining a stable base for transferring kinetic energy from proximal to distal segments." By understanding these patterns, diagnosticians have a standard to assess shoulder movement. "The ability to detect diminished upward rotation of the scapula may aid in preventing and evaluating shoulder impairments. For example, it may help diagnose impairment, such as impingement, or can be used to screen athletes who may be predisposed to shoulder impairment, such as throwers and swimmers." With these patterns measured by degrees ranging from 30 at rest to 120 in an elevated position, "It may be important to assess scapular motion during humeral motion in multiple planes, angles or arcs, and directions of motions." These models can then be used to estimate the likelihood of an injury or to measure the severity of an impingement, such as commonly experienced in the ROTATOR CUFF of tennis players and other upwardly mobile athletes.

After observing a patient's movement in a physical examination and taking a medical history to clarify genetic and athletic tendencies or other contributing factors, a physician may order an X-ray, magnetic resonance imaging (MRI), or ARTHROSCOPY to confirm a diagnosis or explore the particular condition a patient has been shouldering. Common problems include a dislocated joint, separation of the ACROMIOCLAVICULAR JOINT, ADHESIVE CAPSULITIS, BURSITIS, bone FRACTURE, and ARTHRITIS.

If pain continues despite regular treatments with rest, ice, and sometimes HEAT THERAPY, the problem may not be in the shoulder at all. According to *Consumer Reports On Health*, "Ailments of the gallbladder, liver, heart, spine, or neck can all cause referred pain that travels through the nerves to the shoulder." If the shoulder itself proves to have a problem, however, "Nearly all shoulder ailments can be managed through a combination of modified activity, physical therapy, and drugs to reduce inflammation and pain; other noninvasive treatments include electrical stimulation and ultrasound." Although steroid injections may relieve persistent pain, "Injections can eventually weaken tendons and ligaments. So they should be used sparingly (no more than 3 shots per body part per year) and only after other steps have failed." In addition, the *Consumer Report* column stated, "Whatever the treatment, it's important to keep the joint moving. Prolonged immobility can cause scar tissue to form in the joint, freezing it in place."

Such problems occur because the majority of shoulder problems, according to the American Academy of Orthopaedic Surgeons (AAOS), "involve the soft tissues—muscles, ligaments and tendons—rather than bones. And most of these problems fall into three major categories: tendinitis/bursitis, injury/instability, arthritis. Other much more rare causes of shoulder pain are tumors, infection and nerve-related problems." Although JOINT REPLACEMENT surgery more commonly occurs in a knee or hip, ARTHROPLASTY of the shoulder usually meets with fewer complications and "may be recommended if arthritis or degenerative joint disease makes your shoulder stiff and painful or if the upper arm bone is fractured so badly that tissue death may result." Following this procedure, recuperative measures include wearing a sling for the first month and avoiding weight-bearing efforts, such as lifting oneself from a chair. A personalized program of home exercises "4 to 5 times a day for a month or more" also came recommended by AAOS as did this advice, "Don't lift anything heavier than a cup of coffee for the first 6 weeks after surgery. . . . Don't participate in contact sports or do any heavy lifting for at least 6 months." With timely treatment and appropriate therapies, most shoulders will eventually regain a full swing.

American Academy of Orthopaedic Surgeons. "Shoulder Joint Replacement." Available online. URL: http://orthoinfo.aaos.org Downloaded on October 20, 2003.

American Academy of Orthopaedic Surgeons. "Shoulder Pain." Available online. URL: http://orthoinfo.aaos.org Downloaded October 20, 2003.

Borsa, Paul A., Mark K. Timmons, et. al. "Scapular-Positioning Patterns During Humeral Elevation in Unimpaired Shoulders." *Journal of Athletic Training* 38, no. 1 (2003): 12–17.

Consumer Reports on Health. "Joint and Muscle Pain: Shouldering Too Much?" Available online. URL: http://www.consumerreportsonhealth.org Downloaded on July 21, 2004.

National Institutes of Arthritis and Musculoskeletal and Skin Diseases. "Shoulder Problems." Available online. URL: http://www.niams.nih.gov/hi/topics/shoulderprobs/shoulderqa.htm Downloaded on February 18, 2003.

sinuses Not a bone but air-filled pockets within the bones of the FACE and NOSE, the sinuses have names corresponding to their locations. According to Martin J. Citardi, M.D., these sinus cavities include, "Maxillary (one sinus located in each cheek); Ethmoid (approximately 6–12 small sinuses per side, located between the eyes); Frontal (one sinus per side, located in the forehead); Sphenoid (one sinus per side, located behind the ethmoid sinuses, near the middle of the skull)." Since each pocket has an opening or ostium that connects to the nose, one affects the other. For instance, "The lining secretes mucus, a complex substance that keeps the nose and sinuses moist." Keeping the sinuses drained and the nose cleared, however, does not rely on gravity as often supposed but on an active process involving the cilia or hairlike structures that clear blockage in a movement that "is not random; rather it is programmed so that the mucus moves along in a specific pattern." When that movement comes to a halt, however, the congested sinuses can cause more headaches than a traffic jam.

As the fact sheet "Sinus Headaches," from the American Academy of Otolaryngology—Head and Neck Surgery (AAO-HNS), explained, "Sinus headaches are associated with a swelling of the membranes lining the sinuses (spaces adjacent to the nasal passages). Pain occurs in the affected region—the result of air, pus, and mucus being trapped within the obstructed sinuses. The discomfort often occurs under the eye and in the upper teeth (disguised as a headache or toothache). Sinus headaches tend to worsen as you bend forward or lie down." Therefore, "The key to relieving the symptoms is to reduce sinus swelling and inflammation and facilitate mucous drainage from the sinuses." To do this, AAO-HNS recommended moist air, nasal irrigation, and alternating hot and cold compresses with instructions to "place a hot compress across your sinuses for three minutes, and then a cold compress for 30 seconds. Repeat this procedure three times per treatment, two to six times a day." The site also suggested using decongestants, over-the-counter medications to reduce sinus headaches, and alternative remedies, such as mint. Indeed, most herbalists agree that a cup of peppermint tea can do wonders in opening nasal passages.

According to the Centers for Disease Control and Prevention, in the U.S. in the year 2000 alone, "Approximately 32 million persons (18 years and older) were told that they had sinusitis," ultimately resulting in 11.6 million visits to doctors and 1.2 million to outpatient clinics.

The National Institute of Allergy and Infectious Diseases (NIAID) further classified information by saying, "Health care experts usually divide sinusitis cases into Acute, which lasts for 3 weeks or less; Chronic, which usually lasts for 3 to 8 weeks but can continue for months or even years; Recurrent, which is several acute attacks within a year." Since "each sinus has an opening into the nose for the free exchange of air and mucus . . . anything that causes a swelling in the nose—an infection, an allergic reaction, or an immune reaction—also can affect the sinuses." For example, "Air trapped within a blocked sinus, along with pus or other secretions, may cause pressure on the sinus wall. The result is the sometimes intense pain of a sinus attack. Similarly, when air is prevented from entering a paranasal sinus by a swollen membrane at the opening, a vacuum can be created that also causes pain." Just as the location of a sinus region determines its name, so does it clarify which sinus cavity has been affected or infected. "Pain when your forehead over the frontal sinuses is touched may indicate that your frontal sinuses are inflamed. Infection in the maxillary sinuses can cause your upper jaw and teeth to ache and your cheeks to become tender to the touch. Since the ethmoid sinuses are near the tear ducts in the corner of the eyes, inflammation of these cavities often causes swelling of the eyelids and tissues around your eyes, and pain between your eyes. Ethmoid inflammation also can cause tenderness when the sides of your nose are touched, a loss of smell, and a stuffy nose. Although the sphenoid sinuses are less frequently affected, infection in the area can cause earaches, neck pain, and deep aching at the top of your head. Most people with sinusitis, however, have pain or tenderness in several locations, and their symptoms usually do not clearly indicate which sinuses are inflamed."

Those symptoms typically include a fever, tiredness, a cough that worsens at night, and either congestion or a runny nose. Causes may be due to a bacterial infection, fungal infection, or an allergic response to an allergen, such as perfume, foods, mold, dust, and pollen. With so many factors potentially affecting the sinuses, a specialist may be needed to consider the clues and solve the mystery. Then, treatments may include the most appropriate type of antibiotic and, in some cases, surgery to scrape the adjacent bones. As the NIAID explained, "The most common surgery done today is functional endoscopic sinus surgery in which the natural openings from the sinuses are enlarged to allow drainage. This type of surgery is less invasive than conventional sinus surgery, and serious complications are rare."

In reporting on the most likely, albeit infrequent "Complications of Nasal and Sinus Surgery" for the American Rhinologic Society, Dr. Jay M. Dutton of the Rush-Presbyterian-St. Luke's Medical Center in Chicago, Illinois, said, "Surgery on the nasal septum . . . and sinuses is recommended only after it has been determined that medical management has been unsuccessful." Dr. Dutton listed the surgical risks as including post-operative bleeding, complications with anesthesia, subsequent changes in voice or the ability to smell, the onset of infection, scarring that eventually causes a nasal obstruction, numbness, and intracranial complications. In the highly unusual case of the latter, a breech occurs in the area where "the base of the skull forms the roof of the ethmoid and sphenoid sinuses," so that a "leak of cerebrospinal fluid (the fluid that bathes the brain and spinal cord) may occur. . . . This can usually be repaired at the time of the initial surgery, although in rare cases further complications such as meningitis may ensue." Similarly, intraorbital complications can affect the eyes since "The orbit is situated immediately adjacent to several of the paranasal sinuses but is separated by a layer of bone. Because of this close proximity, in rare cases bleeding may occur into the orbit requiring repair at the time of the initial surgery. Visual loss and blindness have been reported but are extremely rare." Despite the risk of these or other complications of surgery, lack of treatment can also cause a BONE INFECTION to occur. Again, this happens only in exceptionally rare instances. Nevertheless, prompt treatment of a sinus condition can help to prevent ill effects on the musculoskeletal system while improving a person's overall health.

American Academy of Otolaryngology—Head and Neck Surgery. "Sinus Headaches." Available online. URL: http://www.entnet.org Downloaded on October 22, 2003.

Citardi, Martin J., M.D. "Brief Overview of Sinus and Nasal Anatomy." Available online. URL: http://www.american-rhinologic.org Downloaded on July 28, 2003.

Dutton, Jay M., M.D. "Complications of Nasal and Sinus Surgery." Available online. URL: http://www.american-rhinologic.org Downloaded on July 28, 2003.

National Center for Health Statistics. "Chronic Sinusitis." Available online. URL: http://www.cdc.gov/nchs Downloaded on October 1, 2003.

National Institute of Allergy and Infectious Diseases. "Sinusitis." Available online. URL: http://www.niaid.nih.gov Downloaded on October 22, 2003.

Sjögren's syndrome With gravelly eyes and a dry swallow being the common symptoms, this chronic autoimmune disorder needs a rheumatologist to head a medical team that most likely includes a dentist and an ophthalmologist. Classified either as a primary disorder or one secondary to another rheumatic condition, such as SYSTEMIC LUPUS ERYTHEMATOSUS, RHEUMATOID ARTHRITIS, or FIBROMYALGIA, Sjögren's syndrome can involve the connective tissue throughout the body. Characteristically though, the syndrome affects the salivary glands that aid digestion and the lacrimal glands that induce tears, thereby putting a damper on their ability to keep dampness at healthy levels in the mouth and eyes. Consequently, various tests to examine ocular and oral function will usually be recommended.

According to a fact sheet from the Sjögren's Syndrome Foundation, those ophthalmologic tests may include a Schirmer test to measure tear production, a rose bengal and lissamine green test with dyes to assess any abnormal cells on the surface of the eye, and a slitlamp exam to measure the volume of tears. In addition, dental tests may include a parotid gland flow to measure the production of saliva, a salivary scintigraphy to measure the function of the salivary gland, and a lip biopsy to confirm lymphocytic infiltration of the minor salivary glands.

A "Sjögren's Syndrome" fact sheet from the American College of Rheumatology (ACR) indicated the need for blood tests too—not to evaluate symptoms but their cause. As ACR stated, "The several factors involved include genetic, immunologic, hormonal, and probably infectious. People with this disease have abnormal proteins in their blood that suggest that their immune system is reacting against their own tissue. The decreased production of tears and saliva is caused when the glands that produce these fluids are damaged.

These glands are attacked by immune cells called lymphocytes. In a small number of people, Sjögren's syndrome is associated with lymphoma, a form of cancer." Although that association may be a rarity, the ACR reported, "Between 1 and 4 million Americans have Sjögren's syndrome. It occurs 10 times more in women than in men." For that reason and also because, "onset can occur at any age, but usually between 45 and 55," hormonal factors may be a presenting factor.

Even though a decrease in estrogen or other hormones can be considered in developing an individualized course of treatment, the initial actions generally taken address the restoration of gland secretion. According to the National Institute of Neurological Disorders and Stroke (NINDS), "Moisture replacement therapies may ease the symptoms of dryness. Nonsteroidal anti-inflammatory drugs may be used to treat musculoskeletal symptoms. For individuals with severe complications, corticosteroids or immunosuppressive drugs may be prescribed." Regarding the latter, NINDS further explained, "Sjögren's can damage vital organs of the body with symptoms that may plateau, worsen, or go into remission. Some people may experience only the mild symptoms of dry eyes and mouth, while others go through cycles of good health followed by severe disease. Many patients are able to treat problems symptomatically. Others are forced to cope with blurred vision, constant eye discomfort, recurrent mouth infections, swollen parotid glands, hoarseness, and difficulty in swallowing and eating. Debilitating fatigue and joint pain can seriously impair quality of life."

By using artificial lubricants to ease dryness and making dietary modifications to assist a person in swallowing, symptoms can often be kept to a minimum. Sensitive patients, however, would be particularly advised to avoid lubricating products containing chemical preservatives or other harsh additives. Similarly, care should be taken in applying liner or other makeup to the eyes. Not only do perfumed cosmetics irritate most people, but powdery eye shadow can easily powder down a pair of already too-dry eyes. Wearing protective UV lenses outside and using lighting that keeps glare to a minimum inside would also be recommended. For protection of the mouth, antimicrobial washes and fluoride treatments may be helpful, or a cup of green tea with honey can offer a natural form that includes a bit of both. To reduce systemic reactions, such as the muscle fatigue associated with Sjögren's syndrome, a natural course of treatment would include supportive NUTRITION and adequate EXERCISE with ample rest and plenty of fresh water to hydrate the entire musculoskeletal system.

American College of Rheumatology. "Sjögren's Syndrome." Available online. URL: http://www.rheumatology.org Downloaded on November 19, 2003.

National Institute of Neurological Disorders and Stroke (NINDS). "NINDS Sjögren's Syndrome Information Page." Available online. URL: http://www.ninds.nih.gov Downloaded on December 27, 2001.

Sjögren's Syndrome Foundation. "Fact Sheet." Available online. URL: http://www.sjogrens.com Downloaded on November 19, 2003.

skeletal bones The adult human skeleton contains 80 AXIAL and 126 APPENDICULAR bones. Interestingly, infants begin with 300 BONES, but eventually fusion takes over, compressing the number to 206. Yet even then, an adult has as many neck vertebrae as a giraffe—just with smaller bones. That and other facts about "Your Gross and Cool Body—Skeletal System" are available on http://yucky.kids.discovery.com which calls itself "The Yuckiest Site on the Internet." According to its sponsor, the Discovery Channel, "Some 97% of critters on earth don't have a backbone or spine. Remarkably enough, of those that do have a backbone, there are lots of similarities: a skull surrounding a brain, a rib cage surrounding a heart, and a jawbone or mouth opening." The Discovery site also added the interesting information that, in humans, the longest bone in the body—the FEMUR or LEG bone—counts "about $^1/_4$ of your height. The smallest is the stirrup bone in the ear which can measure $^1/_{10}$ of an inch."

With bones of all sizes bound by LIGAMENTS or TENDONS and, usually, capped by some kind of CARTILAGE, the skeletal system tallies up to about 20 percent of a person's body weight. Those numbers seem surprisingly small though, considering all that bones can do. The National Cancer Institute's

Surveillance, Epidemiology and End Results (SEER) Program in conjunction with Emory University in Atlanta, Georgia, said, "The living bones in our bodies use oxygen and give off waste products in metabolism. They contain active tissues that consume nutrients, require a blood supply and change shape or remodel in response to variations in mechanical stress. Bones provide a rigid framework, known as the skeleton, that support and protect the soft organs of the body." As if that were not enough to carry, "The skeleton supports the body against the pull of gravity. The large bones of the lower limbs support the trunk when standing." In addition, "Bones work together with muscles as simple mechanical lever systems to produce body movement." Besides getting a person from here to there, "Bones contain more calcium than any other organ." However, "When blood calcium levels decrease below normal, calcium is released from the bones so that there will be an adequate supply for metabolic needs. When blood calcium levels are increased, the excess calcium is stored in the bone matrix. The dynamic process of releasing and storing calcium goes on almost continuously." Thus, bone repair and REMODELING go on too, making the muscle-bound skeleton a living thing, quite unlike the bare-bones model that clicks into being sometime around Halloween.

Discovery Channel. "Your Gross and Cool Body-Skeletal System." Available online. URL: http://yucky.kids.discovery.com Downloaded on October 23, 2003.

National Cancer Institute's Surveillance, Epidemiology and End Results (SEER) Program. "Functions of the Skeletal System." Available online. URL: http://www.training.seer.cancer.gov Downloaded on October 23, 2003.

skeletal muscle As 40–45 percent of a person's body weight, skeletal muscle amasses the greatest total of tissue. According to the University of California–San Diego, "Skeletal muscle comprises the largest single organ of the body." The university defined muscle composition as "single cells or fibers embedded in a matrix of collagen. At either end of the muscle belly, this matrix becomes the tendon that connects the muscle to bone." Once this connection has been made, actin and myosin molecules of protein come into play by way of myofilaments "capable of sliding across each other. To produce force, cross-bridges from the myosin filaments associate with the actin filament, then rotate slightly to pull the filaments across each other (much like the oars of a rowboat pull across the water)." Another article, "Fundamental Functional Properties of Skeletal Muscle," discussed the power of that pull by saying, "In its most basic form, the length-tension relationship states that isometric tension generation in skeletal muscle is a function of the magnitude of overlap between actin and myosin filaments." Regarding the relationship between force and velocity, "The force generated by a muscle depends on the total number of cross-bridges attached. Because it takes a finite amount of time for cross-bridges to attach, as filaments slide past one another faster and faster . . . , force decreases due to the lower number of cross-bridges attached. Conversely, as the relative filament velocity decreases . . . , more cross-bridges have time to attach and to generate force, and thus force increases." With this intensity expanding a muscle, "Higher forces produce greater strengthening. Therefore, exercises performed with muscle activated in a way that allows them to contract at high velocities, necessarily imply that they are also contracting with relatively low force."

See also RESISTANCE TRAINING.

University of California, San Diego. "Fundamental Functional Properties of Skeletal Muscle." Available online. URL: http://muscle.ucsd.edu Downloaded on January 24, 2003.

University of California, San Diego. "Muscle Physiology." Available online. URL: http://muscle.ucsd.edu Downloaded on January 24, 2003.

skull With air-filled SINUSES lightening the weight that might otherwise rest heavily on people's minds, the skull houses and protects the brain and most of the sensory organs. Considered to be the most complex structure in the body, the skull consists of the cranial bones, facial bones, ear bones, and all the others located in the bony HEAD. Some could even call it a block head since, from a side position, the skull extends as high as it does wide, making it fit into a square frame or cube. Within that space, the eight bones comprising the back of the skull or cranium take up about two-thirds of the area with the 14 smaller bones of the FACE making up the other one-third. To hold those bones in place, the skull uses stationary suture JOINTS instead of the more typical ones allowing motion. However, the skull joints of infants do have some mobility or ability to shift, not only to enable the head to fit through the birth canal but, later, to accommodate the rapid and remarkable growth of a young child's brain.

sleep Being asleep does not necessarily mean resting in sweet repose. On the contrary, alternating levels of mental and physical activity occur at various stages of a sleep cycle, influencing the capacity of the RESPIRATORY MUSCLES as well as the motor control of the musculoskeletal system. Since about a third of a person's life will be given to sleep, sweet dreams and easy breathing can help to maintain good health. Unfortunately, sleep disorders adversely affect approximately 10 percent of the population, making this somewhat of a public nightmare. Despite that common concern, medical undergraduates in the U.S. typically receive only about 2.5 hours of training on the subject, while med students from the U.K. reportedly cover it in about 10 minutes. A team from Canada, however, hopes to change this by integrating more instruction on sleep into medical curricula.

Toward this end, Stephen R. Thompson, Uwe Ackermann, and Richard L. Horner investigated "Sleep as a Teaching Tool for Integrating Respiratory Physiology and Motor Control." Their general overview began by discussing how sleep can be measured—with an electroencephalogram (EEG) to measure brain activity and an electromyogram to monitor muscle tone. "On the basis of recordings from such electrodes, two major sleep states have been identified as rapid eye-movement (REM) and non-REM sleep." With these instruments used in recent years to dispel the widespread belief in sleep as a passive process, the evidence continued to show "that sleep is composed of distinct states each actively generated by different brain regions, with each of these sleep states having distinct effects on a variety of physiological processes." For example, "REM sleep occupies ~20% of the total sleep time . . . with generalized heightened brain activity and periodic intense eye movements that give this sleep state its name" of rapid eye movement. "REM sleep is also associated with dreaming and periods of widely fluctuating respiratory and cardiovascular activities." Despite these periods of active or paradoxical sleep similar to the readings of wakefulness shown by an EEG, "Responsiveness to external arousing stimuli such as noise, and even internal signals related to physiological stress such as hypoxia, are markedly reduced in REM sleep compared with non-REM sleep." With muscular movement suppressed, except for occasional twitches, "This absence of skeletal muscle tone in REM sleep is due mainly to processes of motor inhibition resulting in what is commonly likened to sleep 'paralysis'." However, "Breathing, heart rate, and blood pressure are at their most stable in stage IV non-REM sleep compared with REM sleep and wakefulness." With these alternating cycles, "Sleep begins with ~80 min. of non-REM sleep followed by a REM period of ~2–10 min. This 90-min. non-REM-to-REM sleep cycle is then repeated about three to six times during the night," assuming, of course, that nothing throws off the cycle. When interruptions occur on a regular basis, "Sleep deprivation quickly leads to impaired physiological function, deteriorating health, and death." Ironically though, when rest continues full cycle, uninterrupted sleep can also have adverse effects. "For example, the changes in brain neural activity that produce generalized muscle relaxation in sleep also affect the muscles of breathing and these effects can lead to common sleep-related breathing problems." This occurs because "of changes in action potential discharge of the motoneurons that innervate the muscle. The membrane potential of a motoneuron changes across states of wakefulness and sleep because of varying degrees of converging excitatory or inhibitory inputs originating from sleep-wake related cells in the brain stem." Understanding these conditions offers insight—as well as more appropriate treatment therapies—for those patients most apt to experience respiratory distress.

Unfortunately, statistics from the American Medical Association indicate that "only about 30% of those with sleep disruption seek medical care for this problem, relying instead of various self-care strategies." Because musculoskeletal pain can be a major factor in ruining a good night's rest, a team of doctors from the University of North Carolina at Chapel Hill reported on "Self-Reported Arthritis-Related Disruptions in Sleep and Daily Life and the Use of Medical, Complementary, and Self-Care Strategies for Arthritis." The team reported, "Notable clinical, research, and policy implications. When considering that arthritis is the most common cause of disability in those age 65 years and older, that sleep disturbance is present in at least half of individuals in this same age group, and that large proportions of affected individuals with each problem pursue multiple avenues of self-care, medical care, and complementary care for relief of the symptoms, the need for intervention in these 2 common, frequently co-existent, and interrelated conditions in aging becomes apparent. Physicians and other health care providers must be educated about the effect of sleep disturbance, which can be exacerbated by, but is sometimes independent of and wrongly attributed to, arthritis pain. Indeed, it must be concluded that in our study, we cannot know if participants' attribution of arthritis as the cause of their sleep disruption was correct. As such, we cannot determine with certainty whether the sleep disruption itself might have been the factor associated with the use of multiple self-care, complementary, and medical modalities. This is clinically important since relief of arthritis pain may be expected to improve true arthritis-related sleep disruption, but therapy of arthritis alone might not be sufficient to improve either pain or sleep disruption if sleep disruption has been incorrectly attributed to arthritis and other independent and unrecognized causes of sleep disruption coexist untreated. Indeed, physicians and health care providers must recognize that therapy of sleep disturbance may sometimes be required for improved pain. That is, the need for relief of sleep problems and other arthritis-related disruptions in daily life may be at least as important as the need for pain relief." With this in mind, simply gathering information about each patient's quality of sleep could help to awaken the medical community to the seriousness of sleep loss and what can be done to correct the problem, not only for arthritis sufferers but for any patient with fatigue syndromes and musculoskeletal concerns. Undoubtedly, a doctor's routine inquiry into a person's sleep patterns could offer more assistance to patients than their counting only on the help of sheep.

Jordan, Joanne M., Shulamit L. Bernard, et al. "Self-Reported Arthritis-Related Disruption in Sleep and Daily Life and the Use of Medical, Complementary, and Self-Care Strategies for Arthritis." *Archives of Family Medicine: The Journal of the American Medical Association* 9, no. 2 (February 2000): 143–149.

Thompson, Stephen R., Uwe Ackerman, et al. "Sleep as a Teaching Tool for Integrating Respiratory Physiology and Motor Control." *Advances in Physiology Education* 25, no. 2 (June 2001): 29–44.

slipped disk See HERNIATED DISK.

SOMI brace An abbreviation for a sterno-occipital-mandibular immobilizer, this serious-looking brace may be used therapeutically to correct a deformity, provide upper-body support, and/or prevent JOINT movement. Not worn as a permanent device but just long enough to allow the area time to heal, a SOMI brace can immobilize a neck after a WHIPLASH or other severe INJURY. To keep the upper spine inactive, however, necessitates coming at that task from several angles. Therefore, a chin piece props the lower jaw, a headband keeps the forehead strapped into place, another piece along the back of the head stabilizes the base of the skull, and a chest strap provides stability as the entire unit holds the head upright, thereby alleviating stress on the neck. With a penchant for pinching, rubbing, and chafing though, the SOMI can irritate the skin of almost anyone. To avoid this, a white cotton T-shirt can be worn as a protective layer between the brace and the body, also offering a means of soaking up perspiration. If redness, scrapes, or bruising occur—

or, more importantly, if the brace causes any numbness, weakness, or intensification of pain—the patient's physician or an orthopedic specialist will be needed to readjust the device and, when the time has come, remove it.

sore muscle In addition to the DELAYED ONSET MUSCLE SORENESS that commonly occurs at the beginning of a new EXERCISE program, tenderness and achy muscles can result from oxidation. To prevent that potentially harmful process, highly lauded antioxidants, such as vitamins A, C, and E, offer optimal strength, especially when found in fresh fruits, vegetables, and overall good NUTRITION rather than in supplements. Besides this sensible preventative, the February 2003 issue of *Men's Fitness* also suggested the medicinal use of culinary herbs. Medical writer Michael Castleman gave this lively report, "A recent study by the U.S. Department of Agriculture found that common culinary herbs and spices pack a considerably healthy punch. Researchers tested the antioxidant activity of more than three dozen culinary and medicinal herbs. Ounce for ounce, many had more power than fruits and vegetables. Three types of oregano—Mexican, Italian and Greek—showed greater antioxidant activity than vitamin E. Other high scorers were bay, dill, coriander, thyme and rosemary." One advantage, of course, would be the heightened flavor herbs can bring, thus increasing an eater's interest in natural food sources. Besides this tasty value, another interesting point Castleman covered involved the traditional use of herbs in preventing food spoilage. "In fact, in the USDA study, the oregano tested had antioxidant strength comparable to BHA, the standard chemical food preservative." With notable exceptions such as salt soaking and sundrying, the natural measures used to keep foods intact could, conceivably, slow oxidation within the body, thereby protecting the integrity of muscle fibers.

Castleman, Michael. "Herbal Antioxidants: Looking for a Way to Fight Cancer, Heart Disease, High Blood Pressure and Muscle Soreness? Try Your Spice Rack." Available online. URL: http://www.findarticles.com Downloaded on May 20, 2003.

spasm See CRAMP.

spasmodic dysphonia This neurological disorder occurs for unknown reasons, causing the vocal cords to seize up sporadically. Variations in the quality of conversation depend on which muscles of the LARYNX have been affected. The patient's speech patterns can seem choppy or the voice strangled, sometimes sounding like a radio transmission that is breaking up. Although emotional or physical stress can often make the symptoms of spasmodic dysphonia become more severe, a soothing influence—such as song, laughter, or the whisper of a shared confidence—can lessen the tightness and the intensity of these muscle spasms.

spasticity If muscles contract continuously, the results can bring rigidity that inhibits a person's speech—as in SPASMODIC DYSPHONIA—or stiffness that affects general patterns of movement. According to the National Institute of Neurological Disorders and Stroke, some causatives include SPINAL CORD INJURY, MULTIPLE SCLEROSIS, cerebral palsy, head trauma, and metabolic diseases, such as AMYOTROPHIC LATERAL SCLEROSIS (Lou Gehrig's disease). Symptoms may involve increased muscle tightness, contractions, deep-tendon reflexes, fixed joints, and scissoring, a movement pattern defined by involuntarily crossing the legs. From mild stiffness to severe pain, "Spasticity can interfere with rehabilitation in patients with certain disorders, and often interferes with daily activities." Treatments may include suitable medication and/or PHYSICAL THERAPY to stretch the affected muscles and increase the range of motion.

According to the National Parkinson Foundation, "Spastic muscle cells are significantly different than normal muscle cells, and that means spasticity may be more difficult to treat than previously believed." With muscle fibers from healthy participants compared with that from children with cerebral palsy, a recent study revealed "that spastic muscle cells develop passive tension at much shorter lengths and their elastic modulus (a measure of material stiffness) is greater than that found in normal muscle cells." Inadequate information in general "about the mechanical, physiological and biochemical features of spastic muscles" can also make the condition complicated to treat.

In some instances, orthopedic surgery may be needed to reduce the spasticity, increase the range of motion, or reduce pain. As health information from the WE MOVE (Worldwide Education and Awareness for Movement Disorders) Web site explained, a contracture release procedure may be performed surgically to cut and reposition a tendon in a more effective angle. A cast or serial casting would be required later to correct and direct the new growth. Another type of procedure, known as a tendon transfer, has also been used to relocate "the attachment point of a spastic muscle," thus keeping the muscle from pulling the adjacent joint into an awkward or unmanageable position. Still other instances may need an OSTEOTOMY to correct a deformity or ARTHRODESIS to fuse and stabilize the bones adversely affected by spastic movement, thus offering the patient some measure of relief.

National Institute of Neurological Disorders and Stroke. "Spasticity Information Page." Available online. URL: http://www.ninds.nih.gov/health Downloaded on May 27, 2003.

Preidt, Robert. "Spasticity Tougher to Treat than Thought." Available online. URL: http://www.parkinson.org Downloaded on January 14, 2003.

WE MOVE. "Orthopedic Surgery for Spasticity," Available online. URL: http://www.wemove.org Downloaded on February 18, 2003.

spina bifida A type of neural tube defect, spina bifida begins in the first few weeks of life as the spine fails to close during the early stages of fetal development. Often, this serious BIRTH DEFECT will be prevented if the mother herself receives well-balanced NUTRITION prior to pregnancy with a particular emphasis on ample sources of B vitamins—primarily folic acid as naturally found in egg yolks, broccoli, and dark green leafy vegetables, such as mustard greens and kale. For some time, packaged food products like cereals and fruit juices have been fortified with folic acid too. Yet, one in 1,000 newborns in the United States alone will be born with spina bifida each year.

Advanced medical technology enables most children with spina bifida to be surgically treated within the first 24 hours after birth to close the spinal opening and lessen the risk of infection. However, subsequent surgeries also remain likely. Besides these concerns, other complications can bring about permanent paralysis, digestive tract problems, and various types of learning disorders. To aid the awareness necessary for providing a child with optimal care, the Spina Bifida Association of America (SBAA) published "Facts About Spina Bifida." This health information said, "Special attention is needed to identify and treat secondary disabilities." However, a "wide range of neurological damage and mobility impairment" make this especially difficult. With examples of secondary conditions ranging from TENDINITIS to various allergies, such as the commonly occurring allergic reaction to latex products, the SBAA maintained, "Day to day activities should be as normal as possible."

For a child with spina bifida, that normalcy may be hard-won due to an ongoing need for crutches, braces, or wheelchairs to increase a child's mobility and foster his or her ability to manage basic toilet needs. Not to be disheartened, however, the SBAA went on to say, "It is important that health care professionals, teachers, and parents understand the child's physical capabilities and limitations. To promote personal growth, they should encourage children (within the limits of safety and health) to be independent, to participate in activities with their non-disabled peers and to assume responsibility for their own care." Despite the obstacles encountered by youth with spina bifida, "Early intervention can help considerably to prepare the children for school."

Spina Bifida Association of America. "Facts about Spina Bifida." Available online. URL: http://www.sbaa.org Downloaded on October 27, 2003.

spinal cord injury Although the spinal cord belongs to the central nervous system rather than the musculoskeletal system, this foot-and-a-half long cord extends from the base of the brain to the back of the waist, traveling through the protective rungs of the irregularly shaped vertebral bones that comprise the spinal column. The cord does not just slip through like a big threaded needle but sends out nerves that "exit and enter at each vertebral level and communicate with specific areas of the body." An American Association of Neurological Surgeons (AANS) fact sheet explained, "Spinal cord injury (SCI) is damage to the nerves within the spinal canal. Most SCI's are caused by trauma to the vertebral column, thereby affecting the spinal cord's ability to send and receive messages from the brain to the body's systems that control sensory, motor and autonomic function below the level of injury." For example, damage to one or more of the seven cervical vertebrae located in the neck "usually causes a loss of independent breathing and loss of function to the arms and legs, thereby resulting in quadriplegia." When the twelve thoracic vertebrae in the frontal portion of the upper body have been damaged, "Injuries usually affect the chest and the legs and result in paraplegia." If damage occurs in the five vertebrae of the lower back or LUMBAR region, "Injury typically results in loss of control of the legs, bladder, bowel and sexual function." Similarly, sacral damage to the "five vertebrae that run from the pelvis to the end of the spinal column" affects "the nerves emanating from the distal spinal cord conus and typically cause lower motor neuron flaccid paralysis type lesions involving some loss of function in the legs and difficulty with bowel, bladder and sexual control." According to statistics from the AANS, "Approximately 450,000 people in the United States have sustained traumatic spinal cord injuries with more than 10,000 new cases of SCI emerging in the U.S. every year." Of these traumas, 82 percent occur in men with "motor vehicle accidents . . . the leading cause of SCI (44 percent), followed by acts of violence (24 percent), falls (22 percent), sports injuries (8 percent), and other causes (2 percent)." First signs characteristically include extreme pain, pressure, and/or a loss of feeling with prompt treatment imperative in any case. As the AANS reported, "Overall, 85 percent of SCI patients who survive the first 24 hours following injury are alive 10 years later." Also, all instances of SCI do not necessarily mean a completely severed spinal cord. Some may be classified as incomplete, which basically means "some residual motor and sensory function remains below the level of SCI."

The National Institute of Neurological Disorders and Stroke issued a news release based on some earlier studies in animals. It showed that "fetal tissue transplants and neurotrophins can improve regrowth of injured neurons in the adult spinal cord, and that some injured neurons can regrow even after long periods of time." A new study led by Barbara S. Bregman, Ph.D., of Georgetown University Medical Center, indicated that "spinal cord regeneration is actually improved when treatment is postponed until most of the initial injury-related changes in the . . . spinal cord and the surrounding environment have stabilized." With these studies involving laboratory rats "given an experimental therapy several weeks after their spinal cords were severed," the new findings demonstrated "that the window of opportunity for treating spinal cord injury may be wider than previously anticipated."

Although RESEARCH and technological advances increase the hopes of persons with PARALYSIS, other SCI patients indicate more interest in PAIN MANAGEMENT and the relief of CHRONIC PAIN. Diana D. Cardenas, M.D., said, "In a recent study at the UW [University of Washington], 82% of patients with SCI reported persistent, bothersome pain at some time after discharge from their initial inpatient rehabilitation. Post-SCI pain can be so severe and disabling that some patients have said they would give up the possibility of neurological recovery in favor of pain relief." With pain generating discomfort and disability, "Musculoskeletal pain can be caused by injury at the time of SCI, injury following SCI, chronic disorders related to overuse, and problems relating to aging." Described as dull or aching, this typically localized pain "often worsens with activity, diminishes with rest, and responds well to non-steroidal anti-inflammatory drugs (NSAIDs, e.g., ibuprofen), ice, and rest."

As another means of addressing these symptoms, "Massage for Spinal-Cord Injury," in *Massage Magazine*, stated, "Massage benefits people with spinal-cord injuries by increasing their range of motion and muscle strength while decreasing anxiety and depression, according to a recent study." When reporting on those studies performed by a team from the Touch Research Institute at the University of Miami School of Medicine, the article said, "The massage-therapy group received two 40-minute massages per week for five weeks. The exercise group was taught an exercise routine that they performed on their own twice a week for five weeks." At the end of the trial period, "The massage group showed a greater increase in muscle strength than the exercise group on the Manual Muscle Test, designed to assess motor function after spinal-cord injury." In addition, "Range-of-motion tests revealed that both groups improved in shoulder abduction, but the massage group showed greater improvement in wrist extension and flexion." Besides these physical benefits, evidence also indicated that, following these massage and exercise therapies, a subsequent increase in strength and also in flexibility of the participants' musculoskeletal systems enabled the SCI patients to experience less anxiety and less depression too.

American Association of Neurological Surgeons (AANS). "Spinal Cord Injury." Available online. URL: http://www.neurosurgery.org Downloaded on September 23, 2003.

Cardenas, Diana D. "Pain and Spinal Cord Injury: Causes and Treatments." Available online. URL: http://depts.washington.edu/rehab Downloaded on February 28, 2003.

National Institute of Neurological Disorders and Stroke. "Delayed Treatment of Spinal Cord Injury May Improve Recovery." Available online. URL: http://www.nih.gov Downloaded on December 1, 2001.

Staff. "Massage for Spinal-Cord Injury." Available online. URL: http://www.massagemag.com Downloaded on February 14, 2003.

spinal fusion As a treatment for vertebral INJURIES, DEGENERATIVE DISK DISEASE, KYPHOSIS, SCOLIOSIS, and other conditions of the spine, this type of SURGERY fuses two or more small bones in the spinal column, usually with a bone GRAFT or the insertion of a metal rod. Statistics from the American Academy of Orthopaedic Surgeons (AAOS) reported, "About 258,000 spinal fusions were performed in 1999." Of these, "About 119,000 procedures involved the upper (cervical) spine, . . . about 139,000 involved the lower (lumbar) spine." In each of these cases, "The surgery eliminates motion between vertebrae segments, which may be desirable when motion is the cause of significant pain. It also stops the progress of a spinal deformity," but flexibility diminishes correspondingly too.

The August 2003 article "Bone Graft Substitutes for Spinal Fusion," published on the Spine-Health Web site, said, "Significant advances in bone graft substitutes have been made in the last couple of years, and the U.S. Food and Drug Administration (FDA) has approved a number of new products, but much of the ongoing research promises to offer even more options for surgeons and patients looking for alternatives to autograft (patient's own bone)." Although an AUTOGRAFT provides a safer source of grafting material that the body will accept more readily than bone from a donor, high costs and complications can still arise.

To address those obstacles to healing, another Spine-Health article, "Electrical Stimulation for Spinal Fusion," said, "The use of electrical stimulation to improve the effectiveness of lumbar spinal fusion has grown significantly over the past decade." With the procedure initially reported over 25 years ago, "Bone growth stimulators are most typically employed for patients who have a lower likelihood of obtaining a solid fusion," for instance, if multilevel fusions will be needed or if a previous fusion has already failed. Just as "all spinal fusions do not physiologically or biomechanically heal in the same manner," neither do "all electrical stimulation devices work in the same manner." For example, "Internal bone stimulators . . . utilize direct current (DC) electrical stimulation and are implanted at the time of the spinal fusion." In contrast, "External bone stimulators are external devices worn outside the skin . . . as a brace type stimulator or are attached to the skin with pads. . . . The newest type of non-invasive stimulation" is capable of delivering "a constant current to the fusion site." In either case, the goal of an internal or an external stimulator remains the same—to promote vertebral healing and enable the spinal fusion to hold.

Yet another option offers an artificial disk in lieu of fusion. Reporting on "Back in the Swing" for *The Union Leader,* staff writer Katharine McQuaid explained, "As they age, discs between vertebrae lose flexibility, elasticity and shock-absorbing qualities." With spinal fusion, a bone GRAFT "eventually fuses to the vertebrae to become one solid piece of bone," but this procedure stiffens that area of the spine and adds additional stress near the fusion site. Therefore, clinical trials have begun on a new artificial unit called the Maverick with the hope of FDA approval forthcoming. When this transpires, the metal disk now produced by MedTronic may surgically replace worn disks while allowing the patient to retain joint flexibility and regain a natural range of motion.

See also JOINT REPLACEMENT.

American Academy of Orthopaedic Surgeons. "Spinal Fusions." Available online. URL: http://www.orthoinfo.aaos.org/fact Downloaded on July 2001.

McQuaid, Katharine. "Back in the Swing." *The Union Leader* (October 4, 2003): A5.

Spine-Health. "Bone Graft Substitutes for Spinal Fusion." Available online. URL: http://spine-health.com Downloaded on September 26, 2003.

Spine-Health. "Electrical Stimulation for Spinal Fusion." Available online. URL: http://spine-health.com Downloaded on September 26, 2003.

spinal loading A likely place to find an example of spinal loading occurs on school grounds where BACKPACK SAFETY concerns parents whose children shoulder enough weight to induce a permanent shrug. Another likely spot for spinal loading occurs around the yards and corridors of warehouses where hefty loads tax the spines of workers whose jobs involve heaving heavy things from here to there.

In writing about the latter, a research team from the Biodynamics Laboratory of the Institute for Ergonomics, Ohio State University, said, "Low back disorders (LBD) continue to represent the most common and most costly musculoskeletal disorder experienced in the workplace." With LBD accounting for about 16–19 percent of all workers' compensation claims, "These tasks often require the worker to be exposed to several known risk factors including lifting, bending, twisting motions, lateral bending motions, maintenance of static postures, carrying heavy loads, and combinations of these." A major culprit comes in transferring and stacking bags and boxes manually, such as may happen while stocking the shelves in groceries and other stores with heavy sales. Although similar tasks have gone on for centuries, the method still has room for improvement. For instance, the simple addition of "the presence of handles on the boxes had a profound effect of reducing mean maximum . . . compression forces" that "most likely resulted from the decrease in external moments, which indicated that the load was able to be held closer to the body." Besides the use of handles to provide a more sensible means of LIFTING, "The position from which the worker lifted a box on a pallet had the most profound effect on spine loading while the lower level of the pallet represented the greatest loadings on the spine."

Another article from the Ohio State University Department of Industrial, Welding, and Systems Engineering concluded, "Wearing a lumbar back support resulted in no significant differences for any measure of spinal loading as compared with the no-back support condition. . . . Thus, the use of the elastic lumbar back support provided no protective effect regarding spinal loading when individuals were allowed to move their feet during a lifting exercise." The article also reported, "The U.S. Occupational Safety and Health Administration (OSHA), however, does not consider back supports to be personal protective equipment (PPE) for the prevention of LBD," Likewise, "The U.S. National Institute for Occupational Safety and Health (NIOSH) concluded that back supports do not prevent injuries to healthy workers and should not be considered PPE."

A team of doctors from the Biodynamics Laboratory in Ohio worked with the Section of Orthopaedic Surgery and Rehabilitation Medicine of the University of Chicago. They reported, the "first EMG-driven biomechanical evaluation of spine loading" or ELECTROMYOGRAPHY-assessed participants with lower back pain (LBP) because

"Recent studies have suggested that excessive mechanical loading on spinal structures that already are compromised can progressively affect disc degeneration, possibly resulting in chronic LBP. Therefore, it is important to understand the mechanisms by which spine loading occurs in patients with LBP to allow identification of situations that might lead to further spine damage." As the team noted, "However, it is well known that patients with LBP have greater levels of guarding, recruit their muscles in a significantly different manner, move slower, and have altered flexion-relaxation responses, as compared with asymptomatic patients. These facts suggest that patients with LBP may use very different muscle activation patterns to generate internal load support, making deterministic models inappropriate for patients with LBP." With spinal loading a greater risk for those experiencing lower back problems, the researchers found, "Spine loading increased with increasing impairments, primarily as a result of increased trunk muscle coactivation. Although patients with LBP kinematically adjusted their postures to minimize external moment exposure, these compensations did not offset the increased loading resulting from coactivation (guarding) and from the large body mass typical of patients with LBP." Therefore, "The study suggests that most patients with LBP would benefit greatly from reduction in body weight, kinematic conditioning, and efforts to design materials-handling tasks so that lift origins are close to the body and at reasonable lift heights."

The Biodynamics Laboratory of the Institute for Ergonomics, Ohio State University. "Effects of Box Features on Spine Loading During Warehouse Order Selecting." *ERGONOMICS* 42, no. 7 (1999): 980–996.

Department of Industrial, Welding, and Systems Engineering, Ohio State University. "Effect of Foot Movement and an Elastic Lumbar Back Support on Spinal Loading During Free-Dynamic Symmetric and Asymmetric Lifting Exertions." *ERGONOMICS* 43, no. 5 (2000): 653–668.

Marras, W. S., K. P. Granata, et al. "Spine Loading Characteristics of Patients with Low Back Pain Compared with Asymptomatic Individuals." *SPINE* 26, no. 23 (November 23, 2001): 2,566–2,574.

spinal manipulation To manipulate something means to handle it, with or without any hint of exploitation. Nevertheless, that connotation can taint the word, perhaps making an osteopathic or chiropractic spinal adjustment more readily called into question. Indeed, a high-velocity adjustment (HVLA) can create problems, as addressed by Dr. Christopher Kent, president of the Council on Chiropractic Practice. As Dr. Kent explained, "The primary purpose of spinal radiography in chiropractic practice is the analysis of vertebral subluxations," where a shifting of bones occurs without being a fully DISLOCATED JOINT. In category 1, for example, "These patients have no unusual findings that make traditional adjusting techniques hazardous. They have good bone integrity, and thrust (HVLA) adjustments may be safely applied." In category 2, "Patients . . . have weakened or softened bone, or developmental issues that may require the chiropractor to alter the adjusting technique. Adjusting procedures for such persons must be carefully selected." Furthermore, "High velocity adjustments to osteopenic bones should be avoided." Although gentle "judiciously applied" adjustments may be used for this group, Category 3 "persons have unusual findings where the application of high velocity forces to the involved area may be problematic." Therefore, "The chiropractor is encouraged to think in terms of assessing the safety and appropriateness of specific chiropractic techniques in a given case," as, of course, any medical practitioner would do in determining a diagnosis and developing an appropriate course of treatment.

To address spinal manipulation from an objective but traditional medical view, the Mayo Foundation for Medical Education and Research published the 2003 article "Chiropractic Treatment: How Spinal Manipulation Can Reduce Back Pain." Since a 1997 survey had previously shown that 190 million people in the U.S. seek CHIROPRACTIC help each year, Mayo defined such visits as being "based on the philosophy that restricted movement in the spine may lead to reduced function and pain. Spinal adjustment (manipulation) is one form of therapy chiropractors use to treat restricted spinal mobility." With goals "to restore spinal movement, thus improving function and decreasing pain," the article further explained, "Chiropractors manipulate the spine from different positions using varying degrees of force." However, "Manipulation doesn't need to be forceful to be effective. Chiropractors may also use massage and stretching to relax muscles that are shortened or in spasm." In addition, some chiropractors have been trained in the use of an ACTIVATOR to assist in an even gentler form of spinal adjustment. Rather than assuming a person's qualifications though, the Mayo article wisely advised, "Because manipulation has risks, always use properly trained and licensed practitioners."

Although the same should be said about one's choice of doctors or others in the medical field, some remain unconvinced that any amount of training will solve the issue of the therapeutic value of a spinal adjustment. As an exercise in caution, for example, Professor Edzard Ernst in the U.K. addressed "Spinal Manipulation: Its Safety is Uncertain" in a commentary published in the *Canadian Medical Association Journal.* To define general aims or principles, the writer said, "Spinal manipulation entails a range of manual manoeuvres that stretch, mobilize or manipulate the spine, paravertebral tissues and other joints in order to relieve spinal pain and improve locomotor function. Spinal manipulation is practiced by chiropractors, osteopaths, physicians, and physiotherapists, mostly to treat musculoskeletal problems such as back and neck pain." Having noted the large numbers who seek such treatments each year, "7% of people in the United States . . . and as many as 33% in the United Kingdom," the writer concluded, "The safety of spinal manipulation, therefore, is an issue that requires regular and rigorous assessment." Furthermore, "It seems debatable whether the benefits of spinal manipulation outweigh its risks." Since this same debate has continued for decades, many apparently share the professor's concern while others heatedly voice uncompromising opinions that may or may not have a statistical base. Patients in pain may also hold ambivalent views yet want to compare the options before deciding which type of treatment would be most effective and involve the fewest risks.

To put the concept of manipulation into a reasonably balanced perspective, a person might ask whether a need exists to restore a dislodged shoulder or other dislocated joint manually. Similarly, a spinal adjustment attempts to realign vertebrae that have somehow gotten out of place. Although both treatments have their time and place, neither instance will work equally well every time on every person. For example, that dislocated shoulder may eventually require surgery to relocate the joint and hold it in alignment, whereas spinal manipulation gone awry could give a wry neck. More serious problems can also arise if a manipulation involves a highly vulnerable area, such as the cervical vertebrae, especially if cholesterol deposits, a blood clot, or another existing medical condition already impedes the NECK veins. Likewise, a bony protrusion or a projection of some kind pressing against the spinal cord—or evidence of DEGENERATIVE DISK DISEASE—could greatly increase the risk of an adjustment, causing a STROKE or other life-threatening condition. In such circumstances, a patient would do well to consult with an appropriate specialist, such as a neurologist, cardiologist, rheumatologist, or orthopedic surgeon, before proceeding with spinal manipulation. Yet, despite these disclaimers and the abounding controversies, the large numbers of people seeking an adjustment by a chiropractor or an osteopath suggest that most have been helped and/or have nowhere else to turn for improvement of a chronic musculoskeletal condition.

Because spinal manipulation can provide relief of pain as well as realignment of the vertebrae, unbiased studies would be of special value in presenting comparatives, factual data, and recommendations of the optimal conditions for seeking an adjustment. While working toward this effort, the federal Agency for Health Care Policy and Research reported, "Chiropractic care, the most commonly used alternative therapy for back problems, is as effective as medical care alone for reducing disability and pain in patients with low back pain. Adding physical therapy to medical care may be marginally more effective than medical care alone for reducing disability." Before arriving at these conclusions, researchers assigned 681 patients with low back pain "to four treatment groups: medical care with and without physical therapy and chiropractic care with and without physical modalities (heat or cold therapy, ultrasound, and electrical muscle stimulation or EMS). Medical care included proper back care instructions; strengthening and flexibility exercises; prescriptions for pain medicine, muscle relaxants, and anti-inflammatory agents; and recommendations about bed rest, weight loss, and physical activities. Chiropractic care included spinal manipulation or another spinal-adjusting technique and instruction in proper back care. Physical therapy could consist of heat or cold therapy, ultrasound, EMS, soft-tissue and joint mobilization, traction, supervised therapeutic exercise, and strengthening and flexibility exercises." At the end of treatments going from late 1995 through late 1998, "All groups had more than a 3-point reduction (on a 0 to 24 point scale) in disability by 6 months. Patients in the medical and chiropractic care-only groups had similar mean changes in low back pain intensity and disability during each follow-up evaluation."

Since osteopathy can also include spinal adjustments, a group of doctors from the Departments of Orthopedic Surgery and Preventative Medicine at Rush-Presbyterian-St. Luke's Medical Center, Chicago, and the Chicago College of Osteopathic Medicine reported, "Patients in both groups improved during the 12 weeks," with "no statistically significant difference between the two groups in any of the primary outcome measures." However, "The osteopathic treatment group required significantly less medication (analgesics, anti-inflammatory agents, and muscle relaxants)." Therefore, the team of medical researchers concluded, "Osteopathic manual care and standard medical care have similar clinical results in patients with subacute low back pain. However, the use of medication is greater with standard care." For patients with allergies, or even sensitivities to pharmaceuticals, this distinction could make a big difference in determining a personal course of treatment.

Andersson, Gunnar B. J., Tracy Lucente, et al. "A Comparison of Osteopathic Spinal Manipulation with Standard Care for Patients with Low Back Pain." *New England Journal of Medicine* 341, no. 19 (November 4, 1999): 1,426–1,431.

Agency for Health Care Policy and Research. "Chiropractic and Medical Care for Low Back Pain are Comparable in their Effectiveness Over 6 Months of Follow-up." Available online. URL: http://www.ahcpr.gov/news

Ernst, Edzard. "Spinal Manipulation: Its Safety Is Uncertain," *Canadian Medical Association Journal, JAMC* 166, no. 1 (January 8, 2002): 40–41.

Kent, Christopher. "A Systematic Approach to the Evaluation of Plain Spinal Radiographs." Available online. URL: http://www.worldchiropracticalliance.org Downloaded on February 13, 2003.

Mayo Foundation for Medical Education and Research. "Chiropractic Treatment: How Spinal Manipulation Can Reduce Back Pain." Available online. URL: http://www.mayoclinic.com Downloaded on February 21, 2003.

Staff. "Focus Column." *Journal of the American Chiropractic Association.* Available online. URL: http://www.acatoday.com/pdf/focus_May 2002.pdf Downloaded on July 1, 2004.

spinal muscular atrophy This genetic group of neuromuscular diseases progressively disrupts motor neurons controlling voluntary muscle movement yet does not affect involuntary muscles nor the person's hearing and vision. Children diagnosed with spinal muscular atrophy (SMA) often have very high intelligence even though "SMA causes lower motor neurons in the base of the brain and the spinal cord to disintegrate, preventing them from delivering electrical and chemical signals that muscles depend on for normal function." To clarify the characteristics of the three types of SMA, the Muscular Dystrophy Association further explained, "All of the spinal muscular atrophies are caused by one or more gene defects." Although humans have an estimated 100,000 genes, "When genes are defective, they are unable to properly produce proteins that are necessary for a cell to function." Therefore, "A destructive chain of events can be triggered when a protein is absent, when there is too little or too much of it, or if it doesn't work properly for any reason. In the case of spinal muscular atrophy, protein abnormalities prevent the normal functioning of motor neurons, leading to their deterioration and muscle degeneration." Regardless of whether the patient has Type I, II, or III SMA, "All forms affect the skeletal muscles of the trunk and limbs. In general, those muscles closer to the center of the body are more affected than those farther away." In addition, "Respiratory muscles are involved to varying degrees in all forms of the disease."

To define the three types of SMA further, the National Institute of Neurological Disorders and Strokes published the "NINDS Spinal Muscular Atrophy Information Page." Symptoms of Type I can become evident before birth as indicated by "a reduction in fetal movement in the final months of pregnancy." At birth or within the first few months, "Symptoms include floppiness of the limbs and trunk, feeble movements of the arms and legs, swallowing and feeding difficulties, and impaired breathing." In this severest form of SMA, "Affected children never sit or stand and usually die before the age of 2." In Type II SMA, symptoms become apparent between three and 15 months and present "respiratory problems, floppy limbs, decreased or absent deep tendon reflexes, and twitching of arm, leg, or tongue muscles. These children may learn to sit but will never be able to stand or walk. Life expectancy varies." In Type III, the symptoms "appear between 2 and 17 years of age, and include abnormal manner of walking; difficulty running, climbing steps, or rising from a chair; and slight tremor of the fingers." For SMA affecting older adults, the condition may be similar to AMYOTROPHIC LATERAL SCLEROSIS (Lou Gehrig's disease). Symptoms present "progressive limb weakness and weakening of the muscles, difficulty speaking and swallowing, and respiratory problems." For all forms of SMA, supportive care and therapies include "treating pneumonia, curvature of the spine, and respiratory infections, if present. Also, physical therapy, orthotic supports, and rehabilitation are useful. Genetic counseling is imperative."

Because this genetic disorder runs in families, a sibling or first cousin might be another one of the children in every 6,000 births who develops SMA, especially since one of every 40 people is a carrier. To offer information and helpful advice, the Families of Spinal Muscular Atrophy (FSMA) published the booklet *Understanding Spinal Muscular Atrophy: A Comprehensive Guide.* A primary concern, for instance, involves a prompt and accurate diagnosis. "As recently as the fall of 1995, probes that detect deletions in Types I, II, and III SMA were reported. One of these probes is for a gene called Survival Motor Neuron (SMN) and detects the absence of gene sequences in approximately 90–94 percent of SMA patients and is not absent in normal individuals. This information makes this SMN gene test very useful for the diagnosis of SMA." Additionally, a blood test can show indicative levels of creatine phosphokinase, while an electromyograph (EMG) can measure the electrical activity of muscles in the arms or thighs. To determine the severity of the disease, a muscle biopsy may also be suggested. Since this involves an anesthetic and a surgical incision, the FSMA strongly encourages parents to inquire about the less invasive needle biopsy and to ask questions in general.

The organization itself offers some answers regarding what families might expect. For example, the cognitive and emotional development of an infant can be aided by stimulation with balloons and feathers, an advantage being, "Reaching games are a form of physical therapy that can be very helpful." Also, water therapy or other types of professionally determined treatments can offer opportunities for therapeutic exercise. Especially important will be a respiratory therapist's instructions concerning chest physiotherapy to keep the lungs clear. If aspiration of food occurs, parents will need to discuss a choice of gastric tubes with their child's primary care physician while a ventilator may be needed to assist breathing. Seating aids and a body jacket may help too since SMA children usually have some degree of scoliosis that can restrict respiration. Similarly, a standing frame or other walking aid "allows for better respiratory function, greater bowel function, and encourages greater mobility." When possible, "The use of a light weight manual wheelchair can be an exciting addition" that provides SMA children with "mobility, independence and a taste of adventure, while still allowing them to use some of their own strength." However, "for true independence and mobility, a power wheelchair is necessary."

Families of Spinal Muscular Atrophy. "Understanding Spinal Muscular Atrophy." Available online. URL: http://www.fsma.org Downloaded on February 11, 2004.

Muscular Dystrophy Association. "Facts About Spinal Muscular Atrophy." Available online. URL: http://www.mdausa.org/publications Downloaded on February 17, 2003.

National Institute of Neurological Disorders and Strokes (NINDS). "NINDS Spinal Muscular Atrophy Information Page." Available online. URL: http://ninds.nih.gov/health Downloaded on May 27, 2003.

spinal stenosis Marked by a narrowing of the vertebral canal that runs through the backbone, this condition can put a squeeze on the spinal cord and related nerves. Sometimes this happens because of a DEGENERATIVE DISK DISEASE or a bone condition, such as ARTHRITIS, OSTEOARTHRITIS, or PAGET'S DISEASE. At other times, the problem arrives with a tendency inherited at birth. In between, a spinal trauma, bone overgrowth, or less likely, a tumor can constrict the inner spaces of the spine, causing pain, pressure, weakness, or numbness in the affected limbs. If constriction occurs high in the upper neck or cervical vertebrae, the hands may tingle or the arms feel weak. If in the LUMBAR region, the lower back may ache, feet may get clumsy, and leg muscles may cramp or go numb. If left untreated too long, stenosis can cause permanent damage to spinal nerves and various degrees of limited motion or even disability. With proper management, however, its progression can be effectively slowed.

Because other conditions, such as SCIATICA, present related symptoms, a precise diagnosis may require some detective work. In May 2002 the *Journal of The American Chiropractic Association* reported, "Clues should appear in the patient's history. Conditions that might be confused with stenosis, like herniated discs, usually have a rapid and unmistakable onset." Characteristically, "Someone with a herniated disc, then, feels pain at different times and from different types of activity than someone with stenosis." For example, the pain from a herniated disk typically decreases as a patient walks or stands. "Vascular disease may also cause pain, numbness, and weakness in the lower extremities," resulting in leg CRAMPS and LIMPING (claudication), so the likelihood of that condition needs to be eliminated too. "Here again, tracking pain patterns and differentiating clinical findings offer clues." To make this distinction, "Activities like riding a bike and walking up a hill can cause pain in patients with vascular claudication, while they don't tend to cause pain in the stenotic patient. On the other hand, standing makes pain worse for stenotic patients, while it relieves vascular claudication." When musculoskeletal discomfort occurs in the lumbar region, "Spinal stenosis patients generally respond well to soft-tissue management of the low back and any of the classic physical therapies of ultrasound and muscle stimulation to relieve secondary muscle spasms."

The September/October 2003 issue of *Arthritis Self-Management* reported that as many as 400,000 people in the U.S. have been affected by lumbar stenosis. "Since the pain of spinal stenosis typically gets better when people stop walking and sit down, it can easily turn formerly active people into couch potatoes. Yet this painful condition is also treatable. You don't have to take it sitting down." Once other conditions have been ruled out through a physical exam, medical history, and an analysis of the patient's range of motion, X-rays may be used to assess the level of severity. For more detailed imaging, "An MRI [magnetic resonance imaging] is particularly good for detecting damage to the soft tissues, including the disks and ligaments. It also can show the spinal cord, nerve roots, and surrounding spaces." If need be, "A CT [computed tomography] scan can show the spinal canal's size and shape, as well as its contents and the structures around it."

Once a diagnosis of spinal stenosis has been confirmed, most medical specialists, such as the American Academy of Orthopaedic Surgeons (AAOS), suggest conservative treatments. The AAOS recommended patients first try "changes in posture. People with spinal stenosis may find that flexing the spine by leaning forward while walking relieves their symptoms. Lying with the knees drawn up to the chest also can offer some relief." This often helps because "these positions enlarge the space available to the nerves and may make it easier for stenosis sufferers to walk longer distances." Since pressure on the spinal nerves can be caused by swelling, "Nonsteroidal anti-inflammatory medication such as aspirin or ibuprofen may help relieve symptoms." In addition, "Rest, followed by a gradual resumption of activity, also can help. Aerobic activity such as bicycling is often recommended." If the bathroom scale shows that excessive WEIGHT contributes to SPINAL LOADING, a weight reduction program would be advised. However, "When stenosis causes severe nerve root compression, these treatments may not be enough."

To discuss the alternatives, doctors Andrew L. Chen and Jeffrey M. Spivak stated, "In a study of non-operative treatment, most patients who had mild-to-moderate lumbar spinal stenosis remained unchanged after 4 years of follow-up, and no proof of severe deterioration was found. This challenges the notion that early operative intervention is necessary to prevent progression of stenosis and the development of profound neurologic deficits." After using a multifaceted approach, the writers recommended, "The mainstays of non-operative management include anti-inflammatory drugs (NSAIDs), physical therapy with activity modification, bracing, and epidural corticosteroid injection." Rare occasions may require urgent surgery, but in general, "Operative treatment should be considered only when non-operative treatment has failed to improve function or provide adequate pain relief to allow daily activities." At such times, "The main goal in the operative treatment of lumbar spinal stenosis is to decompress the affected neural elements through their entire course from the central canal to their exit. . . . The secondary goal of surgery is to maintain spinal stability or to restore stability in cases of preoperative degenerative instability." Whether stenosis occurs in the lower back or in the upper neck region, a LAMINECTOMY, SPINAL FUSION, or other surgical procedure may be required to bring relief and the resumption of activities.

American Academy of Orthopaedic Surgeons. "Spinal Stenosis." Available online. URL: http://orthoinfo.aaos.org Downloaded on March 6, 2003.

Andrews, Linda Wasmer. "Spinal Stenosis." *Arthritis Self-Management* (September/October 2003): 7–10.

Chen, Andrew L. and Jeffrey M. Spivak. "Degenerative Lumbar Spinal Stenosis: Options for Aging Backs." Available online. URL: http://www.physsportsmed.com Downloaded on September 13, 2003.

spinal tap See LUMBAR PUNCTURE.

spine In a remarkable feat of engineering, the bones of a well-balanced back present a succession of three arcs, bowing at 60 degrees each: in the inward S CURVE of the NECK, the outward SHOULDER curve of the upper back, and the inward curve of the lower back or LUMBAR region. As principles of geometry and physics have proven, these arcs provide the strongest cushioning system for movement and strongest protection against ongoing forces of GRAVITY. Despite the triple triumph of these arcs as seen from the side, when viewed from the back, the well-built backbone gives the appearance of holding a straight—albeit dotted—line. With vertebral bones extending from the base of the SKULL to the PELVIC REGION, a normal spine permits flexible, upright POSTURE without rigidity. Indeed a spine's adaptable RANGE OF MOTION allows forward and backward bending, side-to-side rotation, and the uplifting movement of a stretch. Of course, bones alone can not do this.

An overview, "Spine Anatomy—Muscles and Ligaments," from the New York City–based Hospital for Joint Diseases Spine Center, explained, "In order for the spine to control movement and assume responsibility for balance under the many stresses of physical activity, spinal muscles attach themselves to many different vertebrae and their parts, as well as to the arms and legs, the head, the rib cage, and the pelvis." Furthermore, "Because many spinal muscles overlap in different planes, the spine is well equipped to provide stability during all types and degrees of movement, but there is also ample opportunity for painful events or spasm when any muscle fibers become fatigued or overstretched."

Not surprisingly, those three spinal arcs just mentioned provide three areas for painful encounters, especially since the cervical spine holds up the head, the thoracic vertebrae bear the upper back, and the lumbar vertebrae carry most of the weight and tension of the body. In addition, five bones fuse as one in the SACRUM, with stress also placed on the COCCYX or tailbone during sitting. Should any of these bones be thrown out of alignment, the facets or bony projections of the vertebrae can press on soft tissue and nerves, thus generating numerous sources of pain or numbness.

To describe "Disorders of the Musculoskeletal System" that affect the aching backs of some 20 million Americans, Columbia University College of Physicians and Surgeons provided a "Complete Home Medical Guide." According to information downloaded October 31, 2003, "There are several variations of abnormality that warp the normal shape of the spine. An abnormal kyphosis causes rounded shoulders and a caved-in appearance around the chest. This postural strain on muscles and ligaments often leads to backache. When the normal forward curve of the lumbar spine is exaggerated, a condition termed hyperlordosis, a huge strain builds on the vertebrae and the small joints between them. Lordosis, or swayback, forces the abdomen and buttocks to jut out, weakens muscle tone, and ultimately produces back pain." Aside from BIRTH DEFECTS or inherited tendencies toward SCOLIOSIS, "Years of slouching eventually produce a variety of problems, ranging from back pain to more complicated disorders such as osteoarthritis or disk problems." In addition to postural problems and other causatives of DEGENERATIVE DISK DISEASE, "Traumatic back injuries include any back damage resulting from direct blows to the back, banging into objects, or falling." Such instances can cause a bone FRACTURE or a HERNIATED DISK. When poor NUTRITION causes spine problems, fragile or porous bones usually indicate OSTEOPOROSIS resulting from insufficient calcium. Similarly, lack of bone-strengthening minerals and vitamins, such as citric acid, can produce RICKETS. Other rare conditions affecting the spine include BONE CANCER and BONE INFECTION or OSTEOMYELITIS, while many arthritic conditions, such as ANKYLOSING SPONDYLITIS, can cause rigidity or other types of damage to the spine. As numerous sources attest, however, strong back muscles can prevent a load of problems, including spinal fractures, with RESISTANCE TRAINING and other EXERCISES helping a healthy spine bend, stretch, and reach for the heights of a flexible, mobile life.

Columbia University College of Physicians and Surgeons. "Disorders of the Musculoskeletal System." Available online. URL: http://cpmcnet.columbia.edu Downloaded on October 31, 2003.

Hospital for Joint Disease Spine Center. "Spine Anatomy—Muscles and Ligaments." Available online. URL: http://www.msnyuhealth.org Downloaded on July 8, 2003.

splint From clavicle splints that shoulder the responsibility of good posture to hand-holding devices that cushion the forearm and keep the wrist in a neutral position all the way to the elbow, splints protect and support. Whether made of leather, metal, plastic, or plaster, these various types of ORTHOTICS immobilize one or more joints. According to *Rehab: The Interdisciplinary Journal of Rehabilitation,* "During the rehabilitation process, the use of a splint may change. It may go from being a protective or supportive device to being one that enhances motion or function." How? "Pattern designs are modified or adjusted to suit the particular needs of the patient." For instance, "During the inflammatory and early fibroblastic stages of healing, splints can immobilize the injured area to allow healing, and be removed for basic hygiene and wound care, which can be a major advantage over a cast. Splints are also used to immobilize the limb in the treatment of infections and after trauma or surgery." In addition, "Splints can also be used to protect paralyzed or non-innervated muscle to allow rest and avoid overstretch. This helps maintain a normal muscle length so that when the nerve re-innervates the muscle, it will be better able to function."

Astifidis, Romina P. "Getting the Upper Hand." Available online. URL: http://www.rehabpub.com Downloaded on June 16, 2003.

spondyl- or spondylo- In combination with other forms, this prefix refers to the vertebrae or SPINE. For example, the spondylarthropathies comprise a group of rheumatic diseases that attack the spinal column, such as REITER'S SYNDROME and some types of ARTHRITIS. Spondylitis indicates an inflammation in the vertebral joints, such as occurs in ANKYLOSING SPONDYLITIS. With spondylosis, the spinal column becomes stiff with pain, decreasing the person's mobility.

spongy bone See TRABECULAR BONE.

sports injury See INJURY.

sports medicine This relatively new field of medicine enlists an expert team. Even though physicians need to be up-to-date on diagnostic tools and treatments for STRAINS, SPRAINS, FRACTURES, and other sports-related INJURIES, well-trained therapists may use their knowledge to provide BIOFEEDBACK, electrical stimulation, ULTRASONOGRAPHY, and SPINAL MANIPULATION. Specialties involving BIOMECHANICS, ACUPRESSURE, REPETITIVE MOTION DISORDERS, REHABILITATION, and other considerations for ATHLETES also come into play.

sprain A STRAIN is a pain but worse. A sprain hurts, swells, often looks bruised, and can feel like a broken bone. To contrast the two, the Mayo Foundation for Medical Education and Research explained, "A strain is a stretching or tearing of muscle," whereas, "A sprain is a stretching or tearing of ligaments." Since tough fibrous bands of LIGAMENTS connect one bone to another "to stabilize joints, preventing excessive movement," sprains commonly occur in active areas of the body, such as an ANKLE or KNEE, primarily during "rapid changes in direction or by a collision."

In another article, the Mayo Foundation discussed treatments. "Generally, the greater the pain, the more severe the injury. Expect the sprain to peak in the first 48 hours, then improve daily. For most minor sprains, you can probably treat the injury yourself." Suggestions for self-treatment include PRICE—the RICE METHOD plus a P to "Protect the injured limb from further injury by not using the joint. You can do this using anything from splints to crutches." FIRST AID measures, however, will not be enough if "you hear a popping sound when your joint is injured or you can't use the joint." In such cases, "On the way to the doctor, apply a cold pack." Professional medical assistance will also be needed in the presence of fever or other signs of infection, such as redness or heat in the area. A severe sprain will require medical attention too, especially since "inadequate or delayed treatment may cause long-term joint instability or chronic pain." If a weight-bearing limb, such as an ankle, has been affected, mobility could become unbearable.

In 2002, with cautions about taking nonsteroidal anti-inflammatory drugs immediately after an injury due to the risk of bleeding, Dr. Edward Laskowski explained, "Some sprains involve tissue disruption higher up on the ankle or bone fractures, and these need to be treated in a specific way." Otherwise, even when a sprain has healed and the pain has dissipated, the ankle may be weakened. As active PHYSICAL THERAPY begins, "One exercise is to see how many minutes you can stand on the affected leg." After recommending STANDING exercises to strengthen the ankle and increase overall balance, the doctor explained, "We always like to say that the best brace you can give yourself is your muscle brace. If you develop muscle strength through specific exercises, that's the best protection you can give your ankle."

With ankle sprains the most common injury among sports enthusiasts, "The re-injury rate after lateral ankle sprain has been reported to be as high as 80% among athletes," according to the *Journal of Athletic Training.* According to the authors, Craig R. Denegar and Sayers J. Miller III, on staff at Pennsylvania State University, chronic ankle instability (CAI) occurs because, "Altered joint mechanics during the tissue-repair phase of the healing process may force tissues to heal in elongated positions (producing laxity), expose tissues to excessive forces, create altered afferent feedback to the neuromuscular control system, or result in chronic losses of motion." After reviewing typical strategies aimed to get an athlete quickly back into play, the writers concluded, "We believe that effective management of the acutely injured ankle requires greater protection from stress to healing tissues than is allowed with rapid return to weight bearing, walking, and functional exercises." Nevertheless, "The greatest challenge presented by CAI may not be in treatment but in prevention. To expect therapeutic exercises, external supports, or surgical reconstruction to fully restore the structural and functional integrity of the ankle joints is not reasonable." Although the best ways to keep recurrent sprains from happening cannot be fully answered, these medical writers suggested a sensible approach based on "an understanding of inflammation and lower extremity biomechanics. Through this knowledge, a treatment program that manages the symptoms of inflammation, restores normal joint motion, and gradually applies stress to healing tissues can be offered as a viable alternative to current practices."

Denegar, Craig R., and Sayers J. Miller III. "Can Chronic Ankle Pain Instability Be Prevented? Rethinking Management of Lateral Ankle Sprains." *Journal of Athletic Training* 37, no. 4 (2002): 432.

Mayo Foundation for Medical Education and Research. "Ankle Sprain Rehabilitation: An Interview with a Mayo Clinic Specialist." Available online. URL: http://www.mayoclinic.com Downloaded on September 10, 2002.

Mayo Foundation for Medical Education and Research. "Sprain: First Aid." Available online. URL: http://www.mayoclinic.com Downloaded on January 9, 2002.

Mayo Foundation for Medical Education and Research. "Sprains and Strains." Available online. URL: http://www.mayoclinic.com Downloaded on March 1, 2002.

standing Just standing around can sometimes be more stressful on the joints—and the nerves—than taking an active walk or jogging. Most people want to be able to stand on their own two feet, but standing on one and then the other can offer an interesting exercise in balance. Not only does this strengthen each leg, but balancing on one at a time can show if an existing weakness has gone undetected. If any instability does occur though, the shakiness may not point to the musculoskeletal system but to a circulatory malfunction.

For instance, the Mayo Foundation for Medical Education and Research explained, "The effects of gravity normally cause your blood pressure to drop slightly when you stand up. . . . Blood naturally wants to pool in your leg veins when you change positions from lying or sitting to standing. Your autonomic nervous system typically makes up for this effect by narrowing your blood vessels and increasing your heart rate. This helps blood return to the heart more effectively to maintain blood pressure." If a body fails to make this corrective response, the resulting difficulty in standing may be due to medications, severe dehydration, a dysfunction of the CARDIAC MUSCLE, or other conditions affecting circulation, such as DIABETES. With the curatives depending on the causatives, the person might reassess his or her intake of water and medicines and also discuss the use of support hose or stockings with a cardiologist or primary care physician.

Although most people give little thought to their ability to get themselves into an upright position, patients of all ages with debilitating medical conditions remain keenly aware of the long-standing effect on their daily routines. The August/September 2002 issue of *Rehab: The Interdisciplinary Journal of Rehabilitation* reported, "As rehab professionals, we understand that standing provides an alternative option for positioning and pressure relief for those who use wheelchairs. We realize the positive psychological benefits, particularly in self-esteem, for our clients who use standers." Although health care and government-assisted funding for standing devices may not be currently available, three choices of devices are available: supine, prone, and upright. Reportedly, "Supine standers support the back surface of the body and require the least amount of trunk and head control. Lateral supports are often needed to support the body symmetrically. They can be placed in various degrees of angle from fully horizontal to vertical, and often have trays for upper extremity support or activities." In addition, "Prone standers support the front of the body, while the user is supported in various angles. Lateral supports are combined with pads and straps for positioning the trunk, buttocks, and knees." As a third option, depending on the patient's requirements, "Upright standers are used primarily in the vertical position by individuals who have fair to good trunk and head control. Many rehab professionals believe this is the best way for their non-ambulatory clients to weight bear."

Preventative measures to support and maintain the health of the musculoskeletal system may help to avoid a need for any standing device. With that hope in mind, the American Academy of Physical Medicine and Rehabilitation (AAPMR) took another stance on standing in their online article "Household Chores to Build Functional Fitness." Under the heading "Laundry Toss," for example, the AAPMR said, "It's all in the spin—of your hips—and it will turn the mundane task of laundry into exercise for your abdominal, low back and hip muscles." To test this, "Stand about 10 to 15 feet away from the washing machine . . . with the dirty laundry basket at about waist height on your left side and the washing machine on your right. Pick up pieces of the dirty, dry laundry and, while turning at the hips, pitch the laundry into the open washer." To unload and lift without tossing baskets, "Daily dishes are a great opportunity to stretch side and back muscles. As you take dishes out of the dishwasher, turn your body from side to side, allowing your hips to turn so that your torso twists while you reach to put the clean dishes away on high and low shelves." Whether indoors or out, a "Rake and Twist" movement "works whether you're raking leaves or sweeping the floor. The key is to take long, steady strokes, turning at your hips and raking or sweeping toward your body." By using one side and then the other—from left to right and back—this alternating exercise avoids making the arms do all the work. For a "Standing Side Stretch" exercise, AAPMR suggested taking a common item, such as a carton of milk or a briefcase, and, "Hold a weighted object in either hand while standing up straight with your feet slightly more than a shoulder's width apart, then slowly bend at the waist straight to the side, lowering the hand with the weight down your side as far as it will go. Hold it there and count to 15 or 20 and slowly return to standing up straight," which is, after all, the point.

American Academy of Physical Medicine and Rehabilitation. "Household Chores to Build Functional Fitness." Available online. URL: http://www.aapmr.org Downloaded on November 1, 2003.

Koch, Kay Ellen. "Taking a Stand." Available online. URL: http://www.rehabpub.com Downloaded on April 16, 2003.

Mayo Foundation for Medical Education and Research. "Severe Drop in Blood Pressure on Standing." Available online. URL: http://www.mayoclinic.com Downloaded on May 15, 2003.

statins These cholesterol-reducing drugs may do more than lower fatty deposits in the blood and lessen the likelihood of seismic events affecting CARDIAC MUSCLE. According to medical editor Simeon Margolis, M.D., "Intriguing new research suggests that statins may benefit patients with osteoporosis, Alzheimer's disease, diabetes, or age-related macular degeneration." On the downside, Dr. Margolis reminded readers of the rare but serious side effects statins can have on the liver as toxicity occurs in about 1 percent of patients. Another concern is that, "muscle aches are the most common side effect of statins. About 1 in 1,000 patients develops a muscle condition called myositis; in a very small percentage of these people, this problem progresses to a more dangerous condition called rhabdomyolysis." However, "Stopping statin therapy reverses myositis and prevents rhabdomyolysis." With about 12 million Americans now taking these drugs each day, the numbers will undoubtedly increase as additional criteria from the medical community and new governmental guidelines become available. "Last year," for instance, "the 6,000 people with diabetes in the Heart Protection Study benefited from statin therapy even when their initial LDL [low-density lipoprotein] cholesterol level was below 100 mg/dL." For those patients who have experienced no noticeable benefit, Dr. Margolis said, "The biggest reason for failing is that people are often appropriately started on the lowest statin dose, but the dosage is not increased if their cholesterol doesn't decline enough. Sometimes this happens because the patient doesn't return for monitoring."

Regarding follow-ups, the National Cholesterol Education Program sponsored by the National Heart, Lung, and Blood Institute of the National Institutes of Health said results should be seen in four to six weeks. "After about 6 to 8 weeks, your doctor can do the first check of your LDL-cholesterol while on the medication. A second measurement of your LDL-cholesterol level will have to be averaged with the first for your doctor to decide whether your dose of medicine should be changed to help you meet your goal."

Margolis, Simeon, M.D. "Statins: Celebrating Proven Benefits." *The Johns Hopkins Medical Letter, Health After 50* (November 2003): 6.

National Heart, Lung, and Blood Institute. "Statins." Available online. URL: http://nhlbisupport.com Downloaded on November 1, 2003.

stem cells These cells within everybody's body offer exciting possibilities in medical RESEARCH, especially pluripotent stem cells, such as those found in umbilical cords and placentas, which have the potential of developing into almost any cell that is needed. Although adaptable types of adult stem cells naturally occur in bone marrow and some organs, these multifunctional pluripotent cells have typically come from aborted or miscarried fetuses. With research focusing on this highly versatile yet controversial source, the debates heightened, pressuring the president to establish some guidelines.

On August 9, 2001, President George W. Bush announced standards later outlined by the Department of Health and Human Services of the National Institutes of Health (NIH) in "Information on Eligibility Criteria for Federal Funding of Research on Human Embryonic Stem Cells." The criteria stated, "The stem cells must have been derived from an embryo that was created for reproductive purposes; The embryo was no longer needed for these purposes; Informed consent must have been obtained for the donation of the embryo; No financial inducements were provided for donation of the embryo." In addition to these safeguards, the NIH created a Human Embryonic Stem Cell Registry to keep apprised of the groups devoted to stem cell research, from a company in Athens, Georgia, to university and medical centers in Korea, Sweden, India, and Israel.

In September 2002, the NIH also published *Stem Cells: A Primer,* which explained, "Stem cells have two important characteristics that distinguish them from other types of cells. First, they are unspecialized cells that renew themselves for long periods through cell division. The second is that under certain physiologic or experimental conditions, they can be induced to become cells with special functions such as the beating cells of the heart muscle or the insulin-producing cells of the pancreas." With every fetus in a state of growth, "Stem cells in developing tissues give rise to the multiple specialized cell types that make up the heart, lungs, skin, and other tissues." However, "In some adult tissues, such as bone marrow, muscle, and brain, discrete populations of adult stem cells generate replacements for cells that are lost through normal wear and tear, injury, or disease." Although "adult stem cells typically generate the cell types of the tissue in which they reside," recent experiments "have raised the possibility that stem cells from one tissue may be able to give rise to cell types of a completely different tissue, a phenomenon known as plasticity." Such diverse application may be particularly significant since "today, donated organs and tissues are often used to replace ailing or destroyed tissue, but the need for transplantable tissues and organs far outweighs the available supply. Stem cells, directed to differentiate into specific cell types, offer the possibility of a renewable source of replacement cells and tissues to treat diseases including Parkinson's and Alzheimer's diseases, spinal cord injury, stroke, burns, heart disease, diabetes, osteoarthritis, and rheumatoid arthritis."

Indeed, recent developments give hope to patients with SPINAL CORD INJURY, BIRTH DEFECTS, and muscular concerns, including incontinence. In 2003, *The Taipei Times* reported on the findings of a group of doctors from the Taipei Veterans General Hospital. To explain the premise of this research, the reporter said, "Muscles can become loose and unable to properly regulate bodily functions." However, "Muscle stem cells can bring about contractile activity that can counteract the damage." Although this particular research focused on mice, 80–90 percent of the subjects showed improvement with stem cell treatment.

Other encouraging news of research involving human participants came from HealthDay in 2003. According to the article, a medical team from the University of Frankfurt in Germany discovered that "infusing a patient's own stem cells into a heart artery several days after a heart attack improves the heart's pumping power and speeds the healing process." Since this study of 28 participants only lasted four months, a larger trial has been planned. Meanwhile, "Some patients in the trial got adult stem cells derived from bone marrow, while others got heart-derived cells. Both were equally effective."

Department of Health and Human Services. "Information on Eligibility Criteria for Federal Funding of Research on Human Embryonic Stem Cells." Available online. URL: http://stemcells.nih.gov Downloaded on October 27, 2003.

Department of Health and Human Services. "Stem Cells: A Primer." Available online. URL: http://stemcells.nih.gov Downloaded on November 3, 2003.

Edelson, Ed. "Stem Cell Therapy Helps Heal Damaged Heart." Available online. URL: http://www.healthday.com Downloaded on October 13, 2003.

sterno-occipital-mandibular immobilizer See SOMI BRACE.

sternum The anatomically correct name for the breastbone, this part of the axial skeleton resides in the upper midsection at the front of the chest. Although some say this long, flat bone looks like a dagger or, perhaps, a wide letter opener to the heart, the sternum actually consists of three bones that may or may not fuse into one. Regardless, ARTICULATION occurs on either side with frontal RIBS and the CLAVICLE or collarbone.

Because of its central location over the CARDIAC MUSCLE, various surgical procedures, such as a coronary bypass, may not bypass the breastbone. Although technological advancements no longer require a lengthy incision of the sternum to get to the heart, other surgeries may occur for different reasons. For example, Johns Hopkins University reported on "The Nuss Procedure," which surgically creates "a suspension bridge for the chest." Used to correct "a congenital defect that results in a sunken chest," the Nuss procedure inserts a metal band under the skin, stretching it "across the chest under the sternum," where it is "attached to a rib on either side of the chest cavity. The bar moves sternum and ribs outward and helps take the squeeze off of the heart and lungs." After remaining in place for about two years, the metal band assists the chest in gaining a more normal appearance, which reportedly continues after the bar's removal.

See also TURNER'S SYNDROME.

Johns Hopkins University. "The Nuss Procedure." Available online. URL: http://www.hopkinsmedicine.org Downloaded on November 1, 2003.

steroid See ERGOGENICS.

strain Overstretching a muscle can cause the ACUTE PAIN of a strain. Chronic strain, though, classically results from overuse, such as happens in a REPETITIVE MOTION DISORDER. Taking sensible breaks during physical activity can prevent problems, yet ACCIDENTS still damage the musculoskeletal system as tissue abnormally twists into strained positions.

To compare the often confused, "Sprains and Strains," the American Academy of Orthopaedic Surgeons (AAOS) noted the signs of a SPRAIN as "pain, bruising, and inflammation." AAOS defined the symptoms of a strain by saying, "Typical indications include pain, muscle spasm, muscle weakness, swelling, inflammation and cramping." With strains on the back or on the hamstring muscle mentioned as the most common occurrences, treatments generally consist of the RICE METHOD followed by a conditioning program, stretching EXERCISES, well-balanced NUTRITION, and properly fitted FOOTWEAR. Similar advice came from KidsHealth in "Strains and Sprains Are a Pain." Besides adding that "after 24 hours, it's okay to use warm compresses or a heating pad to soothe aching muscles," the article assured readers that most strains take only a week or so to heal.

American Academy of Orthopaedic Surgeons. "Sprains and Strains." Available online. URL: http://orthoinfo.aaos.org Downloaded on October 31, 2003.

strength training To cut the losses of muscle power that normally occur with aging, this form of RESISTANCE TRAINING can help those with various conditions of the musculoskeletal system as well as children in their growing years. In the September

2003 issue of *The Physician and Sportsmedicine,* doctors Holly J. Benjamin and Kimberly M. Glow of Chicago stated, "Improved muscle coordination gained from strength training can increase athletic performance and help prevent some on-field injuries in sports." Besides suggesting that one adult supervise each group of 10 or fewer children, the authors said, "In a well-run program, exercises begin with simple movements, such as leg extensions, that work one joint at a time. More complex movements that require muscle coordination, such as squats, are learned before speed and power movements like jumping and throwing. Usually, a variety of single- and multiple-joint exercises are done at each session." With the emphasis on correct form and technique rather than competition, the doctors also advised a hazard-free training area, sensible clothing, and realistic goals such as expecting gains in strength while remembering that a child's "muscle size will not increase until after puberty."

In the March 2000 *Saturday Evening Post,* author Carol Krucoff reported, "Numerous studies demonstrate that resistance exercises can help frail elderly people in their 80s and 90s improve their strength to the point where many regain the ability to walk and perform other tasks without assistance." Because the limitations of decreased ACTIVITY often take a person out of his or her own home and put the person into a health care facility, the effects of AGING should not be taken lightly nor lying down. Although it may require "three to four months of doing resistance exercises two or three times a week before muscles are strong enough to start doing moderate aerobic activity," a regular program of strength training can curb muscle and BONE LOSS and lessen the FALLS and IMMOBILIZATION brought on by a weakened musculoskeletal system.

As emphasized in the July 2001 *Current Comment* from the American College of Sports Medicine (ACSM), "Osteoporosis typically begins with an unnoticed decrease in bone mass that leads to structural deterioration of bone tissue and an increased susceptibility to fractures of the hip, spine and wrist." Also in that article, Brendan D. Humphries, Ph.D., stated, "Ultimately, the changes in hormones accompany the changes in bone and muscle strength as well as the other way around." In other words, strength training not only affects muscles and bones directly but also indirectly through its effects on body chemistry which, in turn, affect muscles and bones. "In contrast, physical inactivity has been shown as a contributing factor to the loss of bone, muscle mass and other health risks." Having begun with the approval of a person's primary care physician, "Two important concerns for strength training are intensity and recovery." Then, "A minimum of two sessions a week for 45–60 minutes beginning at 70 percent of the one repetition maximum (1RM) and building to 85 percent 1RM would be appropriate." Regular follow-ups are also suggested to assess a program's effectiveness in recovering and building strength.

Benjamin, Holly J. and Kimberly M. Glow. "Choosing a Strength Training Program for Kids." Available online. URL: http://www.physsportsmed.com Downloaded on September 17, 2003.

Humphries, Brendan D. "Strength Training for Bone, Muscle and Hormones." Available online. URL: http://www.acsm.org/pdf/bonesmscl.pdf Downloaded on November 3, 2003.

Krucoff, Carol. "Strengthening the Elderly." Available online. URL: http://www.findarticles.com Downloaded on February 28, 2003.

stress One of the biggest differences between poetry and prose is not rhyme but stress. With far more stresses—i.e., those accents or emphases heard in reading—a line of verse resounds with a rhythmic beat, thus lifting the writing to a poetic plane. Likewise, conflict creates story as characters care about and resolve issues, perpetuating the plot toward a satisfying end. Real life, however, occasionally plods like poor prose—with stresses overwhelming a person or twisting a musculoskeletal system into episodes offering poor material for reading—on an X-ray or anywhere else.

The winter 2003 issue of *Healthy Living* compared good stress with bad by saying, "Stress can be good for you. But over time, it's mostly bad for your health. It can raise your energy level and help you deal with challenges. But, the wear and tear of stress takes its toll on your heart and blood vessels." With muscles and bones also counting the toll, symptoms include NECK and SHOULDER pain, HEADACHE, BACKACHE, loss of SLEEP, and JAW clenching. However, "The best way to find out what causes stress is to pay attention to what you are feeling—and when you feel it. For example, if you have head, neck and shoulder aches a lot, think about what you've been doing an hour or so before these symptoms start."

Similarly, the National Institutes of Health recommended BIOFEEDBACK and relaxation techniques in a May 2001 release. According to this report, "The study provides the first evidence that chronic tension-type headaches respond to brief behavioral therapy to the same degree as antidepressant medication alone."

One advantage of the modifying behavior, however, is that people may be more open to problem-solving techniques than pharmaceutical intervention. For example, an article in the January 2002 issue of *Successful Farming* reported on managing behavior. With complex family issues, such as dealing with worrisome finances, adapting to the changing roles of gender, and gracefully coping with the ongoing advice of owners-parents, therapists like Ted Matthews of Minnesota have received appointments by the states in which they live to offer aid to farmers. Sometimes this assistance involves multifamily farm corporations and co-ops where "they want to expand, but can't get six personalities . . . to stop fighting." However, with a low-key, nonthreatening approach based on mental health principles rather than mental illness, Matthews said, "We've taken away the stigma with therapy." Therefore, stressed-out patients no longer feel something must be wrong with them if they seek help.

With stresses for all people needing a closer and, often, courageous look, the Mayo Foundation for Medical Education and Research (MFMER) briefly defined it this way, "Stress is a physical response to an undesirable situation." The key, of course, can be identifying and defining what is undesirable. Although the particulars vary from person to person, the MFMER distinguished between short-term and long-term stress by saying, "Acute stress is a reaction to an immediate threat—either real or perceived," whereas, "Chronic stress involves situation that aren't short-lived, such as relationship problems, workplace pressures, and financial or health worries."

Unfortunately, stress can complicate the latter. A report from the National Library of Medicine and the National Institutes of Health said a recent study from New Zealand indicated "that stress affects the portion of the immune system that is involved in setting up the healing process and growing new tissue." This report said, of the 47 participants in the study, "People who were most stressed out before surgery experienced greater pain, poorer recovery and longer recovery time."

Although SURGERY itself can be a distressing event, chronic tension eventually prompts biological changes in body chemistry, complicating matters more. Sometimes though, a single triggering event sets up a succession of physical and emotional reactions. For example, war conflicts have been a primary source of individual and public stress for centuries, but the phenomenon received serious attention only after the Vietnam War. As part of the resultant effort to research and inform, the National Center for Post-Traumatic Stress Disorder, Department of Veterans Affairs offered a fact sheet that stated, "Posttraumatic Stress Disorder, or PTSD, is a psychiatric disorder that can occur following the experience or witnessing of life-threatening events such as military combat, natural disasters, terrorist incidents, serious accidents, or violent personal assault." In many instances then, PTSD does not necessarily cause musculoskeletal problems but frequently begins with them.

With various sources of physical and emotional violence swirling through the news—and people's lives—perhaps the most foundational, groundbreaking treatments reside in intentionally upbuilding the opposite. For example, "It can be helpful to stay connected to natural support systems, whether they are friends, coworkers, family, neighbors, other familiar groups, personal beliefs, or community." That advice from the International Society for Traumatic Stress Studies went on to say, "Taking care of basic needs is important after trauma. This includes trying to get enough sleep, eating well, exercising, drinking enough water and juice, and avoiding alcohol and caffeine." Furthermore, simple matters, such as "keeping to routines and activities if possible, and finding ways to assist someone else, can be helpful for many. And it is particularly important to know you can ask for help." Although, "no single treatment is effective for everyone, and it may take time to find the right treatment," numerous therapies—alone or combined—can help to lighten stress. "For some, medication can be effective. Also, anxiety management, cognitive therapy (focusing on thoughts and beliefs), and exposure therapy (helping the person confront painful memories and situations that are realistically safe although still frightening, through talking about or imaging them) are helpful for reducing PTSD and related reactions. A combination of psychotherapy and medication is often helpful for depression and anxiety following traumatic experiences." With assistance from a family physician, a spiritual adviser, and others who care, stressful events can be turned into a cause for prayer, a healthy incentive to initiate a needed change, the intriguing plot for true story, or the rhythmic stress and rests of a life lived poetically.

Freese, Betsy. "Getting Help with Stress." Available online. URL: http://www.findarticles.com/p/articles/mi_m1204/is_/_/00/ai_82512758 Downloaded on July 21, 2004.

International Society for Traumatic Stress Studies. "What Is Traumatic Stress?" Available online. URL: http://www.istss.org/terrorism Downloaded on November 3, 2003.

Mayo Foundation for Medical Education and Research. "Managing Workplace Stress: Plan Your Approach." Available online. URL: http://www.mayoclinic.com Downloaded on May 16, 2003.

MEDLINEplus. "Stress Slows Wound Healing After Surgery." Available online. URL: http://www.nlm.nih.gov/medlineplus Downloaded on October 31, 2003.

National Center for Post-Traumatic Stress Disorder. "What Is Post-Traumatic Stress Disorder?" Available online. URL: http://www.ncptsd.org Downloaded on May 14, 2003.

National Institute of Neurological Diseases and Strokes. "Drugs and Stress Management Together Best Manage Chronic Tension Headache: Clinical Trial Proves Benefit of Combined Therapies." Available online. URL: http://www.nind.nih.gov/news Downloaded on July 1, 2001.

VHP Community Care. "Dealing with Stress." Available online. URL: http://www.vhptn.com/PDF/Member_Newsletter.htm Downloaded on February 13, 2003.

stress fracture See FRACTURES.

stretching To learn the fine art of stretching, study almost any cat. When aroused from a sedentary position, the back excessively arches—first in one direction, then in another—up and down. The digits of the foot pads flare and widen. The eyelids squeeze together tightly. The mouth yawns a jaw-stretching circle. While at full body length, the limbs extend, expanding the compressed spaces between each vertebra. Although the bravado of nine lives may be open to debate, a cat, nevertheless, displays the importance of flexibility in scatting away from an injury.

How does one state of grace affect another? According to Rice University, "If done properly, stretching increases flexibility, and this directly translates into reduced risk of injury. The reason is that a muscle/tendon group with a greater range of motion, passively, will be less likely to experience tears when used actively. Stretching is also thought to improve recovery and may enhance athletic performance. The latter has not been fully agreed upon in the medical literature, but improved biomechanical efficiency has been suggested as an explanation. Additionally, increased flexibility of the neck, shoulders and upper back may improve respiratory function."

The Mayo Foundation for Medical Education and Research apparently concurs. The benefits of stretching include improved circulation and posture, which assist the RESPIRATORY MUSCLES. In addition, stretching relieves STRESS, enabling a person to breathe easier. With the flexibility that comes from a regularly good stretch, "Daily tasks, such as lifting packages, bending to tie your shoe or hurrying to catch a bus, become easier and less tiring." Also, "Maintaining the full range of motion through your joints keeps you in better balance. Especially as you get older, coordination and balance will help keep you mobile and less prone to injury from falls." Another Mayo article said,

"Stretching your muscles helps you maximize the range of motion of your joints. This allows you to fully contract your muscles. Stretching can also prevent little tears in a muscle or tendon that occur when you force a joint to go through its full range of motion when the tissues are too tight. For example, trying to run uphill with tight calf muscles puts excessive stretch on the Achilles tendon and may injure it," surely something no cool cat would do.

Mayo Foundation for Medical Education and Research. "Stretching: A Key Component of Your Exercise Program." Available online. URL: http://www.mayoclinic.com Downloaded on March 21, 2003.

Rice University. "Introduction to Stretching." Available online. URL: http://www.rice.edu/~jenky/sports/stretching.html Downloaded on November 4, 2003.

stroke Medically known as a cerebrovascular accident (CVA), this condition results from a restriction to the normal flow of oxygen to the brain so that, in one swift stroke, death can occur. More often, however, a patient experiences sudden loss of movement in an arm, a leg, or both limbs, with paralysis or weakened muscles affecting one side of the body, typically the opposite side from which the brain experienced the injury. Speech and mental capacity may also be affected, depending on the level of severity. In any case, medical treatment should be sought immediately since prompt professional care and medication significantly contribute to the patient's ultimate degree of recovery. Those chances are greatly increased when help has been obtained in the first hour or two after the stroke.

With the quality of life on the line for 700,000 people in the United States each year, about two-thirds survive a stroke but require rehabilitation. The National Institute of Neurological Disorders and Stroke also addressed the precipitating factors, saying, "About 80 percent of strokes are caused by the blockage of an artery in the neck or brain; the remainder are caused by a burst blood vessel in the brain that causes bleeding into or around the brain." Although symptoms depend on which area of the brain has been damaged, "Generally, stroke can cause five types of disabilities: paralysis or problems controlling movement; sensory disturbances including pain; problems using or understanding language; problems with thinking and memory; and emotional disturbances." As soon as the patient's condition has stabilized, rehabilitative therapy starts, often within 24 to 48 hours. "The first steps involve promoting independent movement." For example, "Patients are prompted to change positions frequently while lying in bed and to engage in passive or active range-of-motion exercises to strengthen their stroke-impaired limbs." With passive movements aided by OCCUPATIONAL THERAPY or PHYSICAL THERAPY, active participation begins as "patients progress from sitting up and transferring between the bed and a chair to standing, bearing their own weight, and walking, with or without assistance." If language has been affected, as often happens, the medical team will include a speech pathologist as well as a nursing staff that specializes in rehabilitation.

Once a CVA patient has been released from the hospital or nursing facility, home devices can further assist daily activities. For example, propping an arm can relieve pain and shoulder pull while a cane or walker can assist mobility. Velcro-fastened shoes and easy-on clothing make dressing less of a chore. For SAFETY, grab bars on the tub and in a hallway can help to prevent the FALLS that often result from a weakened musculoskeletal system. Recent studies also show, "Stroke survivors who received therapist-supervised, progressive therapy after completing in-hospital rehabilitation, significantly improved their endurance, balance and walking ability." With that information, a medical team reported on "Extended, Progressive Physical Therapy Aids Stroke Survivors' Mobility" in *Stroke: Journal of the American Heart Association.* The team said, "A home-based exercise program that's much more aggressive than what is typically prescribed" helps to assure that "stroke survivors can improve their walking ability, balance, and cardiovascular endurance." With strokes being "the leading cause of disability in older American[s]," continued therapy can assist greater recovery of a patient's musculoskeletal function, helping to regain at least some measure of independence.

subluxation Unlike a DISLOCATED JOINT, subluxation involves the partial, rather than the complete, shifting of bones at the point of ARTICULATION. This may be so subtle that the patient remains unaware that the affected JOINT or SPINE has lost alignment. In other instances, however, pain may be so intense that a FRACTURE, SPRAIN, or STRAIN seems to be the problem. As an example of this possibility, Richard Merritt discussed "Insights into Rare but Devastating Football Hip Injury," stating, "In the first such review of its kind, Duke University Medical Center researchers have analyzed their experiences in treating eight football players with a rare but potentially devastating hip injury." Although, "In a complete dislocation, the 'ball' at the top of the femur which rotates within the hip joint pops completely out" of the socket, "in subluxation, the ball moves in and out of the joint without tearing the capsule surrounding the joint." According to this study, "The researchers said that prompt diagnosis and proper treatment of hip subluxation—which in many cases is dismissed simply as a hip 'sprain' or 'strain'—is important because it appears that up to 25 percent of such injuries may lead to bone death within the hip joint." Detecting this can be a challenge since "standard x-ray exams do not reveal the tell-tale joint fracture characteristic of subluxation; only an obliquely angled x-ray can detect it." The research team also found that MAGNETIC RESONANCE IMAGING can be helpful in obtaining a diagnosis and also in detecting early signs of bone death or NECROSIS. However, with proper treatment and adequate rest of the injured area, most players return to the field.

See also SPINAL MANIPULATION.

American Heart Association. "Extended, Progressive Physical Therapy Aids Stroke Survivors' Mobility." Available online. URL: http://www.americanheart.org Downloaded on September 24, 2003.

Merritt, Richard. "Insights into Rare but Devastating Football Hip Injury." Available online. URL: http://dukemednews.org Downloaded on July 2, 2003.

National Institute of Neurological Disorders and Stroke. "Post-Stroke Rehabilitation Fact Sheet." Available online. URL: http://www.ninds.nih.gov Downloaded on April 21, 2003.

supination The opposite of pronation, this movement of a JOINT can turn up the palms of the hand or the soles of the feet or put the whole body onto its back. As a foot problem in which the arch tilts up, thus wearing down the outer edges of a shoe, supination can often be adjusted through corrective FOOTWEAR or an ORTHOTIC device.

surgery With approaches ranging from conservative to radical, this branch of medicine includes numerous types of procedures to repair INJURIES, remove diseased or damaged tissue, and correct musculoskeletal deformities. The surgeon's skill relies on a focused eye and a well-trained hand in using the most appropriate tool, from a sterilized scalpel to high-tech equipment that can separate parts and zap away tumors or tissue in the flash of a laser light. Although every surgical specialty requires additional medical schooling in the field, potential patients may want to inquire about the number of operations and the success ratio of a surgeon's experiences in the area of surgery that is been recommended.

On the conservative side, SPINAL MANIPULATION and other therapies—from EXERCISE to medication to well-balanced NUTRITION—can often help a patient to avoid or, at least, postpone surgery involving the musculoskeletal system. However, both an osteopath and a chiropractor will certainly make a surgical referral as needed. To discuss the coalition between the latter two fields as well as what best serves the patient, the *Journal of the American Chiropractic Association* said, "Having a cooperative relationship with a neurosurgeon can help the doctor of chiropractic [DC] better determine when a patient can no longer benefit from conservative management and should be referred for surgery. DCs are likely to find that the neurosurgeons in their area share their concern with first using conservative approaches before attempting surgery." To know when that need has arrived, "Three of the key indicators for referral from conservative chiropractic management to surgery include: Persistent, progressive, and/or intractable pain; Progressive neurological deficit to include muscular weakness; Signs and/or symptoms of spinal cord compromises."

Although those concerns primarily consider the SPINE OR SPINAL CORD INJURIES, other surgeries relating to the musculoskeletal system may be as small as a little toe. Fact sheets from the American College of Foot and Ankle Surgeons (ACFAS) addressed the decision-making process by saying, "When the deformity is painful or permanent, surgical correction is recommended to relieve pain, correct the problem, and provide a stable, functional toe." Another option then considers which type of surgery would be the most appropriate. For example, "Tenoplasty and/or capsulotomy refer, respectively, to the release or lengthening of tightened tendons and ligaments that have caused the joints to contract," while "tendon transfer . . . involves the repositioning of a tendon to straighten the toe." In "bone arthroplasty procedures, some bone and cartilage is removed to correct the deformity," whereas other types of ARTHROPLASTY may realign the joint, fuse the joint, or insert an implant. Although the ACFAS fact sheets refer to foot and ankle problems, "Surgery to reconstruct the joint may be needed if arthritis causes chronic problems that cannot be controlled by medications, orthotics or physical therapy, especially if pain is constant," with limited motion restricting normal activities. Then, "In the vast majority of cases, reconstructive surgery can bring improvement." Besides pain relief, "Other benefits may include an improved ability to move the joint, or an improved appearance." Indeed, the "goals of surgery are different for each individual."

With pain again being a major source of motivation toward the choice for surgery, a special report by Brian J. Cole, M.D., and Sudeep Taksali stated, "Patients with severe symptomatic osteoarthritis of the knee who have pain that has failed to respond to medical therapy and have progressive limitations in activities of daily living should be referred for surgical consideration." To outline options that considered the KNEE, the article continued, "Arthroscopy is primarily indicated as a first-line procedure in patients who report an acute or subacute onset in pain. Mechanical symptoms caused by unstable articular cartilage flap tears, meniscal tears or loose bodies are common indications to proceed." As yet another surgical option, "Osteotomy is principally indicated for unicompartmental arthritis and corresponding malalignment or for symptomatic post-traumatic malunions about the knee associated with pain in knee arthritis." In addition, "Unicompartmental knee replacement is primarily indicated for patients who have arthritis of a single compartment, an intact anterior cruciate ligament, and no limb malalignment," but "total knee replacement is indicated in patients who are not candidates for arthroscopy or osteotomy." Other surgical options include marrow-stimulation techniques and restorative techniques, such as implantation and GRAFTING.

With a slightly different focus, pain became the determining factor not for surgery but after it, compelling a team of Canadian doctors to conduct research. After stating the objective, "To examine age-related differences in pain, catastrophizing, and affective distress (depression and anxiety) after athletic injury and knee surgery," the doctors observed that "pain and catastrophizing were greater in adolescents at 24 hours postsurgery. Further, catastrophizing may have mediating effects on the observed pain-score differences between the adolescent and adult samples because controlling for catastrophizing eliminated the group difference for pain." As the doctors anticipated, "Issues of adjustment and pain after sport injury are salient for adolescents because of incomplete development in both the physical and emotional realms and the fact that pain is the most pervasive and debilitating obstacle to effective rehabilitation of sport-related injury." Therefore, with emotions affecting the rapidity and ease of recovery, the growing bodies and minds of youth athletes can be especially vulnerable when an injury requires surgery.

Sometimes there is no question about the need for surgery. "Unfortunately, there are many conditions or diseases that range from trauma to congenital defects that necessitate surgery of the foot and/or ankle." Although the same could be said about other limbs or parts of the musculoskeletal system, this statement came from the American Podiatric Medical Association. As the fact sheet on rearfoot surgery continued, "Reconstructive surgery in many of these cases may require any of the following: tendon repair/transfer, fusion of bone, joint implantation, bone grafting, skin or soft tissue repair, tumor excision, amputation and/or the osteotomy of bone (cutting of bones in a precise fashion). Bone screws, pins, wires, staples, and other fixation devices (both internal and external), and casts may be utilized to stabilize and repair bone in reconstructive procedures."

With numerous bones, surgical options, and methods to consider, typical surgeries involving the musculoskeletal system include arthroplasty, arthrodesis, discectomy, and osteotomy, each of which has a specific purpose and procedure. For example, external fixation may be used to hold a FRACTURE together to assure the proper healing of a broken bone with the aid of a device, such as a pin or plate. For an infected or herniated disk, a LAMINECTOMY may be used to remove the damaged area and relieve compression. If KNEE SURGERY or another type of JOINT REPLACEMENT has failed, fusion may be needed. Depending on the circumstances and location, an implant may also be required with the materials, size, and shape designed for a particular instance. In these and other cases, the surgical approach or process can change as quickly as RESEARCH findings and innovative technology will allow. The February 2003 issue of *Medical Devices & Surgical Technology Week* stated, "This system is intended to promote fusion of the cervical spine and occipito-cervico-thoracic junction affected by degenerative conditions, deformity, trauma, and tumors."

Regarding the latter, BONE CANCER can sometimes present cause for the most radical surgical options. Nevertheless, a 2003 article on bone cancer surgery stated, "Treatment for bone cancer is increasingly successful; even for the more aggressive cancers, survival rates are improving considerably." With a successful outcome often depending on the stage of the cancer and the location of the tumor, "Commonly, treatment for bone cancer involves surgery to remove some or all of the affected limb, as well as some of the surrounding tissue (such as muscle) to ensure that all of the cancer is removed. Surgery is often accompanied by chemotherapy (the use of drugs that kill cancer cells) and radiation (treatment involving high doses of X-rays or other sources of radioactivity) to help shrink the tumor and prevent its spread (metastasis)." Surgical techniques may include removal of bone, insertion of plates or pins, bone grafting, or joint replacement. With arthroplasty used as "limb sparing surgery," the diseased portion of bone may be removed prior to inserting an artificial joint or PROSTHESIS. In young patients, a "growing or expandable joint replacement enables doctors to fit children's growing bones with artificial limbs that can be adjusted as a child grows so that the artificial limb will match the healthy counterpart."

Once surgery of any type has been performed, the recuperative time will depend on the extent of the procedure and the occurrence of complications, such as excessive bleeding, infection, or rejection of the materials used. Although a cast, SPLINT, or other ORTHOTIC may be needed in surgeries affecting the musculoskeletal system, PHYSICAL THERAPY and/or occupational therapy also begin right away. As an example of what to expect from an occupational therapist's assistance, the American Occupational Therapy Association published a tip sheet that explained, "Occupational therapists can help by teaching new ways to move safely during recovery and by providing ingenious equipment for activities such as bathing, cooking, and dressing." For instance, an occupational therapist will provide tools to ease daily tasks and will also instruct the patient in finding a proper seating position, using a walker, and positioning the body while getting in and out of bed. This not only aids a person in regaining mobility and independence as soon as possible but also in maintaining a healthy mental outlook and in fostering physical healing.

A team of doctors from The Center for Sports Medicine and Orthopaedics' Foundation for Research, in Chattanooga, Tennessee, found that although "previous reports have documented a correlation between degree of spirituality and chance of successful recovery from various illnesses or surgical procedures," this study broke new ground in studying "the effects of spirituality on the recovery from spinal surgery." However, the doctors found they "were unable to correlate a patient's level of spirituality with outcome of spinal surgery." Interestingly, the medical team concluded, "A key difference is that in spinal surgery there is often a specific mechanical problem that is responsible for the patient's disorder." Therefore,

"If this mechanical problem is appropriately identified and corrected, the patient's condition should improve. As a result, there is less influence on outside factors as compared with patients in previous studies who were affected by more systemic disorders without a single identifiable and treatable cause." Previously, most studies of the correlation between healing and spirituality focused on patients with debilitating and/or complex conditions marked by unknown factors and unanswerable questions, so that "it is likely that the improvement of these patients is much more dependent on a positive outlook and a strong desire to recover than is found in patients undergoing spinal surgery." Nevertheless, the researchers concluded, "A positive attitude and strong spirituality can provide the patient with the necessary emotional stability and determination to fight to recover from many illnesses. These beliefs should be supported and encouraged by physicians, since they can only be beneficial to a patient's recovery."

American College of Foot and Ankle Surgeons. "Digital Disorders and Treatments." Available online. URL: http://www.acfas.org Downloaded on February 15, 2003.

American Occupational Therapy Association, Inc. "Daily Activities After Hip Replacement Surgery." Available online. URL: http://aota.org Downloaded on February 25, 2003.

American Podiatric Medical Association. "Your Podiatric Physician Talks About Rearfoot Surgery." Available online. URL: http://www.apma.org/topics/rsurgery_printable.htm.

Coady, Catherine, Dean A. Tripp, et al. "Comparing Postoperative Pain Experiences of the Adolescent and Adult Athlete After Anterior Cruciate Ligament Surgery." *Journal of Athletic Training* 38, no. 2 (2003): 154–157.

Cole, Brian J., M.D., and Sudeep Taksali. "Operative Treatment Options for Osteoarthritis of the Knee and Cartilage Defects." Available online. URL: http://www.physsportsmed.com Downloaded on February 28, 2003.

Hodges, Scott D., Craig Humphrey, et al. "Effect of Spirituality on Successful Recovery from Spinal Surgery." *Southern Medical Journal* 95, no. 12 (December 2002): 1,381–1,384.

ISL Consulting Co. "Bone Cancer Surgery." Available online. URL: http://health.yahoo.com Downloaded on November 6, 2003.

Journal of the American Chiropractic Association "Focus." Available online. URL: http://www.amerchiro.org/publications/jaca/back_issues.shtml Downloaded on July 21, 2004.

NewsRX. "FDA Clears its New Altius Spinal Implant System." Available online. URL: http://www.NewsRX.com Downloaded on February 16, 2003.

suture joint Unlike the ARTICULATION of JOINTS that have a specific RANGE OF MOTION to define their movements, these stationary joints occur as various sections of bones come together, forming the SKULL.

swaybacked or swayback Medically known as lordosis, this fairly common malformation of the SPINE results from an excessive curvature of the lower back or LUMBAR region with a corresponding tilt often occurring in the PELVIC REGION too. Depending on the severity, treatments may consist of ORTHOTICS, SPINAL MANIPULATION, rehabilitative EXERCISE, or other therapies. In some instances, a BACKACHE may be relieved by MASSAGE THERAPY.

Jeffrey Burch (a licensed massage therapist in Oregon) said, "An appropriate amount of curve gives the spine springiness." However, "Either too much or too little curve results in poor shock absorption with each footfall. The lumbar portion of the spine can have excessive curve, normal curve, insufficient curve, no curve, or curve in the wrong direction." To determine this, an evaluation can be made by X-RAY or by palpating the spine with a well-trained hand. Movement, RANGE OF MOTION, and the level of pain will also need to be considered. Although helpful information can be obtained by observing a reclining patient, "Lumbar lordosis, like all other features of alignment, must be assessed with the client standing on a level surface, barefoot."

See also POSTURE.

Burch, Jeffrey. "Lordosis: Assessment and Care." Available online. URL: http://www.amtamassage.org Downloaded on February 20, 2003.

swelling Whether caused by an INJURY, an underlying infection, or a medical condition, such as ARTHRITIS, GOUT, PSEUDOGOUT, or RHEUMATOID ARTHRITIS, swelling typically indicates an accumulation of fluids in the soft tissue surrounding a bone or JOINT. If this occurs because of an infection, swelling may be accompanied by redness and localized heat or fever with the potential for serious complications unless a prompt diagnosis and course of antibiotic treatment intervene. If swelling results from a physical trauma, the RICE METHOD generally comes recommended. If due to an ongoing medical condition, a rheumatologist or primary care physician may address the issue with NONSTEROIDAL ANTI-INFLAMMATORY DRUGS, cortisone, or other medication. In some instances, the doctor may also suggest PHYSICAL THERAPY or occupational therapy or prescribe a program of rehabilitative EXERCISE.

swimmer's shoulder See TENDINITIS OR TENDONITIS.

synovial joint This highly mobile type of joint occurs as a BALL-AND-SOCKET, HINGE, PIVOT, or GLIDING JOINT. With the structure of a particular joint reflected in its function, the RANGE OF MOTION depends on which bones meet in ARTICULATION. For example, the synovial joint of the KNEE will obviously not have the same design or purpose as that of the SHOULDER. Both, however, have CARTILAGE and a joint capsule lined with synovial membrane and filled with synovial fluid to cushion the joint from jolts. To keep the bones in place, ligaments acts as a strapping device, quite unlike the SUTURE JOINTS that hold together various sizes and shapes of bone in the jigsaw puzzle of the SKULL.

synovitis This inflammation in the lining of a SYNOVIAL JOINT usually results in pain and SWELLING with causatives including infection, injury, and certain medical conditions, such as RHEUMATOID ARTHRITIS (RA). Indeed, according to the Rheumatoid Arthritis Academy, "All features of chronic synovitis can be observed in early RA." After reporting on the information originally published in the March 2001 issue of *Best Practice & Research Clinical Rheumatology,* this news brief also stated, "However, the contributing factors of synovitis may vary from early onset to late stage RA." Therefore, in instances where RA has been suspected or detected, a rheumatologist can be instrumental in managing synovitis and other symptoms.

RA Academy. "Synovitis and RA." Available online. URL: http://www.raacademy.com Downloaded on November 5, 2003.

systemic lupus erythematosus This chronic inflammatory disease affects the joints and other systems of the body, such as the blood and skin. As explained by the Lupus Foundation of America, "The body's immune system normally makes proteins called antibodies to protect the body against viruses, bacteria, and other foreign materials . . . called antigens." However, "In an autoimmune disorder such as lupus, the immune system loses its ability to tell the difference between foreign substances . . . and its own cells and tissues." Then, as the body directs combative action toward itself, "These antibodies, called 'auto-antibodies,' react with the 'self' antigens to form immune complexes. The immune complexes build up in the tissues and can cause inflammation, injury to tissue, and pain." Although some patients could have serious, even life-threatening complications if vital organs become involved, most have mild cases.

Approximately 500,000 to 1.5 million people in this country have been diagnosed while "More than 16,000 Americans develop lupus each year." Not all of these will actually have lupus, though, since some will receive a false-positive test result, making a second opinion by a rheumatologist crucial in avoiding unnecessary worry. Of those who do have the disease, the category known as systemic lupus erythematosus is the one most commonly referred to as lupus. However, two other types of lupus are identified. "Discoid (cutaneous) lupus is always limited to the skin. . . . Drug-induced lupus occurs after the use of certain prescribed drugs," with symptoms usually fading after the medication has ceased.

Since symptoms can vary greatly from one person to the next, a rheumatologist or primary care physician will take each individual's needs into account prior to prescribing a specific treatment. In general, medications typically include various combinations of NONSTEROIDAL ANTI-INFLAMMATORY DRUGS, corticosteroids, and immunosuppressive drugs with antimalarials sometimes added for skin and joint symptoms. In addition, "Regular monitoring of the disease by laboratory tests can be valuable because noticeable symptoms may occur only after the disease has significantly flared." However, "Changes in blood test results may indicate the disease is becoming active even before the patient develops symptoms of a flare." With early treatment more apt to keep those flare-ups under control, preventative measures also include avoidance of the Sun and regular EXERCISE to "prevent muscle weakness and fatigue."

Lupus Foundation of America, Inc. "Definition." Available online. URL: http://www.lupus.org Downloaded on November 5, 2003.

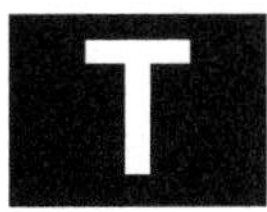

talus bone Commonly known as the ANKLE bone, this protruding short bone articulates with other tarsal bones that, together, connect each lower LEG bone (tibia and fibula) to the FEET. Since the talus adjoins the HEEL, it sees a lot of action with injuries often occurring in the form of a SPRAIN, STRAIN, TENDINITIS, or REPETITIVE MOTION DISORDERS, such as TARSAL TUNNEL SYNDROME. Degenerative conditions of the talus can also come about due to disorders, such as ARTHRITIS and OSTEOARTHRITIS, or those fairly common flaws in BIOMECHANICS that can often be corrected with proper FOOTWEAR or ORTHOTICS.

tarsal bones With the TALUS BONE as the most prominent one, these seven, irregularly shaped bones make up the ANKLE, thereby connecting each foot to the rest of the APPENDICULAR SKELETON to which the tarsals also belong.

tarsal tunnel syndrome Similar to CARPAL TUNNEL SYNDROME, this REPETITIVE MOTION DISORDER affects the TARSAL BONES of the ankle, rather than the carpal bones of the WRIST. As pressure occurs on the tunnel through which the tibial nerve extends into the lower leg, characteristic pain and numbness impinge on the ankle, heel, foot, and toes. Sometimes this happens because of stress on the tarsal area due to FLATFEET, a poor choice of FOOTWEAR, excessive physical activity, lesions within the tarsal tunnel, or the adverse effects of too much WEIGHT. Other pressures affecting the tunnel include edema, circulatory problems, and TENDINITIS. In any case, prolonged STANDING or walking will usually worsen the condition. For most patients most of the time, a conservative course of treatment, such as the self-administered RICE METHOD or the manipulation of bones by a chiropractor or osteopath will alleviate tingling or discomfort. If not, a physician may suggest ORTHOTICS, steroid injections, bracing, or immobilization with a cast. If, in rare cases, these treatments also prove ineffective after ample time has been given for recovery, a referral may be made to a podiatric surgeon.

To explain the surgical procedure occasionally needed, a fact sheet entitled "Tarsal Tunnel Syndrome" from the American College of Foot and Ankle Surgeons (ACFAS) said, "The surgery involves release of the tibial nerve and its branches from the surrounding tight structures along with incision of the laciniate ligament, a structure that forms a roof over the nerve bundle." Aside from possible complications, such as an infection or the continuation of nerve pain and numbness after the SURGERY has been performed, the ACFAS added, "Postoperatively, a period of immobilization followed by protected weight bearing and physical therapy may be prescribed."

American College of Foot and Ankle Surgeons. "Tarsal Tunnel Syndrome." Available online. URL: http://www.acfas.org Downloaded on February 15, 2003.

teeth Not really bones but bony projections extending from the MANDIBLE or JAW, the teeth bite, crush, and grind, depending on their shape, strength, and placement in the MOUTH. They debut from little buds that usually surface one enamel-polished tooth at a time. Eventually, 20 teeth erupt in the first set during childhood and 32 in the secondary set, which are hopefully retained by most adults. Regular dental checkups and good NUTRITION with ample calcium will undoubtedly help that effort. However, when the permanent teeth or dentures do not fit well, a person's bite can be thrown off with reverberations felt throughout the musculoskeletal system. Often, this happens because of radiating pain or general discomfort affecting the whole body, for instance, the loss of SLEEP that occurs in the painfully common TMJ syndrome involving the TEMPOROMANDIBULAR JOINT.

temporal or temporo- With its Latin roots definitely connected to the word *time,* this word and its combinative form somewhat wittily play on the temple region of the HEAD. For example, the temporal bone forms one of a pair of SKULL bones located in front of and slightly above each ear. Temporalis refers to the facial muscles that lift the MANDIBLE in a chewing motion, thus helping to process the food vitally needed for life.

See also TEMPOROMANDIBULAR JOINT.

temporomandibular joint (TMJ) Renowned for the TMJ syndrome that bears its name, this SYNOVIAL JOINT occurs where the TEMPORAL bones of the SKULL articulate with the bones of the lower jaw or MANDIBLE on either side of the face. As a highly mobile joint, this one can also experience problems, such as OSTEOARTHRITIS, commonly known to other active sites. In addition, a fact sheet from the Academy of General Dentistry said that ongoing tension can create problems in the form of "persistent jaw pain, a symptom of TMD (temporomandibular joint disorder)." Besides the tooth-grinding and jaw-clenching symptoms of STRESS that make TMD seem likely, other causatives can be an overbite or a set of poorly fitted dentures that press on nerves with results similar to what happens in CARPAL TUNNEL SYNDROME. However, TMD symptoms differ in that they not only include radiating pain and limited RANGE OF MOTION but an annoying click that occurs with chewing.

As health information from the American Academy of Otolaryngology—Head and Neck Surgery explained, "A small disc of cartilage separates the bones, much like in the knee joint, so that the mandible may slide easily; each time you chew you move it. But you also move it every time you talk and each time you swallow (every three minutes or so). It is, therefore, one of the most frequently used of all joints of the body and one of the most complex." To help patients find the area, the information went on to say, "You can locate this joint by putting your finger on the triangular structure in front of your ear. Then move your finger just slightly forward and press firmly while you open your jaw all the way and shut it. The motion you feel is the TMJ. You can also feel the joint motion in your ear canal." Why is pinpointing it so important? "These maneuvers can cause considerable discomfort to a patient who is having TMJ trouble, and physicians use these maneuvers with patients for diagnosis."

According to the TMJ Association, some predisposing factors for the development of a disorder include migraine headaches, allergies, and abscessed teeth with oral habits, such as tongue thrusting or nail biting, also listed as potential irritants. Another possibility includes the effects of unconscious habits at work or home, for instance, habitually holding a telephone between an ear and shoulder or bending over a book to read. Although differing opinions exist, some also believe poor POSTURE in general can be a causative or at least aggravate the condition.

TMD does not just mean one disorder, however, but three. As defined by the Department of Health and Human Services, National Institutes of Health (NIH), a TMJ disorder will generally fall into one of these categories, "Myofascial pain, the most common form of TMD, which is discomfort or pain in the muscles that control jaw function and the neck and shoulder muscles; internal derangement of the joint, meaning a dislocated jaw or displaced disc, or injury . . . [and] degenerative joint disease, such as osteoarthritis . . . in the jaw joint." Unfortunately, "A person may have one or more of these conditions at the same time." With a variety of indicators, "Pain, particularly in the chewing muscles and/or jaw joint, is the most common symptom. Other likely symptoms include: limited movement or locking of the jaw; radiating pain in the face, neck or shoulders; painful clicking, popping or grating sounds in the jaw joint when opening or closing the mouth; a sudden, major change in the way the upper and lower teeth fit together." In addition, "Symptoms such as headaches, earaches, dizziness, and hearing problems may sometimes be related to TMD."

Regarding therapeutic actions to take, the NIH information said, "The key words to keep in mind about TMD treatment are 'conservative' and 'reversible.'" With noninvasive procedures recommended, self-treatments include "eating soft foods, applying heat or ice packs, and avoiding extreme jaw movements (such as wide yawning, loud singing and gum chewing)." Other conservative home treatments, such as "gentle muscle stretching and relaxing exercises, and short-term use of muscle-relaxing and anti-inflammatory drugs," may also be effective. In some instances, a dentist or orthodontic specialist may suggest an oral splint or a bite plate that fits over the teeth, thus reducing clenching. When considering more invasive treatments, however, the NIH strongly suggested the need for a second opinion since "scientists have learned that certain irreversible treatments, such as surgical replacement of jaw joints with artificial implants, may cause severe pain and permanent jaw damage. Some of these devices may fail to function properly or may break apart in the jaw over time."

Indeed, after having denied approval for or recalling some implant devices, the U.S. Food and Drug Administration (FDA) began revising its handbook, entitled *TMJ Implants—A Consumer Informational Update—1999.* In an interim letter dated April 2001, Dr. David W. Feigal Jr., the director of the Center for Devices and Radiological Health, provided background information about the FDA's regulation of new devices that have entered the market since the 1976 Medical Device Amendments. He then explained that the devices prior to that time had continued to be marketed "without demonstrating safety and effectiveness." Therefore, "In 1993, the Dental Products Advisory Panel reclassified them into Class III—the highest risk category." This meant that "all manufacturers of TMJ devices would be required to submit a Premarket Approval Application . . . demonstrating safety and effectiveness—when called for by the FDA. On December 30, 1998, the FDA called for PMAs from all manufacturers of TMJ implants." Not only did this ruling help to regulate product safety and provide guidelines for use, but patients in need of Class I and Class II devices can be assured, "If there is a lack of information about what makes a device safe and effective, it is put into Class III and the highest level of Premarket review is required." This brings hope for patients who previously encountered a failed product or a failed surgical effort. Besides this group, who may require another round of implants or SURGERY, "The population in need of surgical reconstruction may also include patients with severe trauma to the temporomandibular joint, neoplasms (tumors), congenital deformities, ankylosis or arthritis involving the TMJ, rendering it dysfunctional." Although the FDA maintained that "with more surgeries there is more pain," the overriding concern appeared to be that "patients [need] to understand the limitations of joint replacement surgery." For example, "Patients may need further pain management and physical therapy to achieve improved results." Furthermore, "All implant materials degenerate over time." Nevertheless, surgery offers an existing option with RESEARCH and clinical studies exploring others to come. As the FDA said, "The challenge to the research community is to develop the most functional device from materials that are biocompatible and durable. Future research will include ways to develop biological alternatives, such as implanting cells that will grow new bone and or cartilage."

Academy of General Dentistry. "Fender-Benders: Source of TMD?" Available online. URL: http://www.agd.org Downloaded on November 7, 2003.

American Academy of Otolaryngology—Head and Neck Surgery. "Doctor, What is TMJ?" Available online. URL: http://www.entnet.org/healthinfo/topics/tmj.cfm Downloaded on November 7, 2003.

Department of Health and Human Services. "Temporomandibular Disorders (TMD)." Available online. URL: http://www.nidcr.nih.gov Downloaded on November 7, 2003.

TMJ Association. "TMJ Diseases and Disorders." Available online. URL: http://www.tmj.org Downloaded on November 7, 2003.

U.S. Food and Drug Administration. "TMJ Implants–A Consumer Informational Update—1999." Available online. URL: http://www.fda.gov/cdrh/consumer/tmjupdate.pdf Downloaded on November 7, 2003.

tendinitis or tendonitis This INFLAMMATION of the TENDONS can affect any area where a muscle attaches to a bone, thus making the condition available to virtually every active site in the body. Tendinitis can also arise from an injury or an underlying inflammatory condition, such as GOUT or REACTIVE ARTHRITIS, that is usually treated by a rheumatologist. Some causing factors, however, may be as diverse as each joint's RANGE OF MOTION. One example results from inflammation in the renowned ACHILLES TENDON of the HEEL. However, other types of tendinitis refer to an associated activity as well as a body site. Therefore, the best-known instances descriptively occur as tennis elbow, golfer's elbow, jumper's knee, swimmer's shoulder, runner's knee, and thrower's elbow and/or shoulder. Some, of course, would call these examples of TENDINOSIS, which would certainly be correct when the primary causative does not involves inflammation but, rather, the microscopic tearing of tissue, such as typically occurs from overuse. Then again, people with tennis elbow seldom play tennis.

When discussing that condition, the American Association for Hand Surgery said, "Any activity that over stresses the involved tendon, the extensor carpi radialis brevis, can cause the disorder. These activities include repetitive work, gardening, tennis, and golf." With a medical history, physical examination, and assessment of the range of motion in the affected joint helping to determine a diagnosis, an important distinction must still be made between inflammation and those changes in the tendons due to tissue breakdown or tearing. If inflamed tendons indeed appear to be the problem, treatment then occurs in a staged exercise program often involving rest and NONSTEROIDAL ANTI-INFLAMMATORY DRUGS with later additions of STRETCHING exercises and PHYSICAL THERAPY or occupational therapy. In some cases, SPLINTING may also be required.

When tendinitis involves other joints, such as the ANKLE, ROTATOR CUFF, or KNEE, similar treatments will generally be recommended. The emphasis will be on the cause and what can be done, not only to correct the problem but to prevent it from happening again. For example, STRESS, inadequate NUTRITION, and lack of EXERCISE aggravated by sudden activity may be more of an inflammatory issue than overuse. In any event, an OCCUPATIONAL THERAPIST (OT) can assist.

In 2002, the American Occupational Therapy Association explained an OT will "evaluate the client's injury following care by an orthopedist to coordinate treatment plans and determine the course of intervention" and also "analyze the client's environment at home and work to identify potential barriers to the client's performance." Besides applying "techniques to reduce swelling, prevent further injury, care for wounds, and improve movement," an OT can recommend strengthening exercises to do at home and also show a patient how to complete day-to-day activities, such as dressing and driving, while the injured area rests and heals.

American Association for Hand Surgery. "Lateral Epicondylitis FAQ." Available online. URL: http://www.handsurgery.org/latpicondylitis.pdf Downloaded on November 7, 2003.

American Occupational Therapy Association, Inc. "Intervention for Tendon Injuries." Available online. URL: http://www.aota.org Downloaded on November 8, 2003.

tendinopathy As with TENDINOSIS, the absence of INFLAMMATION distinguishes this condition from TENDINITIS—the name by which many TENDON problems get categorized although most may actually be a type of tendinopathy. To clarify this, an August/September 2002 *Rehab: The Interdisciplinary Journal of Rehabilitation* article by Dr. Louis C. Almekinders—a professor in the Department of Orthopedic Surgery, Sports Medicine Section, at the University of North Carolina at Chapel Hill—explained, "Most forms of tendinopathy develop clear symptomatology in the area where the tendon is affected. Local pain is by far the most common complaint. The pain tends to be most pronounced after a period of rest, e.g., upon arising in the morning, and actually may ease some with continued use." A patient might also experience tenderness in the tendons and "some edema in the tendon sheath whereas mid-substance and insertional tendinopathy may be associated with thickening of the tendon itself. If the diagnosis is not clear, imaging studies can help," particularly of an inaccessible location, such as the ROTATOR CUFF. Then, "MRI [magnetic resonance imaging] and diagnostic ultrasound are the imaging modalities of choice." However, "Apart from recognizing tendinopathy, it is also important not to label chronic pain as tendinitis or tendinopathy." Of equal importance is "explaining to patients that tendinopathy is a chronic, but still temporary condition," which "may take several months or even more than a year . . . to resolve." Since inflammation usually has little bearing on a true tendinopathy, the NONSTEROIDAL ANTI-INFLAMMATORY DRUGS used for tendinitis will seldom be necessary except for the analgesic effect. Instead, more likely treatments include PHYSICAL THERAPY, therapeutic EXERCISE, HEAT THERAPY, COLD THERAPY, ULTRASOUND THERAPY, and electrical stimulation. Although injections may be used to alleviate extreme pain, "The concern of tendon rupture as a result of corticosteroid usage remains unresolved." For unrelenting cases, SURGERY may be needed, which "generally involves a debridement of the involved tendon tissue." This then "converts a chronic, non-healing tendon lesion into an acute tendon injury," so, hopefully, "The response to this acute surgical trauma may evoke a vigorous healing response." Typically, recuperation will then take about four to six months.

Some instances of tendinopathy, however, may resolve relatively quickly. In 2001, a medical team from France evaluated the adverse symptoms of patients receiving STATIN therapy. Although numerous studies have shown statins to be very effective in lowering high cholesterol, "Reported musculoskeletal side effects include myalgia and a few cases of rhabdomyolysis and polymyositis." As a corrective first step in treating these tendinopathies, the medical team withdrew statins from the four participants, thus obtaining an outcome "consistently favorable within 1 to 2 months after discontinuation of the drug."

These findings could prove useful for those who, in a zealous attempt to reduce excess cholesterol and/or body weight, have excluded fats from their diet. If carried to extreme, fat reduction can also remove the protective aspects of that vital substance. As explained by Gayla J. Kirschmann, "Cholesterol is a fat-related substance that is essential for good health. It is a normal component of most body tissues, especially those of the brain, nervous system, liver, and blood. More than nine-tenths of cholesterol ends up in the cells where it performs vital structural and metabolic functions. The unused parts may be harmful in some people, and for this reason high-cholesterol foods containing animal fats should be avoided." However, "In addition to supplying energy and providing valuable nutrients to the body, fats act as carriers for the fat-soluble vitamins, A, D, E, and K. Removing fat from foods also removes these vitamins." Furthermore, "By aiding in the absorption of vitamin D, fats help make calcium available to body tissues and to the bones and teeth." Other functions include lubrication of the connective tissue and assistance in the conversion of carotene to vitamin A. "Fats are beneficial for other reasons as well. Natural oils provide a healthy complexion and nourish the scalp for shiny hair. Our muscles work because the fat that is laced between the fibers carries a constant reserve of energy." Therefore, if strong medication and/or a rigid fat-free diet reduces the body's ability to lubricate and protect the muscles on a cellular level, the results could mean deficiencies in nutrients, loss of energy stores, muscular weakness, and pain.

Almekinders, Louis C. "Breaking with Tradition." Available online. URL: http://www.rehabpub.com Downloaded on April 16, 2003.

Ziza, J. M., P. Chazarain, et al. "Four Cases of Tendinopathy in Patients on Statin Therapy." *Joint Bone Spine* 68, no. 5 (October 2001): 430–433.

tendinosis Unlike the inflammation involved in TENDINITIS, this condition most often occurs with the degeneration of collagen fibers in the tendons or the overuse of a muscle that results in tearing. Therefore, instead of treating tendinosis with the NONSTEROIDAL ANTI-INFLAMMATORY DRUGS used for inflammatory conditions, the emphasis remains on encouraging torn tissue to heal and treating any underlying medical disorder.

As the first of two articles on tendinopathies, Karim M. Khan, M.D., and colleagues said, "If physicians acknowledge that overuse tendinopathies are due to tendinosis, as distinct from tendinitis, they must modify patient management in at least eight areas. These include adaptation of advice given when counseling, interaction with the physical therapist and athletic trainer, interpretation of imaging, choice of conservative management, and consideration of whether surgery is an option." Pathology offers a distinction in that "macroscopically, abnormal tissue examined at surgery shows the tendon to be dull-appearing, slightly brown, and soft," whereas, "Normal tendon tissue is white, glistening, and firm." In either case, inflamed tissue is just not part of the picture, but, in tendinosis, AGING is. "Thus, physicians must shift their perspective and acknowledge that tendinosis is the pathology being treated in most cases and that treatment needs to combat collagen breakdown rather than inflammation. Tendinosis may require a reasonable period of relative rest and attention to strengthening with the aim of first breaking the tendinosis cycle. Once this is done, the patient uses modalities that optimize collagen production and maturation so that the tendon achieves the necessary tensile strength for normal function."

See also NUTRITION.

Khan, Karim M., M.D. "Overuse Tendinosis, Not Tendinitis." Available online. URL: http://www.physsportsmed.com Downloaded on November 8, 2003.

tendon Strong, sinewy, shiny white, and fibrous, these cords of connective tissue attach each muscle to the corresponding bone, enabling the musculoskeletal system to move as MUSCLES contract, relax, and then contract again. Since they are made mostly of collagen or bundles of protein fibers, some tendons, such as those in the hands and feet, have a self-lubricating covering to shield them from friction. When various factors, such as a lack of water or a lack of nutrients, including a small but healthful amount of protective fats, cause the tendon sheath to fail, the resulting inflammation can produce TENDINITIS. In addition, the breakdown of collagen that often occurs with AGING can cause TENDINOSIS. Besides the possibility of these TENDINOPATHIES, the tendons can be pulled, strained, or torn in acute INJURIES—sometimes severely enough to require SURGERY to reestablish the muscular attachment needed to get the affected bone moving again.

tennis elbow See TENDINITIS OR TENDONITIS; TENDINOSIS.

tenosynovitis Similar to TENDINITIS, this inflammatory response lies within the lining of the tendon sheath. As the normally protective sheath becomes inflamed, symptoms typically include pain, tenderness, and SWELLING in the affected joint. In these general instances, treatment emphasizes the relief of pain and inflammation with NONSTEROIDAL ANTI-INFLAMMATORY DRUGS and HEAT THERAPY or COLD THERAPY. SPLINTING or BRACING may also be needed to keep the tendons immobilized during the healing process.

With causes for inflammation as diverse as INJURIES, REPETITIVE MOTION, STRAIN, and underlying medical conditions, such as GOUT or RHEUMATOID ARTHRITIS, yet another possibility concerns infection, which can result from something as simple as an untended cut or as complex as the polluted site of a drug injection. In either case, an infection will usually present symptoms of fever and localized redness or heat with swelling increasing along with the level of seriousness. At such times, tenosynovitis can even become life threatening, thus necessitating surgery to lance the area and rid the body of pus, assuming it has remained confined to a particular locale. A course of antibiotics will also be prescribed with the choice of medication depending on whether the problem occurred from a bacterial or other type of infection. After surgery, patient care then resembles the initial course of general treatment.

tension, muscular See STRESS.

TENS unit See TRANSCUTANEOUS ELECTRONIC NERVE STIMULATOR.

thigh Between the HIP and the KNEE, this portion of the LEG includes the FEMUR or thighbone.

thorax Also known as the chest, this region begins at the base of the NECK and includes the thoracic vertebrae of the BACK and both the STERNUM and RIB cage at the front of the body. The heart and respiratory system are protectively housed in between.

thrower's elbow/shoulder See TENDINITIS OR TENDONITIS.

thumb What would give the HAND a hand without a thumb to count on for opening jar lids, clasping a pencil, or buttoning a button? As the short, thick FINGER that points from the side of either hand, the thumb also differs from the other digits in that it has two phalanges instead of three. Although this means fewer joints to dislocate or lesser ligaments to tear and tendons to pull, this smaller digit keeps up with its counterparts in conditions such as ARTHRITIS, TENDINITIS, TENDINOSIS, SPRAINS, and STRAINS as well as specialized INJURIES, from the INFLAMMATION of a tennis thumb to the SUBLUXATION of a skier's thumb. Of all the available fingers, however, children traditionally favor this one, their mouths apparently doing it no harm with frequent soakings.

tibia Also known as the shinbone, this second longest bone in the body connects with the smaller FIBULA to comprise the lower LEG. At the KNEE, the tibia articulates with the body's longest bone, the FEMUR (or thighbone), then extends distally toward the TALUS, or anklebone Because of these important connections with weight-bearing bones and joints, a fractured tibia keeps a body off its feet to give the bone ample time to heal.

tingling See NUMBNESS.

toe More like an abbreviated THUMB than a FINGER, these digits of the foot normally assist the body in getting a grip on balance. Toes also have an important place in the gait mechanism, particularly in the push-off phase. Without toes, people might be inclined to waddle when they walk. When pointing toward a rheumatic condition, such as GOUT, a swollen toe can become a diagnostic tool, whereas painful toes in general may indicate ARTHRITIS. Tight FOOTWEAR, of course, can put a squeeze on almost anyone, but stroking the sole of a foot usually causes the toes to fan out. Being spread too far while on the move, however, can cause the kind of hard bump that results in a DISLOCATED JOINT in extreme cases or, in lesser ones, a stubbed toe sometimes accompanied by swearing.

tongue Having lent its name to tongue twisters, tongue-and-grove paneling, and tongue-in-cheek humor, this muscular organ usually lies around the floor of the mouth, waiting for something to taste or say. The latter can cause problems in a loose tongue but if strapped too tightly can indicate a congenital defect known as tongue-tied, a physical condition usually correctable by surgery. Comprised of many muscles, the tongue provides taste buds and assists in processing foods, making them more palatable to the digestive tract. These muscles also enable various sounds to shape words into song and language. In a physician's office though, the tongue helps to shape a diagnosis as its coloration often reveals the presence of an illness or disease. For instance, a pale tongue can indicate severe anemia while a bluish tinge may show a circulatory problem or a disease of the cardiac muscle. A coated tongue may mean the presence of too much bacteria and a dry tongue too little water. With numerous possibilities to consider, most doctors have good diagnostic causes to command their patients to give a performance of "Aahh."

torso Also known as the trunk of the body, the torso houses internal organs and locates the muscles of the chest and the abdomen. To strengthen the body overall, torso training often focuses EXERCISES on the chest and ABDOMINAL MUSCLES, thus providing a stronger trunk for packing vital organs, slimming fatty "handles," and balancing muscular limbs.

torticollis Normally, the musculoskeletal system presents a picture of symmetry with a fairly equal distribution of muscle on either side. If, however, an injury at birth or later in life causes muscles around the HEAD, NECK, or upper SHOULDER to tighten significantly, the resulting abnormality can twist the head to one side, restricting range of motion and throwing off the body's well-balanced look. Whether congenital or acquired by factors, such as scarring, RHEUMATISM, or diseases of the cervical vertebrae, torticollis can affect accessory nerves of the spine, causing CONTRACTURES, pain, and muscle SPASMS. Although treatments depend on the cause, immobilization and pain relievers may be used with botulinus toxin (Botox) sometimes needed to restrain the spasms. TRACTION and HEAT THERAPY may also be prescribed.

Regarding wryneck (torticollis), the American Academy of Pediatrics said that other BIRTH INJURIES, such as a dislocated hip, occasionally occur in children with congenital muscular torticollis. In either case, X-RAYS will usually be required for a diagnosis. To treat the wryneck, a pediatrician can show caretakers how to move the child's head, gently, away from the tilt. In addition to doing this several times a day, a sleeping infant can be placed on the back or side with the head turned in the opposite direction of the tilt in a corrective effort to stretch the shortened muscle.

A predisposition for this condition may delay its onset until the young adult or middle-aged years. However, the first symptoms can also appear after an illness, an infection, or an injury to the neck or the head. Certain medications can cause a wryneck, too. To define the condition further, the National Spasmodic Torticollis Association said this "painful and debilitating neurological disorder," also known as cervical dystonia, affects three of every 10,000 people with about 90,000 diagnosed in the U.S. As a movement disorder caused by a dysfunction of the brain, occurrences result in "three distinct varieties of Spasmodic Torticollis: Tonic, in which the head turns to one side; Clonic, which involves the shaking of the head; and Mixed which involves both turning and shaking." The characteristic head turning also has categories, "Rotation, in which the head turns to one side or the other; Laterocollis in which the head is pulled toward the shoulder; Retrocollis in which the head is pulled to the back; or Anterocollis in which the head is pulled forward," with various combinations also possible. Besides medications and, possibly, Botox injections, treatments include PHYSICAL THERAPY, OCCUPATION THERAPY, BIOFEEDBACK, and electrical stimulation. If the muscular spasms or movements seem to lessen during sleep, patients may find it helpful to rest on their backs at intervals throughout the day. In addition, "Touching the opposite side of the face or chin may also cause spasms to cease temporarily." However, if the condition develops prior to age 40 and/or remains mild, "Spontaneous recovery can be found in up to 20 percent of people within five years of the onset of symptoms."

American Academy of Pediatrics. "Wryneck (Torticollis)." Available online. URL: http://www.medem.com Downloaded on November 8, 2003.

National Spasmodic Torticollis Association. "Understanding Spasmodic Torticollis." Available online. URL: http://www.torticollis.org Downloaded on August 1, 2003.

Tourette syndrome Named for the neurologist who first described this inherited neurobehavioral disorder, Tourette syndrome (TS) presents with repeated, sudden, involuntary movements of muscles as facial tics and/or disrupted speech. From very mild to severe, these symptoms usually appear prior to the later teen years with males three to four times more likely than females to experience TS. As additional facts from the Tourette Syndrome Association explained, "In a minority of cases, the vocalizations can include socially inappropriate words and phrases—called coprolalia. These outbursts are neither intentional nor purposeful." Also, "Involuntary symptoms can include eye blinking, repeated throat clearing or sniffing, arm thrusting, kicking movements, shoulder shrugging or jumping."

Information from WE MOVE (Worldwide Education and Awareness for Movement Disorders) stated, "The anatomical locations of motor tics may change over time. Rarely, motor tics evolve to include behaviors that may result in self-injury, such as excessive scratching and lip biting." With this waxing and waning of symptoms, "Tics often subside during absorbing activities such as reading or working, decline during sleep, worsen with stress or fatigue, and may be voluntarily suppressed for brief periods." Although embarrassment and anxiety may cause some patients to withdraw socially, others may have such mild symptoms that no medication is needed. In general, "The goal of therapy in patients with TS is to reduce motor and vocal tics and alleviate associated behavioral problems, such as obsessive-compulsive behaviors . . . and impulsivity." Methods such as BIOFEEDBACK and relaxation techniques to relieve STRESS can be helpful with medications used to address specific symptoms, such as muscle spasm and attention-deficit/hyperactivity disorder.

With an update on ongoing research, the National Institute of Neurological Disorders and Stroke announced, "Investigators are conducting genetic linkage studies in large multigenerational families affected with TS in an effort to find the chromosomal location of the TS gene(s). Understanding the genetics of TS will directly benefit patients who are concerned about recurrence in their families and will ultimately help to clarify the development of the disorder. Investigators also are studying certain neurotransmitters to explore the role they play in the disease process and develop more effective therapies. Others are researching how environmental factors may influence the expression of the disease." Presently, no cure exists. "However, the condition in many individuals improves as they mature. Individuals with TS can expect to live a normal life span. Although TS is generally lifelong and chronic, it is not degenerative. In a few cases, complete remission occurs after adolescence."

National Institute of Neurological Disorders and Stroke (NINDS). "NINDS Tourette Syndrome Information Page," Available online. URL: http://accessible.ninds.nih.gov Downloaded on July 1, 2001.

Tourette Syndrome Association, Inc. "What Is Tourette Syndrome?" Available online. URL: http://www.tsa-usa.org Downloaded on November 10, 2003.

WE MOVE. "Tourette's Syndrome," Available online. URL: http://www.wemove.org Downloaded on January 10, 2003.

trabecular bone With cavernous-looking columns tunneling through the interior, this structural design of the long bones helps to keep a healthy skeletal system lightweight, flexible, and exceptionally sturdy. Too many columns spaced too widely can indicate the absence of balanced NUTRITION or the presence of a degenerative bone condition, such as OSTEOPOROSIS. As living matter, however, these skeletal bones show a capacity for change and, interestingly, a sensitivity to touch.

To study the effects of the latter on BONE MASS, a medical team from the Musculo-Skeletal Research Laboratory of the Department of Biomedical Engineering, State University of New York, Stony Brook, proposed that "Quantity and Quality of Trabecular Bone in the Femur Are Enhanced by a Strongly Anabolic, Noninvasive Mechanical Intervention." The article accompanying that lengthy title stated, "The skeleton's sensitivity to mechanical stimuli represents a critical determination of bone mass and morphology," so that "extremely low level . . . , high frequency . . . , mechanical strains, continually present during even subtle activities such as standing are as important to defining the skeleton as the larger strains typically associated with vigorous activity." With the rear legs of sheep "stimulated for 20 minutes/day using a noninvasive 0.3g vertical oscillation to induce approximately 5 microstrain on the cortex of the tibia," the results a year later showed a 10.6 percent increase of bone mineral content with an 11.3 percent decrease in trabecular spaces, "indicating that bone quantity was increased both by the creation of new trabeculae and the thickening of existing trabeculae." In addition, this low-level stimuli affected bone density with deformations "several orders of magnitude below those peak strains which arise during vigorous activity," thus indicating the potential of therapeutic stimulation as an intervention for osteoporosis and other conditions presenting BONE LOSS.

Rubin, C., A. S. Turner, et al. "Quantity and Quality of Trabecular Bone in the Femur Are Enhanced by a Strongly Anabolic, Noninvasive Mechanical Intervention." *Journal of Bone Mineral Research* 17, no. 2 (February 2002): 349–357.

traction In the ORTHOPEDIC circles encompassing CHIROPRACTICS and OSTEOPATHY, the equipment for traction may look like a torture device yet actually work toward devising therapeutic treatment. For example, if compression in the spinal column induces pain, slightly drawing the vertebrae apart may help to relieve pressure on the spinal nerves. Similarly, elastic wiring by a dentist or orthodontist can apply maxillomandibular traction to correct a malalignment of the JAW or TEETH. A bad break for a long bone can require a hospital stay with traction used to realign, stretch, and/or immobilize the injured arm or leg in an optimal position for healing.

transcutaneous electronic nerve stimulator (TENS) This small electrical stimulatory device has been effectively used to treat pain. Although a transcutaneous electronic nerve stimulator (TENS unit) does not come recommended for pregnant women and patients with a pacemaker, heart condition, or epilepsy, the unit can help a variety of other conditions, such as ARTHRITIS, BURSITIS, OSTEOARTHRITIS, CARPAL TUNNEL SYNDROME, and spinal cord disorders as well as the SPRAINS, STRAINS, and phantom pains of INJURIES.

In the article, "Pulling the Plug on Pain," physical therapist Patrick De Bock of Belgium said, "The treatment of autonomic dysfunction takes time, but leaving the TENS unit on for hours will almost certainly cause adaptation. This, in turn, may cause the treatment to have little or no effect. To prevent adaptation, turning the TENS unit on for 20 minutes and then off for 40 minutes is recommended." The article added, "Intensity (current) is a very important parameter because too high a setting may cause the release of endorphins, which is highly discouraged. On the other hand, if the intensity is too low, there will probably be no effect at all." Therefore, "The best results are obtained using a setting that causes a moderate degree of sensation (slightly above motor level)."

Information from www.spine-health.com further explained, "High frequency stimulation, sometimes called 'conventional,' is tolerable for hours, but the resultant pain relief lasts for a shorter period of time. Low-frequency stimulation, sometimes called 'acupuncture-like,' is more uncomfortable and tolerable for only 20–30 minutes, but the resultant pain relief last longer." To manage these hand-sized or smaller units, "TENS users should experiment with various electrode placements," such as directly over the painful area or immediately surrounding it but also on the opposite side of the body. Trying the unit for several days and placing the electrodes on various spots will help a patient to determine what is most effective over the course of a few weeks.

De Bock, Patrick. "Pulling the Plug on Pain." Available online. URL: http://www.rehabpub.com Downloaded on April 16, 2003.

Spine-Health. "Transcutaneous Electrical Nerve Stimulators (TENS)." Available online. URL: http://www.spine-health.com Downloaded on November 10, 2003.

transverse fracture This type of FRACTURE goes across the bone at a right angle, making the break one of the more severe types.

triceps With three heads attaching this muscle to bone, triceps bring triple strength to the forearm.

Turner's syndrome This congenital disorder of the endocrine system results in the short stature of DWARFISM. In addition to hormone therapy, treatments may include surgical correction of skeletal abnormalities.

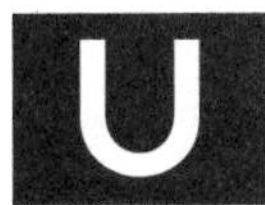

Ullrich congenital muscular dystrophy Evident at birth, this inherited disorder presents mild-to-severe muscle weakness, contractures, and loose joints with symptoms progressively worsening. As a medical team led by Olga Camacho Vanegas from the Department of Internal Medicine at the University of Rome found, "Ullrich Scleroatonic Muscular Dystrophy Is Caused by Recessive Mutations in Collagen Type VI." The team stated, "Ullrich syndrome is a recessive congenital muscular dystrophy affecting connective tissue and muscle" due to the "near total absence of COL6," a type of collagen. Although "the molecular basis is unknown," case studies revealed "more than one sibling affected and a high incidence" of shared genetic ancestry among the healthy parents, "suggesting an autosomal recessive inheritance." Although Ullrich congenital muscular dystrophy occurs very rarely, "Most of the patients die of respiratory failure in the first decade of life," usually as a result of the paralysis that occurs in muscles of the diaphragm. With more investigations such as this RESEARCH from Rome, "Functional studies of the consequences of gene mutations will help in better understanding COL6 function and regulation."

See also MUSCULAR DYSTROPHY.

Vanegas, Olga Camacho. "Ullrich Scleroatonic Muscular Dystrophy Is Caused by Recessive Mutations in Collagen Type VI." *PNAS: Proceedings from the National Academy of Sciences of the United States of America* 98, no. 13 (June 19, 2001): 7,516–7,521.

ulna Of the two long bones in the forearm, this bigger, stronger one resides on the little finger's side, with a thumbs up from the smaller radius bone running parallel in each ARM. Alongside the ulna, the long ulnar nerve extends from fingertip to the spinal column, passing through the humerus region of the ELBOW. There, where the ulna and radius meet the upper arm in ARTICULATION, a bump to this funny bone radiates pain in all directions, but only briefly. Less of a laughing matter would be the bone FRACTURES frequently occurring in the ulna as people of all ages reach out to catch themselves during those unexpected moments of a FALL.

ultrasonography With sounds bouncing off the walls of internal organs and tissues, the differing echoes transmit various qualities of density and elasticity, giving a radiologist a clearer picture of what is going on inside. The resulting images produce an ultrasonogram, a diagnostic tool used to evaluate TENDON tearing, BURSITIS, and other abnormalities of the muscles and JOINTS, such as SYNOVITIS.

When explaining this painless procedure, the Radiological Society of North America said, "An ultrasound image is a useful way of examining the musculoskeletal system of the body to detect problems with muscles, tendons, joints, and soft tissue. Ultrasound images are captured in real time, so they can often show movement, function, and anatomy, as well as enable radiologists to diagnose a variety of conditions and assess damage after an injury or illness." Since "ultrasound has difficulty penetrating bone and therefore can only see the outer surface of bony structures and not what lies within and beyond," the choice of an MRI—MAGNETIC RESONANCE IMAGING—will be more likely "for visualizing bone or internal structure of certain joints." However, "Ultrasound may actually have advantages over MRI in seeing tendon structure." As another advantage, ultrasound scanning is not affected by metal implants, such as plates or pins, and it does not interfere with a pacemaker as an MRI is known to do.

Radiological Society of North America, Inc. "Ultrasound-Musculoskeletal." Available online. URL: http://www.radiologyinfo.org Downloaded on May 13, 2003.

ultrasound therapy Besides its diagnostic use in ULTRASONOGRAPHY, ultrasound provides a tool in PHYSICAL THERAPY by bringing on the heat. With its production of thermal therapeutic effects, ultrasound treats musculoskeletal injuries, such as SPRAINS, INFLAMMATION, scarring, DELAYED ONSET MUSCLE SORENESS, FRACTURES, and damaged JOINTS. "However," Lennart D. Johns, Ph.D., pointed out, "Recent reports demonstrating that ultrasound affects enzyme activity and possibly gene regulation provide sufficient data to present a probable molecular mechanism of ultrasound's nonthermal therapeutic action." In writing for the *Journal of Athletic Training,* Dr. Johns explained, "While clinicians state that ultrasound is used to accomplish heating within deep tissue, there is a common, whispered belief that heating alone cannot account for the clinical effects, especially when ultrasound is delivered at nonthermal settings." Therefore, after reviewing the ultrasound research from the past four decades, the researcher proposed "a molecular mechanism whereby the mechanical properties of ultrasound interact with the molecular and multimolecular complexes within the cell." With a call for more research on the cellular responses to ultrasound that apparently occur without tissue heating, Dr. Johns summarized the hope of raising "awareness that therapeutic levels of ultrasound (1 MHz, 3 MHz, and 45 kHz) stimulate cellular and molecular effects within cells that are centrally involved in the inflammatory and healing processes."

Johns, Lennart D. "Nonthermal Effects of Therapeutic Ultrasound: The Frequency Resonance Hypothesis." *Journal of Athletic Training* vol. 37, no. 3 (2002): 293–299.

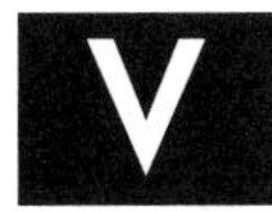

velocity See SKELETAL MUSCLE.

vertebra These 33 bony segments line up the column of the SPINE, making a centrally located and significant part of the AXIAL SKELETON. Each vertebra has the ability to break formation, especially when hit with INJURIES or a degenerative condition of the bones or joints. However, the normal order includes seven cervical, 12 thoracic, five LUMBAR, five sacral (fused into one SACRUM), and two coccygeal vertebrae in one COCCYX or tailbone. When out of line, corrective measures include SPINAL MANIPULATION, various forms of therapy, and/or SURGERY to pull each knobby vertebra into its place of rank while well-balanced NUTRITION and EXERCISE may help to avoid systemic attacks, such as BONE LOSS or OSTEOPOROSIS. In alliance with supportive LIGAMENTS and protective DISKS, each bony segment has the same mission: to protect the spinal cord from injury, to stand at attention with the aid of good POSTURE, and to keep a flexible body on the move throughout life with a well-targeted RANGE OF MOTION.

vertebral compression fracture Unlike the bone FRACTURES resulting from INJURIES, vertebral compression fractures (VCF) occur spontaneously as BONE LOSS, collagen depletion, or underlying medical conditions, such as OSTEOPOROSIS or BONE CANCER, cause weakened vertebrae to compress and collapse. Sometimes this happens with no pain. More typically, though, a band of pain radiates from the spine, encircling the TORSO. Treatment may include pain medication, rest, and supportive devices, such as BRACING. However, if these conservative treatments fail, SURGERY—or the less invasive, nonsurgical procedure of VERTEBROPLASTY—may be recommended.

According to alarming statistics from the University of Maryland Spine Center, "One vertebral compression fracture occurs every 45 seconds." With 1.5 million fractures due to osteoporosis, "Approximately half of these fractures occur in the spine," accounting for "150,000 hospitalizations every year." Furthermore, because of the adverse effects of VCF on the RESPIRATORY MUSCLES involved in pulmonary function, "The five-year mortality rate following a vertebral fracture is significantly higher than in patients without fractures." With complications especially noted for the elderly, "The goal of fracture care should be to restore anatomy, relieve pain, and restore function as rapidly as possible."

To investigate health-related quality of life in patients with VCF, a medical team from Canada studied incident fractures in 2,009 women age 50 years and older who met the study's criteria. They concluded, "Despite improvements in the medical management of osteoporotic fractures, it is clear that fractured patients continue to experience decreased quality of life and that these deficits may often go unnoticed by clinicians. Thus, the challenge for the future is to develop treatment strategies to prevent and also reduce the pain associated with the fractures and to determine how patient satisfaction is impacted when quality of life issues are considered during care."

Adachi, Jonathan D., George Ioannidis, et al. "The Impact of Incident Vertebral and Non-Vertebral Fractures on Health Related Quality of Life in Postmenopausal Women." Available online. URL: http://www.biomedcentral.com/1471-2474/3/11 Downloaded on April 22, 2002.

University of Maryland Spine Center. "Vertebral Osteoporosis and Kyphoplasty." Available online. URL: http://www.umm.edu/spinecenter Downloaded on November 11, 2003.

vertebroplasty With the expertise of a radiologist required instead of a surgeon, this nonsurgical procedure involves the insertion of a gluelike substance to lend stability and strength to a bone collapsed by a VERTEBRAL COMPRESSION FRACTURE. According to the North American Spine Society, "The entire process takes one to two hours, although the actual injection usually takes only about 10 minutes. The cement mixture hardens in about half an hour, and after a short recovery period, the patient is sent home," usually with pain medication for the first couple of days. Obviously, this procedure has advantages over open SURGERY in that it avoids common surgical risks and a more extensive recuperative time. "However, percutaneous vertebroplasty will not correct the bone lost due to osteoporosis; it may only stabilize new fractures."

While staying abreast of such treatments, the U.S. Food and Drug Administration (FDA) Center for Devices and Radiological Health updated an FDA public health notification on April 1, 2003 entitled "Complications Related to the Use of Bone Cement in Treating Compression Fractures of the Spine." It stated, "Complications that relate specifically to the leakage of bone cements include soft tissue damage and nerve root pain and compression. Other reported complications generally associated with the use of bone cements in the spine include pulmonary embolism, respiratory and cardiac failure, abdominal intrusions, . . . and death. Each of these types of complications has been reported in conjunction with use of bone cements in both vertebroplasty and kyphoplasty procedures, two different techniques that employ bone cement to treat spinal compression fractures."

To define the latter, the FDA information continued, "Kyphoplasty, developed in the 1990s, involves introducing a surgical instrument into the vertebral body with the intent to elevate or expand the vertebra. Once this instrument is withdrawn, the space created is then filled with the bone cement mixture. By reducing and fixing the fracture in this way, kyphoplasty procedures may correct deformity and/or restore body height." Although "acrylic bone cements have been used for many years for the fixation of metal and plastic prostheses in joint replacement," these cements "have not been specifically evaluated for the treatment of spinal compression fractures." Because the "existing cements designed for other uses are generally modified for use in treating spinal compression fractures," modification materials and methods can vary from one physician to the next. In addition, "The effects of modified bone cements on the spine and surrounding soft tissues have not been adequately studied to support marketing applications." Therefore, "The Safe Medical Devices Act of 1990 requires hospitals and other user facilities to report deaths and serious injuries associated with the use of medical devices, including bone cement." The FDA also requests that bone cement malfunctions be reported by calling (800) FDA-1088 or writing MedWatch, FDA, HF-2, 5600 Fishers Lane, Rockville, MD 20857.

Center for Devices and Radiological Health. "Complications Related to the Use of Bone Cement in Treating Compression Fractures of the Spine." Available online. URL: http://www.fda.gov/cdrh/safety Downloaded on April 1, 2003.

North American Spine Society. "Percutaneous Vertebral Augmentation." Available online. URL: http://www.spine.org Downloaded on November 11, 2003.

vitamins See NUTRITION.

voice Within the LARYNX or voice box, two bands of smooth muscle tissue form the vocal folds that vibrate as a person sings or speaks. When not producing voice sounds, however, these folds open to ease inhalation. As information from the National Institute on Deafness and Other Communication Disorders (NIDCD) explained, "To produce voice, the brain precisely coordinates a series of events. First, the folds come together in a firm but relaxed way. Once the folds are closed, air from the lungs passes through them, causing vibration and thus making sound. The sound from this vibration then travels through the throat, nose, and mouth (resonating cavities). The size and shape of these cavities, along with the size and shape of the vocal folds, help to determine voice quality." As a further means of distinction between unique speakers, "Variety within an individual voice is the result of lengthening or shortening, tensing or relaxing the vocal folds. Moving the cartilages, or soft, flexible bone-like tissues to which the folds are attached, makes these adjustments possible. For example, shortening and relaxing the vocal folds makes a deep voice; lengthening and tensing them produces a high-pitched voice."

Another NIDCD fact sheet entitled "Statistics on Voice, Speech, and Language" reported, "Approximately 7.5 million people in the United States have trouble using their voices. Disorders of the voice involve problems with pitch, loudness, and quality. Pitch is the highness or lowness of a sound based on the frequency of the sound waves. Loudness is the perceived volume (or amplitude) of the sound, while quality refers to the character or distinctive attributes of a sound. Many people who have normal speaking skills have great difficulty communicating when their vocal apparatus fails. This can occur if the nerves controlling the larynx are impaired because of an accident, a surgical procedure, a viral infection, or cancer." Also according to NIDCD statistics, "Between 6 and 8 million individuals in the United States have some form of language impairment."

As a fact sheet from the American Academy of Otolaryngology—Head and Neck Surgery (AAO—HNS) explained, "Most changes in the voice result from a medical disorder," which may include laryngitis, vocal cord lesions, reflux diseases, vocal cord paralysis, throat cancer, and poor speaking techniques. Regarding the latter, the AAO-HNS said, "Improper or poor speaking technique is caused from speaking at an abnormal or uncomfortable pitch, either too high or too low, and leads to hoarseness and a variety of other voice problems." For example, a trauma to the vocal cords—or an emotional trauma—can cause fatigue of the throat muscles. In addition, "Other factors leading to improper speaking technique include insufficient or improper breathing while talking, specifically breathing from the shoulders or neck area instead of from the lower chest or abdominal area." Thus, "The consequence of this practice is increased tension in the throat and neck muscles, which can cause hoarseness and a variety of symptoms, especially pain and fatigue associated with talking. Voice problems can also occur from using your voice in an unnatural position, such as talking on the phone cradled to your shoulder. This requires excessive tension in the neck and laryngeal muscles, which changes the speaking technique and may result in a voice problem." With STRESS also a factor, voice disorders vary as widely as the people having them. Therefore, treatments differ too, including practices as diverse as speech therapy, the prescription of an antibiotic for a throat infection, the surgical removal of a tumor or polyp, and MASSAGE THERAPY to loosen up the throat muscles, thereby freeing individuals to sing and speak out like themselves again.

American Academy of Otolaryngology—Head and Neck Surgery. "The Most Common Voice Disorders." Available online. URL: http://www.entnet.org/health info/throat Downloaded on July 7, 2003.

National Institute on Deafness and Other Communication Disorders. "Statistics on Voice, Speech and Language." Available online. URL:http://www.nidcd.nih.gov Downloaded on July 7, 2003.

voluntary muscles Being the only one of three types of muscle that people can control does not happen haphazardly. A cooperative effort and tricky timing are needed to get a person to speak, lie down, or run around. While working toward such endeavors, striated bundles of myofibrils first attach themselves with TENDONS to the SKELETAL BONES to round out the musculoskeletal system. This attachment to a corresponding bone then gives each voluntary muscle—and, indeed, the entire body—the capacity to move. For that movement to become intentional means developing a relationship with the brain. Instead of using the tough tendons that tie muscles to bones though, the brain-to-bone connection occurs with motor nerve fibers that weave a highly communicative network system, thus encouraging thought to precede voluntary actions in most of the people most of the time.

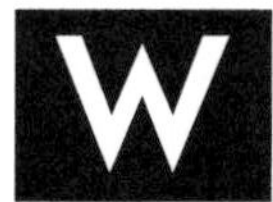

walker With countless designs ready to accommodate an individual's needs, this type of ambulatory device usually has four legs set in a square or rectangular shape with a top bar reaching somewhere around the patient's waistline. As the name implies, the immediate goal is ambulation but with the benefit of helping a person to become more independent, too. For this to be successful, the physician and therapist work with each patient and his or her family to select the right equipment.

As an example, the November 2001 *Rehab: The Interdisciplinary Journal of Rehabilitation* said, "Platform walkers are great for patients who cannot support enough of their weight through their hands and wrists. When the forearm is fully supported and weight bearing, the patient uses less energy for walking and is more stable. The width of the elbows determines the base of support and can make the patient feel very secure." For those not yet ready for a walker, a gait trainer comes recommended to support POSTURE. Reportedly, "Children with severe gross motor dysfunction who are not expected to walk until age 5 or later, if at all, could benefit from using a gait trainer as early as 9–12 months of age. Very young, severely involved children learn to take some of their body weight through their legs as a precursor to assisting with stand pivot transfers, toileting, and perhaps assisted ambulation in later years." Older children and adults may first need upright placement to see if they can tolerate this positioning. However, "If the child has any musculoskeletal deformities (back, hips, knees, and ankles), the orthopedist should be consulted before beginning the program." With medical consent and a patient's proven ability to remain upright for five to 10 minutes, the next step teaches a person to take steps. "This is accomplished by getting on the floor and moving the . . . feet (gently) with your hands." Leaning the patient forward offers another option by stretching and strengthening muscles in the hips and legs, thereby stimulating "some basic reflexes that assist in the performance of stepping reflexes." In either case, "The long-term goal of gait training can vary from reducing flexion contractures and increasing alertness and head control to achieving independent ambulation. By choosing an appropriate gait trainer and teaching the skill of walking, independent functional ambulation can become a reality for many people."

Paleg, Ginny. "Beyond Wheelchairs." Available online. URL: www.rehabpub.com Downloaded on November 12, 2003.

walking More than a form of EXERCISE, the ability to remain mobile without assistance can help to determine a person's quality of life and level of independence. In the presence of DEGENERATIVE JOINT DISEASE, STROKE, PARALYSIS, bone INJURIES, SPINAL CORD INJURY, and musculoskeletal conditions, such as MUSCULAR DYSTROPHY, walking may become impossible or, at least, impaired. IMMOBILIZATION can also occur with AGING as people gradually become more sedentary than they realize, enabling muscles to weaken and, sometimes, ATROPHY. In an attempt to avoid this subtle occurrence, many people find a pedometer helpful in accurately assessing their steps throughout the day.

To encourage older Americans to get more active, the Foot Health Foundation of America—a national health initiative of the American Podiatric Medical Association (APMA)—published "Walking Tips for Seniors." However, most of the suggestions, such as warming up and cooling down, apply to everyone. As the APMA explained, "Stretching improves circulation and decreases build-up of lactic acid—the chemical by-product that causes muscles to ache. It also helps alleviate any muscle stiffness and prevents future muscle strain." Therefore, to warm up muscles, APMA advised, "Before and after walking, allow ample time to perform a few simple movements, stretching the hamstrings, calves, Achilles tendons and shins." With the aid of proper FOOTWEAR, the APMA further suggested, "If possible, walk on grass or dirt paths that are flat, even and well manicured." This not only protects people from FALLING, but "softer ground is more foot-friendly, producing less shock than harder surfaces." To avoid the numbness that can occur in cold weather, "Head to the local mall or walk at an indoor track or exercise facility." In addition, a patient with a circulatory problem, such as DIABETES, should "check your feet daily for redness, blisters or injury. If you experience any numbness, tingling or have wounds or abnormalities of any kind, see a podiatric physician immediately."

With a doctor's approval, most people can slowly increase their pace and/or walking time to get beyond the mild discomforts that may arise. As pointed out by the President's Council on Physical Fitness and Sports, "Some experts say it takes a month of reconditioning to make up for each year of physical inactivity." With patience virtually a key, the activity of walking does not require competition, speed, or high performance yet may require some tips on walking well. To describe an efficient walking style, the site offered these instructions, "Hold head erect and keep back straight and abdomen flat. Toes should point straight ahead and arms should swing loosely at sides. Land on the heel of the foot and roll forward to drive off the ball of the foot. Walking only on the ball of the foot, or in a flat-footed style, may cause fatigue and soreness. Take long, easy strides, but don't strain for distance. When walking up or down hills, or at a very rapid pace, lean forward slightly." With additional advice to "listen to your body when you walk," any symptoms, such as dizziness, pain, or queasiness, signal a cause to stop. Otherwise, "The 'talk test' can help you find the right pace. You should be able to carry on a conversation while walking. If you're too breathless to talk, you're going too fast." Besides, speed is not even necessary. Again according to the President's Council, "Walking burns approximately the same amount of calories per mile as does running, a fact particularly appealing to those who find it difficult to sustain the jarring effects of long distance jogging. Brisk walking one mile in 15 minutes burns just about the same number of calories as jogging an equal distance in 8 $^{1}/_{2}$ minutes." However, elderly persons or those who have been ill may be comfortable walking only a minute or two and then resting before fatiguing begins. For all persons, a relaxed pace and realistic walking time can be slowly established. "After you have been walking for 20 minutes several days a week for one month, start walking 30 minutes per outing. Eventually, your goal should be to get to the place where you can comfortably walk three miles in 45 minutes, but there is no hurry about getting there." Walking should not be the only form of activity. As the site stated, "Walking is good exercise for the legs, heart, and lungs, but it is not a complete exercise program. Persons who limit themselves to walking tend to become stiff and inflexible, with short, tight muscles in the back and the backs of the legs. They also may lack muscle tone and strength in the trunk and upper body." Since these conditions can disturb good POSTURE and become a pain in the back, RESISTANCE TRAINING may help to round out the muscles not used by walking.

Of course, a big problem comes in avoiding a walk. Even when a person has built up strength, boredom with the same old route and routine can become discouraging. To rekindle enthusiasm, the path personally less traveled may be the one to take. Dorothy Foltz-Gray suggested dodging the doldrums by taking walks on a college campus, ambling along a river path or sandy beach, meandering through a zoo or park, and looking for public walking paths converted from out-of-use railroad tracks as listed on www.railtrail.org Likewise, www.ava.org provides the locales of interesting walking trails mentioned by the American Volkssporting Association. For an occasional break, participation in a walkathon offers the added exercise of helping a favorite charity. Then, with a specific sign-up date to jog the memory, walkers may be apt to take that day in stride.

Foltz-Gray, Dorothy. "10 'Can't-Wait' Walks." Available online. URL: http://www.arthritis.org/conditions/exercise/walking/10walks/_5.asp Downloaded on July 21, 2004.

Foot Health Foundation of America. "Walking Tips for Seniors." Available online. URL: http://www.apma.org/seniortips.html Downloaded on February 26, 2003.

President's Council on Physical Fitness and Sports. "Walking for Exercise and Pleasure." Available online. URL: http://www.pueblo.gsa.gov/cic_text/health/walking/walking.htm Downloaded on March 6, 2003.

warm-ups Whether preparing for state championships or getting ready to wash the dog, warming the specific group of muscles that will get a workout improves their flexibility and protects against INJURIES, too. Most of the time, this just means STRETCHING a bit. The American Academy of Orthopaedic Surgeons stated, "Over 58,000 injuries related to ice skating were reported in 2001 according to the U.S. Consumer Product Safety Commission." However, "Orthopaedic surgeons say spending just five minutes stretching before cutting those figure eights can reduce the risk of injury." Otherwise, muscle overuse can occur, especially if cold fibers and tight tendons reduce a person's normal RANGE OF MOTION. To avoid this, warm-ups may include bending one knee with the other leg stretched back for a count of 15. Another option is to "stand with your legs spread far apart. Turn to your left side and slightly bend your left leg. Push on your right hip with your right hand, and hold for a count of 15." Yet another warm-up is to "sit on the floor with your legs spread apart. Keeping your knees straight, extend your left hand and reach to your right heel. Pull your right heel up with your left hand and lean forward. Hold for a count of 15." After doing 10 repetitions of each with one leg, 10 repetitions are done with the other leg. For "toe-ups—Start with your flat feet on the ground and toes pointed straight ahead. Gradually go up on your toes as far as you can and walk on your tiptoes. Repeat 10 times."

As Joe Henderson explained in the March 2001 *Runner's World*, "You don't just step out the door and hit your stride in the first 100 steps. You must shift from one form of inertia (resting) to another (moving), and that transition takes more time than many runners allow." Instead of stretching, however, the writer advised, "A runner warms up best by running." Since runs longer than a half hour generally fall into a normal-, fast-, or long-run category, each has an optimal type of warm-up. For "normal runs: Warm up slowly." For "fast runs: Warm up thoroughly." For "long runs: Warm up well, but not too much." Those who want to take it slower should take up WALKING.

American Academy of Orthopaedic Surgeons. "American Academy of Orthopaedic Surgeons Advises Skaters to Warm Up Before They Go Out on the Ice." Available online. URL: http://www.aaos.org Downloaded on November 27, 2002.

Henderson, Joe. "Joe's Journal: Warming to the Task." *Runner's World* (March 2001): 24.

water workout A self-managed version of HYDROTHERAPY, this EXERCISE program helps the body warm up, increase flexibility and RANGE OF MOTION, and strengthen the musculoskeletal system without encountering the resistance of GRAVITY. This can be especially beneficial in providing a means of exercise for those unsteady on their feet. The water not only cushions a FALL but avoids negative pull on the joints and limbs already stressed by conditions such as ARTHRITIS or DEGENERATIVE DISK DISEASE.

According to the Mayo Foundation for Medical Education and Research, "Done correctly, water workouts can give you the same fitness gains as land workouts, including better balance. And water is hospitable to just about everyone, enabling those with arthritis, disabilities or injuries, those recovering from illness or surgery, and those who are pregnant or overweight to exercise safely and effectively." According to the Mayo Foundation, "Part of the reason for the popularity of water-based workouts is the fact that water's buoyancy supports your weight and significantly reduces stress on your weight-bearing joints, bones and muscles. For those with injuries, the pressure of the water also reduces swelling. If the water is warm, then the heat relaxes muscles and eases joint stiffness." In addition,

"Another benefit of water workouts is the fact that they incorporate resistance training. . . . Simply walking in water with correct posture will work your abdominal muscles." Besides water walking, the exercises of water running and water aerobics can be useful too—an especially interesting challenge since "today, millions of Americans regularly work out in swimming pools, including those who can't swim a stroke."

Mayo Foundation for Medical Education and Research. "Water Workouts: A Cool Way to Exercise Without Stressing Your Joints, Bones or Muscles." Available online. URL: http://www.mayoclinic.com Downloaded on July 8, 2002.

weight, effects of In 2002, the Department of Health and Human Services reported that approximately one-third of American adults have been classified as obese. In addition, about nine million children, ages six to 19, share this category—triple the number reported in 1980. The President's Council on Physical Fitness and Sports said, "Physical inactivity contributes to 300,000 preventable deaths a year in the United States." When put another way, "Some 40% of deaths in the United States are caused by behavior patterns that could be modified." As examples of those modifications, "Significant health benefits can be obtained by including a moderate amount of physical activity (e.g. 30 minutes of brisk walking or raking leaves, 15 minutes of running, or 45 minutes of playing volleyball)."

The article "Exercise and Weight Control" clarified, "Overweight and over-fat do not always mean the same thing. Some people are quite muscular and weigh more than the average for their age and height. However, their body composition, the amount of fat versus lean body mass (muscle, bone, organs and tissue), is within a desirable range. This is true for many athletes." For people in general, "Experts say that body fat for women should be about 20 percent, 15 percent for men." To go by body composition instead of the standard height-weight tables, "An easy self-test you can do is to pinch the thickness of the fat folds at your waist and abdomen. If you can pinch an inch or more of fat (make sure no muscle is included) chances are you have too much body fat." Should loss of weight prove desirable, "Learning how to balance energy intake (calories in food) with energy output (calories expended through physical activity) will help you achieve your desired weight." To accomplish this, "The most powerful formula is the combination of dietary modification with exercise. By increasing your daily physical activity and decreasing your caloric input you can lose excess weight in the most efficient and healthful way." As a general guideline, "Each pound of fat your body stores represents 3,500 calories of unused energy. In order to lose one pound, you would have to create a calorie deficit of 3,500 calories by either taking in 3,500 less calories over a period of time than you need or doing 3,500 calories worth of exercise." However, "It is recommended that no more than two pounds (7,000 calories) be lost per week for lasting weight loss." On the other hand, "If you already have a lean figure and want to keep it, you should exercise regularly and eat a balanced diet that provides enough calories to make up for the energy you expend." To give an idea of how many calories that one hour of exercise might use, the site's energy expenditure chart said that 60 minutes of circuit weight training burns up 756 calories; aerobic dancing 546; tennis 312; swimming 288; light housework 246; ballroom dancing 210; walking at 2 mph, 198; bicycling at 5 mph, 174; and resting or sleeping 90.

To know which activity will work best requires a realistic assessment of one's interests, natural ability, and, most importantly, overall health. For instance, most people can lose around 320 calories playing golf if they carry their own clubs for an hour, but the math is not that simple. In other words, those who weigh more will burn more calories while those who weigh less will use fewer calories because of the variations in energy used to carry one's own poundage. Regardless of an individual's weight or size, however, that same round of golf can exacerbate DEGENERATIVE DISKS in the lower back, annoy a shoulder's ROTATOR CUFF, or aggravate JOINTS already burdened with ARTHRITIS. Similarly, people with LEGS affected by OSTEOARTHRITIS might want to avoid playing basketball to burn calories as that can be like playing with fire at the KNEES. Also, if a body in general has felt the stress of excess weight, the weight-bearing joints may have begun to break down without any signs yet discernible.

As evidence, the *NHS News: The Nurses' Health Study Annual Newsletter* reported, "New data from the Nurses' Health Study suggest that a woman's weight may be the strongest predictor of whether she will need a total hip replacement due to osteoarthritis. Overall, we found that being overweight at a young age was a greater predictor than being overweight later in life. Compared to lean women, those who were obese at age 18 had a five-fold increase in the risk of hip replacement, and those who were obese after menopause had a threefold increase in risk." By contrast, another news brief, "Physical Activity and the Risk of Hip Fractures," on the same page said, "In the Nurses' Health Study, women who walked for at least four hours a week had a 40 percent reduction in risk."

Regarding the impact of weight on muscle, AGING has a bearing too. According to an article in the *Daytona Sun Times,* "As we age there is a natural tendency to lose muscle, and we also are less vigorous in our physical activity, which results in further muscle loss." Then "this loss of muscle tissue results in a decreasing metabolic rate. Lose five pounds of muscle, your calories burned per 24 hours decrease by about 250. While this may not sound like much, it adds up." Which means, "If you continue to eat as you did when you were younger, you will gain a pound of fat in about 14 days. Over a 20-week period you will gain 10 pounds." However, "With a proper exercise stimulus, dormant muscles can be reclaimed. When you get back the muscle that requires 250 calories a day . . . , what used to be an insidious weight-gain problem will become an insidious weight-loss technique."

With stronger muscle power, more activities become possible and more appealing, too. Although this may be important to adults, it is particularly so for children. Avery D. Faigenbaum stated, "In addition to providing youngsters with an opportunity to make friends and have fun, their regular participation in well-designed physical activity programs has the potential to enhance the health and well-being of boys and girls. It helps strengthen bone, reduce body fat . . . and reduce symptoms of anxiety and depression." Healthful activities, however, do not have to mean competitive sports. "While kids do not need to become All-American athletes, all children and adolescents need to participate in physical activities that enhance and maintain cardiovascular and musculoskeletal health." School athletics may well be part of this endeavor, but "we need to encourage kids to run, jump, kick, turn, twist and hop. Focusing on sport-specific skills over fundamental fitness abilities not only discriminates against kids whose motors skills are not as well developed, but may also lead to injury."

Besides the advantage of establishing healthy habits that carry over into the adult years, heightened physical activity among youth can increase BONE MASS, in essence, banking bone from which musculoskeletal strength can be drawn throughout life. This offers one of the best preventatives for OSTEOPOROSIS and other conditions involving bone loss in later years, especially when well-balanced NUTRITION accompanies regular EXERCISE. However, even that sensible approach will not be ideal for all of the people all of the time. According to the Agency for Healthcare Research and Quality (AHRQ), "Weight goals for younger people may not be appropriate for the elderly, for whom weight may be protective." Reporting on the eight-year AHRQ study that "retrospectively analyzed a nationally representative sample of 7,527 community-dwelling people age 70 and older," the article summarized the following interesting facts. "The thin group had the highest mortality rate (54 percent), the obese group the lowest (33 percent), and normal-weight elderly were in the middle (37 percent). Adjustment for demographic factors functional status, and health service use, such as hospitalizations and nursing home visits, still showed that compared with normal-weight older people, obese older people were 14 percent less likely to die, and thin people were 1.5 times more likely to die. Further adjustment for income and medical conditions did not substantially alter these results." Therefore, a protective padding of fat can apparently have a healthful purpose, perhaps by giving reserves to an octogenarian who gets a bad case of flu. For most people though, excess weight has adverse affects on all body systems, including muscles, bones, and joints. To keep up with oneself may involve a frank, ongoing assessment of changing needs, but fortunately, most people can, in time, adapt.

Agency for Healthcare Research and Quality. "Elderly Health." Available online. URL: http://www. ahrq.gov Downloaded on March 4, 2003.

Department of Health and Human Services. "Obesity Still On The Rise, New Data Shown." Available online. URL: http://www.hhs.gov/news/press/2002pres/20021008b.html Downloaded on October 8, 2002.

Faigenbaum, Avery D. "Physical Activity for Youth: Tips for Keeping Kids Healthy and Fit." Available online. URL: http://www.acsm.org/health+fitness/fit_society.htm Downloaded on July 1, 2004.

Nurses' Health Study. "The Impact of Weight on Cancer Risk." *The Nurses' Health Study Annual Newsletter* 10 (2003): 1–2.

President's Council on Physical Fitness and Sports. "Exercise and Weight Control." Available online. URL: http://fitness.gov Downloaded on November 13, 2003.

President's Council on Physical Fitness and Sports. "Physical Activity and Health." Available online. URL: http://fitness.gov Downloaded on November 13, 2003.

Tasso. "Body Fat: Hard Facts About Soft Tissue." *Daytona Sun Times* (March 28/April 3, 2003), p. 13.

weight training See RESISTANCE TRAINING.

wheelchair To assist mobility in nonambulatory patients, one wheelchair size no longer fits all. Once heavy and bulky, this equipment weighed 50 or more pounds in widths that sometimes required removing interior doors from their hinges. Now, compact chairs of lightweight material weighing 25–30 pounds come in widths to accommodate a person's size as well as his or her living quarters. Also, the addition of easy-to-manage features, such as adjustable footrests or padded arms, and the comfort of ERGONOMIC designs further aid patients who need a seated mode of in-house transportation. When outdoors, a collapsible frame fits into the average auto trunk. In fact, automation of the chair itself enables travel without tiring, particularly valuable for patients with weakened arm muscles. To decide which features will be needed, factors such as a person's strength, age, weight, and mental capacity will be considered by the primary physician as well as the physical therapist involved in the patient's treatment to assure a customized fit.

whiplash This descriptive term for an injury to the cervical VERTEBRAE illustrates the moment when the impact of a collision or vehicular accident whips the neck forward and then back with a lash. In some instances, pain occurs immediately. In many instances, though, a whiplash injury may not be apparent for hours later, thus evoking suspicions in matters such as automobile insurance claims. Some contend that people in heavily industrialized nations primarily experience this insurable complaint, but people in nonindustrialized nations rarely ride in cars.

To clarify the conditions concerning this painful topic, the National Institute of Neurological Disorders and Stroke stated, "Whiplash—a soft tissue injury to the neck—is also called neck sprain or neck strain. It is characterized by a collection of symptoms that occur following damage to the neck, usually because of sudden extension and flexion." Commonly resulting from an automobile accident, the disorder "may include injury to intervertebral joints, discs, and ligaments, cervical muscles, and nerve roots." Although pain may delay for several days, "In addition to neck pain, other symptoms may include neck stiffness, injuries to the muscles and ligaments (myofascial injuries), headache, dizziness, abnormal sensations such as burning or prickling (paresthesias), or shoulder or back pain. In addition, some people experience cognitive, somatic, or psychological conditions such as memory loss, concentration impairment, nervousness/irritability, sleep disturbances, fatigue, or depression." Although symptoms vary according to the severity of the accident, so does treatment, which "may include pain medication, nonsteroidal anti-inflammatory drugs, antidepressants, muscle relaxants, and a cervical collar (usually worn for 2 to 3 weeks). Range of motion exercises, physical therapy, and cervical traction may also be prescribed. Supplemental heat application may relieve muscle tension." For the first 24 hours, however, ice may help reduce SWELLING.

Although most patients recover within a few months, some continue to have frequent headaches and neck pain. Assuming no bone FRACTURES or HERNIATED DISKS remain undetected, SPINAL MANIPULATION and MASSAGE THERAPY can sometimes be beneficial as can ULTRASOUND THERAPY, TRACTION, and PHYSICAL THERAPY. Alternating COLD THERAPY with HEAT THERAPY generally helps PAIN MANAGEMENT, too. To be specific though, the symptoms and circumstances of each individual make the advice of a respected therapist or physician crucial in finding an effective course of treatment.

See also SPRAIN; STRAIN.

National Institute of Neurological Disorders and Stroke (NINDS). "NINDS Whiplash Information Page." Available online. URL: http://www.ninds.nih.gov/health Downloaded on July 1, 2001.

wrist Between the HAND and the forearm, eight CARPAL BONES comprise the wrist. Classified as part of the APPENDICULAR SKELETON, these two rows of wrist bones extend into the longer bones of the metacarpals that fan out and frame the palm of each hand, making them prone to FRACTURES in a FALL or to REPETITIVE MOTION DISORDERS, such as CARPAL TUNNEL SYNDROME. Although the carpals may be quite small and non–weight bearing, their high RANGE OF MOTION makes them an active site for temporary flares of INFLAMMATION or ongoing conditions, such as ARTHRITIS, OSTEOARTHRITIS, and RHEUMATISM. With their normally lubricated, intricate system of JOINTS, however, the orchestration of these small bones allows for graceful gestures with the wave of a hand.

wryneck Similar to TORTICOLLIS, this condition occurs as muscle CONTRACTURES produce a painful side tilt to the head. An acute case may result from a cold, a mild trauma, or a muscle cramp that comes from sleeping in an awkward position. Despite the sharp discomfort, this usually passes with heat, time, and neck-cradling rest. A chronic wryneck, however, presents a less temporary problem as a muscle SPASM or irritated spinal nerves require additional treatment, which varies according to the causative and severity.

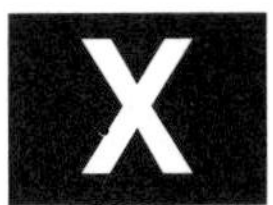

xiphoid process The Greek word for *sword* lends its name to this smallest, lowest part of the STERNUM, while the process itself may refer to the slow ossification of childhood cartilage into adult bone. Although no RIBS attach to this centrally located sword tip, some ABDOMINAL MUSCLES do, with exercise—or the lack thereof—potentially affecting the whole process.

X-ray With short wavelengths of electromagnetic RADIATION penetrating soft tissue, this type of radiography produces lights and shadows on a photographic plate. The May 2003 issue of *Radiology Info* explained, "X-ray imaging is the fastest and easiest way for a physician to view and assess broken bones, cracked skulls and injured backbones. At least two films are taken of a bone, and often three films if the problem is around a joint (knee, elbow, or wrist). X-rays also play a key role in orthopedic surgery and the treatment of sports injuries." With the ability to show hairline FRACTURES, bone chips, and BONE LOSS, such as occurs with OSTEOPOROSIS, "Bone x-rays are an essential tool in orthopedic surgery, such as spinal repair, joint replacements, or fracture reductions." Metal pins or plates from previous SURGERIES, however, will keep a radiologist from performing this procedure as will any possibility of a pregnancy. Otherwise, patients will simply be asked to remove metal objects that can obscure the image. To get a better look at bone density, tumors, and soft tissue though, other diagnostic tools, such as MAGNETIC RESONANCE IMAGING, COMPUTED TOMOGRAPHY or ULTRASONOGRAPHY, offer a more likely choice.

Radiology Info. "Radiography-Bone." Available online. URL: http://www.radiologyinfo.org Downloaded on November 14, 2003.

Z

Z disks This pair of thin, dark lines attach across striated muscle, holding individual fibers together with the unit of contraction known as the sarcomere located in between.

zygomatic arch Great cheekbones usually mean a shapely, pleasing prominence of the zygoma or zygomatic bone, which includes the curve of each lower eye socket as well as the arch of each cheek. In the original Greek, *zygon* referred to the yoke connecting two oxen or other animals to a cart or plow. In the musculoskeletal system, this yoke of facial bones may cart around a case of sinusitis.

APPENDIXES

I. Table of Bone Systems and Disorders
II. Table of Muscle Systems and Disorders
III. Table of Connectors and Joints
IV. Tips on Receiving Quality Health Care
V. Diagnosing Internet Information on Health
VI. National Organizations of Interest
VII. Internet Journals and Magazines
VIII. Related Web Sites

APPENDIX I
TABLE OF BONE SYSTEMS AND DISORDERS

At birth, most people have about 270 bones, many of which later harden or fuse. For instance, in infants, the four or five bones in the sacral region eventually form one sacrum, while another three to five bones gradually become the coccyx. Similarly, the ilium, ischium, and pubis fuse into the pelvic girdle. In addition, as softer tissue and cartilage throughout a child's musculoskeletal system turn into bone during the process of ossification, the fontanels or soft spots of the skull slowly come together as the more stationary suture joints. Sometimes, though, this just does not happen—for example, if joints fail to harden or an overgrowth of bone tissue almost anywhere in the body results in a skeletal deformity. Aside from these rare but potential disorders—and those debilitating accidents or illnesses that can compromise or weaken anybody's bones, most people reach their adult years with a tally of 206 bones well formed and distributed for optimal function in either the axial or the appendicular skeleton:

I. Axial Skeleton—These 80 axial bones include 29 in the head region and 51 in the trunk or torso. With the exception of the spinal column, the axial bones often remain in place and so will usually be less bothered with overuse injuries or repetitive motion disorders. They are more apt to acquire secondary infections as the result of the many types of viruses, bacteria, or allergens that can affect the facial or sinus cavities. Also, the central position of the axial skeleton places the bones out there in front if the body happens to receive a hard blow. Then, as with any bone, a fracture or bone break will be likely with the severity of the condition depending on the force of impact. Bone tumors and bone cancer can occur in the axial skeleton too. However, degenerative bone and joint conditions, such as osteoporosis or osteoarthritis, generally affect the more mobile regions of the appendicular skeleton or those bearing most of the body's weight. Although these disorders can certainly involve the spinal column, most of the vertebrae from the neck to the tailbone characteristically come with fibrous, cartilaginous disks set between each bone to cushion and protect the body from jolts. Then again, these disks may themselves herniate or succumb to wear and tear. However, proper body weight, nutrients, ergonomics, and exercise can usually help a person to maintain the axial skeleton as well as the entire musculoskeletal system.

a. Skull—contains a total of 22 bones with those of the face, cranium, mouth, and ears comprising the full head that protectively houses the brain and locates the body's sensory devices of taste, smell, sound, and sight.

1. Cranial—eight flat bones attached with suture joints having teethlike protrusions to hold the cranium together in the back and side portions of the head

- Frontal bone—seen as the forehead and upper portion fronting the head but also forms the upper part of the eye sockets
- Two parietal bones—forming the top and sides of the head
- Occipital bone—a saucer-shaped bone shaping the back of the head and attaching to the first vertebra in the spinal column
- Two temporal bones—maplike bones on the lower part of either side of the head containing cavities for the ears

- Sphenoid bone—at the base of the skull
- Ethmoid bone—small bone with air spaces between the eye sockets

2. Facial—14 irregular bones that shape the unique face of each individual and that articulate through suture joints, an exception being the mobile synovial joint of the lower jawbone designed to allow a person to speak and eat

- Mandible—large, U-shaped bone of the lower jaw with sockets for securing the lower teeth and with either end projecting upward to provide a mobile joint on either side for ease of movement in eating and vocalizing
- Two maxilla bones—large bones of the upper jaw forming a facial arrowhead shape pointing up with a cavity in the middle to accommodate the nose
- Two zygomatic bones—irregularly shaped and arching to form the prominence of the cheekbones as well as the lower portion of each eye socket
- Two nasal bones—forming a tiny triangle of bone between the maxilla and securing the cartilage of the nose
- Vomer bone—thin, triangle-shaped bone named for the Latin word for plow and separating the lower and back portions of the nasal septum
- Two lacrimal bones—small, fragile bones pertaining to tears and residing in the inner part of the orbital cavity formed to accommodate the eyes
- Two turbinates—from the Latin "turbo," a whorl-shaped bone extending from the ethmoid and covered with mucous membrane along the side wall of the nose
- Two palate bones—forming the hard plate in the roof of the mouth with the soft muscular palate behind

3. Hyoid bone—one small, U-shaped bone located within the throat at the base of the tongue and, therefore, not articulating with other bones in the body

4. Middle ear—six tiny bones also known as ossicles

- Two malleus—small hammerlike or malletlike bones connecting the other two bones of the middle ear
- Two incus—tiny, anvil-shaped bones residing in the midportion of either ear
- Two stapes—shaped like a stirrup and transmitting vibrations from the middle ear ossicles to the inner ear

b. Torso or trunk of the body consists of 51 centrally located bones including the 26 vertebrae, the sternum, and 24 ribs—the latter of which work with the breastbone in protecting the vital organs of the heart and lungs. The flexible spinal column protects the spinal cord and assists the movement of the entire musculoskeletal system. To accommodate these functions, the structure of the spine is itself flexible. For instance, the cervical vertebrae of the neck feature the smallest bones in the spinal column, whereas the lumbar vertebrae of the back present the largest, strongest bones needed to maintain posture. The fused bones of the sacrum have horizontal ridges with openings at the ends to allow easy passage of various nerves and blood vessels vital to movement and bone health. The small, fused bones of the coccyx also have a structure unlike the typical spinal vertebrae, but their simple shell-like ridges provide a place for the muscles of the buttocks to attach.

1. Vertebral column—26 irregularly shaped bones of the spine located within the central part of the skeleton to assist posture, protect the spinal cord, support the head, and provide a connection for the ribs, sternum, and pelvic girdle, thus including the five regions of the spinal column listed below

- Seven cervical vertebrae—irregularly shaped bones of the neck or upper spinal column, each number prefaced by a C, identifying the specific location or function; for instance, the ring-shaped C1 vertebra, known as the atlas, supports the skull; C2, the axis, allows for rotation as the head turns from side to side or back and forth in a nod; and C7, the prominent vertebra, connects the cervical area to the next spinal region

- Twelve thoracic vertebrae—irregular shaped and numbered T1 through T12, located between the cervical vertebrae of the neck and the lumbar vertebrae of the back with attachments for the ribs and the chest (thorax) making up the rib cage or thoracic cage that protects the heart and lungs
- Five lumbar vertebrae—the back part of the body between the ribs and the pelvis with the individual vertebrae identified as L1 through L5 of the spinal column, located between the thoracic and the sacral vertebrae
- Five sacral bones—gradually fusing into one sacrum shaped like a triangle at the back of the pelvis between the hip bones; the large bone connects to L5, the last lumbar vertebra, at its base and points down toward its connection with the coccyx or tailbone
- Two to four coccygeal bones—slowly fusing to form one coccyx or tailbone of the spinal column

2. Ribs—24 curved bones that form the rib cage, which assists respiration and protects and accommodates the vital organs of the heart and lung

- Fourteen true ribs—first seven pairs, which attach to the sternum or breastbone
- Six false ribs—three pairs, which attach to the ribs above rather than directly to the sternum
- Four floating ribs—two pairs, referred to as costa or costal, ending in a bed of muscle

3. Sternum—The long, flat breastbone consists of three parts: the upper manubrium, the middle body of the gladiolus, and the lower xiphoid process. By articulating with the true ribs and clavicle, or collarbone, the sternum provides a place of attachment for various muscles needed for the body to bend, move, and breathe. The breastbone also forms the protective front wall of the chest.

II. Appendicular Skeleton—These 126 bones include 64 in the upper extremities of the arms, wrists, and hands as well as the 62 bones of the lower extremities of the legs, ankles, and feet. At birth, genetic defects and biomechanical flaws may result in the malformation of one or more of these bones. Those conditions will often be correctable with therapeutic exercise, surgery, or orthotic devices. However, as a person becomes more mobile, the strong fibrous ligaments connecting the bones of the appendicular skeleton to one another and to their highly mobile joints can get quite a workout. Then, some possible disorders include pulled or torn ligaments, overuse syndromes, and repetitive motion disorders as well as degenerative conditions. In addition, a sports injury or other type of accident can result in a bone break, fracture, or even the loss of a limb. The possibility of bone cancer, although slim, also exists as does necrosis or bone death, which can result if the blood supply to the bone has been hindered for even a relatively short amount of time. More likely, though, will be the painful effects of arthritis as joints wear with age or under the burden of excess weight, excess usage, or, ironically, lack of use. Indeed, barring a devastating accident or illness, adequate exercise and activity—along with good nutrition—can help the highly flexible appendicular skeleton to regain and retain its remarkable range of motion throughout a person's life.

a. Upper extremities—The 64 bones of the upper region include 10 bones in the shoulder and arm, 16 in the wrist, and 38 in the hand.

1. Pectoral or shoulder girdle—Consisting of a pair of shoulder blades (scapulae) and collarbones (clavicles), this stabilizing part of the appendicular skeleton gives a place

for the upper limbs to attach themselves securely and yet freely swing, enabling the upper body to move with the greatest range of motion.

- Two clavicle bones—pair of rodlike bones extending from either side of the front of the breastbone above the first rib and ending in the prominent projections of the acromion above each shoulder joint, thereby acting as a supportive or stabilizing device
- Two scapulae or shoulder blades—pair of flat, triangular bones extending from either side of the back of the vertebral column into the acromion with bony projections occurring both in the frontal and posterior portions of the skeleton, thereby providing a place for strong muscles to attach to the chest and back

2. Arm—Extending from either shoulder, these upper limbs consist of the forearm and the upper arm with a total of three long bones in each appendage.

- Two humerus—pair of long bones forming the upper arm and cradling into the ball-and-socket joint of each shoulder blade and then fitting into a hinge joint at the elbow to connect the upper arm to the ulna bone in the forearm
- Two ulnas—larger of the two bones in the forearm, articulating with the wrist at one end and with the upper arm in a hinge joint at the elbow, where it also joins with the smaller radius in a pivot joint
- Two radius—smaller, more mobile bone in the forearm located on the side of the thumb with points of articulation in the wrist bones and in the elbow

3. Wrist—Located between the hands and the arms on either side of the appendicular skeleton, these 16 bones come in eight pairs of small carpal bones arranged in two rows of four, a highly mobile, interlinking pattern that allows the bones to slide across one another as they move in activity or gesture.

- Two scaphoid
- Two lunate
- Two triquetrum
- Two pisiform
- Two trapezium
- Two trapezoid
- Two capitate
- Two hamate

4. Hand—With 16 pairs on either side, these 38 bones support a flexible system that includes strong tendons and muscular strapping devices to guide and hold the intricate network of nerves comprising the sense of touch.

- 10 metacarpal bones—five long metacarpals forming each palm and articulating with the wrist carpals at one end and the phalanges at the other
- 28 phalanges or finger bones—three phalanges in each finger and two in each thumb

b. Lower extremities—The 62 bones of the lower extremities include 10 hip and leg bones, 14 ankle bones, and 38 foot bones, each of which more than carries its weight in upholding and mobilizing the body.

1. Pelvic girdle or hips—Originally, the two hip bones consists of three bones, the ilium, ischium, and pubis bones, slowly fused into one pair. Between them, the large, flat sacrum forms a bond, too, with the fused coccyx below completing the strong, supportive system of the pelvic girdle. When viewed on the flattened surface of a photograph, this looks like a large, bone-bleached butterfly. An upper perspective, however, presents the outline of a basin, or perhaps, a fortress, with the posterior walls of the hips, sacrum, and coccyx forming the rear and the pubic bone creating an arch along the front wall.

In males, this design takes on a narrower, more elongated shape. In females, the pelvis widens to accommodate childbirth. In either sex, various cavities and surface ridges in and around the bones provide a gripping design and also a sturdy edifice for snugly attaching strong muscles and the highly mobile lower limbs.

2. Leg—These eight bones come in four pairs distributed in two appendages or lower limbs on either side of the body. Not only do the legs uphold the body's weight, they allow movement as a person learns to crawl, walk, run, jump, skip, or kneel—often in that chronological order.

- Two femurs or thighbones—longest bone in the body, singly upholding each upper leg with a ball-and-socket joint attaching it to the acetabulum, the cupped hollow of the hip bone, at one end while a hinge joint makes a connection with the lower leg at the knee
- Two patellas or kneecaps—small, triangle-shaped flat bones capping the front of the leg joints and enabling movement by their connection with the thigh muscle in the upper leg and their attachment (with the help of securing ligaments) to the tibia of the lower leg
- Two tibias or shinbones—the larger of the two bones in each lower leg with two articulating facets in the knee joint and an attachment to one tarsal in the ankle joint
- Two fibulas—the smaller of the two bones in each lower leg, located on the outside with the lower end forming part of the ankle joint and the upper end articulating with the tibia rather than making a direct connection with the knee

3. Ankle—With seven pairs occurring between the leg and foot on either side, these 14 interlinking bones consist of chunky tarsals, the largest pair being the calcaneus or heel bones to which the calf muscles of each leg attach, thereby providing liftoff during locomotion.

- Two talus
- Two calcaneus or heel bones
- Two navicular
- Two cuboid
- Two internal cuneiform
- Two middle cuneiform
- Two external cuneiform

4. Foot—Similar in design to the hand, these 38 bones are smaller still with 19 sets on either side. Although they literally form the lowest bones of the appendicular skeleton, their health holds a key position in determining a person's mobility and independence as the feet bear the weight of the entire body.

- 10 metatarsals—five long pairs, extending from the tarsals of the ankle to the phalanges of the toes in the form of an arch that enables the feet to sustain the body's weight
- 28 phalanges—short toe bones with 14 in either foot consisting of the two phalanges of the big toe and three in each of the other toes

APPENDIX II

TABLE OF MUSCLE SYSTEMS AND DISORDERS

The skeleton provides a frame for the body, but the muscles present the picture. Not only do they reveal a person's overall health and fitness by their tautness or laxity, but their performance can show a motion picture or a still life. When in good working order, muscles usually move in pairs by opposition, such as occurs in flexion and extension or push and pull. They enable a person to lift a bag of groceries, raise an eyebrow, and lift a finger. Without muscles, the bones would fold like an umbrella. With them, a body can maintain upright posture, mobility, continence, and the dignity of daily activity. If a part refuses to move, the resulting disorder often indicates a flawed or severed connection of some kind. This may be due to the tearing of a tendon in an accident or sports injury that disconnected a particular muscle from its corresponding bone. Disruption of movement can also occur because of interference in the nerve impulses from brain to muscle to bone, such as happens in multiple sclerosis. Other conditions, such as muscular dystrophy, can cause muscle wasting or atrophy—as can a relentless lack of activity. Conversely, too much activity and too little hydration, rest, or nutrition can result in muscle fatigue. In general though, unless an injury, illness, or genetic disorder dictates otherwise, muscles were meant to be used—not necessarily for show but as part of a living picture shaped by sensible choice and exercise.

MUSCLES OF THE HEAD AND NECK

aryepiglottic assists in closing the larynx
auricularis moves the ear
buccinator facilitates movement in the cheek and enables the mouth to close
corrugator supercilii creases the brow or forehead
cricothyroid elongates and tightens the vocal cords
depressor anguli oris turns down the mouth
depressor labii inferioris pulls down the lower lip
digastric lifts the hyoid bone and lowers the mandible to allow swallowing
frontalis lifts the brow
genioglossus withdraws the tongue
geniohyoid lifts the hyoid bone and lowers the mandible
hyoglossus lowers the tongue
inferior constrictor muscle of pharynx assists swallowing
inferior oblique aids eye movement
inferior rectus lowers the eye
intrinsic muscles of tongue allows the movement needed to speak, eat, and swallow
lateral cricoarytenoid adducts and assists the larynx
lateral pterygoid allows the mandible to lower
lateral rectus abducts the eye
levator anguli oris lifts the lips in a smile
levator labii superioris lifts the upper lip
levator labii superioris alaeque nasi lifts the upper lip and flares the nostrils
levator palpebrae superioris lifts the upper eyelid
levator veli palatini elevates the soft palate of the mouth
longus capitis allows the neck to flex
longus colli flexes and rotates the neck
masseter lifts the mandible and allows the mouth to close
medial pterygoid allows flexible movement in the mandible
medial rectus adducts the eye
mentalis lifts and creases the chin in a pout

middle constrictor muscle of pharynx assists swallowing
mylohyoid elevates the hyoid and floor of the mouth
nasalis flexes the nostrils
oblique arytenoid adducts cartilage in the larynx
obliquus capitis inferior rotates the axial joint and allows head movement
obliquus capitis superior allows flexion of the upper cervical vertebrae
omohyoid lowers the hyoid and larynx
orbicularis oculi closes the eye and assists tearing with a blink
orbicularis oris purses the lips
palatoglossus lifts the back of the tongue and aids swallowing
palatopharyngeus lifts the larynx and assists swallowing
platysma draws the mouth down and wrinkles the chin
posterior cricoarytenoid abducts and rotates cartilage around the larynx
procerus allows the forehead to express a frown
rectus capitis anterior flexes the upper neck
rectus capitis lateralis allows joint flexion near the jugular
risorius pulls back the mouth
salpingopharyngeus assists the auditory canal during swallowing
scalenus anterior aids inhalation
scalenus medius aids inhalation
scalenus minimus assists the upper membrane of the lungs
scalenus posterior aids inhalation
semispinalis capitis extends, rotates, and moves the head to one side
splenius capitis rotates the neck and holds the head up high
splenius cervicis extends and rotates the neck
stapedius assists the middle ear
sternocleidomastoid flexes the neck, rotates the head, and raises the sternum
sternohyoid lower the hyoid bone
sternothyroid lowers the larynx
styloglossus lifts and pulls back the tongue
stylohyoid elevates the hyoid bone and moves the larynx to aid swallowing
stylopharyngeus assists swallowing
superior constrictor muscle of pharynx assists swallowing
superior oblique varies movement in the eye
superior rectus lifts the eye
temporalis closes the jaw
temporoparietalis moves the scalp
tensor tympani aids the ossicles of the ear
tensor veli palati tightens the soft palate
thyroarytenoid shortens and relaxes the vocal cords
thyroepiglottic helps the larynx to close
thyrohyoid lifts the larynx and lowers the hyoid bone
transverse arytenoid adducts cartilage in the larynx
uvulae forms the soft mass hanging from the back roof of the mouth
vocalis shortens and relaxes the vocal cords
zygomaticus major lifts the corners of the mouth
zygomaticus minor lifts and turns the upper lip

MUSCLES OF THE THORAX

diaphragm aids respiratory function
external intercostal lifts the ribs to aid breathing
innermost intercostal assists respiration
internal intercostal lifts the ribs and assists respiration
levatores costarum elevates the ribs
pectoralis major adducts and rotates the arm and flexes the elbow
pectoralis minor lifts the ribs and pulls the scapula down and forward
serratus posterior inferior aids exhalation
serratus posterior superior aids inhalation
subcostal lowers the lower ribs
transversus thoracis lowers the upper ribs

MUSCLES OF THE BACK

deltoid abducts and rotates the upper arm
erector spinae lengthens the spine
iliocostalis lumborum flexes and lengthens the spine
infraspinatus rotates the arm and stabilizes the shoulder

interspinales allows the spine to extend
intertransversarii flexes the spinal column
latissimus dorsi assists breathing and varied movements in the arms and ribs
levatores costarum lifts the ribs
levator scapulae raises the shoulder
longissimus thoracis lengthens the spine
multifidus rotates the spinal column
rectus capitis posterior major extends and rotates the upper neck
rectus capitis posterior minor extends the upper neck joint
rhomboid major draws up and rotates the shoulder
rhomboid minor draws up and rotates the shoulder
rotatores allows the spinal column to rotate
semispinalis lengthens and flexes the spine
serratus posterior inferior aids exhalation
serratus posterior superior aids inhalation
spinalis thoracis allows flexion of the spine
splenius capitis lengthens and rotates the neck vertebrae
splenius cervicis lengthens and rotates the neck
supraspinatus abducts the arm and offers shoulder support
teres major adducts the arm and stabilizes the shoulder joint
teres minor rotates the arm and strengthens the shoulder
transversospinalis extends the spinal column
trapezius raises the arm and rotates the shoulder

MUSCLES OF THE ABDOMEN

diaphragm assists breathing
external oblique supports the abdomen, aids exhalation, and rotates the torso
internal oblique abducts, supports, and rotates the torso and assists respiration
psoas major rotates and flexes the hips
psoas minor provides some support of the torso
pyramidalis supports the rectum
quadratus lumborum flexes the torso
rectus abdominis enables the torso to flex
transversus abdominis assists breathing and upholds the abdominal wall

MUSCLES OF THE PELVIC REGION

adductor brevis abducts the hip
adductor longus abducts and rotates the hips
adductor magnus abducts and rotates the hips, affecting the hamstring
bulbospongiosus assists in urination and, in males, ejaculation
coccygeus provides pelvic support
cremaster pulls in the testes
dartos wrinkles the skin of the scrotum
deep transverse perineal upholds the organs in the pelvic floor
gluteus maximus extends, rotates, and supports the hips
gluteus medius abducts and rotates the hips and tilts the pelvis on ambulation
gluteus minimus abducts and rotates the hips
iliacus flexes and rotates the hips from the spine
iliococcygeus provides pelvic support
inferior gemellus assists stability and rotation of the hips
ischiocavernous facilitates an erection of the penis
levator ani provides pelvic support
obturator internus stabilizes the hips and allows lateral hip rotation or sway
pectineus rotates the hips side to side
piriformis stabilizes and rotates the hips laterally
pubococcygeus provides pelvic support
puborectalis strengthens the rectal area
pubovaginalis gives pelvic support
sphincter ani assists in the work of the rectum
sphincter urethrae prevents incontinence
superficial transverse perineal assists the vaginal opening
superior gemellus provides stability and allows the hips to rotate

MUSCLES OF THE UPPER LIMBS

abductor digiti minimi of hand abducts the little finger
abductor pollicis brevis abducts the thumb

abductor pollicis longus abducts and extends the thumb
adductor pollicis adducts the thumb joint
anconeus abducts the ulna, somewhat extends the elbow
articularis cubiti lifts the joint capsule from the elbow
biceps brachii turns up the forearm and flexes the elbow and shoulder
brachialis flexes the elbow
brachioradialis flexes and turns the forearm at the elbow
coracobrachialis flexes and slightly adducts the upper arm
deltoid abducts the upper arm and assists rotation
dorsal interosseous of hand abducts and flexes the middle finger
extensor carpi radialis brevis abducts and extends the hand
extensor carpi radialis longus abducts and extends the hand
extensor carpi ulnaris adducts and extends the hand
extensor digiti minimi extends the little finger
extensor digitorum extends the finger joints
extensor indicis points or lengthens the index finger
extensor pollicis brevis stretches the thumb joint
extensor pollicis longus extends the thumb
flexor carpi radialis abducts and flexes the wrist
flexor carpi ulnaris adducts and flexes the wrist
flexor digiti minimi brevis of hand flexes the little finger
flexor digitorum profundus flexes all fingers but the thumb
flexor digitorum superficialis flexes all joints but the thumb
flexor pollicis brevis flexes the midjoint of the thumb
flexor pollicis longus flexes the end joint of the thumb
infraspinatus rotates the arm and lends stability to the shoulder
latissimus dorsi adducts and rotates the arm
lumbrical of hand extends and flexes all but the thumb
opponens digiti minimi rotates and flexes the little finger
opponens pollicis rotates and flexes the thumb
palmar interosseous adducts and flexes the middle finger
palmaris brevis draws in the skin of the palm to aid the hand in gripping
palmaris longus flexes the wrist and tenses the palm
pronator quadratus turns the forearm downward
pronator teres turns the forearm and flexes the elbow
serratus anterior allows rotation in the scapula
subclavius lowers the shoulder
subscapularis assists rotation and stabilization of shoulder joint
supinator turns the forearm
supraspinatus abducts the arm and offers shoulder support
teres major adducts the arm and stabilizes the shoulder joint
teres minor rotates the arm and strengthens the shoulder
triceps brachii stabilizes the shoulder and extends the upper arm

MUSCLES OF THE LOWER LIMBS

abductor digiti minimi of foot flexes and abducts the fifth toe and assists the foot's arch
abductor hallucis flexes and abducts the big toe and assists the foot's lengthwise arch
adductor hallucis abducts and flexes the big toe with cross support of the arch
articularis genu retracts the suprapatellar bursa as the knee extends
biceps femoris flexes and rotates the knee
dorsal interosseous of foot abducts the middle toes
extensor digitorum brevis spreads out the toes
extensor digitorum longus stretches the toes
extensor hallucis longus points the big toe
flexor digiti minimi brevis of foot flexes the little toe
flexor digitorum brevis flexes all but the big toe and upholds the length of the arch

flexor digitorum longus flexes all but the big toe and strengthens across the arch
flexor hallucis brevis flexes the big toe and strengthens the longitudinal arch
flexor hallucis longus flexes the big toe and supports across the arch
gastrocnemius flexes the knee and foot
gracilis flexes and rotates the knee
lumbrical of foot four muscles that extend and flex all toes but the big toe
peroneus brevis bends the foot and supports the length of the arch
peroneus longus turns and flexes the foot and supports the arch
peroneus tertius turns and extends the foot
plantar interosseous adducts the middle toes
plantaris flexes the knee and foot
popliteus unlocks the kneecap and allows rotation
quadratus femoris rotates and stabilizes the hips
quadratus plantae flexes the toes
rectus femoris flexes and extends the thigh
sartorius abducts and rotates the thigh
semimembranosus extends the hip and allows for rotation of the knee
semitendinosus extends the hip and rotates the leg at the knee
soleus flexes the foot and assists circulation in the leg
tensor fasciae latae abducts the hip and extends the knee
tibialis anterior inverts the foot and assists the arch
tibialis posterior inverts the foot and supports the arch
vastus intermedius lengthens the knee
vastus lateralis extends the knee
vastus medialis extends the knee and strengthens the kneecap

APPENDIX III
TABLE OF CONNECTORS AND JOINTS

Compiled by Dr. Lori B. Siegel

BURSAS

The 260 or more bursas in the body function as friction reducers as muscles and tendons slide over each other and over bone. When irritated or overworked, the bursas become enlarged and inflamed, causing bursitis. Some common bursas are listed.

Upper extremity:

- Subcutaneous olecranon bursa (elbow)
- Subdeltoid bursa
- Subacromial bursa

Lower extremity:

- Trochanteric bursa
- Iliopsoas (iliopectineal) bursa
- Ischial bursa (ischiogluteal)
- Prepatellar bursa
- Deep infrapatellar bursa
- Suprapatellar bursa
- Anserine bursa
- Pre/post calcaneal bursa
- Achilles bursa

TENDONS

Tendons and ligaments, where the muscles insert onto bone, may also become inflamed or strained with overuse or when not used in a biomechanically correct fashion. Some common tendonitis syndromes are listed.

Upper extremity:

- Rotator cuff tendinitis
- Bicipital tendonitis
- Lateral epicondylitis (tennis elbow)
- Medial epicondylitis (golfer's elbow)
- De Quervain's tenosynovitis
- Wrist tenosynovitis

Lower extremity:

- Popliteal tendonitis
- Patellar tendonitis
- Achilles tendonitis
- Plantar faciitis
- Posterior tibial tendonitis
- Peroneal tendonitis

JOINTS

Joints also are connectors between bones and are covered by a synovial lining. Many types of arthritis may involve different parts of the joint capsule or underlying tissue. Anatomically, joints fall into categories based on histological features and range of motion. Different types of joints are involved in different diseases. Some are affected by physical stresses, while others are autoimmune-induced problems.

Types of joints:

- *Synarthroses:* These joints form the suture lines of the skull.
- *Amphiarthroses:* Because they are surrounded by flexible fibrocartilage, these joints have modest

movement. They are found in the pubic symphysis and sacroiliac joints. A subclass of this joint is also found in the spine between vertebral bodies and intervertebral disks.

- *Diarthroses:* These are the most mobile joints. These joints contain a synovial membrane and synovial fluid. These joints are further classified into four different groups.
    - Ball-and-socket joint (hip)
    - Hinge joint (interphalangeal)
    - Saddle joint (first metacarpal—thumb)
    - Plane joint (patellofemoral)

Diseases of joints:

- Wear and tear—osteoarthritis
- Infectious arthritis
- Autoimmune arthritis
    - Rheumatoid arthritis
    - Systemic lupus erythematosus
    - Spondyloarthritis
    - Vasculitis-associated arthritis
- Crystalline arthritis
    - Gout (monosodium urate crystals)
    - Pseudogout (calcium pyrophosphate crystals)
    - Hydroxyapatitie-associated arthritis
- Malignancy-associated arthritis—other site versus intra-articular
- Endocrine-associated arthritis

APPENDIX IV
TIPS ON RECEIVING QUALITY HEALTH CARE

To guide patients into finding quality care and individualized treatment, the Department of Health and Human Services Agency for Healthcare Research and Quality (AHRQ) publishes a number of helpful tip sheets on their Web site, http://www.ahrq.gov.

The AHRQ Publication No. 01-0004, October 2000, "Improving Health Care Quality," suggested individuals gather information from his or her state department of health. To obtain quality reports regarding certification, credentials, registries, and/or the accreditation awarded to various medical personnel, hospitals, and other health care facilities by independent groups, the publication also mentioned the following.

The National Committee for Quality Assurance
http://www.ncqa.org

Joint Commission on Accreditation of Healthcare Organizations
http://www.jcaho.org

American Accreditation HealthCare Commission/URAC
http://www.urac.org

Community Health Accreditation Program
http://www.chapinc.org/chap-consumer.htm

When a reputable doctor or health facility has been found, another AHRQ Publication, No. 01-0040a, "Quick Tips—When Talking with Your Doctor," current as of May 2002, advised, "The single most important way you can stay healthy is to be an active member of your own health care team. One way to get high-quality health care is to find and use information and take an active role in all of the decisions made about your care."

To become better equipped to do this, the AHRQ suggested, "Give information. Don't wait to be asked! You know important things about your symptoms and your health history. Tell your doctor what you think he or she needs to know." As a reminder of those important points, an updated list or health history can be useful in helping the physician arrive at a diagnosis or early detection.

Since new medication may need to be prescribed, the AHRQ strongly advised, "Always bring any medicines you are taking or a list of those medicines (include when and how often you take them) and what strength. Talk about any allergies or reactions you have had to your medicines." Besides prescription pharmaceuticals, this list includes herbal products and other alternative treatments. Also, if X-rays or other test results have been completed by another source, copies of those will be useful in giving the new doctor or medical facility a more complete picture of the patient's health.

In addition to providing information and answering questions that help a doctor know what to be aware of, the patient should ask questions. This will help the patient clarify and recall detailed instructions later. Doing this has great significance, even helping someone follow a medical course of action. Therefore, getting the facts correct will be made easier by the patient writing down a list of questions beforehand, asking the doctor the questions, and duly noting the doctor's answers. If there is too much to write down—or if explanations, terminology, or instructions remain confusing—the patient can request written information from the physician to act as a guide. Often, relevant brochures and tapes will be available from a doctor's office or nearby clinic, too.

When the primary care physician or health care specialist recommends medical tests, such as blood work, X-rays, or other diagnostic tools, the AHRQ Publication No. 01-0040b, May 2002, "Quick Tips—When Getting Medical Tests," advised patients to ask how the test is done and what kind of information it will provide. Questions about the test's benefits, risks, accuracy, procedure, and length of time can be especially helpful in making a decision about whether to proceed. After a test has been completed, the AHRQ further advised, "Do not assume that no news is good news. If you do not hear from your doctor, call to get your test results."

If surgery offers the best course of treatment, the AHRQ Publication No. 01-0040d, May 2002, "Quick Tips—When Planning for Surgery," reminded readers that "No surgery is risk free." However, "Research has shown that patients who are informed about their procedure can better work with their doctors to make the right decisions." With a second opinion almost always advisable, helpful questions include asking what type of operation this will be, why it's important, whether any alternatives exist, and where and how it will be done. Again, questions about the benefits, risks, and specifics of an actual procedure will help patients come to the decision that's right for them.

In the rare event that a condition offers no known or satisfactory course of treatment, participation in a clinical trial provides yet another option. To find out about the requirements for being part of a research effort or an upcoming clinical trial, the Web site http://www:clinicaltrials.gov posts up-to-date listings and locations, criteria about patient qualification, and other necessary information.

APPENDIX V

DIAGNOSING INTERNET INFORMATION ON HEALTH

Some people have a bone to pick with the Internet. By typing the word *bones* into the search box, 650 links came up on one search engine while another offered even more choices—2,440,000 to be exact. For people faced with a pressing health concern, this response not only overwhelms but defeats the purpose of gaining immediate access to medical information and answers.

One practical-sounding solution suggested being more specific in the choice of wording for a search. For example, by typing *fractured bones* into the overkill engine's box, the choices narrowed to 29,700 links. The first page, however, mainly mentioned sports stars who had had a bad break and the law firms addressing those particular types of accidents or injuries.

Other hot links went to sites made for ordering unusual music, scary books, and horror flicks with an emphasis on bones. Undoubtedly, those offerings eventually included voluminous contemporary poems with bleached bones freely littering their lines.

In yet another attempt toward precision, the phrase *first aid for broken bones* offered 75,440 links. The first page actually gave reliable sites, including one with instructions for setting the broken bone of a dog. For a hurried search, however, this method does not necessarily locate the most relevant choices as many people apparently—and, sometimes, desperately—want to do.

In the article "Hunting for Health," published in the November 17, 2003 issue of *U.S. News & World Report,* pages 48–50, writer Katherine Hobson reported, "A recent study by the Pew Internet & American Life Project found that some 93 million people, or 80 percent of adults who use the Internet, have used it to learn about at least one major health topic." To avoid millions of Web responses, however, the article suggested, "You can save a lot of time by starting your search from a health gateway site like the federal government's Healthfinder (http://www.healthfinder.gov) or with NOAH (http://www.noah-health.org), a New York–based group of health and science libraries. These groups have, for general medical information, vetted some generally reliable sites. The Medical Library Association has also come up with a Top 10 list of the most useful Web sites (http://www.mlanet.org/resources/medspeak/topten.html), including disease-specific resources like http://www.cancer.gov. It has links to everything from the latest studies to clinical trial information and other clearinghouse sites like http://www.medem.com, which links to information from medical societies like the American Academy of Pediatrics."

As the Internet source for this book, each day's online research usually began with a visit to MEDLINEplus Health Information from the National Library of Medicine (NLM), located at http://www.nlm.nih.gov/medlineplus. Still another favorite from the NLM came from the Web site of PubMed Central, http://www.pubmedcentral.com. In either instance, excellent links arose, assisting a focused search for valuable information on almost any medical topic. Besides those generous offerings, the Web sites of medical schools or college research centers, such as those from the University of Miami, Johns Hopkins, Duke, and Harvard, offered reliable information that has been professionally reviewed and frequently updated. Sites from a highly reputable medical facility, such as the Mayo Clinic, or a very respected company that produces medical guides, such as *The Merck Manual,* provide sound and thorough medical advice, too.

Another possibility for locating information includes Web sites for the many professional associations of doctors, nurses, and therapists—most of which offer patient information online. To obtain current articles that could be timely or of great value, however, most of these Web sites require the payment of membership dues or fees per copy to access the professional journals made available on the Internet. In addition to those costs, patients may find a somewhat slanted perspective in the presentation of the "facts." Understandably, each profession professes a particular area of expertise that comes with a unique medical stance or belief that can, albeit inadvertently, result in bias. One might expect this, say, in the product information from a manufacturer. However, the opposite proved to be more likely simply because the Food and Drug Administration requires each company to list the potential side effects or risks involved in the products they make, which, almost automatically, creates a more balanced view.

Some useful Web sites, however, have come into being to provide Internet health care information and may not exist apart from that function. Although these sites may have advertising banners or products to sell, they also provide a means of quickly locating health information that, in general, seems to be thorough and reasonably balanced. For instance, WebMDHealth, located on http://www.webmd.com, offers a newsletter, news of medical alerts, and information about symptoms, diseases, drugs, herbs, diet, and nutrition as well as providing a medical dictionary. On http://health.yahoo.com, Yahoo! Health offers similar information. Additionally, Virtual Hospital: A Digital Library of Health Information offers some excellent professional medical resources, patient handbooks, fact sheets, and teaching aids about the body, including the conditions affecting the musculoskeletal system on their Web site, http://www.vh.org/index.html Undoubtedly, other sites of a comparable quality and nature presently exist with new ones quite likely to come.

To assist the consumer further is the article "Assessing the Quality of Internet Health Information," current as of June 1999, came from the Web site of the Department of Health and Human Services Agency for Healthcare Research and Quality (AHRQ), http://www.ahrq.gov. According to this summary, the "Criteria for Evaluating Internet Health Information" consists of the following suggestions as quoted in full in the list below:

- *Credibility:* includes the source, currency, relevance/utility, and editorial review process for the information.
- *Content:* must be accurate and complete, and an appropriate disclaimer provided.
- *Disclosure:* includes informing the user of the purpose of the site, as well as any profiling of collection of information associated with using the site.
- *Links:* evaluated according to selection, architecture, content, and back linkages.
- *Design:* encompasses accessibility, logical organization (navigability), and internal search capability.
- *Interactivity:* includes feedback mechanisms and means for exchange of information among users.
- *Caveats:* clarification of whether site function is to market products and services or is a primary information content provider.

Besides those important guidelines, an Internet search might also take into account the clarity of a Web page presentation and its ease of use. Some Web sites, for instance, employ enough graphics and pop-ups to overload an older computer system as well as the newer computer user. Not only does the technological wizardry present a colorful overkill of information, it often generates eyestrain. At the opposite end of the spectrum though, a Web page with lengthy text and/or difficult language can equally defeat the purpose of producing reliable information as quickly as possible in a highly accessible form. Therefore, some useful sites with highly readable information for adults may be those especially aimed for children, such as the government's healthfinder for kids on http://www.healthfinder.gov/kids, the Department of Health and Human Services on http://www.hhs.

gov/kids, or U.S. Food and Drug Administration (FDA) information located on http://www.fda.gov/oc/opacom/kids.

To assist readers further, appendixes have been provided below with links to government sites, universities, organizations, support groups, clinical trials, and other topics of interest. With those sites used as a port of entry, a search can then be narrowed by typing in the topic of interest, again, being as specific as possible. For example, on the FDA site provided above, a search for *growth charts for children* produced a link, http://www.fda.gov/ohrms/dockets/ac/02/briefing/3903b1-04.pdf to a 21-page brochure entitled *The Use of NCHS and CDC Growth Charts in Nutritional Assessment of Young Infants.* After using the same search phrase, a visit to the American Academy of Pediatrics site provided a list of links from which to choose, depending on the age and sex of a child, http://search.aap.org/AAP/query.html?col=aapsites+bookstor+pedjobs&qc=aapsites+bookst or+pedjobs&ql=&qt= growth+charts+for+children. From the Centers for Disease Control and Prevention (CDC), the National Center for Health Statistics gave comprehensive information on the healthy growth of children—in English, Spanish, or French—in the "2000 CDC Growth Charts: United States," located on November 22, 2003 on http://www.cdc.gov/growthcharts.

Since a child's growth depends on many factors, such as heredity, nutrition, and economics, a present emphasis concerns not how tall a boy or girl will be at a particular age but how heavy or slim. Therefore, the CDC now provides information on assessing the body mass index (BMI) in "Using the BMI-for-Age Growth Charts" on the Web site http://www.cdc.gov/nccdphp/dnpa/growthcharts/training/modules/module1/text/into.htm. For adults, a number of groups, such as AARP or Weight Watchers, offer online information to help people determine their BMI. In addition, the Department of Health and Human Services, National Heart, Blood, and Lung Institute offers an "Obesity Education Initiative" Web page on http://www.nhlbi.nih.gov/about/oei/index.htm with an online BMI calculator to aid individuals on http://www.nhlbisupport.com/bmi and a comparative chart of the "Body Mass Index Table" on http://www.nhlbi.nih.gov/guidelines/obesity/bmi_tbl.htm. The search may take a little time and focus to find the specific helps, information, or answers wanted in each instance. However, whatever the musculoskeletal concern may be, someone has most likely addressed that very topic on the Internet.

APPENDIX VI
NATIONAL ORGANIZATIONS OF INTEREST

Most national organizations freely offer useful information concerning prevention and treatment, statistical data, and fact sheets as well as local contacts or family support groups. Additionally, some organizations fund research projects, present certification programs and scholarships, or, for typically reasonable fees, provide workshops, journals, and member directories. To assist you in finding out about an organization, the following list includes Web sites, phone numbers, and mailing addresses for group headquarters or another primary contact point. These organizations may be involved in ongoing research or can refer you to clinical trials. To learn about or participate in government-sponsored research, see the Web site http://www.clinicaltrials.gov for up-to-date information.

AbleData
8630 Fenton Street
Suite 930
Silver Spring, MD 20910
(800) 227-0216
http://www.abledata.com

Resources on assistive devices and rehabilitation equipment products compiled by the National Institute on Disability and Rehabilitation Research

Aerobics and Fitness Association of America
15250 Ventura Boulevard
Suite 200
Sherman Oaks, CA 91403
(877) YOUR-BODY or (877) 968-7263
http://www.afaa.com

Fitness educator offering certification

AMC Cancer Research Center
1600 Pierce Street
Denver, CO 80214
(800) 321-1557 or (303) 233-6501
http://www.amc.org

Research institute dedicated to the prevention of cancer and other chronic diseases

American Academy of Family Physicians
P.O. Box 11210
Shawnee Mission, KS 66211-2672
(800) 274-2237 or (913) 906-6000
http://www.aafp.org

Professional organization with news, articles, and patient information

American Academy of Orthopaedic Surgeons
6300 North River Road
Rosemont, IL 60018-4262
(800) 346-AAOS or (847) 823-7186
http://www.aaos.org

Professional organization with patient/public information and educational materials

American Academy of Pediatrics
National Headquarters
141 Northwest Point Boulevard
Elk Grove Village, IL 60007-1098
(847) 434-4000
http://www.aap.org

Profession organization with safety tips and resources for parents

American Academy of Physical Medicine & Rehabilitation
One IBM Plaza
Suite 2500
Chicago, IL 60611-3604
(312) 464-9700
http://www.aapmr.org

National medical society with information about musculoskeletal conditions

American Academy of Podiatric Sports Medicine
(888) 854-FEET
http://www.aapsm.org

Professional organization with emphasis on prevention and biomechanics with helpful lists, fact sheets, and newsletter

American Alliance for Health, Physical Education, Recreation, and Dance
1900 Association Drive
Reston, VA 20191-1598
(800) 213-7193
http://www.aahperd.org

Professional organization with programs and publications

American Association for Cancer Education
610 Walnut Street
256 WARF Building
Madison, WI 53726
(608) 263-9515
http://www.aaceonline.com

Founded in 1947 by professional coordinators from medical and dental schools with mission of fostering education throughout world

American Association for Hand Surgery
20 North Michigan Avenue
Suite 700
Chicago, IL 60602
(312) 236-3307
http://www.handsurgery.org

Professional organization with educational emphasis on research, grants, and online information for the public

American Association of Hip and Knee Surgeons
704 Florence Drive
Park Ridge, IL 60068-2104
(847) 698-1200
http://www.aahks.org

Educational opportunities for members and information for patients

American Back Society
St. Joseph's Professional Center
2647 International Boulevard
Suite 401
Oakland, CA 94601
(510) 536-9929
www.americanbacksoc.org

Health care professionals with online articles

American Board of Physical Medicine and Rehabilitation
21 First Street SW
Suite 674
Rochester, MN 55902-3092
(507) 282-1776
http://www.abpmr.org

Professional certification and online newsletter

American Cancer Society
(800) ACS-2345
http://www.cancer.org

Medical news, statistical information, online resources, and patient support groups

American Chiropractic Association
1701 Clarendon Boulevard
Arlington, VA 22209
(800) 986-4636
http://www.amerchiro.org

Professional organization with media facts and patient information

American Chronic Pain Association
P.O. Box 850
Rocklin, CA 95677-0850
(800) 533-3231 or (916) 632-0922
http://www.theacpa.org

International support system with sales catalog

American Cleft Palate Association
1504 East Franklin Street, Suite 102
Chapel Hill, NC 27514-2820
(919) 933-9044
http://www.acpa-cpf.org

International, interdisciplinary professional medical society with journal, research, and educational information

American College of Foot and Ankle Surgeons
515 Busse Highway
Park Ridge, IL 60068
(800) 421-2237
http://www.acfas.org

Professional medical society with conferences, ongoing research, excellent health information, and educational materials online for patient and public use

American College of Radiology
1701 Pennsylvania Avenue, NW
Suite 610
Washington, DC 20006
(800) ACR-LINE
http://www.acr.org

Accrediting body providing patient information and professional guidelines, publications, medical news, and resources

American College of Rheumatology
1800 Century Place
Suite 250
Atlanta, GA 30345
(404) 633-3777
http://www.rheumatology.org

Professional organization with research interests, online fact sheets, and other materials for public education

American College of Sports Medicine
P.O. Box 1440
Indianapolis, IN 46206-1440
(317) 637-9200
http://www.acsm.org

Worldwide organization with grants and research initiatives, certification, and excellent health and fitness information online for public use

American Counsel for Headache Information
19 Mantua Road
Mt. Royal, NJ 08061
(856) 423-0258
http://www.achenet.org

Patient health professional partnership with publications and interests in public education

American Counsel on Exercise
4851 Paramount Drive
San Diego, CA 92123
(800) 825-3636 or (858) 279-8227
http://www.acefitness.org

Largest fitness certification and education provider in the world in this field

American Fibromyalgia Syndrome Association
6380 E Tanque Verde
Suite D
Tucson, AZ 85715
(520) 733-1570
http://www.afsafund.org

Organization with dedication to research, education, and patient advocacy

American Fitness Professionals & Associates
P.O. Box 214
Ship Bottom, NJ 08008
(609) 978-7583
http://www.afpafitness.com

International fitness company providing seminars, conferences, certification, and continuing education

American Heart Association
National Center
7272 Greenville Avenue
Dallas, TX 75231
(800) AHA-USA-1 or (800) 242-8721
http://www.americanheart.org

Organization with educational resources for the public and professionals

American Juvenile Arthritis Association
P.O. Box 7669
Atlanta, GA 30357-0669
(800) 283-7800
http://www.arthritis.org/cummunities/juvenile_arthritis

Council serving children, youth, and their families with advocacy, information, support, research, and other resources

American Massage Therapy Association
820 Davis Street
Evanston, IL 60201
http://www.amtamassage.org

Professional organization with publications and educational materials

American Medical Association
515 N State Street
Chicago, IL 60610
(312) 464-5000
http://www.ama-assn.org

Professional medical association with publications, news, media information, and other online resources for public awareness

American Occupational Therapy Association
4720 Montgomery Lane
P.O. Box 31220
Bethesda, MD 20824-1220
(301) 652-2682
http://www.aota.org

Professional group offering tip sheets for the public and continuing education courses and articles online for professional use

American Orthopaedic Foot and Ankle Society
2517 Eastlake Avenue E
Seattle, WA 98102
(206) 223-1120
http://www.aofas.org

Orthopedic professionals with research, grants, educational funds, media information, publications, and excellent online fact sheets for patients and public

American Orthopaedic Society for Sports Medicine
6300 N River Road
Suite 500
Rosemont, IL 60018
(847) 292-4900
http://www.sportsmed.org

National organization with emphasis on research, education, health care, and rehabilitation relating to sports interests and injuries

American Osteopathic Foundation
142 East Ontario Street
Chicago, IL 60611
(800) 621-1773 or (312) 202-8000
http://www.aof-foundation.org

Professional group with research, scholarships, and educational supports

American Pain Foundation
201 N Charles Street
Suite 710
Baltimore, MD 21201-4111
(888) 615-PAIN
http://www.painfoundation.org

Support advocates speaking for people in pain and connecting to online news, articles, and other helps

American Pain Society
4700 W Lake Avenue
Glenview, IL 60025
(847) 375-4715
http://www.ampainsoc.org

Multidiscipline organization advancing pain-related research, education, treatment, and professional practice

American Paraplegia Society
75-20 Astoria Boulevard
Jackson Heights, NY 11370
(718) 803-3782
http://www.apssci.org

Organization founded in 1954 to promote awareness and improve quality in medical care for persons with spinal cord injuries

American Physical Therapy Association
1111 North Fairfax Street
Alexandria, VA 22314-1488
(800) 999-2782 or (703) 684-APTA
http://www.apta.org

National professional organization with publications and other educational helps

American Podiatric Medical Association
9312 Old Georgetown Road
Bethesda, MD 20814
(800) ASK-APMA or (301) 571-9200
http://www.apma.org

Medical group with journal, foot facts, and health information

American Running Association
4405 East West Highway
Suite 405

Bethesda, MD 20814
(800) 776-2732 or (301) 913-9517
http://www.americanrunning.org

Membership group with journal, brochures, newsroom, fitness links, and helpful online articles

American Senior Fitness Association
P.O. Box 2575
New Smyrna Beach, FL 32170
(800) 243-1478 or (386) 423-6634
http://www.seniorfitness.net

Professional resources, training, certification programs, and distance education

American Spinal Injury Association
2020 Peachtree Road, NW
Atlanta, GA 30309-1402
(404) 355-9772
http://www.asia-spinalinjury.org

Multidisciplinary organization with journal and research interests

American Volkssport Association
1001 Pat Booker Road
Suite 101
Universal City, TX 78148
(800) 830-WALK or (210) 659-2112
http://www.ava.org

Club for walkers sponsoring publications and events

Amputee Coalition of America
900 East Hill Avenue, Suite 285
Knoxville, TN 37915-2568
(888) 269-5669
http://www.amputee-coalition.org

National amputee consumer education organization with information center and support groups

Arthritis Foundation
P.O. Box 7669
Atlanta, GA 30357-0669
(800) 283-7800
http://www.arthritis.org

Organization with journal, events, programs, and excellent online health information

Arthritis Research Institute of America
300 South Duncan Avenue
Suite 240
Clearwater, FL 33755
(727) 461-4054
http://www.preventarthritis.org

National charity group focusing on prevention, research, education, and online newsletter

Association for Advancement of Automotive Medicine
P.O. Box 4176
Barrington, IL 60011
(847) 844-3880
http://www.carcrash.org

Multidisciplinary professional organization dedicated to understanding and preventing motor vehicle crash injuries

Cancer Care
275 7th Avenue
New York, NY 10001
(800) 813-HOPE
http://www.cancercare.org

Organization offering counseling, education, referrals, news, and other information

Center for Food Safety and Applied Nutrition
5100 Paint Branch Parkway
College Park, MD 20740-3835
(888) SAFE-FOOD
http://www.cfsan.fda.gov

News and information provided by the U.S. Food and Drug Administration

Centers for Disease Control & Prevention
1600 Clifton Road
Atlanta, GA 30333
(800) 311-3435 or (404) 639-3311
http://www.cdc.gov

Federal agency for protecting people at home and abroad with travel information, news updates, statistical data, and other health facts

Cervical Spine Research Society
6300 N River Road
Suite 727
Rosemont, IL 60018-4226
(847) 698-1628
http://www.csrs.org

Multidisciplinary organization offering research, studies, newsletter, and online health information

Charcot-Marie-Tooth Association
2700 Chestnut Street
Chester, PA 19013-4867
(800) 606-CMTA (2682)
http://www.charcot-marie-tooth.org

Association involved in research, resources, and support groups

Christopher Reeve Paralysis Foundation
500 Morris Avenue
Springfield, NJ 07081
(800) 225-0292
http://www.christopherreeve.org

Organization committed to providing information and funding research on spinal cord injury and other disorders of the central nervous system

Department of Health and Human Services
200 Independence Avenue, SW
Washington, DC 20201
(877) 696-6775 or (202) 619-0257
http://www.hhs.gov

Nation's guide to safety and wellness with information on policies, laws, regulations, research, grants, Medicaid, health insurance, and concerns for patients of all ages

Disabled Sports USA
451 Hungerford Drive
Suite 100
Rockville, MD 20850
(301) 217-0960
http://www.dsusa.org

National organization with sports rehabilitation programs and other resources

Dystonia Medical Research Foundation
One East Wacker Drive
Suite 2430
Chicago, IL 60601-1905
(312) 755-0198
http://www.dystonia-foundation.org

International partnership offering research, patient helps, publications, and worldwide conferences every two years

Families of Spinal Muscular Atrophy
P.O. Box 196
Libertyville, IL 60048-0196
(800) 886-1762
http://www.fsma.org

Resource center with information on support groups, fund-raising, clinical trials, news updates, and other educational helps for patients and their families

Guillain-Barré Syndrome Foundation International
P.O. Box 262
Wynnewood, PA 19096
(610) 667-0131
http://www.guillain-barre.com

International organization with online helps and discussion

Health Research and Services Administration
U.S. Department of Health and Human Services
Parklawn Building
600 Fishers Lane
Rockville, MD 20857
(888) ASK-HRSA
http://www.hrsa.gov

Information on resources and referrals, primarily for low-income, uninsured individuals and those with special health needs

Huntington's Disease Society of America
158 West 29th Street
7th Floor
New York, NY 10001-5300
(800) 345-HDSA
http://www.hdsa.org

National voluntary health agency emphasizing research, advocacy, information, and awareness

International Association of Infant Massage
1891 Goodyear Avenue
Suite 622
Ventura, CA 93003
(888) 488-9489 or (805) 644-9272
http://www.iaim-us.com/

Organization with training helps and certification for caretakers of infants

International Osteoporosis Foundation
http://www.osteofound.org

Nongovernmental organization with French and Swiss offices supporting awareness and prevention

International Society of Arthroscopy, Knee Surgery, and Orthopaedic Sports Medicine
145 Town Country Drive
Suite 106
Danville, CA 94526-3063
(925) 314-7920
http://www.isakos.com

Membership group promoting relevant charitable, scientific, and literary works

The Leukemia and Lymphoma Society
1311 Mamaroneck Avenue
White Plains, NY 10605
(914) 949-5213
http://www.leukemia-lymphoma.org

Voluntary health organization focusing on science, research, patient services, and disease information

Leukemia Research Foundation
820 Davis Street
Suite 420
Evanston, IL 60201
(847) 424-0600
http://www.leukemia-research.org

Foundation with dedication to research, scientific developments, and education

March of Dimes Birth Defects Foundation
1275 Mamaroneck Avenue
White Plains, NY 10605
http://www.marchofdimes.com

Organization devoted to prevention of birth defects through research, education, and other supportive resources

Multiple Sclerosis Association of America
706 Haddonfield Road
Cherry Hill, NJ 08002
(800) 532-7667
http://www.msaa.com

Organization offering information

Movement Disorder Society
611 Wells Street
Milwaukee, WI 53202
(414) 276-2145
http://www.movementdisorders.org

International professional society with journal, newsletter, and continuing education resources

Muscular Dystrophy Association
3300 E Sunrise Drive
Tucson, AZ 85718
(800) 572-1717
http://www.mdausa.org

Voluntary health agency promoting research, grants, news, updates, and helpful online facts

Muscular Dystrophy Family Foundation
2330 North Meridian Street
Indianapolis, IN 46208-5730
(800) 544-1213 or (317) 923-6333
http://www.mdff.org

Organization providing emotional support and news

Myasthenia Gravis Foundation of America
5841 Cedar Lake Road
Suite 204
Minneapolis, MN 55416
(800) 541-5454 or (952) 545-9438
http://www.myasthenia.org

National volunteer health agency funding research and providing patient information, news, and numerous educational helps

Myositis Association
1233 20th Street, NW
Suite 402
Washington, DC 20036
(202) 887-0082
http://www.myositis.org

Organization providing news, publications, events, and patient support

National Amputee Foundation
40 Church Street
Malverne, NY 11565
(516) 887-3600
http://www.nationalamputation.org

Originally founded in 1919 to help war veterans with services and later expanded to include civilian amputees too

National Association for Sport and Physical Education
American Alliance for Health, Physical Education, Recreation & Dance
1900 Association Drive
Reston, VA 20191-1598
(800) 213-7193
http://www.aahperd.org

Alliance to support creative and healthy lifestyles by increasing knowledge and sound medical practices

National Birth Defects Center
40 Second Avenue
Suite 520
Waltham, MA 02451
(781) 466-9555
http://www.thegenesisfund.org

Organization dedicated to raising funds for children with birth defects and genetic diseases

National Cancer Institute
Public Inquiries Office
Suite 3036A
6116 Executive Boulevard
MSC8322
Bethesda, MD 20892-8322
(800) 4-CANCER or (800) 422-6237
http://www.cancer.gov

Federal government's principal agency for cancer research, trials, training, and education with statistical data and FAQ sheets for public information, part of the National Institutes of Health

National Center for Biotechnology Information
National Institutes of Health
Building 38A
8600 Rockville Pike
Bethesda, MD 20894
(301) 496-2475
http://www.ncbi.nlm.nih.gov

National resource for research and public databases

National Center on Birth Defects and Developmental Disabilities
http://www.cdc.gov/ncbddd

Health information with Web form supplying contacts for help with birth defects, human development, and disabilities

National Chronic Fatigue and Fibromyalgia Association
P.O. Box 18426
Kansas City, MO 64133
http://www.ncfsfa.org

Offers links to information and patient resources

National Chronic Pain Outreach Association
P.O. Box 274
Millboro, VA 24460
(540) 862-9437
http://www.chronicpain.org

Organization emphasizing education and awareness of chronic pain and its management

National Dysautonomia Research Foundation
1407 W Fourth Street
Suite 160
Red Wing, MN 55066-2108
(651) 267-0525
http://www.ndrf.org

Advocacy foundation with discussion forums, research database, and online educational health information

National Fibromyalgia Association
2200 N Glassell Street
Suite A
Orange, CA 92865
(714) 921-0150
http://fmaware.org

Organization with resources dedicated to public and media awareness

National Headache Foundation
820 N Orleans
Suite 217
Chicago, IL 60610
(888) NHF-5552 or (773) 388-6399
http://www.headaches.org

Organization helping headache sufferers and professionals participate in clinical trials, stay abreast of news, and become better informed

National Institute for Occupational Safety and Health
1600 Clifton Road
Atlanta, GA 30333
(404) 639-3311 or (800) 311-3435
http://www.cdc.gov/niosh

Federal agency conducting research, making recommendations, and offering facts sheets and news updates

National Institute of Arthritis and Musculoskeletal and Skin Diseases
National Institutes of Health
Building 31, Room 4C02
31 Center Drive
MSC 2350
Bethesda, MD 20892-2350
(301) 496-8190
http://www.niams.nih.gov

Health information, outreach, coalition, patient registries, and research devoted to musculoskeletal conditions

National Institute of Child Health and Human Development
National Institutes of Health
P.O. Box 3006
Rockville, MD 20847
(800) 370-2943
http://www.nichd.nih.gov

National biomedical research with statistical data, news, and educational information

National Institute on Aging
Building 31, Room 5C27
31 Center Drive, MSC 2292
Bethesda, MD 20892
(301) 496-1752
http://www.nia.gov

Part of the National Institutes of Health, with ongoing research programs, health information, funding of studies, and news

National Institutes of Health
9000 Rockville Pike
Bethesda, MD 20892
http://health.nih.gov

Steward of medical and health research for the nation and agency under the auspices of the Department of Health and Human Services, sponsors events, research, and excellent online health information and news releases

National Institutes of Health Osteoporosis and Related Bone Diseases National Resource Center
1232 22nd Street, NW
Washington, DC 20037-1292
(800) 624-BONE or (202) 223-0344
http://www.osteo.org

Part of the Department of Health and Human Services' National Institutes of Health, provides excellent online information, news releases, and fact sheets

National Marfan Foundation
22 Manhasset Avenue
Port Washington, NY 11050
(800) 8-MARFAN or (516) 883-8712
http://www.marfan.org

Voluntary health organization supporting research and offering timely information to patients, families, and health care groups

National Marrow Donor Program
Suite 500
3001 Broadway Street Northeast
Minneapolis, MN 55413-1753
(800) MARROW2 or (800) 627-7692
http://www.marrow.org

Facilitator bringing patients and donors together and providing informational publications to help raise awareness

National Multiple Sclerosis Society
733 Third Avenue
New York, NY 10017
(800) FIGHT-MS or (800) 344-4867
http://www.nmss.org

Nationwide network promoting research, news, information, education, and advocacy

National Osteoporosis Foundation
1232 22nd Street, NW

Washington, DC 20037-1292
(202) 223-2226
http://www.nof.org

Leading resource for those seeking news and information

National Parkinson Foundation
1501 NW 9th Avenue
Bob Hope Road
Miami, FL 33136-1494
(305) 547-6666
http://www.parkinson.org

Institution housing therapeutic centers and offering patient information

National Safety Council
1121 Spring Lake Drive
Itasca, IL 60143-3201
(630) 285-1121
http://www.nsc.org

Founded in 1913 and chartered by Congress in 1953 as the nation's advocate for safety, health, and environmental policies

National Scoliosis Foundation
5 Cabot Place
Stoughton, MA 02072
(800) NSF-MYBACK
nsf@scoliosis.org
http://www.scoliosis.org

Organization with educational resources for children, care-takers, and health care providers

National Spasmodic Dysphonia Association
One East Wacker Drive
Suite 2430
Chicago, IL 60601-1905
(800) 795-NSDA
http://www.dysphonia.org/nsda

Organization funding research and offering support and information

National Spasmodic Torticollis Association
9920 Talbot Avenue
#233
Fountain Valley, CA 92708
(800) HURTFUL or (714) 378-7837
http://www.torticollis.org

Organization promoting research and providing information, advocacy, and support

National Spinal Cord Injury Association
6701 Democracy Boulevard
Suite 300-9
Bethesda, MD 20817
(800) 962-9629
http://www.spinalcord.org

Civilian organization dedicated to improving the quality of life for those with spinal cord injury or disease and their families

North American Spine Society
22 Calendar Court
2nd Floor
LaGrange, IL 60525
(877) SPINE-DR
http://www.spine.org

Organization providing workshops, research, advocacy, and other informational helps

Office of Cancer Complementary and Alternative Medicine
National Cancer Institute
6116 Executive Plaza North
Suite 600, MSC 8339
Bethesda, MD 20852
http://www.cancer/gov/occam

Supporting research and educational information, including conferences and clinical trials

Orthopaedic Research Society
6300 N River Road
Suite 727
Rosemont, IL 60018
(847) 698-1625
http://www.ors.org

Organization promoting research in surgery, diseases, and other aspects of the musculoskeletal system with journal and mentoring of scientists

Orthopaedic Trauma Association
6300 N River Road
Suite 727
Rosemont, IL 60018-4226
(847) 698-1631
http://www.ota.org

Educational group with courses, research grants, Internet studies, and other online helps

Osteogenesis Imperfecta Foundation
804 W Diamond Avenue
Suite 210
Gaithersburg, MD 20878
(800) 981-2663 or (301) 947-0083
http://www.oif.org

National voluntary health organization with emphasis on education, research, medical treatments, support groups, and other means of helping people to cope

The Paget Foundation
120 Wall Street
Suite 1602
New York, NY 10005-4001
(800) 23-PAGET or (212) 509-5335
http://www.paget.org

National voluntary health agency with information and physician referrals by email

Paralyzed Veterans of America
801 Eighteenth Street, NW
Washington, DC 20006-3517
(800) 424-8200
http://www.pva.org

Congressionally chartered veterans service organization founded in 1946 providing advocacy, research, and information regarding spinal cord injuries and musculoskeletal dysfunctions resulting in immobility

Post-Polio Health International
4207 Lindell Boulevard #10
St. Louis, MO 63108-2915
(314) 534-0475
http://www.post-polio.org

Research, advocacy, support, and educational group

Scoliosis Association
P.O. Box 811705
Boca Raton, FL 33481-1705
(561) 994-4435
http://www.scoliosis-assoc.org

Volunteer nonmedical organization with information lines and support groups

Scoliosis Research Foundation
611 East Wells Street
Milwaukee, WI 53202-3892
(414) 289-9107
http://www.srs.org

Professional organization with online information for medical and personal use

Shriners Hospitals for Children
2900 Rocky Point Drive
Tampa, FL 33607-1460
(800) 237-5055
http://www.shrinershq.org

Headquarters with 22 hospitals around the country and in Canada with expert staff and facilities devoting no-cost orthopedic, spinal cord injury, and burn care services to children under 18

Sjögren's Syndrome Foundation
8120 Woodmont Avenue
Suite 530
Bethesda, MD 20814
(800) 475-6473
http://www.sjogrens.com

National voluntary health agency providing information and coping strategies through education and research

Spina Bifida Association of America
4590 MacArthur Boulevard, NW
Suite 250
Washington, DC 20007-4226
(800) 621-3141 or (202) 944-3285
http://www.sbaa.org

Group offering excellent online information for patients, including medical updates

Spinal Injury Foundation
11080 Circle Point Road
Westminster, CO 80020
(866) 5SPINE5
http://www.spinalinjuryfoundation.org

Advocacy group providing information and funding research

Spondylitis Association of America
P.O. Box 5872
Sherman Oaks, CA 91413

(800) 777-8189
http://www.spondylitis.org

Sponsor of international conferences, support groups, and informational awareness

Tourette Syndrome Association
42-40 Bell Boulevard
Bayside, NY 11361
(718) 224-2999
http://www.tsa-usa.org

National voluntary membership organization with research, news, educational information, international contacts, and support groups around the world

Turner Syndrome Society of USA
14450 TC Jester
Suite 260
Houston, TX 77014
(800) 365-9944 or (832) 249-9988
http://www.turner-syndrome-us.org

National organization providing assistance, support, and education

WE MOVE (Worldwide Education and Awareness for Movement Disorders)
204 W. 84th Street
New York, NY 10024
(800) 437-MOV2
http://www.wemove.org

Internet resource informing patients, public, and professionals about clinical advances, treatment options, and other educational needs

Wheelchair Sports USA
10 Lake Circle
Suite G19
Colorado Springs, CO 80906
(719) 574-1150
http://www.wsusa.org

Begun in 1956 as an organization to encourage activities among those with paralysis by offering sports events, publications, news updates, and other resources

APPENDIX VII

INTERNET JOURNALS AND MAGAZINES

In addition to the fact sheets, health information, journals, newsletters, bulletins, or other publications made available by most of the organizations listed in Appendix VI, the following sites offer online resources and/or archived articles.

www.americanscientist.org
American Scientist—The magazine of Sigma Xi, The Scientific Research Society

www.worldchiropracticalliance.org/tcj/this.htm
The Chiropractic Journal—A publication of the World Chiropractic Alliance

www.clinicalanatomy.org/journal.html
Clinical Anatomy, Journal of the American Association of Clinical Anatomist

www.primusweb.com/fitnesspartner
Fitness Jumpsite

www.fitnessmagazine.com
Fitness Magazine

www.fitpregnancy.com
Fit Pregnancy magazine

www.jama.ama-assn.org
JAMA: Journal of the American Medical Association

www.ejbjs.org
Journal of Bone & Joint Surgery

www.jci.org
The Journal of Clinical Investigation

www.japmaonline.org
Journal of the American Podiatric Medical Association

www.naturalmuscle.net
Natural Muscle Magazine

www.physsportsmed.com/personal.htm
The Physician & Sports Medicine journal

www.shapemag.com
Shape magazine

APPENDIX VIII
RELATED WEB SITES

Activator.com
http://www.activator.com
Information about activator methods and use with a directory of qualified practitioners

Alternative Medicine Channel
http://www.alternativemedicinechannel.com
Glossary, forum, and educational information on various conditions

Centers for Disease Control and Prevention
http://www.cdc.gov/growthcharts
Growth charts for children provided by the CDC National Center for Health Statistics
http://www.cdc.gov/nasd7/docs/d000701-d000800/d000799/d000799.html
NASD (National Agriculture Safety Database): Basic First Aid

Graston Technique.com
http://www.grastontechnique.com
Information about the Graston technique with a directory of qualified practitioners

Groupe International Cotrel Dubousset
http://www.gicd.org
Nonprofit international organization devoted to the latest advances in spine surgery

Health Finder
http://www.healthfinder.gov
Reliable sources of health information compiled by the Office of Disease Prevention and Health Promotion, Department of Health and Human Services

The Hypermobility Syndrome Association, England
http://www.hypermobility.org
Health information and membership site

Johns Hopkins Medicine
http://www.hopkinsmedicine.org
News and informational articles

Mayo Clinic
http://www.mayoclinic.com
Educational information from the Mayo Clinic

National Bone and Joint Decade, 2000–2010
http://www.boneandjointdecade.org/us
U.S. site with an extensive list of facts, health care, and patient information

National Certification Board for Therapeutic Massage & Bodywork
http://www.ncbtmb.com
Information on locating certified professionals

National Heart, Lung, and Blood Institute
http://nhlbisupport.com/bmi
Calculate your body mass index with online assistance from the National Heart, Lung, and Blood Institute of the National Institutes of Health

Occupational Safety & Health Administration (OSHA)
http://www.osha.gov
Information on job safety and ergonomics plus publications from this governmental agency
www.osha.gov/SLTC/ergonomics
OSHA ergonomics page

Office of Minority Health
http://www.omhrc.gov
Data, statistics, information, publications, and health links

Podiatry Network
http://www.podiatrynetwork.com
Excellent articles and information on foot problems and health

President's Council on Physical Fitness and Sports
http://www.fitness.gov
Government sponsored site encouraging physical activity

Safe USA.org
http://www.safeusa.org
Alliance of major public and private groups devoted to safety with informational helps, fact sheets, and statistical data

Spinal Stenosis.org
www.spinalstenosis.org
Spinal stenosis Web site with extensive information on care and treatment

Spine-Health.com
www.spine-health.com
Newsletter, information, and announcements of research

Spine & Sport
www.spineandsport.com
Ongoing research projects

Spine Surgery
www.spine-surgery.com
Articles on surgeries of the spine

Spineuniverse.com
www.spineuniverse.com
Article and resources

Department of Pain Medicine and Palliative Care at Beth Israel Medical Center
www.stoppain.org
Site of Beth Israel Medical Center in New York City whose Department of Pain Medicine and Palliative Care was the first of its kind in the country

Typing Injury FAQ
www.tifaq.com
Answers to frequently asked questions and articles

Virtual Hospital
www.vh.org
Sponsored by the University of Iowa with a wealth of online atlases, articles, and educational materials

Washington University in St. Louis
http://spine.wustl.edu
Site of Washington University in St. Louis where actor Christopher Reeve received rehabilitative treatment after the 1995 spinal injury that left him paralyzed

University of Alabama
http://www.spinalcord.uab.edu
Spinal cord injury information network sponsored by the University of Alabama

University of Miami School of Medicine
http://www.med.miami.edu
Medical information from the University of Miami School of Medicine

BIBLIOGRAPHY

Baggaley, Ann, ed. *Human Body, First U.S. Edition.* New York, N.Y. Dorling Kindersley Publishing, Inc., 2001.

Balch, James F., M.D., and Phyllis A. Balch. *Prescription for Nutritional Healing, Second Edition.* Garden City Park, N.Y.: Avery Publishing Group, 1997.

Beers, Mark H., M.D., et al., eds. *The Merck Manual of Medical Information, Second Home Edition.* Whitehouse Station, N.J.: Merck Research Laboratories, 2003.

Brueninger, Cynthia C., and Pat Wittig, eds. *Diseases, Third Edition.* Springhouse, Pa.: Springhouse Corporation, 2001.

Burne, Hogarth. *Dynamic Anatomy.* New York, N.Y.: Watson-Guptill Publications, 1990.

Carter, Daniel, and Michael Courtney. *Anatomy for the Artist.* Bath, U.K.: Parragon Publishing, 2002.

Cassell, Dana K., and Noel Rose, M.D. *The Encyclopedia of Autoimmune Diseases.* New York, N.Y.: Facts On File, Inc., 2003.

D'Ambrosia, Robert D., M.D. *Musculoskeletal Disorders: Regional Examination and Differential Diagnosis, Second Edition.* Philadelphia, Pa.: J. P. Lippincott Company, 1986.

Graedon, Joe, and Teresa Graedon. *The People's Pharmacy Guide to Home and Herbal Remedies.* New York, N.Y.: St. Martin's Press, 2001.

Klag, Michael J., M.D., et al., eds. *Johns Hopkins Family Health Book.* New York, N.Y.: HarperCollins Publishers, 1999.

Komaroff, Anthony L., M.D., ed. *Harvard Medical School Family Health Guide.* New York, N.Y.: Simon & Schuster Source, 1999.

Kunz, Jeffrey R. M., M.D., ed. *The American Medical Association Family Medical Guide.* New York, N.Y.: Random House, 1982.

Lach, William, ed. *Ultimate Visual Dictionary of Science, First American Edition.* New York, N.Y.: DK Publishing, Inc., 1998.

Larson, David E., M.D., ed. *Mayo Clinic Family Health Book, Second Edition.* New York, N.Y.: William Morrow and Company, Inc., 1996.

Murray, Michael T., and Joseph E. Pizzorno. *Encyclopedia of Natural Medicine.* Rocklin, Calif.: Prima Publishing, 1991.

Patton, Kevin, and Gary Thibodeau, et. al., eds. *Mosby's Handbook of Anatomy Physiology.* St. Louis, Mo.: Mosby, Inc., 2000.

Rothenberg, Mikel A., M.D., and Charles F. Chapman. *Dictionary of Medical Terms for the Nonmedical Person, Third Edition.* Hauppauge, N.Y.: Barron's Educational Series, Inc., 1994.

Segen, Joseph C., M.D., and Joseph Stauffer. *The Patient's Guide to Medical Tests.* New York, N.Y.: Facts On File, Inc., 1998.

Thibodeau, Gary A., and Kevin T. Patton. *Structure & Function of the Body, Tenth Edition.* St. Louis, Mo.: Mosby-Year Book, Inc., 1997.

Thomas, Clayton M.D., et al., eds. *Taber's Cyclopedic Medical Dictionary, Edition 18.* Philadelphia, Pa.: F.A. Davis Company, 1997.

ACUPRESSURE

Gach, Michael Reed. *Acupressure's Potent Points: A Guide to Self-Care for Common Ailments.* New York, N.Y.: Bantam Books, 1990.

BIRTH DEFECTS

Wynbrandt, James and Mark D. Ludman, M.D. *The Encyclopedia of Genetic Disorders and Birth Defects, Second Edition.* New York, N.Y.: Facts On File, Inc., 2000.

BONE CANCER

Altman, Robert, and Michael J. Sarg, M.D. *The Cancer Dictionary, Revised Edition.* New York, N.Y.: Facts On File, Inc., 2002.

FIRST AID

The Official Government First Aid Manual. Woodbury, N.Y.: Platinum Press, Inc., 2000.

HERBS

Bestic, Liz. *A Guide to Natural Home Remedies.* Bath, U.K.: Parragon Publishing, 2002.

Bremness, Lesley. *Eyewitness Handbooks: Herbs, First American Edition.* New York, N.Y.: Dorling Kindersley, Inc., 1994.

Buchman, Dian Dincin. *Herbal Medicine.* Avenel, N.J.: Wings Books, 1996.

Fetrow, Charles W., and Juan R. Avila. *The Complete Guide to Herbal Medicines.* New York, N.Y.: Pocket Books, 2000.

Fleming, Thomas, et. al., eds. *PDR for Herbal Medicines.* Montvale, N.J.: Medical Economics Company, Inc., 1998.

Mowrey, Daniel B. *Herbal Tonic Therapies.* Avenel, N.J.: Wings Books, 1996.

Simonetti, Gualtiero and Stanley Schuler, eds. *Simon & Schuster's Guide To Herbs and Spices.* New York, N.Y.: Fireside, 1990.

Tenney, Louise. *Today's Herbal Health, Third Edition.* Provo, Utah: Woodland Books, 1992.

Williams, Jude C., M.H. *Jude's Herbal Home Remedies.* St. Paul, Minn.: Llewellyn Publications, 1997.

MASSAGE THERAPY

Harrold, Fiona. *The Complete Body Massage, First U.S. Edition.* New York, N.Y.: Sterling Publishing Company, Inc., 1992.

MEDICAL ALTERNATIVES

O'Mathúna, Dónal and Walt Larimore, M.D. *Alternative Medicine: The Christian Handbook.* Grand Rapids, Mich.: Zondervan Publishing House, 2001.

Tkac, Debora, et. al., eds. *The Doctors Book of Home Remedies.* Emmaus, Pa.: Rodale Press, Inc., 1990.

Tkac, Debora, et. al., eds. *LifeSpan-Plus.* Emmaus, Pa.: Rodale Press, Inc., 1990.

Wagner, Edward M. and Sylvia Goldfarb. *How to Stay out of the Doctor's Office.* New York, N.Y.: Instant Improvement, Inc., 1993.

Whorton, James C. *Nature Cures: The History of Alternative Medicine in America.* New York, N.Y.: Oxford University Press, 2002.

NUTRITION

Blaylock, Russell L., M.D. *Excitotoxins: The Taste that Kills.* Santa Fe, N.M.: Health Press, 1997.

Cassell, Dana K. *Food for Thought: The Sourcebook for Obesity and Eating Disorders.* New York, N.Y.: Checkmark Books, 2000.

Cassell, Dana K., and David H. Gleaves. *Encyclopedia of Obesity and Eating Disorders, Second Edition.* New York, N.Y.: Facts On File, Inc., 2000.

Cheraskin, E., M.D., W. M. Ringsdorf Jr., and J. W. Clark. *Diet and Disease.* New Canaan, Conn.: Keats Publishing, Inc., 1995.

Cichoke, Anthony J. *Enzymes and Enzyme Therapy.* New Canaan, Conn.: Keats Publishing, Inc., 1994.

Colbin, Annemarie. *Food and Healing.* New York, N.Y.: Ballantine Books, 1996.

Haas, Elson M., M.D. *Staying Health with Nutrition.* Berkeley, Calif.: Celestial Arts Publishing, 1992.

Harris, Ben Charles. *Better Health with Culinary Herbs.* New York, N.Y.: Weathervane Books, 1971.

Harris, Ben Charles. *Kitchen Medicines.* Barre, Mass.: Barre Publishers, 1968.

Hausman, Patricia, and Judith Benn Hurley. *The Healing Foods.* Emmaus, Pa.: Rodale Press, 1989.

Howell, Edward. *Enzyme Nutrition: The Food Enzyme Concept.* Wayne, N.J.: Avery Publishing Group, Inc., 1985.

Kirschmann, Gayla J., and John D. Kirschmann. *Nutrition Almanac, Fourth Edition.* New York, N.Y.: McGraw-Hill, 1996.

Lipski, Elizabeth. *Digestive Wellness.* New Canaan, Conn.: Keats Publishing, Inc., 1996.

OSTEOPOROSIS

Nelson, Miriam E. and Sarah Wernick. *Strong Women, Strong Bones.* New York, N.Y.: G. P. Putnam's Sons, 1999.

PAIN MANAGEMENT

Griffith, H. Winter, M.D., et. al. *1999 Edition Complete Guide to Prescription and Nonprescription Drugs.* New York, N.Y.: Perigee Books, 1998.

Sifton, David W., ed. *The PDR Pocket Guide to Prescription Drugs, Fifth Edition.* New York, N.Y.: Pocket Books, 2002.

SPORTS MEDICINE

Fortin, Francois. *Sports: The Complete Visual Reference.* Buffalo, N.Y.: Firefly Books (U.S.), Inc., 2000.

Sobell, Sheila. *Smart Guide to Sports Medicine.* New York, N.Y.: Cader Company, Inc., 1999.

INDEX

Boldface page numbers indicate major treatment of a subject.

A

B

C

F

I

K

L

M

P

Q

R

S

U

V

ABOUT THE AUTHORS

A freelance and assignment writer for three decades and a writing instructor for two, Mary Harwell Sayler has herself remained a lifelong student. With particular interests in poetry, health, and nature—from wildlife to all aspects of human life—her formal studies focused on nutrition. An avid reader and researcher, her published works include more than 1,000 short pieces, including nonfiction articles, regular columns on various topics, word games, and numerous poems. She has also had over two dozen books of nonfiction and fiction published with her first book of poems, first book of children's poetry, and course book on poetrywriting to be released in 2004.

As assistant dean in education affairs, Lori Siegel, M.D., F.A.C.P., F.A.C.R., oversees the four-year curriculum for the Chicago Medical School. After obtaining a degree in French, she graduated from the Medical College of Wisconsin and then did her residency in internal medicine prior to receiving a fellowship in rheumatology at Georgetown University in Washington, D.C. Her work at the Chicago Medical School has since given her the opportunity to direct the opening of a state-of-the-art education and evaluation center that allows for use of standardized patients in the medical school curriculum. In addition to directing the freshman and sophomore physical diagnosis course and writing medical reviews and articles, Dr. Siegel has a busy practice in rheumatology.